Clinical Manual of

MEDICAL-SURGICAL NURSING

CONCEPTS AND CLINICAL PRACTICE

Based on material from

MEDICAL-SURGICAL NURSING

CONCEPTS AND CLINICAL PRACTICE

FIFTH EDITION

EDITED BY

WILMA J. PHIPPS, PhD, RN, FAAN

Professor Emeritus of Medical-Surgical Nursing
Frances Payne Bolton School of Nursing
Case Western Reserve University
Cleveland, Ohio

VIRGINIA L. CASSMEYER, PhD, RN, CS

Associate Professor and Academic Coordinator
School of Nursing, University of Kansas Medical Center
Kansas City, Kansas

JUDITH K. SANDS, EdD, RN

Associate Professor and Director of Undergraduate Studies
School of Nursing
University of Virginia Health Sciences Center
Charlottesville, Virginia

†MARY KAY LEHMAN, MSN, RN

Doctoral Candidate, Director Student Services
Frances Payne Bolton School of Nursing
Case Western Reserve University
Cleveland, Ohio

†Deceased.

Clinical Manual of
MEDICAL-SURGICAL NURSING

CONCEPTS AND CLINICAL PRACTICE

JUDITH K. SANDS, EdD, RN
Associate Professor and Director of Undergraduate Studies
School of Nursing
University of Virginia Health Sciences Center
Charlottesville, Virginia

PAMELA E. DENNISON, MSN, RN
Clinician IV, Heart Center
University of Virginia Health Sciences Center
Charlottesville, Virginia

THIRD EDITION

with 232 illustrations

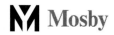 Mosby

St. Louis Baltimore Boston Carlsbad Chicago Naples New York Philadelphia Portland
London Madrid Mexico City Singapore Sydney Tokyo Toronto Wiesbaden

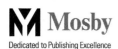
Mosby
Dedicated to Publishing Excellence

A Times Mirror
Company

Publisher: Nancy L. Coon
Editor: Michael S. Ledbetter
Senior Developmental Editor: Teri Merchant
Project Manager: Patricia Tannian
Production Editor: Melissa Mraz
Senior Book Designer: Gail Morey Hudson
Cover Designer: Jeanne Wolfgeher
Manufacturing Supervisor: Betty Richmond

A NOTE TO THE READER:
The author and publisher have made every attempt to check dosages and nursing content for accuracy. Because the science of pharmacology is continually advancing, our knowledge base continues to expand. Therefore we recommend that the reader always check product information for changes in dosage or administration before administering any medication. This is particularly important with new or rarely used drugs.

THIRD EDITION
Copyright © 1995 by Mosby–Year Book, Inc.

Previous editions copyrighted 1991, 1987

Printed in the United States of America
Composition by Carlisle Communications, Ltd.
Printing/binding by Von Hoffmann Press, Inc.

Mosby–Year Book, Inc.
11830 Westline Industrial Drive
St. Louis, Missouri 63146

Library of Congress Cataloging in Publication Data

Sands, Judith K.
    Clinical manual of medical-surgical nursing: concepts and
    clinical practice. — 3rd ed./ Judith K. Sands, Pamela E. Dennison.
       p.   cm.
    Includes bibliographical references and index.
    ISBN 0-8016-7889-7
    1. Nursing—Handbooks, manuals, etc.   2. Surgical nursing—
Handbooks, manuals, etc.   I. Dennison, Pamela E.   II. Title.
III. Title: Medical-surgical nursing.
    [DNLM: 1. Nursing—handbooks.   2. Surgical Nursing—handbooks.
WY 49 S221c 1995]
RT51.P46 1995
610.73—dc20
DNLM/DLC
for Library of Congress   95-1131
                                                                    CIP

95 96 97 98 99 / 9 8 7 6 5 4 3 2

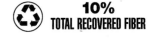
10%
TOTAL RECOVERED FIBER

This book is dedicated
with love and thanks to the "guys" who make it all worthwhile

David and Eric Sands
Peter, Mark, and Geoffrey Dennison

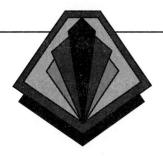

Preface

The third edition of the *Clinical Manual of Medical-Surgical Nursing* has been greatly expanded but is still designed to meet its original purposes. It is not intended to be a full textbook or a specialist reference. Rather, it is designed to be a concise yet thorough clinical resource book that presents an overview of the essential nursing care involved in the management of most common medical and surgical conditions. The manual still serves as an excellent reference book for nursing students at all levels of education, new graduates, and practicing nurses in virtually all medical-surgical practice settings.

All of the content in the book has been revised and updated, and it has also been expanded in several significant ways. Each body systems chapter now begins with an overview of the appropriate health history, physical assessment, and diagnostic tests in common use in that area. The focus of this content is on essential data that the nurse can incorporate into bedside assessment or patient teaching concerning diagnostic efforts. A consistent logo is used throughout the book to draw attention to this material. Two new chapters have been added. Chapter 3 presents an overview of substance abuse, a problem that complicates the admission and management of a significant percentage of patients on every medical-surgical unit. Chapter 17 on the immune system is also new. It incorporates data concerning the management of HIV/AIDS and the patient undergoing transplant. Both of these areas are making a significant impact on the practice of nursing in acute care facilities.

Several new features have also been added throughout the book. The care of the elderly is highlighted, first in the assessment sections of each chapter and then with each appropriate medical or surgical condition. This material has been placed in boxes and identified with a consistent logo to make it readily recognizable and easily accessible. Another new feature, technologies, reflects the increasing complexity of care delivery in all settings. Com- monly used technologies are highlighted in boxes and identified with a consistent logo. The focus again is on making this material as practical and user friendly as possible. The final added feature involves home care. When specific teaching information is critical to provide for a patient situation, the home care aspects of management have been boxed and labeled with a home care logo.

The book is again organized to present the most comprehensive information possible in a minimum of space. Three approaches are used in covering the material. Some conditions are presented in a simple paragraph that provides an overview of the condition and its management. Others are presented in paragraph form with a section devoted to each of the following: Etiology/Epidemiology, Pathophysiology, Medical Management, and Nursing Management. Major conditions are presented in modified outline format incorporating the use of the entire nursing process. The NANDA taxonomy is used for the presentation of all nursing diagnoses. The 1994-1995 list of NANDA diagnoses is included on the inside back cover. Liberal use has again been made of boxes and tables to highlight core content, present additional related material, and provide the reader with easy access to relevant information. Numerous new illustrations have been added to enhance the clarity of the material.

Managed care is becoming a fact of life in most inpatient practice settings. It is critical for all caregivers to be delivering focused and efficient patient care. Protocols and critical pathways are governing increasing aspects of care. To reflect these changes in the practice environment, critical pathways from the Phipps, Cassmeyer, Sands, and Lehman text have been incorporated into the manual to augment the more traditional care plans. Both are included in most situations to provide a basis for comparison. Numerous guidelines boxes summarize the care required in a wide variety of patient care situations. The approach throughout is both practical and practice oriented, and it should provide a useful resource for both planning and delivering patient care.

The world of nursing practice is changing rapidly, and numerous stresses are being placed on both students and professionals to be creative, to adapt, and to evolve into new roles and find new approaches to old challenges. It is our hope that the *Clinical Manual of Medical-Surgical Nursing* will serve as a practical resource for helping nurses to meet the challenges of nursing in the 90s. We would like to thank the editorial staff at Mosby–Year Book for their support and assistance in the preparation of the third edition, particularly Terry Van Schaik, who encouraged us to expand our dreams for the book, and Teri Merchant, who has helped it become a practical reality.

Judith K. Sands
Pamela E. Dennison

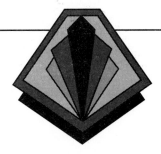

Contents

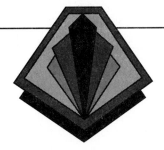

Cancer

Few diseases evoke greater feelings of anxiety and fear than cancer. Its physiologic and psychologic impact on patients and families is profound. Despite significant progress in cancer care and control, the diagnosis still signifies pain, mutilation, and death to many. Nurses are products of their society and may share many of its negative attitudes toward the disease. Cancer nursing challenges every aspect of a nurse's creativity, skill, and commitment.

ETIOLOGY/EPIDEMIOLOGY

Cancer is an umbrella term used to describe a large group of diseases that involve uncontrolled cellular growth, destruction of healthy tissue, and the risk of death. Despite significant advances in treatment, cancer remains the second leading cause of death in the United States. It is estimated that one out of every three to four Americans develops some form of cancer during his or her lifetime. Cancer occurs in all age-groups, both sexes, and all races, although the incidence statistics vary among groups. The incidence of all forms of cancer increases with age, and 52% of all cancers occur in persons over 65 years of age. Figure 1-1 shows the incidence by involved organs for both cancer and cancer deaths for males and females.

The etiology of cancer is clearly believed to be multicausal, involving the complex interplay of a wide variety of factors. Heredity plays a major role, and the extensive variations that exist in the geographic distribution of certain cancers point to an equally clear environmental role. Major known or suspected risk and predisposing factors are summarized in Box 1-1.

PATHOPHYSIOLOGY

All body tissues are derived from primitive stem cells that develop specialized functions as they grow. The process by which differentiation occurs is unknown. Multiplication takes place by the orderly process of mitosis in response to body needs. The cell cycle has several distinct phases that progress in a predictable fashion. Contact inhibition prevents overlap and disorderly growth.

Abnormal cell growth may result in benign growths from hyperplasia (an increase in cell number) or, hypertrophy (an increase in cell size but not number). Dysplasia refers to changes in individual cell size and shape. Malignant growth is characterized by cells whose basic structure and activity are uncontrolled by normal regulatory mechanisms.

Characteristics of cancer cells include the following:
- Anaplasia: succeeding generations of cells increasingly lose their similarity to the parent tissue
- Uncontrolled growth pattern: diminished or absent resting phase of the cell cycle
- Metastasis: ability to spread via blood, lymph system, or local invasion
- Presence of larger and irregularly shaped nuclei
- Disorderly growth: less contact inhibition
- Unencapsulated: may directly invade adjacent and surrounding tissue

The complex process of carcinogenesis begins with *initiation,* the exposure of normal cells to carcinogens. They promote cellular mutation. The second step is *promotion,* which may last for years. Promoting agents such as tobacco and alcohol act on the mutation for years. *Progression* involves the uncontrolled growth of a malignant tumor capable of metastasis. The initiating cellular changes are believed to be irreversible. The rate of tumor growth is affected by the rate of cell replication, amount of the total population replicating, and the rate of cell loss from death and exfoliation.

TUMOR CLASSIFICATION

Tumors may be classified via several criteria. The degree of cellular malignancy may be estimated by histologic criteria or grades. A grade 1 tumor is most like the parent tissue, whereas a grade 4 is highly anaplastic. The grading criteria are used to estimate likelihood of response to various types of treatment. Clinical staging classifies on the basis of disease spread from stage 0 for cancer in situ to stage IV for evidence of metastasis. The TNM classification is used worldwide to describe the nature and extent of cancer spread and evaluate treatment protocol outcomes (Box 1-2).

The clinical manifestations of cancer are diverse and may affect multiple systems. The effects may be local and/or systemic (Box 1-3).

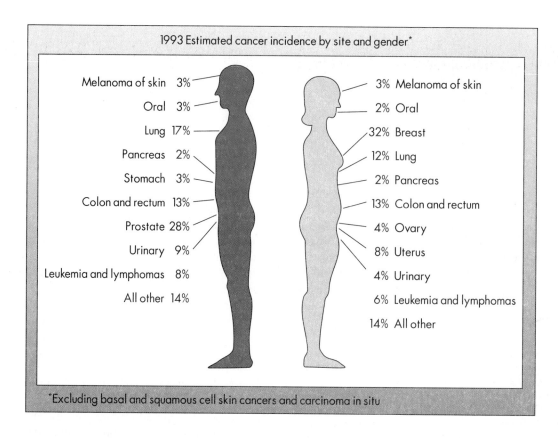

1993 Estimated cancer incidence by site and gender*

Male		Female
Melanoma of skin	3%	3% Melanoma of skin
Oral	3%	2% Oral
Lung	17%	32% Breast
Pancreas	2%	12% Lung
Stomach	3%	2% Pancreas
Colon and rectum	13%	13% Colon and rectum
Prostate	28%	4% Ovary
Urinary	9%	8% Uterus
Leukemia and lymphomas	8%	4% Urinary
All other	14%	6% Leukemia and lymphomas
		14% All other

*Excluding basal and squamous cell skin cancers and carcinoma in situ

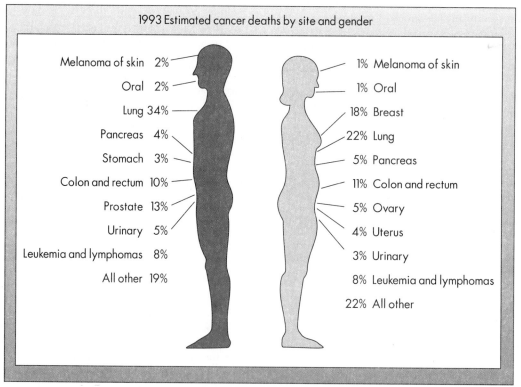

1993 Estimated cancer deaths by site and gender

Male		Female
Melanoma of skin	2%	1% Melanoma of skin
Oral	2%	1% Oral
Lung	34%	18% Breast
Pancreas	4%	22% Lung
Stomach	3%	5% Pancreas
Colon and rectum	10%	11% Colon and rectum
Prostate	13%	5% Ovary
Urinary	5%	4% Uterus
Leukemia and lymphomas	8%	3% Urinary
All other	19%	8% Leukemia and lymphomas
		22% All other

FIGURE 1-1 Comparison of cancer incidence and deaths by site and sex, 1993 estimates. (Modified from *CA,* Jan/Feb 1993.)

BOX 1-1   Major Predisposing or Risk Factors Affecting Host Susceptibility to Cancer

HOST FACTORS

Genetics

Family history is important in many cancers, but a few are directly related to a chromosomal change or genetic defect; for example, Wilms' tumor, retinoblastoma, some breast cancer, and familial polyposis.

Hormones

Although not believed to be direct carcinogens, hormones seem to play a permissive role in some cancers, such as estrogen and breast, uterine, and hepatic tumors.

Immune Deficiency

Natural or induced immune deficiency is associated with a significant-rise in cancer incidence of many types.

Drug Effects

List includes immunosuppressives, oral contraceptives, anabolic steroids, cytotoxic agents, and phenacetin-containing over-the-counter (OTC) analgesics.

ENVIRONMENTAL FACTORS*

Occupational Hazards

A wide variety of agents and additives such as nitrosamines, polycyclic hydrocarbons, asbestos, and dyes have been clearly identified as carcinogenic. The safe limits for exposure have not been established, however.

Ionizing Radiation

High-dose radiation exposure clearly alters cell chemistry and behavior and increases the incidence of cancer. Safe limits are unknown, and the exposure is cumulative.

Sun Exposure

Effects are related to ultraviolet B radiation and increased risk of skin cancers.

Radon

Radon is produced by the ground decay of uranium. Alpha particles released show a clear link to lung cancer development.

Electromagnetic Fields

A weak but persistent link is seen between high voltage and the incidence of leukemia.

Air and Water Pollution

Long-term consequences are unclear. Greatest concerns exist over depletion of the ozone layer and accumulation of gases such as carbon dioxide, methane, and fluorocarbons that increase the risk of lung cancer.

LIFE-STYLE FACTORS

Smoking/Tobacco Use

Moderate and heavy cigarette smoking is clearly linked with lung cancer incidence. Effects of second hand smoke are being heavily researched. Smokeless tobacco is implicated in oral cancer.

Diet

Research indicates strong correlations between diet components and cancer. High-fat intake appears clearly related to colon cancer, and a high-fiber diet may have some protective effect.

Alcohol

A significant relationship exists between high alcohol consumption and oral, esophageal, and bladder cancers. The effect rises when combined with heavy smoking.

Sexual Practices

Cervical cancer rates are associated with multiple sex partners and presence of sexually transmitted diseases (STDs).

Life Stressors

Some evidence exists that immune response can be influenced consciously by the individual.

_____
*Estimated to account for up to 90% of cancers seen today.

MEDICAL MANAGEMENT
EARLY DETECTION

With our current level of knowledge about cancer, early detection offers the best approach to the reduction of the incidence of cancer deaths. The seven warning signs of cancer (Box 1-4) should be reinforced to the public at every opportunity. The American Cancer Society's current guidelines for cancer screening are summarized in Table 1-1. The importance of risk factor reduction and early detection in cancer is also reflected in the *Healthy People 2000* health status objectives. Objectives related to cancer are presented in Box 1-5.

A wide variety of diagnostic tools may be used in diagnosing cancer. These include all standard tests plus a few that are uniquely targeted toward identifying cancerous cells. Categories and examples include the following:

1. Laboratory tests: elevations of enzymes such as acid and alkaline phosphatase.
2. Cytology: examination of cells for dysplasia or evidence of malignant changes.
3. X-rays and scans: organ mapping plays an important role in cancer diagnosis.
4. Radioisotope studies: tumors typically either fail to pick up the isotope or heavily concentrate it. Both "hot spots" and "cold spots" are useful diagnostically.
5. Biopsy: the only definitive means to diagnose cancer. It may involve aspiration, excision, or needle biopsy.
6. Endoscopy: allows for direct visualization of suspected sites and usually is accompanied by biopsy.

BOX 1-2	TNM Staging Classification System

TUMOR

T_0	No evidence of primary tumor
T_{is}	Carcinoma in situ
T_1, T_2, T_3, T_4	Ascending degrees of tumor size and involvement

NODES

N_0	No evidence of disease in lymph nodes
N_{1a}, N_{2a}	Disease found in regional lymph nodes; metastasis not suspected
N_{1b}, N_{2b}, N_3	Disease found in regional lymph nodes; metastasis suspected
N_x	Regional nodes cannot be assessed clinically

METASTASIS

M_0	No evidence of distant metastasis
M_1, M_2, M_3	Ascending degrees of metastatic involvement of the host, including distant nodes

BOX 1-3	Clinical Manifestations of Cancer

Obstruction of function
Pressure on surrounding tissue
Infiltration and destruction of surrounding tissue
Hemorrhage
Infection and ulceration
Pain: not always present, not an early sign
Cachexia syndrome: anorexia, weight loss, tissue wasting, hypermetabolism—usually a late sign

BOX 1-4	Seven Warning Signs of Cancer

Change in usual bowel or bladder function
A sore that does not heal
Unusual bleeding or discharge
Thickening or lump in the breast or elsewhere
Indigestion or dysphagia
Obvious change in a wart or mole
Nagging cough or hoarseness

7. Cancer markers: secreted enzymes, proteins, or hormones whose increased presence may represent a malignant process. Examples include carcinoembryonic antigen (CEA), chorionic gonadotropin, alpha fetoprotein (AFP), and prostate-specific antigen (PSA).

■ ■ ■

Research concerning the most appropriate and effective medical management for cancer is ongoing but revolves around four major forms of intervention: surgery, radiotherapy, chemotherapy, and immunotherapy. These interventions are usually employed in combination to reduce the associated toxic effects and increase the chances of destroying the malignant cells.

SURGERY

Surgery is the oldest and still most common form of treatment. Surgery may be used for diagnosis and staging, palliation, pain control, and reconstruction. Its most common use, however, is in the attempt to cure through the removal of all cancerous tissue before it metastasizes. Cancer surgery attempts to ensure a margin of healthy tissue and frequently results in significant loss of function as well as body image disturbance. Care of patients undergoing surgery for cancer is discussed with the presentation of each body system.

RADIOTHERAPY

Radiotherapy is the use of ionizing radiation to cause damage and destruction to cancerous cells during their replicative cycles. Radiotherapy can be delivered externally, by exposing the patient to rays generated by machines, or internally, by placing radioactive material within the tissues or a body cavity.

Radiotherapy may be given as a primary treatment or as adjuvant therapy after surgical removal of all identifiable cancer tissue. It works at the cellular level and is aimed at the control of micrometastases. All body tissue is affected to some degree, and rapidly dividing cells are affected first. Radiosensitivity is a measure of the potential susceptibility of cells to injury by radiation. Tumor resistance to radiation is a major problem believed to be largely related to tissue hypoxia. Hypoxic cells require three times as much radiation to destroy them as do well-oxygenated cells. Tumor cells may become increasingly hypoxic as they become distanced from their capillary blood supply by rapid growth.

External radiation treatments are just a few minutes in length. They are often "split" with periods of rest in between to allow normal cells to recover. The precise target area is carefully established and marked with ink or tatoos.

There is no pain associated with external radiotherapy, but some degree of skin reaction and bone marrow suppression is expected. In addition, most patients experience some degree of radiation syndrome, which includes fatigue, headache, anorexia, nausea, and vomiting. Specific reactions unique to the tissue being treated may also occur.

Brachytherapy is the placement of radioactive substances on or directly into a tumor. The source may be sealed or unsealed and may present a significant hazard to staff and visitors. A radiation safety officer has responsibility for informing all caregivers concerning specific risks and precautions to be followed.

Radioactive substances may be used in the form of molds, capsules, seeds, wires, and other applicators. Exact positioning is critical to minimize the exposure of adjacent tissues. Time of treatment may range from

TABLE 1-1 American Cancer Society Guidelines for Cancer Screening

TEST OR EXAMINATION	SEX	AGE (YR)	TESTING INTERVALS
Papanicolaou test (Pap test)	Female	Over 20; under 20 if sexually active	q 3 yr after two initial negative tests 1 yr apart
Pelvic examination	Female	18-40	q 1-3 yr with PAP test
		Over 40 or at menopause	Yearly
Endometrial tissue sample	Female	At menopause if high risk	High risk: history of infertility, obesity, failure of ovulation, abnormal uterine bleeding, estrogen therapy
Breast self-examination	Female	Over 20	Monthly
Breast physical examination	Female	20-40	q 3 yr
		Over 40	Yearly
Mammogram	Female	35-40	One baseline mammogram
		40-49	q 1-2 yr
		Over 50	Yearly
Stool guaiac slide test	Male and female	Over 50	Yearly
Digital rectal examination	Male and female	Over 40	Yearly
Sigmoidoscopic examination or colonoscopy	Male and female	Over 50	q 3-5 yr based on advice of physician
Prostate: digital rectal examination	Male	Over 40	Yearly
Prostate-specific antigen	Male	Over 50, high risk, and after treatment	Yearly

---

BOX 1-5 *Healthy People 2000:* Cancer-Related Objectives

REDUCTION IN DEATH RATES

1. Reverse the rise in cancer deaths to achieve a rate of 130/100,000 persons.
2. Slow the rise in lung cancer deaths to a rate of no more than 42/100,000 persons.
3. Reduce breast cancer deaths to no more than 20.6/100,000 women.
4. Reduce deaths from cancer of the uterine cervix to no more than 1.3/100,000 women.
5. Reduce colorectal cancer deaths to no more than 13.2/100,000 persons.

CANCER RISK REDUCTION

1. Reduce cigarette smoking to a prevalence of no more than 15% among persons aged 20 or older.
2. Reduce dietary fat intake to an average of 30% of calories or less and average saturated fat intake to less than 10% of calories among persons aged 2 and older.
3. Increase complex carbohydrate and fiber-containing foods in the diets of adults to five or more daily servings for vegetables and fruits and to six or more daily servings for grain products.
4. Increase to 60% of the general population those who limit sun exposure, use sunscreens and protective clothing when exposed to sunlight, and avoid artificial sources of ultraviolet light (sun lamps, tanning booths).

EARLY DETECTION GOALS

1. Increase to 75% the proportion of care providers who routinely counsel patients about tobacco cessation, diet modification, and cancer screening recommendations.
2. Increase to 80% the proportion of women aged 40 and older who have received a clinical breast examination and mammogram, and to 60% of those aged 50 and older who have received them within the preceding 1 to 2 years.
3. Increase to 95% the proportion of women aged 18 and older with uterine cervix who have ever had a Pap test, and to 85% the number who had a Pap test within the preceding 1 to 3 years.
4. Increase to 50% the number of persons aged 50 and older who had fecal occult blood testing within the preceding 1 to 2 years and to 40% those who have ever had a proctosigmoidoscopic examination.
5. Increase to 40% the number of persons aged 50 and older visiting a primary care provider in the preceding year who had oral, skin, and digital rectal examinations during one such visit.

From US Department of Health and Human Services. Public Health Service: *Healthy people 2000: Summary report,* Boston, 1992, Jones & Bartlett.

---

hours to days. Cervical, endometrial, prostate, breast, and head and neck tumors are frequently treated through brachytherapy.

Brachytherapy may also be used in select situations in an unsealed or "atomic cocktail" form. If the isotope emits gamma particles the risk of exposure for others is extremely high. Unsealed sources are frequently eliminated in the urine, feces, vomitus, perspiration, and sputum. All excretions and linens will require special handling. Principles of staff protection during brachytherapy are outlined in the Guidelines box.

Patients may also experience delayed reactions to the radiotherapy months or years after therapy. They include fibrotic tissue changes, ulceration, stricture, fistula, or perforation. No adequate explanation exists at present for their development. Late effects are usually permanent. Radiotherapy does itself also have carcinogenic potential for the future.

Guidelines for Radiation Therapy and Protection of Staff

- Radiation applied externally can cause injury only during the time the treatment is being administered.
  NOTE: Patient is never radioactive.
- Radiation with alpha or beta rays applied internally creates little hazard to staff, since these rays cannot pass through the patient's skin. Substances emitting gamma rays cause the patient to transmit gamma radiation.
- Each radiation substance has its own half-life: the period of time in which half its radioactivity is dissipated and the dangers of radiation are reduced.

To protect staff from the effects of radiation, the following factors should be considered:

AMOUNT OF EXPOSURE TO RADIATION SOURCES

Radiation doses are cumulative. Limit interactions with patients with internal radiation therapy to 15 minutes per visit; group activities to maximize use of time.
Each nurse must wear his or her own film badge when in contact with source to monitor cumulative exposure levels.

STRENGTH OF RADIATION SUBSTANCE

Radiation safety officer can and should provide data about substance—its half-life, nature of rays, and ways it may be excreted from the body, if any, such as in urine, sweat, or saliva.

DISTANCE FROM RADIATION SOURCE

Rays are more numerous and concentrated at close range. Exposure risks decrease sharply with distance.

TYPE AND DEGREE OF SHIELDING IN USE

Lead-lined container and long-handled forceps must always be in room to contain source if dislodged.
Proper receptacles for linens and excreta should be used if needed (necessary only when source is not sealed).
Lead aprons should be used by nursing staff if indicated.

RISK TO STAFF

Patient is placed in a private room with a radiation hazard sign on the door.
Rotate nursing care among nurses who are at least risk from radiation hazard; pregnant nurses should not provide care. Follow restrictions on time at bedside carefully.

NURSING MANAGEMENT: Radiotherapy

◆ ASSESSMENT
Subjective Data

Knowledge of:
    Goals of treatment (cure, palliation)
    Radiation treatment protocol (duration, frequency)
    What to expect during treatment
    Common side effects and their management
Prior experience with radiotherapy, misconceptions

Objective Data

General health status
Tissue integrity in treatment field

◆ NURSING DIAGNOSES

Possible nursing diagnoses for the person receiving radiotherapy may include, but are not limited to, the following:
    Knowledge deficit (related to radiotherapy and radiation precautions)
    Skin integrity, high risk for impaired (related to effects of radiation)
    Nutrition, altered: less than body requirements (related to the anorexia, nausea, and vomiting of radiation syndrome)
    Infection, high risk for (related to immunosuppressive effects of radiation)

◆ EXPECTED PATIENT OUTCOMES

1. Patient will correctly describe components of radiation treatment plan.
2. Patient will identify effects of radiation on the skin and measures to minimize adverse effects.
3. Patient will ingest sufficient balanced nutrients to meet daily needs and maintain stable body weight.
4. Patient will identify effects of radiation on the bone marrow and measures to prevent infection and bleeding.

◆ NURSING INTERVENTIONS
Teaching About Treatment Protocol

Teach patient about the nature of radiotherapy (see Guidelines boxes at left and below). Reassure patient about concerns over becoming "radioactive" and a danger to family or friends.
Teach patient about how the treatment is administered—setting, equipment, positioning, markings.
Inform patient about expected side effects.
Prepare patients for general symptoms of radiation syndrome—fatigue, anorexia, nausea. Encourage patient to space activities and plan for additional needed rest.

Guidelines for Nursing Care of the Patient Receiving Internal Brachytherapy

Teach patient about rationale for therapy, side effects, and reasons for required safety precautions.
Place patient in private room with signs that identify nature and extent of radiation hazard.
Restrict visitors to 15-minute visits per day.
Counter effects of isolation by frequent visits from doorway and encourage use of radio or television for stimulation.
Promote comfort measures.
Ensure that a lead container and long-handled forceps are present in the room at all times.
Reinforce the importance of activity restrictions.
Utilize the principles of distance, time, and shielding for all bedside care delivery.
For cervical implants explain rationale for enforced bed rest, Foley catheter, and diet restrictions.

Minimizing Skin Reactions

Teach patient to do the following:

Wash irradiated skin daily with tepid water. Use mild soap if cleansing is required.

Avoid removing skin markings.

Avoid exposure to sun, wind, and extremes of temperature.

Avoid tight, constrictive clothing over treatment port.

Avoid commercial cosmetics, perfumes, lotions, or powders over treatment area. Commercial products frequently have heavy metal bases.

Consult radiation oncologist if skin problems develop. Cornstarch, A&D ointment, and Vaseline may be approved.

Promoting Adequate Nutrition

Prepare patient for likelihood of anorexia and nausea.

Encourage small frequent meals throughout the day.

Explore use of high-protein, high-carbohydrate, low-fat meals. Sweet foods are frequently better tolerated.

Encourage patient to rest before and after meals.

Avoid use of "empty calorie" foods. Offer enriched supplements to meet nutritional needs.

Administer antiemetic medications as ordered before onset of nausea.

Assist patient to redistribute nutrients throughout the day to maximize nausea-free periods. Enrich breakfast nutrients if appropriate.

Encourage patient to avoid eating or drinking immediately before or after treatment.

Check and record weight weekly.

Preventing Infection and Injury

Monitor weekly blood tests.

Have patient avoid crowds and individuals with upper respiratory infections.

Monitor vital signs.

Observe bleeding precautions if patient is thrombocytopenic.

Encourage patient to plan for fatigue and rest at intervals throughout the day.

Teach patient importance of careful personal hygiene and regular oral hygiene. Report development of bruising, nosebleeds, blood in urine or stool, bleeding gums, or mouth ulcers.

♦ EVALUATION

Successful achievement of expected outcomes for the patient receiving radiotherapy is indicated by the following:

Accurate description of purpose of radiation therapy, nature of the treatment and side effects, and actions to be taken to manage side effects

Intact skin without evidence of erythema or dryness

Ingestion of balanced nutrients and maintenance of stable body weight

Absence of fever, stomatitis, or bleeding

CHEMOTHERAPY

Cancer chemotherapy is based on the actions of certain drugs that create changes in the cell cycle phases as the cells replicate. They particularly affect rapidly dividing cells, both cancerous and noncancerous. Chemotherapy is used for both cure and palliation of symptoms. It is also used as adjuvant treatment after radiation or surgery to destroy residual micrometastasis not detectable with current screening tools. Drugs are frequently given in combination to attack the tumor cells simultaneously from different points of the cell cycle and prevent the development of tumor resistance. Drugs are chosen on the basis of tumor size and rate of growth and may be administered orally, intravenously (IV), arterially, intrathecally, and by regional perfusion. Chemotherapy is more effective with relatively small but rapidly growing tumors. Several courses of chemotherapy are typically ordered. Chemotherapy agents are theorized to kill a certain proportion of tumor cells with each administration, such as 90%. Several administrations would be required to bring the cell numbers down to a level that can be successfully destroyed by the immune system. Table 1-2 summarizes many of the drugs in current use for cancer chemotherapy.

Since chemotherapeutic drugs are significantly toxic, concern exists over the risks of exposure for health care professionals in their preparation and administration. The major points from the U.S. Occupational Safety and Health Administration (OSHA) safe handling guidelines are summarized in the Guidelines box.

Chemotherapy always results in some degree of injury to normal cells. The bone marrow, gastrointestinal (GI) epithelium, hair follicles, and reproductive tract are the most vulnerable. Numerous other toxicities occur related to the use of specific agents.

Bone marrow suppression may be life threatening. Blood counts are evaluated before therapy and at intervals to identify the nadir (low) point of suppression. Patients may become severely anemic and are vulnerable to infection and bleeding. Transfusions of packed

Guidelines for Handling Chemotherapeutic Agents

1. Drugs should be prepared in strict laminar flow environments.
2. Surgical gloves and a long-sleeved, closed-front gown should be worn during preparation of drugs.
3. Wash skin areas thoroughly with soap and water in the event of skin contact with drugs.
4. Dispose of all needles and IV materials carefully in appropriately labeled containers.
5. Wash hands thoroughly before and after giving drugs.

TABLE 1-2 Drugs Used in Cancer Chemotherapy

AGENT	MECHANISM OF ACTION	MAJOR TOXIC MANIFESTATIONS
ALKYLATING AGENTS		
Chlorambucil (Leukeran)	Interfere with DNA replication by attacking DNA synthesis throughout cell cycle (cell cycle nonspecific)	Bone marrow depression with leukopenia, thrombocytopenia, and bleeding; cyclophosphamide may cause alopecia and hemorrhagic cystitis
Melphalan (Alkeran)		
Cyclophosphamide (Cytoxan)		
Myleran (Busulfan)		
Triethylenethiophosphoramide (Thiotepa)		
Mechlorethamine (nitrogen mustard)		
ANTIMETABOLITES		
Methotrexate (MTX)	Structural analogs of essential metabolites and therefore interfere with synthesis of these metabolites (cell cycle specific)	Bone marrow depression; oral and gastrointestinal ulceration
6-Mercaptopurine (6-MP)		
5-Fluorouracil (5-FU)		
Arabinosylcytosine (Cytosar, Ara-C)		
6-Thioguanine (Thioguan)		
Floxuridine (FUDR)		
ANTIBIOTICS		
Doxorubicin (Adriamycin)	Interfere with DNA or RNA synthesis, varying with the drug (cell cycle nonspecific)	Stomatitis, gastrointestinal disturbances, and bone marrow depression
Bleomycin (Blenoxane)		Doxorubicin and daunorubicin cause cardiac toxicity at cumulative doses over 500 mg/m^2
Dactinomycin (Cosmegan)		
Daunorubicin (Cerubidine)		
Plicamycin (Mithramycin, Mithracin)		Bleomycin can cause alopecia and pulmonary fibrosis but only minimal bone marrow depression
Mitomycin (Mutamycin)		
Mitoxantrone (Novantrone)		
PLANT ALKALOIDS		
Vinblastine (Velban)	Interfere with mitosis (cell cycle specific)	Alopecia, areflexia, bone marrow depression
Vincristine (Oncovin)		Neurotoxicity with ataxia and impaired fine motor skills, constipation and paralytic ileus
STEROID HORMONES		
Androgens (Halotestin, Drolban, Teslac)	Alter host environment for cell growth (cell cycle nonspecific)	Specific for the actions of the hormone
Estrogens (DES, Estinyl)		
Progestins (Prodox, Megace, Provera)		
Adrenocorticosteroids (prednisone, dexamethasone, Solu-Medrol, Solu-Cortef)		
Antiestrogens (Tamoxifen, Leuprolide)		
OTHER		
L-Asparaginase (Elspar)	Inhibits protein synthesis	Fever and hypersensitivity
Cisplatin (Platinol)	Inhibits DNA, RNA, and protein synthesis	Renal damage
Procarbazine (Matulane)	As above	CNS depression reaction
Carmustine (BCNU)		Bone marrow depression
Lomustine (CCNU)		Bone marrow depression
Mitotane (Lysodren)		Skin eruptions, diarrhea
Dacarbazine (DTIC-Dome)	Inhibits protein synthesis	Bone marrow depression

Modified from Porth C: *Pathophysiology: concepts of altered health states,* ed 4, Philadelphia, 1993, Lippincott.

red blood cells (RBCs) and platelets may be needed, and every effort is made to prevent infection.

Nausea and *vomiting* are generally recognized as the most distressing aspects of chemotherapy. They may occur with treatment, after treatment, or in anticipation of subsequent treatment. Nutritional concerns are worsened by severe anorexia and the development of stomatitis in the mouth and throat, which parallels the fall in white blood cells (WBCs).

Alopecia does not occur with all drugs, but it is usually a traumatic problem for the patient. Several patterns occur, including drying, thinning, and hair root atrophy, which causes the hair to come out in clumps. All body hair has the potential to be affected.

Chemotherapy reaches the reproductive organs during treatment and may cause transient or permanent sterility and the potential for genetic abnormalities. Effects vary with drugs and doses, but pregnancy is not recommended for at least 2 years after treatment.

Administering Chemotherapy

Chemotherapy may be administered by virtually any route, although IV is the most common. Intrathecal administration allows the agent to bypass the blood-

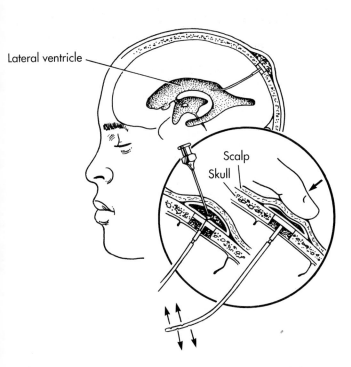

FIGURE 1-2 Ommaya reservoir for administration of chemotherapy. (Modified from Ratcheson RA, Ommaya AK: *N Engl J Med* 279:1025-1031, 1968.)

Lateral ventricle

Scalp

Skull

brain barrier (Figure 1-2), and intracavitary routes provide high local concentrations while minimizing systemic effects. Centrally placed venous access devices and ports are a standard part of chemotherapy today. They allow for intermittent or continuous infusion of chemotherapy, blood products, antibiotics, antiemetics, analgesics, and total parenteral nutrition (TPN) if indicated. Options for establishing central access are described in Chapter 4. "Tunneled" catheters are popular for chemotherapy, since they reduce bacterial growth and access along the tract. Most catheters and access ports are adaptable for home management. External or implantable infusion pumps also allow for delivery of chemotherapy in the community.

NURSING MANAGEMENT: Chemotherapy

◆ ASSESSMENT
Subjective Data

Patient's understanding of the nature and goals of chemotherapy—drugs to be used, expected side effects and their management

Prior experience with chemotherapy or other cancer treatment

Support persons and resources available

Objective Data

Body weight, general health, and nutritional status

Status of venous system

◆ NURSING DIAGNOSES

Possible nursing diagnoses for the person receiving chemotherapy may include, but are not limited to, the following:

Knowledge deficit (related to chemotherapy and its effects)

Nutrition, altered: less than body requirements (related to anorexia, stomatitis, nausea, or vomiting)

Infection or injury, high risk for (related to immunosuppression)

Mucous membrane, altered oral (related to cell destruction)

Body image disturbance (related to alopecia)

◆ EXPECTED PATIENT OUTCOMES

1. Patient will be knowledgeable about drugs to be used and the management of their expected side effects.
2. Patient will maintain an adequate and nutritious oral intake and maintain a stable body weight.
3. Patient will be free of infection and not develop bleeding.
4. Patient will maintain intact mucous membranes.
5. Patient will maintain social interactions and make positive references to self.

◆ NURSING INTERVENTIONS
Teaching About Chemotherapy

Teach patient names of drugs, expected side effects, and management of side effects.

Encourage patient to maintain self-care and usual activities, as tolerated.

Remind patient of importance of close follow-up if outpatient treatment is given.

Maintaining Nutrition

Prepare patient for anorexia or nausea if expected with drugs.

Administer antiemetics as prescribed. Administer drugs *before* anticipated nausea so oral forms may be used (usually 30 to 45 minutes before therapy).

Determine from patient best time for food and fluid intake in relation to treatment. Avoid food at time of treatment.

Avoid empty-calorie foods. Offer enriched supplements to meet nutritional needs if they can be tolerated.

Experiment with food groups useful during periods of nausea: dry bulky foods, sweet foods, clear liquids, soft bland foods. Avoid dairy products and red meats.

Keep environment clean and odor free.

Maintain fluid intake, and offer frequent mouth care.

Teach relaxation and distraction techniques if appropriate.

Weigh patient twice weekly.

Preventing Infection, Bleeding, or Injury

Monitor daily or weekly blood counts. Be aware of expected nadir (low point). Neutrophil count below 1000/mm³ indicates moderate risk of infection.

Monitor vital signs and assess oral mucous membranes and lungs regularly for early signs of infection.

Teach patient signs of infection and thrombocytopenia.

Avoid use of acetaminophen (Tylenol) or aspirin products, which may mask the signs of infection.

Teach patient importance of scrupulous personal hygiene; for example, bathing and changing clothing regularly, performing mouth care and perineal care, and keeping fingernails short. Emphasize the importance of frequent careful handwashing.

Use creams and lotions to prevent drying and cracking of skin.

Instruct family and friends with colds or flu not to visit. Avoid all sources of infection.

Institute reverse isolation if prescribed. Follow scrupulous aseptic technique for all care.

Give no enemas or rectal medications; do not take rectal temperatures. Be sure family has and can read a thermometer.

Institute bleeding precautions: give no intramuscular injections, inspect for bruises, test stool and urine for blood.

Administer packed red blood cells and platelets as ordered.

Avoid fresh fruits and vegetables and foods with active cultures such as yogurt. Serve well-cooked foods.

Maintain meticulous aseptic technique for IV changes and dressings.

Teach home-based patient to use water-soluble lubricant for intercourse and avoid anal penetration.

Monitor all infusions carefully. Ensure that IV is patent before beginning drug administration.

Know which drugs cause widespread tissue necrosis, for example, vincristine, nitrogen mustard, and doxorubicin. Monitor these infusions continuously.

If extravasation occurs, immediately discontinue infusion and apply ice to site.

Encourage patient to use and exercise arms between treatments if possible but to avoid injury.

Maintaining Intact Oral Mucous Membranes

Inspect mouth carefully for signs of irritation or ulceration at least twice daily.

Encourage frequent oral hygiene with soft toothbrush and mild mouthwashes such as saline, baking soda, or dilute peroxide solutions. Use a water pik if platelets are low.

Stimulate the flow of saliva with gum and hard candies.

Use artificial saliva as needed (Salivart, Ora-lub).

Assess frequently for *Candida* infection. Use nystatin tablets or suspension for prevention.

Use rinses and viscous lidocaine (Xylocaine) before meals for analgesia. Apply mineral oil or KY jelly to cracked lips. Avoid use of lemon and glycerin swabs, which dry.

Adjust diet toward bland, mechanically soft foods.

Supporting a Positive Body Image

Teach patient about hair loss—when it will occur and to what degree. NOTE: All body hair is affected.

Reassure patient that drug-induced hair loss is not permanent but new hair growth may be different in color, texture, and thickness. NOTE: Not all drugs cause hair loss (Box 1-6).

Plan with patient in advance of hair loss for the acquisition and use of wigs, scarves, and cosmetics.

Avoid frequent shampooing and hair care with hot combs and so on.

Encourage patient to express feelings about hair loss.

Employ ice caps if prescribed and patient desires. NOTE: Ice caps are not employed for patients with leukemia or other blood-borne cancers because cancer cells are sequestered from effects of drugs.

◆ EVALUATION

Successful achievement of expected outcomes for the patient receiving chemotherapy is indicated by the following:

Accurate description of purpose of chemotherapy, drugs to be used, expected side effects, and their management

Maintenance of a stable body weight and ingestion of sufficient nutrients to meet basic body needs

Afebrile and does not experience bleeding, injury, or infection

Intact mucous membranes and veins

Maintenance of normal social interactions and choice of satisfactory method to deal with alopecia

IMMUNOTHERAPY/BIOTHERAPY

The role of the immune system in the development of cancer is being intensely studied. It is theorized that a

BOX 1-6	Chemotherapeutic Agents Most Responsible for Hair Loss	
Bleomycin	5-Fluorouracil
Cyclophosphamide	Hydroxyurea
Cytosine arabinoside	Methotrexate
Dactinomycin	Mitomycin-C
Daunorubicin	Mitoxantrone
Doxorubicin	Melphalan
Etoposide	Vincristine

natural immunity to cancer exists that normally destroys cancerous cells as fast as they develop. The development of clinical cancer may represent a failure of immune regulation, and immunotherapy attempts to stimulate the patient's own immune system to recognize cancer cells as "nonself" and destroy them. The cells involved in the immune response interact and exchange signals at the cellular and hormonal levels. At present immunotherapy is used primarily as a supportive therapy after surgery, radiation, or chemotherapy has removed the bulk of the tumor.

Immunotherapy or biotherapy attempts to manipulate the immune system to modify the body's response to cancer or cancer therapy. Both specific and nonspecific agents are being investigated. Options include several different types of biologic response modifiers, such as (1) agents that attempt to restore or strengthen the immune response (interferons [INFs]); (2) cells with direct antitumor activity (tumor necrosis factor [TNF] or natural killer cells [NKs]); and (3) agents that may affect cell growth and differentiation (colony-stimulating factors [CSFs], granulocyte macrophage CSF). Research is ongoing in all areas. Commonly encountered side effects of biotherapy are summarized in Table 1-3.

CANCER PAIN
ETIOLOGY/EPIDEMIOLOGY

Pain is one of the most feared aspects of cancer. Contrary to popular belief, pain is rarely a problem in early stages of cancer, but it is a significant challenge for 60% to 90% of patients with disease in an advanced stage with metastasis.

Cancer pain is commonly characterized as being early, intermediate, or late stage and typically has different causes at different times. Early pain is often related to diagnostic and surgical procedures and is acute but short term. Intermediate pain may occur from scar retraction, nerve entrapment, and pressure of the growing tumor resulting in tissue ischemia and inflammation. Late pain is chronic and may be progressively worsening. Destruction of bone by metastasis is the most common cause as well as increasing tissue ischemia,

pressure, and obstruction. The patient's response to the pain is clearly tied to the cancer diagnosis itself and the threat of loss or death.

MEDICAL MANAGEMENT

The ultimate goal of management involves the relief of pain so the patient may carry on with his or her daily life-style. The physician will first attempt to deal with treatable causes such as relief of obstruction, radiation to shrink the tumor mass, or nerve blocks to interrupt pain transmission pathways.

Pharmacologic management involves a few basic principles. Nonnarcotics (usually nonsteroidal antiinflammatory drugs [NSAIDs]) are most appropriate for mild pain and can be administered orally. However, research indicates that undertreatment is a significant problem and pain relief is the most important goal. Other principles include the following:

1. As-needed (PRN) administration is ineffective for managing chronic severe pain.
2. Intramuscular (IM) administration and subcutaneous (SQ) administration are usually inappropriate in the presence of tissue wasting and bleeding tendencies.
3. When narcotic analgesics are used, both tolerance and physical dependence will inevitably occur.
   a. Doses will need to be adjusted upward as tolerance builds.
   b. *Addiction* is not a concern in cancer pain management.
   c. Equianalgesic doses must be used when drugs are changed.
4. If pain is constant, around-the-clock administration is appropriate. Consider use of patient-controlled analgesia (PCA) to handle breakthrough pain.
5. The use of adjuvant drugs such as antidepressants, neurolytics, or corticosteroids should be explored.

NURSING MANAGEMENT

The nurse works with the patient to implement the overall pain program and serves as a patient advocate to ensure adequate and appropriate drugs, doses, and methods of administration. Ongoing pain assessment is

TABLE 1-3 Common Side Effects of Biotherapy	
TYPE	SIDE EFFECTS
Interferons (INFs) (alpha, beta, gamma)	Flulike symptoms of fatigue, fever, chills, myalgias, headache, anorexia, nausea and vomiting, diarrhea, rash, hypotension, CNS manifestations (confusion, depression, somnolence, parethesias)
Interleukin-2 (IL-2)	Fever, chills, malaise, nausea and vomiting, anorexia, arthralgias, myalgias, hypotension
Growth factors	
G-CSF	Mild medullary bone pain
GM-CSF	Mild myalgias, low-grade fever, headache, flushing, bone pain (lumbar, sacral, sternal)
(EPO)	Hypertension, coldness, sweating, bone pain
Tumor necrosis factor (TNF)	Chills, fever, myalgias, arthralgias, malaise, anorexia, nausea and vomiting, hypotension, pain at tumor site

Home Management of Cancer Pain

Ineffective pain management has been a common reason for advanced cancer patients to be unable to remain in their home setting. Advances in analgesic delivery should make remaining at home a feasible goal for more patients. Success is built around these principles:

- Reassure patient and family about differences among dependence, tolerance, and addiction. Addiction is *not* an outcome of cancer pain treatment.
- Use sustained release oral analgesics if possible. Do not hesitate to increase doses in response to pain levels.
- Tolerance develops to respiratory effects of narcotics as well as the analgesic effects.
- Experiment with equianalgesic combinations of drugs and doses to achieve maximal pain relief with minimal side effects.
- PCA pumps can be effectively used in the home.
- Epidural catheters can be safely used and allow a constant level of pain relief with fewer side effects.
- Be sure that patient and family have telephone numbers for contact persons who can assist if problems arise.

critical to adequately document the pain experience and patient response to it. Home care management of cancer pain is discussed in the accompanying home care box.

The nurse also helps the patient develop and implement behavioral strategies for augmenting pain management. These may include relaxation, distraction, meditation, and imagery. Maintaining nutrition and promoting rest and sleep are also important. If narcotics are being used, it is also critical to develop strategies to prevent ongoing complications such as severe constipation or drowsiness. See Chapter 2 for a more indepth discussion of pain management.

CANCER REHABILITATION

As the 5-year survival rate for cancer has approached 50% it has become increasingly important to focus on cancer rehabilitation and the task of *living* with cancer. Emphasis is placed on quality of life rather than simply duration. Activities such as promoting good nutrition, exercise, stress management, and social support may be included.

Patients and families should also be informed about the resources and services available through the American Cancer Society, Medicare/Medicaid, and the National Cancer Institute. Peer support groups are also sponsored in most communities and include services to

mastectomy, ostomy, and laryngectomy patients as well as bereavement support. If cancer recurs it may also be important for families to know of the services provided through home health agencies and hospice organizations.

SELECTED REFERENCES

Baird SB, McCorkle R, Grant M: *Cancer nursing: a comprehensive textbook,* Philadelphia, 1991, WB Saunders.

Caliendo G, Joyce D, Altmiller M: Nursing guidelines and discharge planning for patients receiving recombinant interleukin-2, *Semin Oncol Nurs* (3, suppl 1):25-31, 1993.

Campbell-Forsyth L: Patient's perceived knowledge and learning needs concerning radiation therapy, *Ca Nurs* 13(2):81-89, 1990.

Carey PJ et al: Appraisal and caregiving burden in family members caring for patients receiving chemotherapy, *Oncol Nurs Forum* 18(8): 1341-1348, 1991.

Carnevallid DL, Reiner AC: *The cancer experience: nursing diagnosis and management,* Philadelphia, 1990, Lippincott.

Cartmel B, Loescher LJ, Villar-Werstler P: Professional and consumer concerns about environment, lifestyle, and cancer, *Semin Oncol Nurs* 8(1):20-29, 1992.

Dorr RT, Von Hoff D, editors: *Cancer chemotherapy handbook,* ed 2, Norwalk, CT, 1994, Appleton & Lange.

Dow KH, Hilderly LJ: *Nursing care in radiation oncology,* Philadelphia, 1992, WB Saunders.

Edwards JN et al: Comparison of patient-controlled and nurse-controlled antiemetic therapy in patients receiving chemotherapy, *Res Nurs Health* 14:249-257, 1991.

Ferrell B et al: Effects of controlled-release morphine on quality of life for cancer pain, *Oncol Nurs Forum* 16(4):521-528, 1989.

Frank-Stromberg M, Rohan K: Nursing's involvement in the primary prevention and secondary prevention of cancer: nationally and internationally, *Ca Nurs* 15(2):79-108, 1992.

Groenwald SL et al, editors: *Cancer nursing: principles and practice,* ed 3, Boston, 1993, Jones and Bartlett.

Laizner AM et al: Needs of family caregivers of persons with cancer, *Semin Oncol Nurs* 9(2):114-120, 1993.

Lewis FM: Psychosocial transitions and the family's work in adjusting to cancer, *Semin Oncol Nurs* 9(2):127-129, 1993.

O'Connor L, Blesch K: Life cycle issues affecting cancer rehabilitation, *Semin Oncol Nurs* 8(3):174-185, 1992.

Olson SJ, Frank-Stromberg M: Cancer prevention and early detection in ethnically diverse populations, *Semin Oncol Nurs* 9(3):198-209, 1993.

Reville B, Almadrones L: Continuous infusion chemotherapy in the ambulatory setting: the nurse's role in patient selection and education, *Oncol Nurs Forum* 16(4):529-538, 1989.

Strohl RA: The nursing role in radiation oncology: symptom management of acute and chronic reactions, *Oncol Nurs Forum* 15(4):429-438, 1988.

Travaglini J, Nevidjon B: Complications related to cancer therapy, *Clin Adv Oncol Nurs* 2(2):1-13, 1990.

Watson PG: Cancer rehabilitation: an overview, *Semin Oncol Nurs* 8(3):167-173, 1992.

White LN, Spitz MR: Cancer risk and early detection, *Semin Oncol Nurs* 9(3):188-197, 1993.

Whitman HH, Gustafson JP: Group therapy for families facing a cancer crisis, *Oncol Nurs Forum* 16(4):539-546, 1989.

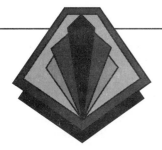

Pain

The experience of pain is universal, but no phenomenon in health care is more elusive. Pain is an entirely subjective feeling that can be described only by the person experiencing it. It is a learned process that is inextricably interwoven with the personal, social, cultural, and religious situation of the individual. What is experienced as pain varies widely among people and even may differ in the same person from one time to another.

Pain serves an important role. It warns us of the presence of environmental danger, causes us to rest and allow injured parts to heal, and stimulates us to seek help for dealing with organ disease or tissue damage. Not all pain, however, has apparent meaning, and its presence frequently persists long after its warning purpose has been achieved. Pain is the most dreaded aspect of the diagnosis of cancer, and in most individuals facing surgery it arouses primitive fears. As pain management strategies have, of necessity, become more holistic, nurses have assumed an integral role in its management.

The successful management of pain is one of the greatest challenges confronting health care professionals today, and the track record of successful achievement is not impressive. Research indicates that significant numbers of hospitalized patients experience moderate pain that is unrelieved by treatment. Health professionals today commonly verbalize a commitment to successful pain management, but the belief often does not significantly influence practice. The presence of pain is frequently either denied by health professionals or tolerated as an accepted norm.

TYPES OF PAIN

Pain is an abstract concept that defies accurate definition. Margo McCaffery's classic definition that "pain is whatever the experiencing person says it is and exists whenever he says it does" provides the most useful framework for nursing. There are, however, several different types of pain, each of which challenges the nurse and patient in different ways. One common classification of pain is based on the length of time it has persisted:

Acute pain is pain that generally lasts a few days. It is typically caused by tissue injury and can be expected to end when the tissue heals.

Subacute pain is similar in nature to acute pain but persists from days to weeks or even several months.

Recurrent acute pain involves episodic bouts of what is typically acute pain. The pathologic condition underlying the pain may or may not be known.

Chronic pain is pain that persists for longer than 6 months.

The major features of acute and chronic pain are compared in Table 2-1.

Some research further subdivides the large chronic pain category into three categories: ongoing cancer pain, chronic benign pain, and chronic intractable pain in which the person is completely immobilized by the pain experience. Pain may also be classified by its presumed physiologic source. These categories are summarized in Box 2-1.

TABLE 2-1 Comparison of Acute and Chronic Pain		
CHARACTERISTIC	**ACUTE PAIN**	**CHRONIC PAIN**
Source	External agent or disease process	Often unknown; if known, treatment is ineffective
Onset	Usually sudden	May be either sudden or insidious
Duration	Days to weeks: no longer than 6 mo	Greater than 6 mo; may be years
Localization	Painful areas usually clearly defined	Painful areas less clearly differentiated
Pattern	Self-limiting or readily corrected	Continuous or intermittent intensity; may vary or remain constant
Purpose	Warning that something is wrong	Meaningless, no purpose
Clinical signs	Accompanied by signs of sympathetic overactivity and visible distress	Few overt signs, response patterns vary
Prognosis	Strong likelihood of complete eventual relief	Complete relief of pain unlikely

<table>
<tr><td>**BOX 2-1**</td><td>**Types of Pain (Classified by Physiologic Cause)**</td></tr>
</table>

Somatic pain: Pain that originates in the superficial structures (skin and subcutaneous tissue) or in deeper structures (muscles or bones). It may be experienced as sharp and well localized, dull and diffusely aching, or poorly localized, depending on the fibers involved in transmission.

Visceral pain: Pain that originates in the viscera. It is usually poorly localized and is frequently accompanied by nausea, vomiting, and other autonomic symptoms. It frequently radiates or is referred.

Referred pain: Pain that is felt in areas other than those stimulated. It appears to occur most commonly in response to visceral injury. Although the mechanism is not well understood, the pattern of referral has been well documented and is fairly constant.

Psychogenic pain: Pain that appears to have no physiologic basis, originating in the mind of the patient. No adequate explanation exists at present.

Phantom limb pain: Pain perceived to be occurring in an extremity that has been amputated. The process is poorly understood.

Neuralgia: Pain that has a segmental or peripheral nerve distribution.

Headache: Although many forms have a clear physiologic basis, it is not yet possible to explain the nature of migraine or cluster headaches fully.

PHYSIOLOGY OF PAIN

Our understanding of the physiology of pain is still evolving. Each piece that is unraveled simply serves to reinforce the understanding that the process of pain perception and transmission is even more complex than originally recognized.

Pain receptors, or *nociceptors,* are free nerve endings of usually unmyelinated afferent neurons. They are located extensively in the skin and mucosa, and it is estimated that 50% of all sensory fibers have this property. They are also found in varying concentrations in deeper structures and organs. These nociceptors respond to potentially harmful thermal, mechanical, and chemical stimuli. Chemical pain stimuli include histamine, serotonin, bradykinin, prostaglandins, H^+ ions, and substance P, all of which have excitatory effects.

Pain impulses are transmitted to the spinal cord by two types of fibers: (1) A-delta fibers (thinly myelinated and fast conducting) and (2) C fibers (unmyelinated and slower conducting). Impulses conducted on myelinated, larger-diameter A-beta and A-alpha fibers appear to have an inhibitory effect on those transmitted via smaller nerve fibers. Fibers enter the spinal cord through the dorsal root and synapse in the dorsal horn (Figure 2-1). Substance P is released at the synapses and acts as a

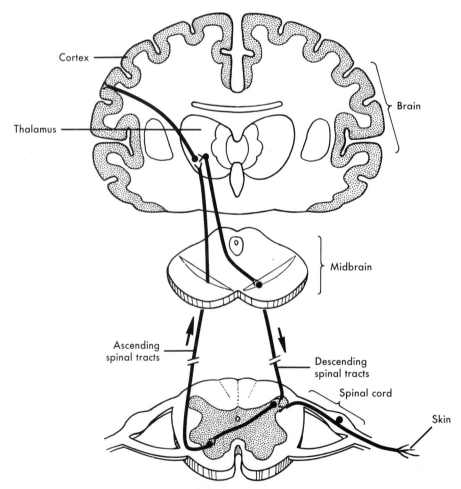

FIGURE 2-1 Pathways of pain transmission to and from cortex.

major pain transmitter. Impulses cross the spinal cord and connect with ascending spinal pathways. They travel through the midbrain to the thalamus and eventually to the cortex.

The transmission and perception of pain can also be inhibited by several powerful factors. Both the brain and spinal cord have receptor sites to which opiate compounds bind. Endogenous morphinelike polypeptides (endorphins and enkephalins) have been identified that inhibit conduction of pain impulses or inhibit release of pain transmitters such as substance P. The descending spinal pathways conduct nociceptive inhibitory impulses that may be stimulated by the A-delta fibers.

Theories concerning pain transmission continue to evolve as research is ongoing. No one theory at present adequately explains this complex process.

Specificity theory outlines the process of nociceptor pain stimulus and transmission via the pain fibers and their pathways to the brain. It does not explain the psychologic aspects of pain perception or the large variation in individual response.

Pattern theory contends that pain results from the combined effects of stimulus intensity and summations of impulses in the dorsal horn. It again does not account for psychologic aspects.

Gate control theory theorizes that pain impulses can be at least partially controlled by a "gating mechanism" in the dorsal horn of the spinal cord. Factors influencing the gate include stimulation by fast- or slow-conducting fibers, chemical modulators, and the inhibitory effects of the descending pathways.

EXPERIENCE OF PAIN

The pain experience of any individual involves both the perception of the pain sensation and the individual's response. The perception of pain takes place in the cortex and is both physiologic and relatively consistent among different individuals if the nervous system is intact. Pain tolerance, however, is extremely variable among individuals and within the same individual at different times. Pain tolerance is a reflection of culture, family influences, personality, past experience, and the meaning of the pain to the individual. It can be influenced in the same person by distraction, fatigue, anxiety, and conditioning. People also respond to pain in a myriad of ways from the stoic to the overtly demonstrative.

ASSESSMENT OF PAIN

Pain assessment is a collaborative effort among patients, physicians, and nurses. It is important to remember that although careful and thorough data collection and documentation are important, the pain experience is essentially subjective and can be truly described only by the patient.

Numerous tools have been developed in recent years to help health care personnel gather accurate and detailed data concerning pain. Figure 2-2 is an example of a detailed pain assessment tool. Simple tools can be easily used at the bedside and maintained by either the nurse or the patient. They provide an efficient way to track a patient's pain experience or response to medication over time. Examples of several scales that can be easily adapted for this purpose are contained in Boxes 2-2 and 2-3. Initial pain assessment will also involve the collection of both subjective and objective data.

Subjective Data

Characteristics and description of the pain
    Site   Type
    Severity   Intensity
    Duration   Changes over time
    Location
Measures that relieve the pain
Factors that worsen the pain
Usual coping strategies and their effectiveness
Expectations of health care team in regard to the pain
Interference of the pain with preferred life-style
    Impact on activities of daily living
    Social impact
    Occupational impact
    Impact on family and sexual life

Objective Data

Medications being taken for pain
    Dose
    Frequency
    Success in pain control or relief

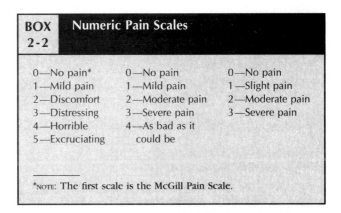

BOX 2-2	Numeric Pain Scales	
0—No pain*	0—No pain	0—No pain
1—Mild pain	1—Mild pain	1—Slight pain
2—Discomfort	2—Moderate pain	2—Moderate pain
3—Distressing	3—Severe pain	3—Severe pain
4—Horrible	4—As bad as it could be	
5—Excruciating		

*NOTE: The first scale is the McGill Pain Scale.

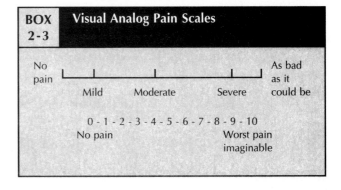

BOX 2-3   Visual Analog Pain Scales

No pain |———————|———————|———————| As bad as it could be
      Mild   Moderate   Severe

0 - 1 - 2 - 3 - 4 - 5 - 6 - 7 - 8 - 9 - 10
No pain   Worst pain imaginable

PAIN ASSESSMENT TOOL

Name _____

Age _____ Diagnosis _____

Physician _____ Date first seen _____

Medications for pain _____

Location

Have patient point to or trace the area of pain

_____

_____

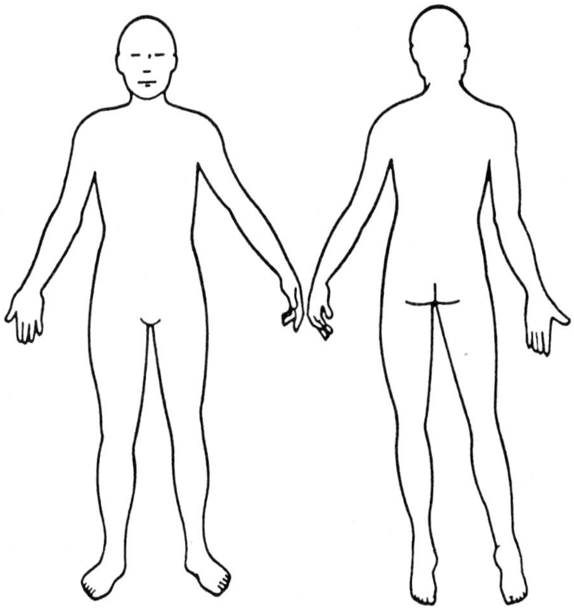

Intensity

Rate pain on a 0 to 5 scale (0 = no pain,
5 = worst pain imaginable):

At present: _____

1 hour after medication: _____

Worst it gets: _____

Best it gets: _____

Comfort

Rate comfort on a 0 to 5 scale (0 = no relief,
5 = complete relief:

At present: _____

1 hour after medication: _____

Worst it gets: _____

Best it gets: _____

Quality

Have patient describe pain in his words: _____

Chronology

When did the pain start? _____

What time of day does it occur? _____

How often does it appear? _____

How long does it last? _____

Is it constant or intermittent? _____

Has the intensity changed? _____

Patient's view of pain

What makes the pain better? _____

What makes the pain worse? _____

Any associated symptoms? _____

Does pain disturb the patient's sleep? _____

How does the pain affect the patient's mood? _____

What has helped control pain in the past? _____

What is the pain preventing the patient from doing that he would like to do? _____

_____

Signature of person performing assessment _____

FIGURE 2-2 Sample pain assessment tool. (From Beare PG, Myers JL: *Principles and practice of adult health nursing,* ed 2, St Louis, 1994, Mosby.)

Physiologic indicators of acute pain

Tachycardia	Pallor and diaphoresis
Tachypnea	Dilated pupils
Increased blood pressure (both systolic and diastolic)	Muscle tension
	Nausea and vomiting

Behavioral indicators of acute pain

Restlessness and irritability	Frowning
Clenched teeth or fists	Crying or moaning
Rigid body posture	

Accurate documentation of the pain experience is a critical and often overlooked aspect of pain assessment. A simple flowchart such as that illustrated in Figure 2-3 is an excellent tool. It presents a graphic record of the pain, pharmacologic and nonpharmacologic interventions, and their perceived effectiveness. It can provide much needed objective data on which to base modifications of the pain management plan.

MEDICAL MANAGEMENT OF PAIN
PHARMACOLOGIC APPROACHES
Analgesics

Two groups of analgesics are the cornerstone of pain management. Nonopioid drugs (e.g., aspirin, NSAIDs) block impulses primarily in the periphery by inhibiting the synthesis of prostaglandins. Opioid or narcotic analgesics (e.g., morphine) act mainly on the central nervous system to alter the perception of pain. Commonly used analgesics are summarized in Table 2-2.

Salicylates and acetaminophen

Although their specific action is unknown, salicylates and acetaminophen block prostaglandin synthesis. They are the most widely used analgesics for mild pain and have an additive effect when administered with a narcotic. Acetaminophen has no antiinflammatory effect. Aspirin inhibits platelet aggregation and slightly increases bleeding time and is therefore not given when coagulation is a concern.

Nonsteroidal antiinflammatory drugs

NSAIDs are a broad group of drugs that possess both analgesic and antiinflammatory effects. They act primarily by inhibiting prostaglandin synthesis. Gastric irritation is a common side effect, and NSAIDs should be buffered with food or antacid.

Narcotics

Opium alkaloids and synthetic narcotics such as meperidine (Demerol) are narcotic agonists that have an affinity for certain receptor sites in the brain and suppress the cells involved in pain perception. The mixed agonist-antagonist group, which includes pentazocine, buprenor-

phine, and butorphanol, share many of the pain-relieving properties of the narcotic agonists but are less likely to induce respiratory depression and tolerance.

Narcotics are the most effective analgesics for the relief of moderate to severe pain. Narcotic side effects include constipation, the most common side effect. A bowel program of stool softeners or laxatives should be promptly initiated. Nausea and vomiting are experienced by some patients, but they are usually responsive to antiemetics. Sedation and drowsiness are common in the first 24 to 72 hours of narcotic use, but patients then develop a tolerance to these effects. Respiratory depression and hypotension are rarely severe with standard doses and can be easily reversed with naloxone (Narcan) if needed.

The proper use of analgesics depends on the correct drug being administered in an adequate dose by an appropriate route at appropriate intervals. Not all drugs are equally effective in all forms. Table 2-2 compares common oral analgesics, and Table 2-3 compares the oral and parenteral effectiveness of several commonly used analgesics.

Much attention has been paid to the danger of addiction in the use of analgesics, often to the detriment of the patient. Studies have repeatedly shown that the danger of addiction from the hospital administration of narcotics is minimal. It is important that the differences among the following terms be clearly understood:

Tolerance is the need for a larger dose of a drug or increased frequency of administration to achieve the same degree of pain relief. If the level of pain remains unchanged, tolerance will *always* develop.

Physical dependence is the body's physiologic adjustment to the ongoing presence of narcotics. It will develop in *anyone* who receives consistent doses of narcotics over a period of 5 to 7 days and should be anticipated. The use of the drugs must be tapered.

Addiction refers to the overwhelming involvement of the individual with acquiring and using a drug. It should not be a factor with hospitalized patients whose pain is effectively managed.

In recent years, new options have been developed for the administration of analgesics. Continuous IV infusion, subcutaneous infusion pumps, and the development of sustained-release forms of oral morphine have added several alternatives. Perhaps the most significant of the new approaches is patient-controlled analgesia (PCA), in which the patient self-activates a syringe pump with narcotic attached to an IV line on an as-needed basis. Patients using PCA report improved pain relief and often use fewer total analgesics than patients receiving narcotics by traditional methods.

Epidural administration allows for pain relief without diminishing CNS function. It can be used postoperatively as well as for the home management of severe or intractable pain (see Guidelines boxes).

FLOW SHEET—PAIN

Patient _____ Date _____

*Pain rating scale used _____

Purpose: To evaluate the safety and effectiveness of the analgesic(s).

Analgesic(s) prescribed: _____

Time	Pain rating	Analgesic	R	P	BP	Level of arousal	Other†	Plan & comments

*Pain rating: A number of different scales may be used. Indicate which scale is used and use the same one each time. For example, 0-10 (0 = no pain, 10 = worst pain).

† Possibilities for other columns: bowel function, activities, nausea and vomiting, other pain relief measures. Identify the side effects of greatest concern to patient, family, physician, nurses.

FIGURE 2-3   Flow sheet for monitoring patient's response to pain. (From McCaffery M, Beebe A: *Pain: clinical manual for nursing practice,* St Louis, 1989, Mosby.)

TABLE 2-2 Commonly Used Analgesics

NAME	USUAL DOSAGE*	ROUTE	ONSET	PEAK	DURATION
NARCOTICS (OPIATE AGONISTS)					
Morphine sulfate	5-20 mg q 3-4 hr	SQ, IM	5-10 min	60 min	4-6 hr
Codeine sulfate	15-60 mg q 3-4 hr	SQ, oral	5-30 min	30-60 min	3-4 hr
Hydromorphone hydrochloride (Dilaudid)	2-4 mg q 4-6 hr	IV, IM, SQ, oral	5-15 min	1 hr	4-6 hr
Meperidine hydrochloride (Demerol)	50-150 mg q 3-4 hr	IV, IM, SQ, oral	10-15 min	30-60 min	2-4 hr
Methadone (Dolophine)	2.5-10 mg q 3-4 hr	IM, SQ, oral	10 min	1-2 hr	4-6 hr
Fentanyl (Sublimate)	50-100 mg/kg q 1-2 hrs	IV	1-2 min	3-5 min	0.5-1½ hr
MIXED AGONIST-ANTAGONISTS					
Buprenorphine (Buprenex)	0.3-0.6 mg q 6-8 hr	IM	15 min	1 hr	6 hr
Butorphanol (Stadol)	1-4 mg q 3-4 hr	IM	10-30 min	1 hr	4 hr
	0.5-2.0 mg q 3-4 hr	IV			
Nalbuphine (Nubain)	10 mg q 3-6 hr	IV, IM, SQ	2-15 min	1 hr	3-6 hr
Pentazocine (Talwin)	15-30 mg q 3-4 hr	IV, IM	10-30 min	1 hr	2-3 hr
	50-100 mg q 3-4 hr	Oral			
NONNARCOTICS					
Acetylsalicylic acid (aspirin)	300-1000 mg q 3-4 hr	Oral	15-30 min	1 hr	3-4 hr
Acetaminophen (Tylenol, Datril)	325-650 mg q 4-6 hr	Oral	15-30 min	1-2 hr	4-6 hr
Ibuprofen (Motrin, Advil, Nuprin)	200-600 mg q 4-6 hr	Oral	15-30 min	1-2 hr	3-4 hr
Ketorolac (Toradol)	10 mg q 4-6 hr	Oral	15-30 min	1-2 hr	4-6 hr
	30-60 mg q 6 hr	IM	10 min	0.75-1.5 hr	4-6 hr

*Must be individualized.

SQ, Subcutaneous; *IM,* intramuscular; *IV,* intravenous.

TABLE 2-3 Equianalgesic Doses of Commonly Used Narcotics

NAME		IM/SQ DOSE (MG)	ORAL DOSE (MG)
Morphine	(MS, Contin)	10	20-30
Hydromorphone	(Dilaudid)	2	7.5
Meperidine	(Demerol)	80-100	300
Codeine		120	200
Levorphanol	(Levo-Dromoran)	2	4
Methadone	(Dolophine)	8-10	20
Oxycodone	(Roxicodone)	—	30

Analgesic adjuncts

Numerous drugs have been administered over the years in attempts to augment pain relief or deal with concurrent problems and thus relieve pain. They are not classified as analgesics but may be used alone to treat problems such as sleep disturbances or in combination with an analgesic. Their appropriate use is based on careful assessment of the individual. Specific options are summarized in Table 2-4.

Tricyclic antidepressants—Amitriptyline (Elavil), imipramine (Tofranil), and doxepin (Sinequan) were initially administered in chronic pain situations to promote restful sleep and thereby improve quality of life. They also appear to stimulate the activity of endogenous opiates by increasing the levels of serotonin, a neurotransmitter. Subclinical doses are administered at bedtime.

TABLE 2-4   Analgesic Adjuncts

DRUGS	USES	COMMENTS
Major tranquilizers (phenothiazines, chlorpromazine)	Nausea, anxiety	Little justification for use in pain management
Benzodiazepines (diazepam, chlordiazepoxide)	Muscle spasm, alcohol withdrawal	Not recommended for chronic pain because they cause depression
Tricyclic antidepressants (amitriptyline, doxepin, imipramine)	Chronic pain, cancer pain, phantom limb pain	Direct analgesic effect and may potentiate narcotics
		Block reuptake of serotonin and when given at bedtime can be a sleep aid
Antihistamines (hydroxyzine)	Nausea, anxiety	Have some analgesic effects (50 mg intramuscularly = 5 mg of morphine)
		Give deep intramuscularly because injections are extremely painful and irritating

Anticonvulsants—Phenytoin (Dilantin) and carbazepine (Tegretol) are frequently employed to deal with nerve pain such as trigeminal neuralgia or phantom limb pain.

Sedatives—The use of sedatives, particularly the phenothiazines, has been a common approach in the attempt to promote analgesic effectiveness by inducing relaxation and drowsiness. This approach is no longer recommended. Research has indicated that these drugs have no analgesic effect but do increase the narcotic-related sedation, hypotension, and respiratory depression. The most effective way to promote relaxation is to adequately treat the patient's pain. *Sedation does not equal pain relief.*

Potentiators—It has been a relatively common practice to administer so-called narcotic potentiators in the attempt to augment analgesia without raising narcotic doses. Promethazine (Phenergan) and hydroxyzine (Vistaril) have been most widely used. Hydroxyzine does have some independent analgesic effect that is additive to that of the prescribed narcotic. Its proven antiemetic properties make it useful in the postoperative period. When given intramuscularly, however, it is extremely painful and tissue irritating.

Promethazine, however, has no independent analgesic effect, does not potentiate narcotics, and may even *increase* the perceived intensity of the pain. It also lacks proven effectiveness as an antiemetic. Its use in pain management is questionable at best.

Patient-controlled analgesia

Patient-controlled analgesia (PCA) has rapidly evolved into the strategy of choice for managing acute pain. An infusion pump delivers the desired amount of medication through an IV catheter, an implantable SQ catheter, or an epidural catheter. The device is programmed to deliver a specified amount of drug (usually morphine) at specified minimum intervals or via continuous infusion. Locked reservoirs and syringe systems prevent accidental overdosage. The patient controls the number of medication boluses delivered. PCA bypasses environmental variables such as nurse availability and the perceptions of other caretakers (Figure 2-4). Research with PCA clearly indicates the following:

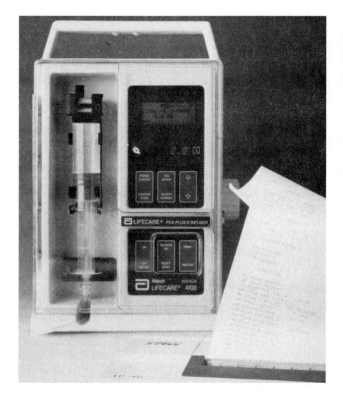

FIGURE 2-4   Patient-controlled analgesia (Life Care PCA Plus II infuser). (Courtesy Abbott Laboratories, Abbott Park, IL.)

- Patient satisfaction with pain relief is higher.
- Overall pain relief is more effective.
- Patients use no more total medication than with nurse-controlled administration.

NOTE: Patients are found to use *more* medication in the early hours and days but less later.

Patient education is the key to PCA success. Ideally the patient should be alert enough to understand and comply with the directions. A patient will not do well with PCA if he or she cannot understand it (see accompanying Guidelines box).

Epidural analgesia

Epidural analgesia has been increasing dramatically in popularity. It involves the administration of a narcotic or local anesthetic into the epidural space (Figure 2-5). A narcotic administered epidurally can control pain

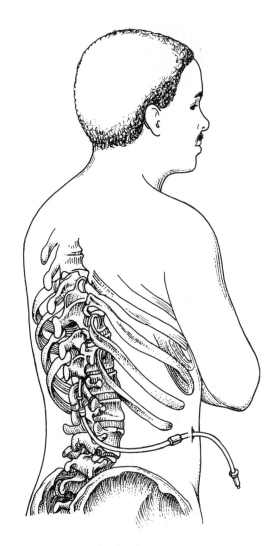

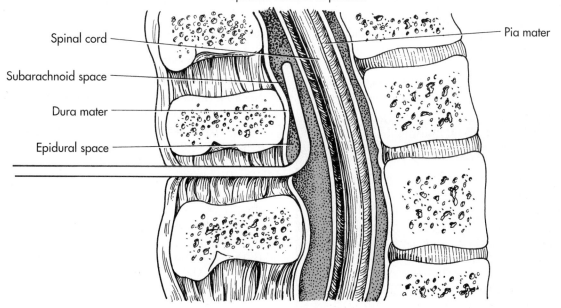

Epidural catheter in position

Spinal cord

Subarachnoid space

Dura mater

Epidural space

Pia mater

FIGURE 2-5   Epidural catheter.

Guidelines for Teaching Patients About Patient-Controlled Analgesia

- Explain how the pump works and precisely how to increase the dose.
- Explain the importance of using PCA *before* the pain becomes severe, since bolus doses are small.
- Explore the patient's fears and concerns over use of the pump or dependency on narcotics.
- Reinforce the lock-out safeguards that are in place to prevent accidental overdosage.
- Include family members in teaching plan if possible. Address their concerns.
- Secure the cord with bolus button within easy access of the patient.
- Keep side rails up and monitor for orthostatic hypotension when moving the patient.
- Monitor respiratory rate during initial administration to determine patient response.

Guidelines for Changing from IM/IV to PO Administration

The conversion to oral analgesic administration must be skillfully handled to prevent a return of pain and loss of faith by the patient in the effectiveness of oral drugs. A gradual changeover reduces the risk of potential overdosage or underdosage. Principles include the following:

1. Begin administering a nonnarcotic on a regular basis.
2. Select the equianalgesic dose of the oral narcotic to replace the current IM/IV dose.
3. Decrease the IM/IV dose by 10% to 33% and calculate the PO dose needed to replace it and administer both.
4. Assess the effectiveness and adjust the PO dose up or down as needed.
5. When analgesia is effective, reduce the IM/IV dose again by the same amount (10% to 33%) and replace with the correct amount of PO narcotic.
6. Continue to follow this procedure until the entire parenteral dose is replaced. Continue to monitor the effectiveness with the patient throughout the change.

Modified from McCaffery M, Beebe A: *Pain—clinical manual for nursing practice*, St Louis, 1989, Mosby.

originating anywhere below the cranial nerves. There are opiate receptors located all along the spinal cord. The drug diffuses slowly through the dura mater into the cerebrospinal fluid (CSF), which carries it directly to the cord, bypassing the blood-brain barrier. The narcotic acts directly on the receptors of the dorsal horn, producing localized analgesia without motor blockade. Lower doses can be used, and systemic effects are minimized. Patients are more alert, respiratory depression is rare, and adverse reactions are few. Analgesics may be administered via a needle or a temporary or permanent catheter. The drug itself is either directly injected or continuously infused (see accompanying Guidelines box).

NONPHARMACOLOGIC APPROACHES

Nonpharmacologic approaches may be used instead of or in addition to analgesics in pain management.

Cutaneous Stimulation

Applications of heat and cold are forms of cutaneous stimulation and utilize the principles of the gate control

Guidelines for Epidural Catheter Care

Infection is the greatest concern. Basic care for an epidural catheter includes the following:

- Teaching patient and family about epidural administration, its benefits and side effects
- Cleansing the insertion site and changing the dressing as ordered using aseptic techniques (weekly if covering is dry and intact)
- Assessing the site daily for inflammation or infection
- Assessing for side effects: nausea, temporary urinary retention, and itching from histamine release (NOTE: Itching may be troublesome and unresponsive to antihistamines.)
- Monitoring respirations during first 24 hours to assess individual response to narcotic

pain theory. Beside their effectiveness in controlling and resolving inflammation they also are able to modify the sensory input at the site of pain. Massage is the classic form of cutaneous stimulation and is used spontaneously by most individuals who experience mild to moderate discomfort. Pressure and vibration may also be used.

The effects of cutaneous stimulation are variable and unpredictable, but in general the pain is eliminated or decreased in intensity during and/or after the stimulation. Guidelines for cutaneous stimulation are found in the box on p. 23.

Electrical Nerve Stimulators

Nerve stimulators attempt to modify pain stimuli by blocking them or altering them with other stimuli. This approach uses the gate control theory. The transcutaneous electrical nerve stimulator (TENS) is the most common form. It uses a battery-powered stimulator attached to two or more electrodes that are applied around or near the pain site. The patient regulates the power source and electrode placement to achieve the best effect.

Principles for use of TENS are outlined in the Guidelines box, p. 23. Spinal cord stimulators are similar to TENS but involve placement of the electrodes directly on or near the spinal cord.

Nerve Blocks

Nerve blocks involve the injection of local anesthetic agents or neurolytic agents close to nerves to block pain impulse conduction. They are indicated for pain con-

Guidelines for Cutaneous Stimulation

The results of cutaneous stimulation are unpredictable. Involve the patient in the planning and experimentation at every step. Encourage an open mind to the application of stimulation proximal or distal to the painful area, at known trigger points, and even contralateral to the painful spot.

- Cutaneous stimulation is recommended for intervals of 20 to 30 minutes.
- Experiment with the technique; for example, try dry and moist heat or different weights and pressure for massage.
- Try different forms, such as heat versus cold, or alternate them either at different times or rhythmically during one treatment interval (contrast baths).
- Use more than one method at a time, such as a cold pack over menthol.
- Ensure patient safety with all uses of superficial heat and cold, especially in elderly persons:
  - Hot water bottles (wrap to prevent burns)
  - Heating pads (do not lie directly on)
  - Hydrocollator packs (wrap and do not lie on directly)
  - Ice packs (always wrap to prevent tissue injury)
- Use what appears to work best for the patient unless contraindicated.
- Do not use heat if bleeding and swelling are present.
- Do not use either heat or cold if patient has impaired sensation or anesthetic areas.
- Consider ice massage (direct application of ice to the skin) for sports injuries, for muscle spasms, for tooth pain, and before venipunctures. It is used for brief intervals and never for more than 10 minutes.

Guidelines for Using TENS

Follow manufacturer's directions carefully because units vary.
Apply electrodes to clean, unbroken skin directly over the area of pain, at trigger points on nerve pathways, or in the same dermatome.
Observe skin daily for signs of irritation.
Make sure the device is turned off before applying or removing electrodes. Remove and clean electrodes daily.
Tape electrodes to the skin using hypoallergenic tape.
Adjust the controls so that the impulse is a comfortable, pleasant sensation. If muscle contraction occurs, turn down the intensity. Pins and needles feelings are expected.
Placement of electrodes should never be over the eyes, hair, carotid sinuses, throat, or abdomen during pregnancy.
Contraindications for TENS use
People with demand cardiac pacemakers
Patients with a history of cardiac dysrhythmias or myocardial infarction
Pregnancy in the first trimester (may have some benefit for back labor during delivery)
Confused or elderly patients with decreased sensory perception

fined to a specific area or nerve distribution. They can provide short-term pain relief or be designed to physically damage or destroy the affected nerve. Spinal administration is the most common, and patients are carefully monitored for motor and sensory function following the procedures. Repeated blocks may be used and often produce progressively longer periods of pain relief.

Neurosurgical Approaches

Relentless intractable pain may be reduced or abolished by the use of one of the following surgical procedures:

Neurectomy: Nerve fibers to affected area are severed from the cord. Also sacrifices the fibers controlling movement and position sense. Peripheral fibers may regenerate.

Rhizotomy: A posterior nerve root is resected just before it enters the spinal cord. May be employed to relieve painful spasticity. It interferes with the ability to perceive heat and cold.

Cordotomy: The pain pathways in the spinothalamic tract of the spinal cord are severed, producing a wide sense of analgesia while preserving other sensory and motor functions.

Acupuncture

Acupuncture is an ancient method of pain relief that has only recently been used in Western societies. It involves the insertion and manipulation of small needles at specific body points, producing often immediate and ongoing pain relief. Lasers are also being utilized instead of needles.

Cognitive Strategies

Relaxation exercises, rhythmic breathing, distraction, and visual imagery are all techniques that attempt to deal with the anxiety that frequently surrounds the pain experience. Reducing fear and anxiety assists patients to remain in control of their overall situation. Not all of these techniques are effective with every patient, but they can help in restoring a sense of power and self-mastery. Being overwhelmed by pain can be terrifying.

Biofeedback and Autogenic Training

Some persons can be taught to modify their body functions through mental concentration. Biofeedback training uses an electroencephalogram (EEG) machine to measure brain wave activity. The individual gradually learns to concentrate on slowing brain wave activity to a state of complete relaxation.

Relaxation can also be learned without the reinforcement of a machine. Practiced meditation may enable the individual to achieve an astonishing degree of concentration and self-control. External hypnosis or self-hypnosis may be taught to alter the perception of pain through the acceptance of positive suggestions.

NURSING MANAGEMENT: Pain

♦ ASSESSMENT
Subjective Data

History of the pain experience, precipitating and aggravating factors

Beliefs about pain origins and causes

Description of the pain (character, quality, duration)

Strategies in use for dealing with pain and their effectiveness

Impact of pain on activities of daily living, job, social activities

Medications in use and their side effects—constipation, depression, gastric acidity

Sleep and rest pattern—complaints of fatigue or insomnia

Impact of pain on mobility

Usual coping patterns and effectiveness

Knowledge of and attitudes concerning nonpharmacologic pain management strategies

Objective Data

General appearance

Vital signs—presence of tachycardia, tachypnea, or elevated blood pressure

Restless, anxious, irritable behavior; tense muscles

Moist skin or pallor

♦ NURSING DIAGNOSES

Nursing diagnoses for the person with pain may include, but are not limited to, the following:

Pain, acute or chronic (related to the disease process, surgery, trauma, or other cause)

Anxiety (related to inability to control the pain experience)

Knowledge deficit (related to nonpharmacologic pain control strategies)

Constipation (related to the side effects of analgesics)

♦ EXPECTED PATIENT OUTCOMES

Patient will experience a decreased and manageable level of pain or state that pain is eliminated.

Patient will express confidence that the pain can be successfully controlled.

Patient will be knowledgeable about the overall pain plan:

Correct use of all analgesics

Use of nonpharmacologic strategies

Patient will reestablish a regular pattern of bowel elimination.

♦ NURSING INTERVENTIONS
Relieving/Reducing the Pain

Establish a bedside tool to monitor pain and evaluate the effectiveness of interventions. Teach patient how to properly use the tool.

Administer analgesics and adjuncts as prescribed. Monitor vital signs.

Assess level of consciousness and maintain patient safety.

Administer an adequate dose—assess for effectiveness of drug.

Use pain relief measures *before* pain becomes severe:

Start with a high dose and work back slowly as control is established.

Offer analgesics for acute pain around the clock rather than as needed.

Explore use of PCA with physician.

Combine analgesic and nonpharmacologic strategies when possible.

Assess and record the effectiveness of all analgesics:

Explore the use of adjuncts with physician if pain control remains inadequate.

Follow equianalgesic tables when converting from parenteral to other forms of administration.

Reassure patient concerning issue of addiction.

Assess for signs of tolerance with prolonged administration: increased complaints of pain, shorter duration of relief, anxiety, preoccupation with medication schedule.

Collaborate with physician to safely increase doses to maintain adequate analgesia.

Relieving Anxiety

Reassure patient that control of pain is possible.

Teach patient about the cause and expected duration of the pain and measures immediately available for dealing with it.

Involve patient in all plans concerning pain management, activity, and medications.

Maintain consistency in assignments if possible.

Encourage patient to seek assistance and support from pain clinics, counseling, and religious beliefs as appropriate.

Explore patient concerns related to addiction.

Teaching About Nonpharmacologic Methods

Apply cutaneous stimulation if appropriate. Teach patient techniques for safe use of heat and cold at home.

Discuss with patient the use of distraction techniques—TV, visitors, music, activity. Avoid overfatigue.

Avoid social isolation and sensory overload.

Teach or reinforce relaxation and rhythmic breathing techniques—use positive visual imagery if patient is receptive.

Assist patient to find positions that promote comfort. Encourage frequent position changes.

Move patient gently, using support to affected areas.

Use pressure-relieving aids to augment comfort.

Offer gentle back rubs with position changes.

Maintain or establish a pleasant environment.

Assist patient with hygiene, fresh clothes, and linens.

Maintain comfortable temperature, eliminate odors.

Plan activities and needed care for pain-free intervals if possible. Plan for additional rest periods.

Provide for uninterrupted nighttime sleep if possible.

Schedule needed medications and treatments to avoid awakening patient.

Time analgesics to support needed sleep.

Preventing Narcotic-Related Constipation

Promote optimal nutrition.

Offer small, frequent meals attractively served.

Prevent constipation through diet modification or use of stool softeners.

Encourage a liberal fluid intake.

Encourage patient to be active during pain-free intervals.

♦ EVALUATION

Successful achievement of expected outcomes for the patient with pain is indicated by the following:

Manageable pain levels or pain-free state

Feeling of control over pain experience and management of protocol

Appropriate utilization of nonpharmacologic pain management strategies

Regular pattern of bowel elimination

SELECTED REFERENCES

Carr E: Postoperative pain: patients' expectations, *J Adv Nurs* 15:89-100, 1990.

Dolan MB, Robinson JH, Roberts S: When the doctor delays pain relief, *Nurs 93* 23(4):46-49, 1993.

Ferrell B, McCaffery M, Grant M: Clinical decision making and pain, *Ca Nurs* 14:289-297, 1991.

Ferrell BR, McCaffery M, Rhiner M: Pain and addiction: an urgent need for change in nursing education, *J Pain Symptom Manage* 7(2):117-122, 1992.

Fulton JS, Johnson GB: Using high dose morphine to relieve cancer pain, *Nurs 93* 23(2):34-39, 1993.

Hansberry JL, Bannick KH, Durkan MJ: Managing chronic pain with a permanent epidural catheter, *Nurs 90* 20(10):53-55, 1990.

McCaffery M, Beebe A: Giving narcotics for pain, *Nurs 89* 19(10):161-165, 1989.

GERONTOLOGIC PATIENT CONSIDERATIONS FOR PAIN MANAGEMENT

Research consistently indicates that many hospitalized patients, especially elderly ones, are undermedicated for pain. The fear of overdosage causes many elders to suffer needlessly. Narcotics are generally well tolerated by elders, but their initial responses must be monitored more closely. Age is not significant in determining doses, but it is often important in determining the frequency of administration, since drugs tend to be cleared more slowly from elders' bodies. Doses should be based on the therapeutic response and the presence of undesirable side effects, if any. It is important to carefully review other medications the elder may be taking to prevent adverse drug interactions.

McCaffery M, Beebe A: Managing your patients' adverse reactions to narcotics, *Nurs 89* 19(10):166-168, 1989.

McCaffery M, Beebe A: *Pain: clinical manual for nursing practice,* St Louis, 1989, Mosby.

McCaffery M, Ferrel B: Do you know about narcotic when you see one? *Nurs 90* 20(6):62-63, 1990.

McCaffery M, Ferrell BR: Does the gender gap affect your pain control? *Nurs 92* 22(8):48-51, 1992.

McCaffery M, Ferrell BR, O'Neil-Page E: Does lifestyle affect your pain control decisions? *Nurs 92* 22(4):58-61, 1992.

McGuire L: Administering analgesics: which drugs are right for your patient? *Nurs 90* 20(4):34-41, 1990.

Mueller R: Cancer pain: which drugs for which patient? *RN* 55(4):38-45, 1992.

Noah VA: Preop teaching is the key to PCA success, *RN* 53(5):60-63, 1990.

Pasero C, McCaffery M: Unconventional PCA: making it work for your patient, *Am J Nurs* 93(9):38-41, 1993.

Relieving pain: an analgesic guide: principles of analgesic use, *Am J Nurs* 88:815-826, 1988.

Turnage G, Clark L, Wild L: Spinal opioids: a nursing perspective, *J Pain Symptom Manage* 5:154-162, 1990.

Vandenbosch TM: How to use a pain flow-sheet effectively, *Nurs 88* 18(8):50-51, 1988.

Walker M, Wong DL: A battle plan for patients in pain, *Am J Nurs* 91(6):33-36, 1991.

Wild L: Pain management, *Crit Care Clin North Am* 2(4):537-547, 1990.

Wild L, Coyne C: Epidural analgesia: the basics and beyond, *Am J Nurs* 92(4):26-36, 1992.

Woodin LM: Cutting postop pain, *RN* 56(8):26-33, 1993.

Wright S: The use of therapeutic touch in the management of pain, *Nurs Clin North Am* 22(3):705-714, 1987.

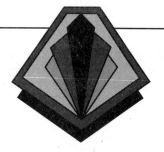

Substance Abuse

Substance abuse (chemical dependency) is being increasingly recognized as a major social and health problem in the United States. Substance abuse encompasses a complex set of behaviors involving physical and psychologic dependence on one or more substances and overwhelming preoccupation with obtaining and using the substance. It is increasingly recognized that chemical dependency severely complicates the admissions of many individuals in the acute care setting.

Common terms used to describe substance abuse and chemical dependency are defined in Box 3-1.

> **BOX 3-1** **Definitions of Terms Related to Chemical Dependency**
>
> Physical dependence: physical adaptation of the body to the chronic use of a substance. A withdrawal syndrome will occur if the substance is suddenly stopped.
> Tolerance: present when a given dose of a substance fails to produce the same effect and larger doses are required.
> Chemical dependency/addiction: a problem characterized by compulsive use of substances for nonmedical reasons, loss of control over the circumstances of substance use, continued use despite adverse consequences, frequent relapses after periods of abstinence, and the inability to voluntarily decrease use (psychologic dependence).

ALCOHOLISM
ETIOLOGY/EPIDEMIOLOGY

Alcoholism is by far the most common form of chemical dependency. It is variously estimated that 9 to 10 million persons are alcoholic and that alcoholism adversely affects the lives of 30 million other friends and relatives. The abuse of alcohol is directly linked to motor vehicle accidents and fatalities, suicides, homicides, and home accidents. Alcohol-related problems are estimated to cost over $70 billion annually in medical costs, lost wages, and so on. The vast majority of alcoholics have been assumed to be men, but research is identifying increasing numbers of women, who are more likely to hide their drinking.

Alcoholics do not exhibit one single pattern of drinking behavior or response to the disease. Some alcoholics are classic daily heavy drinkers, others drink episodically in binges, whereas still others drink infrequently but in an uncontrolled manner. It is important to distinguish drinking alcohol abusively from alcoholism. An individual may drink large amounts for years without becoming alcoholic. The chemical dependence of alcoholism reflects a progressive intake, increasing tolerance and physical dependence, and compulsive focusing on obtaining and using alcohol, even in the face of serious personal consequences. Blackouts may occur.

Theories concerning the etiology of alcoholism have changed over time, and no single theory explains all its aspects. Research indicates that the key etiology involves a genetically determined biochemical defect, possibly augmented by minor defects in the body's response to and metabolism of alcohol. The incidence of alcoholism is high in at-risk families. Distinct cultural variations also exist. Theories concerning moral faults or sins are no longer accepted, but a moral tone still exists in how societies deal with and respond to the alcoholic person.

PATHOPHYSIOLOGY

Alcohol affects every organ system of the body. It does not require digestion and is absorbed directly from both the stomach and intestine. After absorption, alcohol is distributed throughout the body fluids and crosses all membranes. Alcohol is not converted to glycogen, and it cannot be stored (Figure 3-1). One ounce of alcohol contains 200 kilocalories. It is metabolized by the liver at a rate of 6 to 10 g/hr.

Alcohol is a central nervous system (CNS) depressant that inhibits the action of specific neurotransmitters. Its initial stimulating effects are related to suppression of higher centers governing judgment and self-control. As

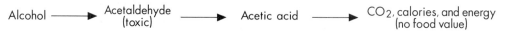

Alcohol ⟶ Acetaldehyde (toxic) ⟶ Acetic acid ⟶ CO_2, calories, and energy (no food value)

FIGURE 3-1   Metabolism of alcohol.

BOX 3-2 **Effects of Alcohol on Body Organs**

CENTRAL NERVOUS SYSTEM

Depression leading to loss of memory and difficulty concentrating
Loss of self-control and judgment

CARDIOVASCULAR SYSTEM

Increased pulse rate
Dilation of cutaneous blood vessels

IMMUNOLOGIC SYSTEM

Increased susceptibility to infection

GI TRACT

Stimulation of gastric secretions
Direct irritation of mucosa
Decreased vitamin absorption in bowel

KIDNEY

Diuretic effect

BOX 3-3 **Alcohol and Pregnancy**

Women who drink during pregnancy have a higher incidence of children with birth defects, and the risk increases with the frequency and quantity of drinking. Fetal alcohol syndrome is a devastating complex of symptoms including the following:

Mental retardation   Facial abnormalities
Microcephaly   Skeletal, urogenital, and cardiac
Growth deficiencies   abnormalities

Even moderate drinking can increase the risk of births of infants with significant lags in mental and motor development.

BOX 3-4 *Healthy People 2000:* **Goals Related to Alcohol Use**

1. *Reduce deaths caused by alcohol-related motor vehicle crashes to no more than 8.5 per 100,000 people from an age-adjusted baseline of 9.8 per 100,000 in 1987. Special target populations for this goal include young adults aged 15-24 and American Indian/Alaskan men.*
2. Reduce cirrhosis deaths to no more than 6 per 100,000 people from an age-adjusted baseline of 9.1 per 100,000 in 1987.
3. Reduce the proportion of high school seniors and college students engaging in heavy drinking of alcohol to no more than 28% of high school seniors and 32% of college students. Baseline was 33% of high school seniors and 41.7% of college students in 1989.
4. Reduce alcohol consumption by people aged 14 and older to an annual average of no more than 2 gallons of alcohol per person.

From US Department of Health and Human Services, Public Health Service: *Healthy people 2000: national health promotion and disease prevention objectives,* Washington, DC, 1990, US Government Printing Office.

---

alcohol accumulates, unconsciousness may set in, and the brain may be so overwhelmed that it stops functioning permanently. Typical systemic effects of alcohol are summarized in Box 3-2. Effects of alcohol on the fetus during pregnancy are summarized in Box 3-3.

MEDICAL MANAGEMENT

Medical management of alcoholism usually focuses on the management of individuals during acute withdrawal followed by referral for ongoing rehabilitation. Prevention rarely plays a major role in alcoholism, since the disease is genetically predisposed once the person begins alcohol consumption of any kind. Complete abstinence is the only prevention and the only treatment. Prevention is critical in the broader area of alcohol abuse, however, and is reflected clearly in the *Healthy People 2000* goals (Box 3-4). Prompt diagnosis and treatment referral are essential in identifying alcoholics who can be helped to recovery before their lives fall into complete disarray.

Managing Alcoholic Withdrawal

An alcoholic develops a steadily increasing tolerance to and dependence on alcohol. Withdrawal affects motor control, mental status, and body functions and in rare cases can even be fatal. It may be mild or severe and is influenced by increasing age and coexisting illnesses and nutritional deficiencies.

Mild withdrawal is characterized by hand tremor, restlessness, anxiety, insomnia, anorexia, and tachycardia.

Moderate withdrawal is characterized by a worsening of all symptoms. Vague transient hallucinations may occur, and seizures are possible.

Severe withdrawal (delirium tremens [DTs]) is characterized by a pathologic state of consciousness caused by interference with brain metabolism. Marked confusion and auditory hallucinations are common and are accompanied by acute restlessness, shaking, and intense anxiety. Excessive sweating and elevated vital signs are present. Untreated cases carry a greater than 15% mortality. Severe withdrawal can occur from 3 to 7 days after the last drink.

Management of withdrawal includes nutritional support and sedation as indicated by the patient's condition. High-calorie diets are administered if tolerated, and all patients receive aggressive multivitamin supplementation. If needed, tranquilizing agents such as chlordiazepoxide (Librium), diazepam (Valium), or paraldehyde may be administered. Seizures are prevented or treated through the use of phenytoin (Dilantin) or magnesium sulfate. Medication should be administered at the first sign of withdrawal symptoms and used liberally during the first several days to ensure patient safety.

BOX 3-5 **Wernicke-Korsakoff Syndrome**

Wernicke-Korsakoff syndrome is a consequence of long-term abuse of alcohol and may be seen in elderly patients or patients in long term–care facilities. Alcohol plays a role, but long-term nutritional deficiency, particularly of thiamine, is the primary cause. Symptoms include the following:

Ocular disturbances, such as nystagmus
Ataxia
Apathy, confusion, and psychosis
Memory problems

Treatment is supportive, and the prognosis is uncertain.

BOX 3-6 **Diagnostic Test Findings in Alcoholism**

Some abnormalities occur in routine blood tests that are directly related to alcoholism. Common abnormalities include the following:

Elevated liver enzymes (aspartate aminotransferase [AST], alanine aminotransferase [ALT], bilirubin)
Hypoalbuminemia
Hypomagnesemia
Anemia: increased mean corpuscular volume (MCV)

BOX 3-7 **Disulfiram (Antabuse)**

Disulfiram (Antabuse) is an aversive agent that may be used as an adjunct to the treatment of alcoholism. Metabolically, the drug blocks the enzymatic action necessary to metabolize alcohol. Even a small sip of alcohol can cause severe nausea, vomiting, palpitations, and general prostration. It may be used to reinforce an initial period of sobriety or as an adjunct to other treatment. It is not primary therapy and can cause very serious general reactions.

REHABILITATION

The painful process of alcoholic withdrawal accomplishes little if the individual does not proceed to active rehabilitation and make a commitment to recovery. Abstinence is the only way to control alcoholism, and social drinking is not an option. Relapse is common, and there is no approach with uniform effectiveness. Behavior modification, psychoanalysis, and group therapy have all been used, but the self-help approach of Alcoholics Anonymous (AA) has had the most consistent success. AA is composed of self-acknowledged alcoholics whose purpose is to stay sober and help others achieve and maintain sobriety. Recognizing that recovery is a lifelong process, the approach focuses on remaining sober today and facing one day at a time.

BOX 3-8 **Impaired Professionals**

It is estimated that one in six to seven nurses will become dependent on drugs or alcohol during their work lives. Most states now have outreach programs to assist the impaired professional. This represents a major change from the punishment mode common in the past. Peer assistance programs focus simultaneously on protecting the public and rehabilitating the person if possible.

 GERONTOLOGIC PATIENT CONSIDERATIONS FOR ALCOHOLISM

Both alcoholism and other chemical dependencies are common problems in elderly persons, but they are frequently unacknowledged. The issue of loneliness frequently exacerbates what may have been a hidden or "closet" problem. Nurses need to be alert to substance abuse as a possible contributing factor to confusion, falls, or other injuries. The principles of treatment are the same and must include social support.

NURSING MANAGEMENT

◆ ASSESSMENT

Subjective Data

Drinking patterns: amount, type, frequency, and duration; date and time of last drink
Other substances used
Family history of alcoholism
Past experience with treatment, efforts at sobriety
Problems related to drinking
    Occupational, family, legal, sexual
    History of blackouts, hallucinations
Medications in use, prescription and over the counter (OTC)
Normal diet and eating pattern

Objective Data

Mental functioning
    General behavior and affect
    Memory loss, difficulty concentrating
    Presence and severity of tremor
Presence of anorexia, nausea/vomiting
Vital signs
Body weight
    Presence of ascites
    Symptoms of vitamin deficiency

The remainder of the nursing management of a patient with acute alcoholism is summarized in the nursing care plan. A sample critical pathway on managing detoxification is also included.

CRITICAL PATHWAY	**Alcohol/Drug Detoxification Without Inpatient Rehabilitation**

DRG #: 435 Expected LOS: 4

	Day of Admission Day 1	Day 2	Day 3	Day of Discharge Day 4
Diagnostic Tests	Complete blood count, urinalysis, SMA/18,* drug screen			
Medications	Chlordiazepoxide, 10 mg PO q 4 hr PRN for agitation; antiemetic q 4 hr PRN; antacid PRN; vitamins daily: B_{12} IM; thiamine, 100 mg	Chlordiazepoxide, 10 mg PO q 4 hr PRN for agitation; antiemetic q 4 hr PRN; antacid PRN; vitamins daily: thiamine, 100 mg	Chlordiazepoxide, 10 mg q 4 hr PRN for agitation; antiemetic q 4 hr PRN; antacid PRN; vitamins daily	Vitamins daily
Treatments	Vital signs (VS) q 2 hr; intake and output (I&O) q 8 hr; neurochecks q 2 hr; provide protective environment	VS q 2 hr; I&O q 8 hr; neurochecks q 2 hr; participates in individual and group activities	VS q 4 hr; disc I&O; neurochecks q 4 hr; participates in individual and group activities and counseling	VS q 8 hr; participates in outpatient individual or group counseling
Diet	Clear liquids; advance diet as tolerated: force fluids	Regular diet: force fluids	Regular diet: force fluids	Regular diet
Activity	Up as tolerated: protect from falls if unstable: minimize stimulation	Up as tolerated: protect from falls if unstable: minimize stimulation	Up ad lib	Up ad lib
Consultations	CD counselor, neurologist, psychiatrist	CD counselor	CD counselor	

NOTE: Acknowledge that patients recover at varying rates; therefore specified daily actions should be based solely on patient need.
*Serum calcium, phosphorus, triglycerides, uric acid, creatinine, BUN, total bilirubin, alkaline phosphate, aspartate aminotransferase (AST, formerly serum glutamic oxaloacetic transaminase [SGOT]), alanine aminotransferase (ALT, formerly serum glutamic oxaloacetic transaminase [SGPT]), lactic dehydrogenase (LDH), total protein, albumin, sodium, potassium, chloride, total CO_2, glucose. *CD,* Chemical dependency.

DRUG ABUSE

Since alcohol is a drug, it is rightly incorporated into any discussion of chemical dependency, but the abuse of other drugs does have unique features. There is also an increasing tendency for persons to abuse a mixture of both drugs and alcohol.

No reliable statistics exist on drug use nor is there even substantial agreement as to what constitutes drug abuse. Some consider it the ongoing use of any drug, whereas others restrict the definition to drugs that lead to psychologic or physical dependence. The basic categories of drugs of abuse include stimulants, depressants, hallucinogens, and narcotics. The various drug categories and their effects are summarized in Table 3-1.

The approach to the management of drug abuse is similar in most ways to that described for alcoholism. The person is assisted to withdraw from the substance, offered nutritional support, and encouraged to pursue ongoing treatment and peer support in abstinence from groups such as Narcotics Anonymous. Success is not assured, and relapses are common.

CHEMICAL DEPENDENCY AND PAIN MANAGEMENT

Few situations are more challenging and frustrating than managing acute or chronic pain in known or suspected substance abusers. Yet, based on the prevalence of both pain and chemical dependency, it is reasonable to expect the two challenges to coexist frequently in acute care settings. Addicts typically generate many hostile feelings from health care workers, including beliefs about their irresponsibility, lack of contribution to society, and self-destructive behavior. Conflicts arise between the desire to meet the patient's needs and fears of worsening the abuse or being duped into supporting the abuse pattern. At the same time the patient realizes that he or she has lost control over his or her own pattern of substance use and experiences considerable anxiety and fear. Principles of care are outlined in the Guidelines box.

NURSING CARE PLAN

FOR PERSON WITH ACUTE ALCOHOLISM

■ NURSING DIAGNOSIS

Injury, high risk for (related to cognitive deficits and lack of awareness of environmental hazards)

Expected Patient Outcome	Nursing Interventions
Patient will complete detoxification without physical injury.	Monitor vital signs q 2-4 hr for first 48 hr.
	Medicate as ordered with chlordiazepoxide (Librium) or other agents. Initiate medication as soon as symptoms of withdrawal are evident.
	Keep side rails up while patient is in bed.
	Maintain seizure precautions. Monitor for seizure activity and hallucinations.
	Clear environment of obvious hazards. Ensure patient safety. Utilize restraints only if needed.
	Keep environmental stimulation at a low level.
	Reorient the patient as needed.
	Reassure family about reversibility of symptoms, and limit number of outside visitors.

■ NURSING DIAGNOSIS

Nutrition, altered: less than body requirements (related to alcohol consumption and poor nutritional intake)

Expected Patient Outcome	Nursing Interventions
Patient will ingest a nutritionally balanced diet and reverse deficiencies.	Offer balanced diet as tolerated.
	Provide multivitamin supplements.
	Offer liberal fluids.
	Provide candy and sweet foods if cravings develop.
	Record intake and output.
	Monitor weight daily.
	Provide antacids or antiemetics as needed.

■ NURSING DIAGNOSIS

Sleep pattern disturbance (related to withdrawal stimulation)

Expected Patient Outcome	Nursing Interventions
Patient will gradually return to a normal sleep pattern with no more than two nighttime awakenings.	Keep evening stimulation at a low level.
	Teach use of cognitive and progressive muscle relaxation strategies.
	Avoid use of caffeine, particularly in the evening.
	Encourage active daytime physical activity.
	Avoid daytime napping.
	Avoid all use of sleeping aids.

NURSING CARE PLAN

FOR PERSON WITH ACUTE ALCOHOLISM

■ NURSING DIAGNOSIS

Home maintenance management, high risk for altered (related to intense anxiety, return to alcoholic life patterns)

Expected Patient Outcomes	Nursing Interventions

Patient will verbalize acceptance of powerlessness over alcohol:
  Admit the impact of alcohol on life pattern and family
  Verbalize understanding of alcoholism and need for lifelong abstinence
	Encourage patient to establish a daily routine with planned exercise.
	Discuss disease/genetic basis of alcoholism.
	Instill hope but recognize the frustrations of early recovery.
	Encourage patient to verbalize and grieve for:
	  Needed life-style changes
	  Loss of alcohol
	  Needed changes in friendship and social patterns
	Encourage involvement with AA. Initiate first contact with patient.
	Plan strategies for dealing with periods of intense cravings.
	Reinforce importance of approaching sobriety one day at a time.
	Refer family members for support through Al-Anon to increase awareness of codependence and enabling behaviors.
	Caution patient to avoid all OTC medicines containing alcohol.

TABLE 3-1 Major Drugs of Abuse

CATEGORY/EXAMPLES	EFFECT	MAJOR CLINICAL MANIFESTATIONS
STIMULANTS (NATURAL AND SYNTHETIC)	Strong stimulating effect on CNS, speeding up activity of heart and brain	Tachycardia and hypertension Increased alertness and concentration, decreased fatigue Insomnia Agitation, restlessness, and anxiety Lack of appetite, weight loss Severe fatigue and depression during withdrawal

Amphetamines
  Dextroamphetamine (Dexedrine)
  Methamphetamine (Methedrine)
  Amphetamine (Benzedrine)
  Bennies, speed, crystal, meth, whites, pep pills
	Repeated use causes tolerance and intense psychologic dependence	

Cocaine
  Crack: free base foundation of cocaine hydrochloride
  Blow, snow, coke, crack, dust, flake, toot, nose candy
	Acts as CNS stimulant, blocking neurotransmitters and prolonging action of dopamine and norepinephrine
	Both tolerance and dependence occur with ongoing use; physical withdrawal with abrupt cessation
		Acute tachycardia and hypertension
		Fatal disrhythmias possible in sensitive people
		Feelings of energy, power, confidence, and euphoria
		Trembling and insomnia
		Appetite suppression
		NOTE: The "high" achieved with crack is even more intense but of extremely short duration.
		Severe letdown effect or crash as drug wears off

DEPRESSANTS
Sedatives
  Methaqualone (Quaalude)
  Ludes, lemons, love drug, wallbangers
	Synthetic drugs that depress CNS
	Slow CNS and impair coordination
	Repeated use produces tolerance, physical and psychologic dependence
	Withdrawal requires medical intervention
		Relaxed, mellow feeling of well-being
		Drowsiness
		When combined with alcohol, respiration may be severely or terminally suppressed

Barbiturates
  Pentobarbital (Nembutal)
  Secobarbital (Seconal)
  Amobarbital (Amytal)
  Phenobarbital (Luminal)
  Yellow jacket, red devil, phennie, blue heaven, downers, goof balls
	Synthetic drugs that depress CNS, slowing physical and mental reflexes
	Ongoing use causes tolerance, physical and psychologic dependence
		Relief from anxiety
		Feeling of well-being, drowsiness, lethargy effect potentiated by alcohol; may cause overdose

Tranquilizers
  Chlordiazepoxide (Librium)
  Diazepam (Valium)
  Oxazepam (Serax)
  Lorazepam (Ativan)
  Alprazolam (Xanax)
	Slow activity in CNS and relax muscles
	Physical and psychologic dependence with long use; tolerance may develop
		Sense of relaxed well-being
		Drowsiness
		Most widely prescribed drugs in world
		Anxiety rebounds as drugs wear off

HALLUCINOGENS
  Lysergic acid diethylamide (LSD)
  Mescaline
  Psilocybin
  3,4-methylene-dioxyamphetamine (MOA)
  Buttons, mesc, magic mushroom, love drug, acid, dots, blotter
	Natural and synthetic drugs that affect mind and produce changes in thinking and perception; effects primarily psychologic
	Tolerance develops quickly, and cross tolerance occurs among drugs
		Amplify and distort user's experience of environment
		Increased sensory awareness
		Fantasies, illusions, hallucinations
		Anxiety
		"Bad trips" with possibility of psychotic breaks do occur

Phencyclidine (PCP) *Angel dust, crystal, dust, hog*	Synthetic drug that produces different effects at different doses Psychologic dependence occurs Physical dependence unclear	Low doses: hallucinations and sense of euphoria plus increases in blood pressure and tachycardia Incidence of "bad trips": 5 times that of LSD Extremely violent and combative behavior and prolonged psychosis possible with overdoses

Street names for drugs are indicated by italics.

TABLE 3-1 Major Drugs of Abuse–Continued

CATEGORY/EXAMPLES	EFFECT	MAJOR CLINICAL MANIFESTATIONS
NARCOTICS Heroin Morphine Codeine Meperidine (Demerol) *"H," horse, junk, smack, scag*	Drugs derived from opium poppy or produced synthetically Decrease cortical perception of pain and depress CNS Physical and psychologic dependence and tolerance develop rapidly with ongoing use Withdrawal requires medical supervision	Drowsiness and lethargy Feeling of well-being, euphoria Loss of concentration, judgment
CANNABIS (MARIJUANA) *Joint, reefer, Mary Jane, pot, grass, weed* Hashish: resinous extract of leaves and flowers; more concentrated	Comes from Indian hemp plant Used medically to control chemotherapy-related nausea and vomiting and to treat glaucoma Depresses higher brain centers and releases inhibitory impulses Psychologic dependence possible but not tolerance or physical dependence	One of most popular and commonly used drugs Stimulates appetite Alters perception of time, sight, sound, touch Feeling of well-being Confusion and reality distortion possible

Street names for drugs are indicated by italics.

Guidelines for Nursing Care for Managing Pain in Chemically Dependent Patients

Identify the chemically dependent patient as quickly as possible and begin to draft a care plan.

Identify and involve available specialists, such as pain and substance abuse nurse specialists.

Designate one physician to write medication orders. Utilize team meetings.

Prevent or minimize the occurrence of withdrawal symptoms.

Pain is an innately subjective experience. Accept the patient's reports of pain presence and severity.

Accept that patient's reports of pain may be exaggerated. Avoid adversarial confrontations.

Utilize a consistent pain rating scale for assessment and monitoring, such as 0 to 10 with 0 being no pain.

Administer sufficient narcotics to relieve or control the pain. Tolerance also develops to side effects such as respiratory depression, making high doses safe.

Administer drugs by continuous drip, by patient-controlled analgesia (PCA), or at regular intervals to avoid conflicts associated with asking for medication.

CAUTION: Never administer a mixed agonist/antagonist agent, such as pentazocine (Talwin), butorphanol (Stadol), buprenorphine (Buprenex), or nalbuphine (Nubain), to an opium-addicted patient, because it will precipitate acute withdrawal.

Contract with patient concerning behavior limits.

Manage drug, dosage, and route of administration changes carefully with advice from a pain specialist.

Explore readiness to undergo detoxification and treatment. Refer to area resources as appropriate.

CAUTION: Never use placebos in the pain plan. Avoid use of sedatives and so-called narcotic additives or potentiators.

Retain a commitment to adequate pain relief for all patients.

SELECTED REFERENCES

Belcaster A: Caring for the alcohol abuser, *Nurs 94* 24(2): 56-59, 1994.

Bell K: Identifying the substance abuser in clinical practice, *Orthop Nurs* 11(2):29, 1992.

Covello B: Codependency taints nursing's goals, *RN* 54(4):132, 1991.

Eels M: Strategies for promotion of avoiding harmful substances, *Nurs Clin North Am* 26(4):915, 1991.

Felblinger D: Substance abuse in women: a growing challenge for nurses, *Med-Surg Nurs Q* 1(1):101-109, 1992.

Flandermeyer A et al: Nursing care of women who abuse alcohol, *Med Surg Nurs Q* 1(1):122-139, 1992.

Green P: The chemically dependent nurse, *Nurs Clin North Am* 24(1):81-94, 1989.

Hall S, Wray L: Codependency: nurses who give too much, *Am J Nurs* 89(11):1456, 1989.

Herrick C: Codependency: characteristics, risks, progression, and strategies for healing, *Nurs Forum* 27(3):12-19, 1992.

House M: Cocaine, *Am J Nurs* 90(4):40, 1990.

Hughes T: Models and perspectives of addiction: implications for treatment, *Nurs Clin North Am* 24(1):1-12, 1989.

Jacques J, Snyder M: Newborn victims of addiction, *RN* 54(4):47, 1991.

Johnson L: How to diagnose and treat chemical dependency in the elderly, *J Gerontol Nurs* 15(12):22-26, 38-39, 1989.

Joyce C: The woman alcoholic, *Am J Nurs* 89(10):1314-1318, 1989.

Krach P: Discovering the secret: nursing assessment of elderly alcoholics in the home, *J Gerontol Nurs* 16(11):32, 1990.

Levy G, Hickey J: Fighting the battle against drugs, *RN* 54(4):44, 1991.

Lippman H: Addicted nurses: tolerated, tormented, or treated? *RN* 55(4):36, 1992.

McCaffery M, Vouraokis C: Assessment and relief of pain in chemically dependent patients, *Orthop Nurs* 11(2):13-25, 1992.

Miller H: Addiction in a coworker: getting past the denial, *Am J Nurs* 90(5):72, 1990.

Nuckols C, Greenson J: Cocaine addiction: assessment and intervention, *Nurs Clin North Am* 24(1):33-44, 1989.

Parette H: Nursing attitudes toward the geriatric alcoholic, *J Gerontol Nurs* 16(1):26, 1990.

Pires M: Substance abuse: the silent saboteur in rehabilitation, *Nurs Clin North Am* 24(1):291-296, 1989.

Williams E: Strategies for intervention, *Nurs Clin North Am* 24(1):95, 1989.

Wilson S: Can you spot an alcoholic patient? *RN* 57(1):46-50, 1994.

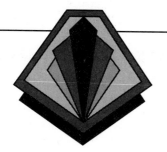

Fluid, Electrolyte, and Acid-Base Imbalance

FLUID AND ELECTROLYTE IMBALANCE

Fluid and electrolyte balance may be threatened or upset by virtually any medical or surgical disorder or therapy. Imbalances are commonly categorized as specific excesses or deficits, although multiple imbalances may be present in a given clinical situation.

PRIMARY FLUID IMBALANCES

Approximately 60% of adult body weight consists of fluid (Box 4-1). It is distributed between the intracellular (ICF), interstitial (IF), and intravascular (IVF) fluid compartments. Total body water content varies with fat content, sex, and age. Fat cells contain little water, and women have proportionately more body fat. Elderly persons also typically have less lean body tissue.

Body fluids are in constant motion. The ICF remains quite stable, but the extracellular fluid (ECF) interacts with and is modified by the external environment. Regulation of fluid movement is accomplished by osmosis, diffusion, filtration, and the sodium-potassium pump. The kidneys, heart, and blood vessels, skin, lungs, and gastrointestinal (GI) tract play major roles in maintaining homeostasis. Table 4-1 summarizes the daily intake and output of fluid for an average adult.

TABLE 4-1	Approximate Daily Fluid Intake and Output for an Adult Eating 2500 Calories		
INTAKE		**OUTPUT**	
METHOD	AMOUNT (ML)	METHOD	AMOUNT (ML)
Water in food	1000	Skin	500
Water from oxidation	300	Lungs	350
Water as liquid	1200	Feces	150
		Kidneys	1500
TOTAL	2500	TOTAL	2500

Isotonic Fluid Volume Deficit

Fluid volume deficit occurs when both water and electrolytes are lost in an isotonic fashion. It almost always results from loss of body fluids, typically from the GI tract, or as the result of fever, polyuria, sweating, decreased intake, and third spacing (Box 4-2). Isotonic volume loss does not disturb serum osmolality and is restricted to the ECF compartment, but it can deplete ECF volume rapidly and lead to vascular collapse. Table 4-2 summarizes clinical manifestations.

Medical management

Treatment consists of identifying and correcting the underlying cause of fluid loss and then replacing the fluids and electrolytes that have been lost with appropriate isotonic fluids or blood products.

BOX 4-1	Total Body Fluid Distribution and Physiologic Changes with Aging

BODY FLUID DISTRIBUTION

Intracellular fluid: 40% of body weight
Extracellular fluid: 20% of body weight
   Interstitial fluid (15%)
   Intravascular fluid (5%)
Total body fluid: 60% of body weight

PHYSIOLOGIC CHANGES WITH AGING

40-60 years
   Men: 55%
   Women: 47%
Over 60 years
   Men: 52%
   Women: 46%

BOX 4-2	Third Spacing of Body Fluids

Third spacing refers to a shift of fluid from the vascular space to body spaces, where it is trapped and unavailable for functional use. It can be sequestered in potential spaces (pleura, peritoneum), trapped in the bowel by obstruction, in inflamed tissue, or in the interstitial space.

Third space losses cannot be observed or measured. Although fluid is lost, the patient may actually gain weight as losses are replaced intravenously. Initial symptoms mimic isotonic losses. As the condition resolves, fluid returns to the intravascular space and may create a transient hypervolemia. It is then excreted by the kidney.

TABLE 4-2	Clinical Manifestations of Hypovolemia and Hypervolemia	
HYPOVOLEMIA	**HYPERVOLEMIA**

SKIN AND SUBCUTANEOUS TISSUE

Dry, less elastic	Warm, moist, pitting edema or shiny, tight

FACE

Sunken eyes (late)	Periorbital edema

TONGUE

Dry, coated (early) Fissured (late)	Moist

THIRST

Present	Not significant

SALIVA

Scanty, thick	Excessive, frothy

VITAL SIGNS
Temperature

May be elevated	Not significant

Pulse

Rapid, weak, thready	Rapid, bounding

Respirations

Rapid, shallow	Rapid, dyspnea, moist rales, frothy cough

BLOOD PRESSURE

Low, orthostatic hypotension (early)	Normal to high

WEIGHT

Loss	Gain (best early sign)

URINE OUTPUT

Low; increased specific gravity	Increased or normal; decreased specific gravity

Isotonic Fluid Volume Excess

An isotonic volume excess occurs in conditions in which both extracellular water and electrolytes are retained by the body. Volume is increased, but the osmolality remains in the normal range. It is always secondary to an increase in total body sodium content. It may be caused by simple fluid overloading or a failure in the homeostatic regulatory mechanisms. Congestive heart failure, overuse of isotonic fluids such as normal saline, and excessive ingestion of sodium chloride or other salts in the body are possible causes.

Medical management

Treatment is directed at correcting the underlying condition if possible. If correction is impossible, treatment is aimed at symptomatic management through restriction of dietary sodium, fluid restrictions, and use of diuretics.

Hyperosmolar Fluid Volume Deficit: Dehydration

An extracellular water deficit occurs when the amount of water is decreased in proportion to the amount of solute in the water, causing the osmolality to exceed 300 mOsm/L. Hyperosmolality causes water to move from the cells to the vascular compartment to help maintain the circulating blood volume. Osmotic diuresis occurs as the kidneys attempt to excrete the excess solute. Dehydration worsens as a result of the loss of fluid used to flush out solutes in the urine. If the problem is not recognized and corrected:

The ICF compartment becomes depleted, markedly impairing cell function. NOTE: Brain cells are particularly sensitive, and mental status changes may be among the first signs.

ECF losses impair circulation, further interrupting cellular metabolism and possibly leading to vascular collapse.

Hyperosmolar fluid deficits occur with the intake of hyperosmolar fluids such as tube feedings and when solutes accumulate in the body secondary to conditions such as renal failure or diabetic ketoacidosis. Blood values show increased sodium and hematocrit and higher osmolality of fluids.

Medical management

Medical management consists of replacing lost fluids plus supplying current daily needs. The amount of fluid loss can be estimated from weight loss: 1 kg of body weight equals 1 L of fluid. The method of fluid delivery may be oral, IV, or both. Initial fluid replacement is frequently glucose and water, supplemented by electrolyte solutions once the patient's renal function is ensured. Replacement may take place over several days to avoid overtaxing the heart.

Hypoosmolar Fluid Volume Excess: Water Intoxication

An extracellular water excess occurs when the amount of water is increased in proportion to the amount of solute in the water, causing the osmolality to fall below 275 mOsm/L. This imbalance is uncommon but can occur when intake of water exceeds the ability of the kidneys to excrete it.

Extracellular water excess rapidly becomes intracellular water excess as fluid moves into the cells to equalize the solute concentration, causing the cells to swell. NOTE: Brain cells are particularly sensitive to water increases, and the most common symptoms are changes in the patient's mental status.

Water excess rarely occurs under normal conditions since a falling osmolality usually suppresses the antidiuretic hormone (ADH), allowing the excess water to be excreted by the kidney. The imbalance can occur with continuous irrigation or administration of hypoosmolar fluids by mouth (PO) or IV. Tap water enemas and bladder irrigations are potential causes. Blood values show decreased sodium and hematocrit and lower fluid osmolality.

Medical management

Most patients respond well to simple water restriction. If severe symptoms are present, the patient may be treated with the infusion of hypertonic saline IV plus the administration of furosemide (Lasix) in addition to fluid restriction.

NURSING MANAGEMENT: Primary Fluid Imbalances

◆ ASSESSMENT
Subjective Data

Disease process affecting fluid balance, such as diabetes, renal disease, bowel obstruction
Medication use, such as diuretics, steroids
Dietary changes or restrictions, such as fluids, sodium
Ability to acquire or swallow fluids orally
Presence and degree of thirst

Objective Data

24-hr intake and output totals
Urine appearance and specific gravity
Body weight
Skin and mucous membrane appearance, moisture, turgor
Presence, location, and severity of edema
Vital signs
Neck vein filling
Level of consciousness

◆ NURSING DIAGNOSES

Possible nursing diagnoses for the person with a fluid imbalance may include, but are not limited to, the following:
Fluid volume deficit (related to disturbances in intake or failure of regulatory mechanisms)
Fluid volume excess (related to excessive fluid intake or failure of regulatory mechanisms)

◆ EXPECTED PATIENT OUTCOMES

Patient will replace lost fluids and return to a normal hydration status.
Patient will safely eliminate excess fluids and return to a normal hydration status.

◆ NURSING INTERVENTIONS
Collaborative Interventions: Monitoring

Monitor IV fluid rates closely.
Monitor daily AM weights. NOTE: 500 ml = 1 lb.
Monitor urine output, intake and output (I&O) balance, and urine specific gravity.
Assess vital signs, mental status, skin turgor, and mucous membranes.
Monitor hematocrit, BUN/creatinine, and serum sodium.

Replacing Lost Fluids

Offer small amounts of oral fluids frequently.
Explore patient's likes and dislikes.
Keep fluids available at the bedside.
Assess adequacy of gag reflex and swallowing ability before offering oral fluids.
Offer or provide frequent mouth care.
Administer IVs or tube feedings if unable to meet needs PO.
Monitor urine response to increased fluids.
Teach patient about adjusting fluid intake in response to exercise, heat, and humidity.

Eliminating Excess Fluid

Review instructions and encourage adherence to sodium or fluid restrictions. Emphasize importance of reading labels.
Administer diuretics as ordered and monitor response.
Restrict IV and PO fluids as ordered.
Teach patient importance of self-monitoring of body weight.
Turn and reposition frequently.
Inspect skin for pressure and breakdown.
Elevate dependent parts to assist venous return.
Avoid prolonged bed rest.

◆ EVALUATION

Successful achievement of expected outcomes for the patient with a fluid imbalance is indicated by the following:
Parameters indicating normal fluid balance:
Electrolytes, hematocrit, and serum osmolality within normal limits
Intake and output balanced; urine specific gravity 1.010 to 1.020
Stable body weight
Absence of peripheral edema

ELECTROLYTE IMBALANCE

The body electrolytes are substances that develop an electrical charge when dissolved in water. Those developing positive charges are called anions, and those developing negative charges are cations. The electrolyte content of the body fluid compartments varies significantly, and a great deal of energy is expended in maintaining these balances by means of the cell membrane pumps (Table 4-3). Electrolytes are essential to the transmission of nerve impulses, and imbalances are often reflected in the functioning of the body's muscles.

Sodium Imbalance

Sodium is the primary extracellular cation, and it has a primary role in controlling water distribution and ECF volume. A loss or gain of sodium is usually accompanied

BOX 4-3	Imbalances Related to Heat Stress

Physiologic imbalances resulting from heat exposure may range from mild to severe. They usually involve both fluid and sodium imbalances.

HEAT CRAMPS

Heat cramps are painful muscle cramps after strenuous activity in a hot environment. Conditioned athletes are often most vulnerable. Cramps may be triggered by sodium depletion in the muscle. Cramps are usually relieved by salt ingestion before or during exercise.

HEAT EXHAUSTION

Heat exhaustion is a common yet nonspecific clinical entity related to either primary salt depletion or primary water depletion.

Salt depletion occurs when large volumes of sweat are replaced by adequate water volume but inadequate salt. Weakness, headache, anorexia, and nausea may occur. Treatment involves salted liquids by mouth.

Water depletion occurs when sweat losses are not replaced. Intense thirst, weakness, and impaired judgment may occur. Temperature elevation and weight loss are typical. Treatment involves slow replacement of water losses, orally if possible.

HEATSTROKE

Heatstroke involves life-threatening elevations of body temperature (106° to 108° F) from reduced circulatory volume brought on by excessive sweat losses or the effects of hyperthermia on the brain. Sweating-induced heatstroke primarily affects athletes, whereas classic heatstroke may strike elderly persons in chronic heat stress. Treatment involves lowering the body temperature and careful fluid replacement.

TABLE 4-3 Values of Electrolytes in Plasma vs. Intracellular Fluids

ELECTROLYTE	PLASMA VALUE (mEq/L)	INTRACELLULAR VALUE (mEq/L)
CATIONS		
Sodium (Na^+)	142	10
Potassium (K^+)	5	150
Calcium (Ca^{2+})	5	Negligible
Magnesium (Mg^{2+})	2	40
ANIONS		
Chloride (Cl^-)	103	Negligible
Bicarbonate (HCO_3^-)	26	10
Phosphate (PO_4^{2-})	2	150
Sulfate (SO_4^{2-})	1	150
Proteinate	17	40

by a loss or gain of water. ECF concentration of sodium has a profound effect on body cells. Low levels produce a dilute ECF, and water is drawn into the cells. Higher concentrations in the ECF allow water to be drawn *out* of the cells.

Hyponatremia (sodium deficit)

A serum sodium level below 138 mEq/L can result from either a sodium loss or a water excess creating a relatively greater concentration of water than sodium. Even if there is no excess of body water, the decreasing osmolality creates a condition similar to water excess; water moves into the cell by osmosis, leaving the extracellular compartment depleted. Both circulatory functioning and cellular functioning are impaired. The brain's ability to expand is severely limited by the skull, and generalized cellular edema can create severe neurologic compromise. Possible causes of this complex imbalance are summarized in Box 4-4. Clinical manifestations include the following:

Anorexia and nausea

Muscle weakness

Irritability, personality changes (NOTE: If the hyponatremia evolves rapidly, the neurologic changes are often more dramatic.)

Seizures or coma if sodium below 110 to 115 mEq/L

Medical management—Lost sodium and water are replaced by the rapid administration of saline solution (0.9% NaCl) plus plasma expanders if the patient is in shock. Other electrolytes are replaced as need is established by blood values. Treatment is aimed at correcting the underlying cause. Salt or salty foods may be added to the diet.

Hypernatremia (sodium excess)

A serum sodium level greater than 145 mEq/L exists when there is an excess of sodium in relation to water in the ECF. The body normally protects itself from hypernatremia through stimulation of thirst and release of ADH. Hypernatremia is not seen in alert persons with access to fluids. Osmolality increases, and water leaves

BOX 4-4	Possible Causes of Hyponatremia

Sodium loss from gastrointestinal tract
   Vomiting or diarrhea
   GI suction
   GI drainage: fistulas, biliary, ileostomy
Profuse perspiration
   Fever
   Exercise
Excess diuretic effect
Shift of body fluids
   Massive edema—ascites
   Burns
   Small bowel obstruction
Drugs, conditions, or tumors producing syndrome of inappropriate antidiuretic hormone (SIADH)
   Chemotherapeutic drugs, tranquilizers
   Head injury
   Brain tumor, oat cell lung tumor, leukemia

BOX 4-5	Possible Causes of Hypernatremia

Deprivation of water, lack of access
Hypertonic tube feedings
Excessive sodium ingestion: oral, IV
Greatly increased insensible fluid loss
Inability to excrete sodium
    Excess aldosterone production, renal failure
Saltwater drowning

BOX 4-6	Possible Causes of Hypokalemia

Decreased potassium intake
    NPO
    Severe dieting/fasting
    Failure to adequately replace losses
Increased potassium loss
    GI losses
    Vomiting or diarrhea
    Draining fistulas
    Potassium wasting diuretics (thiazide diuretics)
    Losses from cellular trauma, such as burns
Cellular shifts of potassium
    Acidosis
    Alkalosis

the cells by osmosis to dilute the ECF, leaving the cells water depleted and disrupting their function.

Cellular shrinkage in the brain causes most of the neurologic symptoms. In slowly evolving states the brain is gradually able to compensate and restore its fluid content. Rapidly evolving cases can result in death. Possible causes are summarized in Box 4-5. Clinical manifestations include the following:

Thirst (usually strong enough to prevent imbalance)
Dry, sticky mucous membranes
Muscle weakness and irritability
Restlessness, disorientation, delusions, stupor

NOTE: Neurologic changes are dramatic if condition evolves rapidly.

Medical management—Plasma sodium values are gradually reduced over a minimum of 48 hours to prevent rebound cerebral edema and permanent neurologic damage. Free water may be given orally or in hypotonic IV fluids (D5W or 0.45% NaCl). The patient's cardiac function and renal function are carefully monitored during fluid replacement.

Potassium Imbalances

Potassium is the primary intracellular cation. It has a direct effect on muscle and nerve excitability, maintains intracellular osmotic pressure, and helps maintain acid-base balance. It is continuously moving in and out of cells.

Potassium enters the cells during anabolism and glucose conversion to glycogen; potassium leaves the cell during cellular breakdown resulting from either trauma or catabolism. The body conserves potassium less effectively than it conserves sodium, excreting potassium through the kidneys even when the body needs it.

Potassium must be replaced daily in the range of 40 to 60 mEq/day. Disturbances in potassium balance are common and associated with a number of diseases and conditions.

Hypokalemia (potassium deficit)

A serum potassium level below 3.5 mEq/L alters the polarization of cells, causing them to be less excitable. This loss of excitability can be life threatening when it occurs in cardiac muscle. Possible causes are summa-

rized in Box 4-6. Clinical manifestations include the following:

Neuromuscular changes (cardiac, striated, and smooth muscle)
    Fatigue, weakness, cramps
    Anorexia, decreased peristalsis, ileus
Cardiac changes
    Ventricular dysrhythmias
    Hypotension
    Electrocardiogram (ECG) changes: flattened T waves, ST depression
    Increased sensitivity to digitalis
Neurologic changes
    Paresthesias
    Dizziness and confusion

NOTE: Symptoms are not usually present until potassium falls below 3.0 mEq/L.

Medical management—Although the best treatment is prevention, medical management consists of prompt administration of potassium either orally or by IV infusion. Oral administration may be by foods rich in potassium (Box 4-7) or by oral potassium preparations. IV infusions of potassium ideally should not exceed 10 to 20 mEq/hr and should be extremely diluted (40 mEq/L) to control peripheral vein irritation and sclerosing. Concentrations greater than 60 mEq/L should not be administered by peripheral IV line. Potassium is *never* administered by IV push.

Hyperkalemia (potassium excess)

A serum potassium level above 5.5 mEq/L rarely occurs in the presence of normal renal function. Excess potassium decreases the membrane potential of cells, causing them to become more excitable.

Hyperkalemia is less common than hypokalemia but more dangerous because of the associated risk of cardiac arrest. Possible causes are summarized in Box 4-8. Clinical manifestations include the following:

BOX 4-7 Foods Rich in Potassium

FRUITS	VEGETABLES*	PROTEIN FOODS	BEVERAGES
Apricots	Asparagus	Beef	Cocoa
Bananas	Dried beans	Chicken	Cola drinks
Grapefruit	Broccoli	Liver	Dry instant tea and coffee
Melon	Cabbage	Pork	Milk
Honeydew	Carrots	Veal	
Cantaloupe	Celery	Turkey	
Dried fruits	Mushrooms	Nuts	
Figs, dates, raisins	Dried peas	Peanut butter	
Oranges	Potatoes, white and sweet		
	Spinach		
	Squash		

*Most raw vegetables contain potassium, but it is frequently lost in cooking.

BOX 4-8 Possible Causes of Hyperkalemia

Decreased potassium loss
  Renal failure
  Adrenal insufficiency
  Potassium-sparing diuretics
Cellular shifts of potassium
  Trauma
  Metabolic acidosis
Malignant cell lysis with chemotherapy
Excess potassium intake
  Dietary excess (in presence of renal insufficiency)
  Excessive IV administration
Improper use of oral potassium supplements

Cardiac effects
  Tall peaked T waves
  Widened QRS complex and P-R interval
  Ventricular dysrhythmias and cardiac arrest
  NOTE: Cardiac effects become significant at 7 mEq/L or greater.
Neuromuscular effects
  Weakness progressing to flaccid paralysis
  Paresthesias of face, tongue, hands
GI effects
  Nausea
  Abdominal colic or diarrhea

Medical management—In nonacute situations treatment may be limited to restriction of dietary potassium and discontinuing any contributing drugs. If it is necessary to actively remove excess potassium, a cation exchange resin such as sodium polystyrene sulfonate (Kayexalate) may be given. It removes potassium by exchanging it for sodium in the intestinal tract and may be given orally or as a retention enema. It is commonly administered with an osmotic agent such as sorbitol, which stimulates bowel motility. Oral doses can be repeated every 4 to 6 hours, and enemas every 2 to 4 hours.

Dialysis may be employed in renal failure. In emergency situations, concentrated glucose may be administered with regular insulin to facilitate movement of potassium into the cells. Sodium bicarbonate will effect a temporary shift of potassium into the cells, and calcium gluconate may be administered to temporarily block the action of potassium on the heart. The patient must be monitored carefully during any of these interventions.

Calcium Imbalances

Calcium is present in the blood in two forms: ionized and bound to plasma proteins. Only the ionized calcium is physiologically active. It functions to support blood clotting; smooth, skeletal, and cardiac muscle function; and nerve function. Both parathyroid hormone (PTH) and vitamin D are necessary for normal absorption of calcium from the GI tract.

Because many factors affect calcium balance there are multiple causes of calcium imbalances and they are relatively common in acutely ill persons.

Hypocalcemia (calcium deficiency)

A serum calcium level below 4.5 mEq/L affects cell membrane chemistry. In hypocalcemia, depolarization takes place more easily, producing increased excitability of the nervous system and the skeletal, smooth, and cardiac muscles. It can lead to muscle spasms, tingling sensations, and even tetany if severe. Possible causes are identified in Box 4-9. Clinical manifestations may vary widely depending on the severity and duration of the imbalance. Patients with mild hypocalcemia are often asymptomatic. Classic manifestations include the following:
  Neuromuscular excitability
    Numbness, tingling around the mouth and fingertips (circumoral paresthesia) or in the hands and feet

BOX 4-9	Possible Causes of Hypocalcemia

Inadequate intake, malabsorption
Hypoparathyroidism or post thyroidectomy
Acute pancreatitis (calcium salts bind with fatty acids, and PTH secretion is inadequate)
Renal failure: hyperphosphatemia triggers a reciprocal drop in serum calcium
Burns, draining wounds, fistulas
Transfusion with citrated blood (citrate combines with calcium and removes it from circulation)

Muscle spasms in face or extremities
Muscle cramps, tetany, laryngeal spasm
Positive Chvostek's sign (tapping over facial nerve elicits a grimace)
Positive Trousseau's sign (carpal spasm induced by inflating blood pressure [BP] cuff on the upper arm)
Irritability, depression, and seizures (may be first sign)
Decreased cardiac output, dysrhythmias
GI cramping, nausea, diarrhea

Medical management—The treatment is ideally directed at relieving the cause. Medical management includes administration of oral calcium salts and a high calcium diet. It is usually sufficient to supplement with 1 to 2 g of elemental calcium daily in divided doses. Vitamin D supplements may also be necessary. Acute hypocalcemia is a medical emergency necessitating IV administration of calcium, usually as calcium gluconate. Diluting the calcium salt and infusing it over several hours reduces the venous irritation and cardiac irregularities.

Hypercalcemia (calcium excess)

A serum calcium level above 5.8 mEq/L affects cell membrane chemistry by inhibiting depolarization and depressing the function of nerves and skeletal, smooth, and cardiac muscles. Any condition causing immobility results in calcium leaving the bone and concentrating in the extracellular fluid. Excess calcium passing through the kidneys can cause precipitation and stone formation, especially in the presence of urine alkalinity.

The prevalence of hypercalcemia in hospitalized patients is 0.6% to 3.6%, and if severe, it carries a high mortality. Common causes of hypercalcemia are outlined in Box 4-10. Clinical manifestations vary significantly with the severity and duration of the imbalance but may include the following:

Reduction in neuromuscular excitability
   Muscle weakness
   Depressed deep tendon reflexes
Decreased GI motility: constipation, anorexia, nausea
Increased gastric acid secretion (action of calcium on parietal cells of stomach)

BOX 4-10	Possible Causes of Hypercalcemia

Malignancy, especially bone metastasis
Hyperparathyroidism
Thiazide diuretic use (increases PTH effect)
NOTE: 98% of cases of hypercalcemia can be attributed to one of these causes.
Immobility: increased bone resorption
Excess use of calcium-containing antacids

Subtle personality changes to acute psychosis: impaired memory
Polyuria and polydipsia (action of calcium on tubules)
Kidney stones, bone pain, pathologic fractures
Hypertension and ECG changes if severe

Medical management—Treatment is directed toward eliminating the excess calcium through the kidneys or blocking bone resorption and calcium absorption. General measures include ensuring a high fluid intake, dietary restrictions, elimination of drugs contributing to the imbalance, and preventing immobility. The urine may also be acidified to prevent the formation of stones. Administration of IV saline (physiologic flushing) followed by furosemide (Lasix) promotes calcium excretion with the sodium. Administration of inorganic phosphate, mithramycin (Mithracin), or glucocorticoids increases calcium excretion.

NURSING MANAGEMENT: Electrolyte Imbalances

The nursing role with patients experiencing electrolyte imbalances involves collaborative monitoring of all at risk patients. This will standardly include baseline vital signs, intake and output, and daily weights. The patient will be instructed about specific risk factors and the prevention of imbalances through diet modifications, increasing oral fluid intake, and the safe use of all medications.

IV FLUIDS

The main objectives of fluid therapy are to replace losses and keep up with ongoing needs. IV fluids are selected to match deficits in various body fluid compartments. Many patients require only maintenance fluids while NPO or otherwise PO restricted. Trauma and fever dramatically alter those needs.

ISOTONIC FLUIDS

Isotonic fluids are distributed in the ECF compartment and do not enter the ICF. They are used to correct ECF deficits. Examples of isotonic fluids are 0.09% sodium chloride and lactated Ringer's solution (balanced physiologic solution).

HYPOTONIC FLUIDS

Hypotonic fluids include 5% dextrose in water and 0.45% sodium chloride. The former is distributed in both the ECF and ICF compartments, with roughly two thirds moving to the ICF. The dextrose makes it nearly isotonic on administration but is then metabolized to CO_2 and H_2O leaving the distilled water. It is used to replace total body water rather than restore the ECF.

A second hypotonic fluid, 0.45% sodium chloride, contains half the electrolytes of normal saline plus additional free water. It is often used for maintenance fluid requirements or in hypovolemia when fluid deficits exceed those of sodium.

HYPERTONIC SOLUTIONS

Hypertonic solutions are rarely used and are potentially dangerous. They may be administered slowly in small volumes in severe hyponatremia. They cause rapid fluid shifts into the intravascular compartment and can cause rapid volume overload, congestive heart failure, and pulmonary edema. 5% dextrose in 0.45% sodium chloride is initially hyperosmolar and can induce slight shifts from the IF and ICF spaces to the vascular to reduce edema. As the dextrose is metabolized, the solution reduces in osmolality.

Examples of hypertonic solutions are 3% sodium chloride, 5% sodium chloride, and 5% dextrose in 0.45% sodium chloride.

IV THERAPY

Provision of IV therapy is a standard part of nursing responsibilities in all areas of practice. The available technology has proliferated rapidly and extensively over the last decades.

INFUSION SYSTEMS

Infusion systems may be plastic or rigid, closed or open. Plastic containers are most popular, because they are flexible and collapsible, contain no vacuum, and thus do not require coring or air venting. The risks of contamination are therefore reduced.

ADMINISTRATION SETS

Regular or *macro sets* come with and without in-line filters. The drop factor varies by manufacturer.

Micro sets contain drip tubes of much smaller diameter. Sets standardly deliver 50 to 60 gtt/ml.

Check valves contain in-line, pressure-sensitive valves that prevent mixing of fluids given "piggyback." Rate of flow is established by the primary set.

Nonpolyvinyl chloride sets are used with lipid emulsions and drugs that are absorbed into the walls of standard PVC tubing.

Filters may be add-ons or part of the set; 0.22 μm filters are felt to be absolutely bacteria retentive and air

eliminating. Controversy exists over their use.

FLOW CONTROL DEVICES

A wide range of controllers and pumps are available to ensure more accurate administration of fluids and drugs.

Controllers regulate IV flow rates and rely on gravity rather than pressure. They are appropriate for most routine situations.

Pumps are set to deliver a specific volume of fluid per designated time period and are used where accuracy of delivery is crucial. They operate on positive pressure and adjust to overcome resistance within preset limits. Multiple programmable systems are now available. Manufacturers' directions should be carefully followed.

PERIPHERAL INTRAVENOUS CATHETERS

The *scalp vein needle (butterfly)* consists of a metal cannula with two flexible wings attached to the hub. A short length of plastic tubing is attached with either an adaptor or resealable injection site at the end (Figures 4-1 and 4-2).

In *over- and through-the-needle catheters* a needle is used to make the venipuncture and then a flexible catheter is left in the vein and the needle is removed. They can be threaded through a needle or manufactured with the needle inserted in the middle.

CENTRAL VENOUS CATHETERS

A variety of catheters are available to meet the need for long-term venous access and administration of hyperosmolar solutions. They are placed in the central veins by the physician.

Single-lumen or *multilumen catheters* typically are 8 to 12 inches in length and inserted percutaneously. Multiple lumens allow for the administration of different and possibly incompatible drugs and solutions.

GERONTOLOGIC PATIENT CONSIDERATIONS FOR VENIPUNCTURE

Veins often appear prominent under the skin of elderly persons, but the veins are fragile and lack collagen support. Hematomas form easily, and infiltration occurs as the lack of elasticity prevents the vessel from sealing around the catheter.

1. Healthy veins feel soft and resilient. Avoid veins with a hard or "corded" feel.
2. Avoid hand veins, because they lack superficial tissue for support and infiltrate easily. Consider the cephalic vein on thumb side of wrist or the basilic vein on posterior aspect of forearm. Avoid also the palm side of wrist, antecubital fossa, and lower extremity. Infiltration at the antecubital site eliminates use of any site distal to the damaged vessel. Begin distally and work up.
3. Use an over-the-needle catheter of small size.
4. Maintain traction on the skin during venipuncture.
5. Make tape selections carefully. Protective skin preps can be helpful.

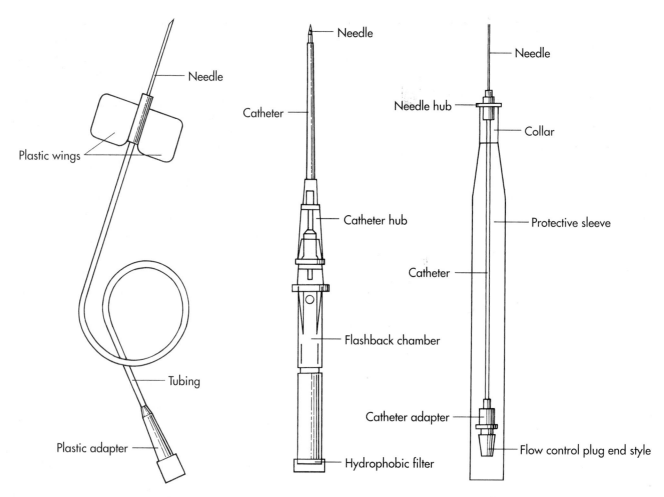

FIGURE 4-1 Peripheral IV needles/catheters. **A,** Scalp vein needle (butterfly). **B,** Over-the-needle catheter. **C,** Through-the-needle catheter.

Guidelines for Accessing an Implanted Port

Gather all needed equipment and place the patient comfortably on his or her back. Wash hands carefully and put on gloves and mask.

1. Attach Huber needle to extension tubing.
2. Draw up 10 ml of sterile saline, and attach syringe to the extension tubing. Flush the tubing.
3. Prepare the site with alcohol. Allow to dry. Clean with povidone-iodine, and allow to dry.
4. Palpate the port, and stabilize with thumb and forefinger.
5. Insert Huber needle perpendicularly to the septum.
6. Aspirate to ensure patency, and then flush with saline. Attach lines as needed.
7. Dress site with a transparent dressing. Stabilize Huber needle with a folded 2 × 2 gauze under it and one on top.
8. Heparinize the port if not in continuous use.

Tunneled catheters are implanted surgically. A subcutaneous tunnel is formed from the venous insertion site to a point usually near the nipple line. Dacron cuffs are found midway in the tunnel and as fibrous tissue adheres to the cuff, the risk of infection is minimized. The catheter, single lumen or multilumen, may be used continuously or intermittently and may remain in place for months. Hickman and Broviac catheters are commonly used examples (Figure 4-3).

The *Groshong catheter* is similar to the Hickman but with a unique feature, a pressure-sensitive valve near the tip (the tip itself is closed). It opens inward with aspiration and outward with infusion but closes when not in use, reducing the risk of air embolism or clotting. It does not require clamping. Normal saline irrigation is performed vigorously (Figure 4-4).

Implantable devices (ports) are totally implanted under the skin, which minimizes both the maintenance and risk of infection. There are two components: a Silastic catheter and an injection port. They are accessed by means of a noncoring Huber point needle (Figure 4-5).

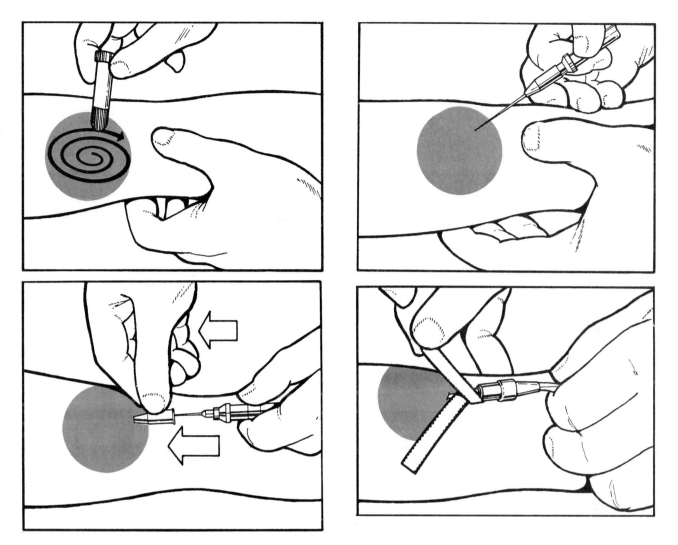

FIGURE 4-2   Peripheral IV insertion. **A,** Cleanse venipuncture site. **B,** Insert catheter, bevel side up, at 30- to 45-degree angle. **C,** Advance catheter until blood flashback is seen. **D,** Anchor catheter. Label insertion site with date and time. (From LaRocca JC, Otto SE: *Pocket guide to intravenous therapy,* ed 2, St Louis, 1993, Mosby.)

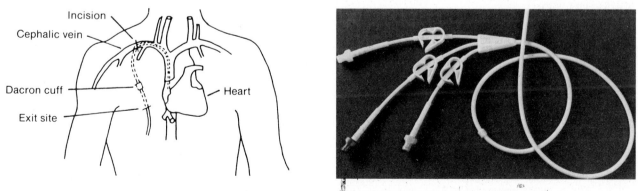

FIGURE 4-3   Placement of a tunneled catheter. **A,** Tunneled catheter. **B,** Hickman catheter. (**A** from LaRocca JC, Otto SE: *Pocket guide to intravenous therapy,* ed 2, St Louis, 1993, Mosby; **B** courtesy CR Bard, Inc, Cranston, RI.)

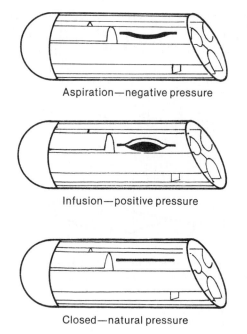

Aspiration—negative pressure

Infusion—positive pressure

Closed—natural pressure

FIGURE 4-4 Three-position Groshong valve. (Courtesy CR Bard, Inc, Cranston, RI.)

PICC lines, originally developed for use with neonates, are peripherally inserted central catheters that may be appropriate for some patients. They are nonsutured, are inserted through the antecubital area, and terminate in the subclavian vein or superior vena cava. They require daily site care and coverage with an occlusive transparent dressing. Nurses are inserting PICC lines in many ICU settings (Figure 4-6).

ACID-BASE IMBALANCES

The body is able to maintain its plasma pH within the narrow range of 7.35 to 7.45 in most situations. It does so by means of its chemical buffering mechanisms and through the kidneys and lungs. The regulation of body pH is vital because even slight deviations from the normal range will cause significant changes in the rate of cellular chemical reactions.

The body's primary chemical buffer system is bicarbonate (HCO_3)/carbonic acid (H_2CO_3). The body maintains 20 parts of HCO_3 for every part of H_2CO_3 (20:1 ratio). If this ratio is upset, the pH will change. The chemical buffers work continuously and instantaneously. The kidneys regulate the HCO_3 level in the ECF by excretion or retention of H^+ ions and HCO_3. These adjustments may take hours. The lungs control the CO_2 (and H_2CO_3) content of the ECF by adjusting ventilation in response to the amount of CO_2 in the blood. Respiratory adjustments require minutes to hours. In a disease state in which normal acid-base balance is upset, the lungs and kidneys attempt to compensate for the imbalance by initiating appropriate changes in blood CO_2 and bicarbonate levels.

The best way to evaluate acid-base balance is by measuring arterial blood gases. Normal values are summarized in Box 4-12.

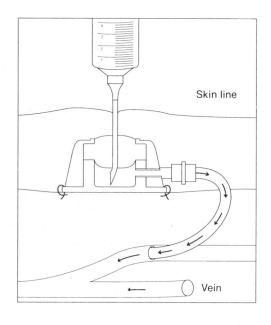

Skin line

Vein

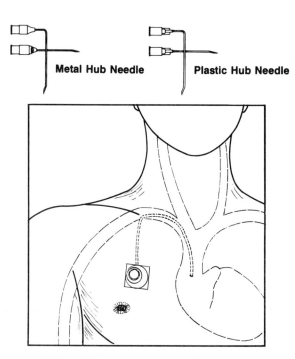

Metal Hub Needle   Plastic Hub Needle

FIGURE 4-5 Implantable ports and Huber needles. **A,** Cross section of implantable port with needle access. **B,** Huber needles. **C,** Placement of implantable venous access device. (**A** and **B** courtesy Pharmacia Deltec, Inc, St Paul, MN; **C** from LaRocca JC, Otto SE: *Pocket guide to IV therapy,* ed 2, St Louis, 1993, Mosby.)

BOX
4-11

BOX 4-11	Common IV Complaints

COMMON PROBLEMS

Infiltration
The most common complication; cannula may slip out completely or be dislodged so only the tip remains in the vein
  Signs: coolness, leaking at site, swelling, and tenderness; if infiltration is partial, blood return may still be present
  Treatment: remove IV line and reinsert at a distant site

Phlebitis
Indicates vein is irritated from catheter, drugs, or IV fluids; may develop after IV line is removed
  Signs: redness, tenderness, and swelling near site and palpable hardness; red line may be apparent above insertion site; blood return and infusion may be normal
  Treatment: remove IV line and restart at distant site; warm soaks may be applied for comfort

Clot Formation
Usually accompanied by some phlebitis and results from excess catheter movement or poor anchoring
  Signs: infusion runs sluggishly and site appears phlebitic
  Treatment: aspirate before attempting to irrigate to prevent release into bloodstream; restart if cannot aspirate

Site Infection
Serious risk with patients who are elderly, have an existing infection, or are immunocompromised
  Signs: site painful, red, and hot but not hard or swollen; flow rate may be sluggish; may proceed to systemic sepsis
  Treatment: antibiotics; prevention includes strict asepsis and changing wet or contaminated dressings

PREVENTING IV PROBLEMS

Preventing Infection
Change parenteral fluid containers, primary intermittent sets, and TPN sets every 24 hours.
Change peripheral and central sets every 48 hours.
Change gauze dressings over sites every 48 hours. Reapply antimicrobial ointment after careful inspection.
Change transparent semipermeable dressings at intervals established by institution.
Date and label all equipment accurately.

Site Rotation
Change peripheral lines every 48-72 hours if condition of veins permits.

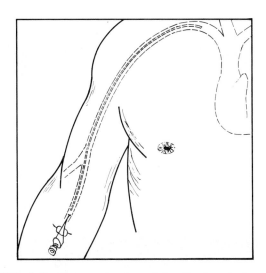

FIGURE 4-6 Placement of peripherally inserted central venous catheter. (From LaRocca JC, Otto SE: *Pocket guide to intravenous therapy*, ed 2, St Louis, 1993, Mosby.)

BOX 4-12	Arterial Blood Gas Values	
pH	7.35-7.45	Reflects H+ ion concentration
P_{O_2}	80-100 mm Hg	Partial pressure of oxygen in arterial blood
P_{CO_2}	35-45 mm Hg	Partial pressure of carbon dioxide in arterial blood
HCO_3	22-28 mEq/L	Bicarbonate concentration in blood plasma
Base excess (BE)	$^-2$-$^+2$ mEq/L	Reflects metabolic excess (+) or deficit (−) of bicarbonate

METABOLIC ACIDOSIS

Metabolic acidosis is characterized by a low pH and a low plasma bicarbonate level. The lungs hyperventilate to decrease the P_{CO_2} concentration. Its classic causes include diabetic ketoacidosis, lactic acidosis, and renal failure. Clinical manifestations include the following:
  Headache, confusion, drowsiness
  Increased respiratory rate and depth (Kussmaul breathing in diabetes with a fruity odor)
  Abdominal cramping, nausea
  Warm, moist skin

Medical management
Treatment is directed at correction of the underlying imbalance. If imbalance is severe, sodium bicarbonate may be administered cautiously. Imbalances in potassium may be evident as the condition resolves.

METABOLIC ALKALOSIS

Metabolic alkalosis is characterized by a high pH and a high plasma bicarbonate level. The lungs hypoventilate to maintain or increase the P_{CO_2} concentration. The most common cause is vomiting or gastric suction with accompanying loss of acids. It may also accompany hypokalemia or occur from excess alkali ingestion (use of bicarbonate-containing antacids, such as Alka-Seltzer). Clinical manifestations include the following:

BOX 4-13	Expected Directional Changes With Acid-Base Imbalances		
	pH	**HCO₃**	**Pco₂**
Respiratory Acidosis			
Uncompensated	↓	Normal	↑
Partly compensated	↓	↑	↑
Compensated	Normal	↑	↑
Respiratory Alkalosis			
Uncompensated	↑	Normal	↓
Partly compensated	↑	↓	↓
Compensated	Normal	↓	↓
Metabolic Acidosis			
Uncompensated	↓	↓	Normal
Partly compensated	↓	↓	↓
Compensated	Normal	↓	↓
Metabolic Alkalosis			
Uncompensated	↑	↑	Normal
Partly compensated	↑	↑	↑
Compensated	Normal	↑	↑

Symptoms of calcium ionization, such as numbness or tingling of mouth and fingers, hypertonic muscles, spasms

Decreased respiratory rate

Dizziness

Medical management

Treatment is aimed at reversal of the underlying etiology. Sodium, potassium, or ammonium chloride may be administered to restore balance.

RESPIRATORY ACIDOSIS

Respiratory acidosis is characterized by a low pH and a high plasma Pco_2 level. It may be acute or chronic. In chronic states the kidneys compensate by increasing the bicarbonate concentration. It is virtually always the result of failure to excrete CO_2 from the lungs. Acute acidosis accompanies pulmonary edema, pneumothorax, and severe pneumonia. Chronic acidosis is associated with chronic obstructive pulmonary disease (COPD). Clinical manifestations include the following:

Mental cloudiness, dizziness, headache (CO_2 is a direct CNS depressant)

Warm, flushed skin

Hypoventilation

Tachycardia

Guidelines for Interpreting Arterial Blood Gases

pH
  Reflects H⁺ ion concentration
  7.40: electrochemically neutral
  Normal range 7.35-7.45 (below 6.8 or above 7.8 usually considered to be incompatible with life)
Pao₂
  Partial pressure of oxygen dissolved in arterial blood
  Normal range: 80-100 mm Hg
Paco₂
  Partial pressure of carbon dioxide dissolved in arterial blood
  Normal range: 35-45 mm Hg
HCO₃
  Bicarbonate buffer
  Normal range: 22-28 mEq/L (20:1 ratio)

STEPS FOR ANALYSIS
  1. Evaluate pH.
    a. Label as normal, acidosis, or alkalosis.
    b. Initially label all values that deviate from the neutral 7.4.
  2. Evaluate ventilation.
    a. Compare Pco₂ value with normals.
    b. Above 45 mm Hg represents respiratory acidosis or a process of compensation.
    c. Below 35 mm Hg represents respiratory alkalosis or a process of compensation.
  3. Evaluate bicarbonate buffer.
    a. Compare HCO₃ with normals.
    b. Above 28 mEq/L represents metabolic alkalosis or a process of compensation.
    c. Below 22 mEq/L represents metabolic acidosis or a process of compensation.

  4. Determine primary vs. compensatory disorder (occurs in presence of a primary imbalance plus the body's attempt to compensate).
    a. **The pH indicates the primary problem.** If both Pco₂ and HCO₃ are elevated, an acidotic pH (↓7.40) tells you the primary disorder is respiratory acidosis with retention of HCO₃ to compensate. If both Pco₂ and HCO₃ are low, an acidotic pH (↓7.40) tells you the primary disorder is metabolic acidosis with excretion of Pco₂ to compensate.
    b. Compensation may be (1) noncompensation (e.g., only Pco₂ *or* HCO₃ is abnormal, not both), (2) partial compensation (e.g., both Pco₂ *and* HCO₃ are abnormal and so is pH), or (3) compensation (e.g., both Pco₂ *and* HCO₃ are abnormal but pH is normal).
  5. Evaluate oxygenation.
    a. Normal is 80-100 mm Hg.
    b. Mild hypoxemia is 60-80 mm Hg.
    c. ↓60 is moderate to severe hypoxemia.
NOTE:
Metabolic imbalances: pH and HCO₃ values go in the same direction, such as:
  Acidosis: pH↓, HCO₃↓
  Alkalosis: pH↑, HCO₃↑
Respiratory imbalances: pH and Pco₂ go in opposite directions, such as:
  Acidosis: pH↓, Pco₂↑
  Alkalosis: pH↑, Pco₂↓

Guidelines for Drawing Blood for Arterial Blood Gas Analysis

SITE SELECTION

- First choice: radial artery; easily accessible and away from major nerves and other vessels
- Second choice: brachial artery; good collateral but less accessible and near other structures
- Third choice: femoral artery; large but poor collateral circulation exists, risk of bleeding high, and other structures vulnerable to injury

ALLEN'S TEST FOR CIRCULATION

1. Occlude both radial and ulnar arteries by pressure.
2. Have patient make a fist and open slowly (palm will be blanched).
3. Release pressure on the ulnar artery and observe for flushing in 3-6 seconds; indicates adequate perfusion with the radial artery occluded.

EQUIPMENT

- Heparinized syringe with rubber stopper or 5 ml syringe and ampule of heparin
- 22-gauge, 1-inch needle for radial or brachial; 20-gauge, 1½-inch needle for femoral
- Ice
- TB syringe with 0.1-0.3 ml of 1% lidocaine

PROCEDURE

1. Position site with wrist dorsiflexed, supported on a roll.
2. Prepare site with alcohol followed by povidone-iodine using aseptic technique. Leave on skin for 1 minute, and wipe off with alcohol.
3. Anesthetize the site with lidocaine (not standard in all settings).
4. Coat the syringe with heparin and expel the excess.
5. Isolate and stabilize the artery with two fingers.
6. Insert needle, bevel up, at a 45-degree angle (60 degrees for brachial and 90 degrees for femoral). Advance until blood appears in the syringe. Do not pull back. Arterial blood will pulsate.
7. Collect 1.5-3 ml of blood and withdraw.
8. Apply firm pressure with 2 × 2 sponges for 5 minutes, 10 minutes for femoral. Get assistance for this step.
9. Invert needle to expel any air bubble in syringe against a gauze square. Seal with rubber cap or cork, and rotate to mix with the heparin.
10. Immerse in ice, label, and deliver promptly to laboratory.

Medical management

Treatment is directed at improving ventilation, although specific interventions depend on the cause. Vigorous pulmonary care, bronchodilators, and increased fluids may be used to open the airway and improve alveolar gas exchange.

RESPIRATORY ALKALOSIS

Respiratory alkalosis is characterized by a high pH and a low plasma Pco_2 level. It is virtually always the result of hyperventilation, and it may be acute or chronic. The kidneys attempt to compensate by lowering the plasma bicarbonate level. Extreme anxiety is the most common cause, but it may also accompany fever and sepsis, excessive rate or sighs with mechanical ventilation, and hypoxemia. Clinical manifestations include the following:

Lightheadedness

Symptoms of calcium ionization, such as numbness or tingling of mouth and fingers, muscle spasms

Tinnitus

Tremulousness and blurred vision

Nausea

Seizures

Medical management

If the cause of respiratory alkalosis is anxiety, treatment is directed at helping the patient slow and control his or her breathing. The patient may breathe into a paper bag or even require sedation to regain control. Treatment for other forms is directed at the underlying cause.

NURSING MANAGEMENT: Acid-Base Disorders

The nursing role is primarily collaborative and involves careful ongoing monitoring and data collection. Independent nursing interventions are primarily related to airway management, such as encouraging deep breathing and coughing as needed to prevent CO_2 accumulation, particularly with persons on bed rest, postsurgical patients, the obese, and those with COPD.

SELECTED REFERENCES

Anderson S: Six easy steps to interpreting blood gases, *Am J Nurs* 90(8):42-45, 1990.

Bowman M et al: Effect of tube-feeding osmolality on serum sodium levels, *Crit Care Nurse* 9(1):22-28, 1989.

Brenner M, Welliver J: Pulmonary and acid-base assessment, *Nurs Clin North Am* 25:761-770, 1990.

Craft K: Do you really know how to handle sharps? *RN* 53(8):33-34, 1990.

Cullen L: Interventions related to fluid and electrolyte balance, *Nurs Clin North Am* 27(2):569-597, 1992.

Felver L, Pendarvis J: Electrolyte imbalances: intraoperative risk factors, *AORN J* 49(4):992-1008, 1989.

Finke CT: How to draw ABG specimens, *Nursing* 19(9):32k-32o, 1989.

Gasparis L, Murray EB, Ursomanno P: IV solutions: which one is right for your patient? *Nurs 89* 19(4):62-64, 1989.

Gershan JA et al: Fluid volume deficit: validating the indicators, *Heart Lung* 19(2):152-156, 1990.

Gonsoulin SM, Broussard PC: Shedding light on IV therapy, *Nurs 91* 21(12):62-64, 1991.

Hadaway LC: IV tips, *Geriatr Nurs*, pp 78-81, March/April 1991.

Handerhan B: Computing the anion gap, *RN* 54(7):30-31, 1991.

Howard MP, Eisenberg PG, Gianino MS: Dressing a central venous catheter, *Nurs 92* 22(3):60-61, 1992.

Hurray J, Saver C: Arterial blood gas interpretation, *AORN J* 55(1):180-185, 1992.

Janusek LW: Metabolic acidosis: pathophysiology and the resulting signs and symptoms, *Nurs 90* 20(7):52-53, 1990.

Janusek LW: Metabolic alkalosis: pathophysiology and the resulting signs and symptoms, *Nurs 90* 20(6):52-53, 1990.

Lindell KO, Wesmiller SW: Using arterial blood gases to interpret acid-base balance, *Orthop Nurs* 8(3):31-34, 1989.

Masoorli S, Angeles T: PICC lines: the latest home care challenge, *RN* 53(1):44-51, 1990.

Mathewson M: Intravenous therapy, *Crit Care Nurs* 9(2):21-23, 26-28, 30-36, 1989.

McAfee T, Garland LR, McNabb TS: How to draw blood safely from a vascular access device, *Nurs 90* 20(11):42-43, 1990.

Meares C: PICC and MLC lines, *Nurs 92* 22(10):52-55, 1992.

Messner RL, Pinkerman ML: Preventing a peripheral IV infection, *Nurs 92* 22(6):34-41, 1992.

Metheny NM: Why worry about IV fluids? *Am J Nurs* 90(6):50-57, 1990.

Metheny NM: *Fluid and electrolyte balance: nursing considerations,* ed 2, Philadelphia, 1992, Lippincott.

Millam DA: Starting IV's, *Nurs 92* 22(9):33-46, 1992.

Mims BC: Interpreting ABGs, *RN* 54(3):41-47, 1991.

Rountree D: The PIC catheter, *Am J Nurs* 91(8):22-25, 1991.

Sherman JE, Sherman RH: IV therapy that clicks, *Nurs 89* 19(5):50-51, 1989.

Sidebottom J: When it's hot enough to kill, *RN* 55:30-35, 1992.

Sommers M: Rapid fluid resuscitation: how to correct dangerous deficits, *Nurs 90* 20(1):52-59, 1990.

Taylor DL: Respiratory alkalosis: pathophysiology, signs, and symptoms, *Nurs 90* 20(8):60-61, 1990.

Taylor DL: Respiratory acidosis: pathophysiology, signs and symptoms, *Nurs 90* 20(9):52-53, 1990.

Teplitz L: Arterial line disconnection, *Nurs 90* 20(5):33, 1990.

Thomason SS: Using a Groshong central venous catheter, *Nurs 91* 21(10):58-60, 1991.

Viall CD: Your complete guide to central venous catheters, *Nurs 90* 20(2):34-41, 1990.

Weber BB: Timely tips on adhesive tape, *Nurs 91* 21(10):52-53, 1991.

Whitney RG: Comparing long term central venous catheters, *Nurs 91* 21(4):70-71, 1991.

Wiggins MS, Sesin P: Guidelines for administering IV drugs, *Nurs 90* 20(4):145-152, 1990.

Workman ML: Magnesium and phosphorus: the neglected electrolytes, *AACN Clin Issues Critical Care* 3(3):655-663, 1992.

Young M, Flynn K: Third-spacing: when the body conceals fluid loss, *RN* 51(8):46-48, 1988.

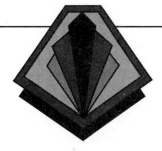

Disorders of the Heart

◆ ASSESSMENT

Health history
  Past medical history and family history
    Sudden death or death from heart disease of family
      member before 50 years of age
    Previous cardiac problems, hospitalizations, sur-
      gery
    Past and current medication use
    Diabetes
    Hyperlipidemia
    Hypertension
    Congenital heart defects
    Acute rheumatic fever

Cardiovascular symptoms
  Chest pain or discomfort (onset, manner of onset,
    duration, precipitating factors, location/radia-
    tion, quality, intensity, chronology/frequency,
    associated symptoms, aggravating factors, allevi-
    ating factors)
  Dyspnea, dyspnea on exertion, orthopnea, parox-
    ysmal nocturnal dyspnea
  Edema, weight gain
  Syncope
  Palpitations
  Unusual or persistent fatigue
Symptom variations in elderly persons
  Confusion, blackouts, syncope

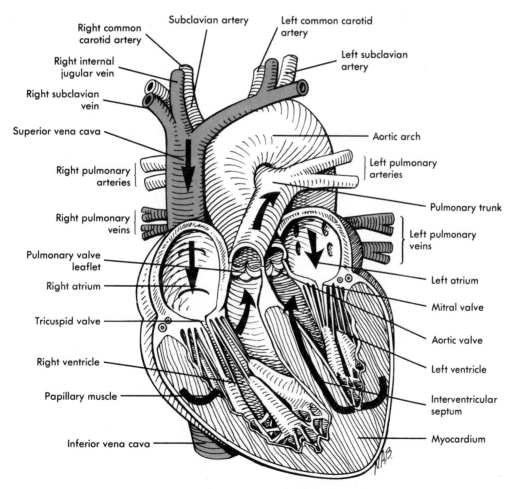

FIGURE 5-1   Major structures of the heart.

Palpitations
Cough, especially at night
Shortness of breath
Leg edema (pattern, time of day most pronounced)
Chest pain or tightness
Fatigue

PHYSICAL ASSESSMENT

Inspection
    Skin color
        Pallor
        Cyanosis (central, peripheral, circumoral)
    Visible pulsations
    Point of maximal impulse (PMI)/apical impulse
    Respiratory rate and character
    Presence of edema
    Nail clubbing
Palpation
    PMI/apical impulse
    Thrills (palpable murmur), thrusts, heaves
    Peripheral pulses
        Bilateral examination of absence or presence, rate, rhythm, amplitude, quality, equality
    Capillary refill
Percussion
    Technique of limited value in cardiac assessment
    Outlining border of cardiac dullness can be helpful in orientation for cardiac and pulmonary examinations
    Actual size and contour of heart more accurately determined by other diagnostic examinations (chest x-ray, echocardiogram)
Auscultation
    Heart rate
    Heart rhythm (regular, irregular)
    Heart sounds (presence, absence, location) (Figures 5-2 and 5-3)
        Listen first with diaphragm of stethoscope in all areas, then the bell; diaphragm best for picking up relatively high-pitched sounds (S_1, S_2); bell more sensitive to low-pitched sounds (S_3, S_4)
    S_1: first heart sound; produced by almost simultaneous closures of mitral and tricuspid valves; signals onset of ventricular systole; loudest at apex
    S_2: second heart sound; produced by almost simultaneous closures of aortic and pulmonic valves; loudest at base
    Splitting of S_1 or S_2: may be a normal or pathologic occurrence caused by enhanced transmission of right side heart sounds, mitral and pulmonic valves, respectively; best heard at peak of inspiration
    Extra heart sounds
        S_3: ventricular diastolic gallop; produced by rapid ventricular filling; indicates increased volume or decreased ventricular compliance; normal finding in healthy children and young adults; pathologic sign in older persons indicating elevated left ventricular filling pressures associated with congestive heart failure (CHF), mitral regurgitation, and constrictive pericarditis; use bell at apex with patient in left lateral recumbent position
        S_4: atrial diastolic gallop; produced by decreased ventricular compliance; pathologic sign associated with hypertensive cardiovascular disease, Idiopathic hypertrophic subaortic sclerosis (IHSS), angina pectoris, myocardial infarction (MI); use bell at apex with patient supine or semilateral
    Murmurs: audible vibrations of heart and great vessels that occur because of turbulent blood flow produced by hemodynamic events or structural alterations; auscultate with stethoscope diaphragm except for low-pitched murmur of mitral stenosis; characterized by timing (position in cardiac cycle), intensity, quality, pitch, location and direction of radiation

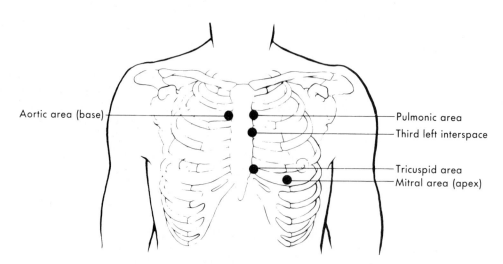

Aortic area (base) — Pulmonic area
— Third left interspace
— Tricuspid area
Mitral area (apex)

FIGURE 5-2 Cardiac auscultatory areas. (From Kinney M et al: *Comprehensive cardiac care,* ed 7, St Louis, 1991, Mosby.)

A Pulmonic and aortic areas (Base)

a

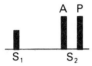

S_1 S_2

Tricuspid and mitral areas (Apex)

b

S_1 S_2

c Normal physiological splitting of S_2
(best heard at pulmonic area during inspiration)

A P

S_1 S_2

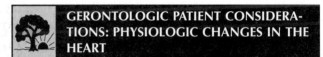

FIGURE 5-3 **A,** Heart sounds. *A,* Aortic; *P,* pulmonic. **B,** Relationship of ECG, cardiac cycle, and heart sounds. (From Lewis SM, Collier IC: *Medical-surgical nursing,* St Louis, 1992, Mosby.)

Categories

    Innocent: systolic, without evidence of physiologic or structural abnormality

    Functional: associated with physiologic alterations of high cardiac output states, such as thyrotoxicosis, anemia, increased blood volume during pregnancy; may or may not involve heart disease

    Pathologic: always caused by a structural abnormality of the heart

Pericardial friction rub: extra heart sound originating from pericardial sac, associated with inflammation, infection, or infiltration and occurs as heart moves; sound clearest at apex

Bruit: murmur or unexpected sound; auscultation over an artery for a bruit indicated when following radiation of a murmur or looking for evidence of local obstruction; usually low pitched and relatively hard to hear; sites at which to auscultate for a bruit are carotid, jugular, temporal, abdominal, aortic, renal, and femoral arteries

Blood pressure

    Usually measured in arm and should be measured in both arms at least once

---

✍ DIAGNOSTIC TESTS
LABORATORY (BLOOD AND URINE) TESTS

Major blood and urine tests for the cardiovascular system are summarized in Table 5-1.

GERONTOLOGIC PATIENT CONSIDERATIONS: PHYSIOLOGIC CHANGES IN THE HEART

The presence of atherosclerosis in most older adults makes it difficult to separate the normal physiologic consequences of aging from changes related to pathologic conditions. Some specific changes associated with aging have been identified; however, overall the heart is able to function adequately into advanced age unless adversely affected by concurrent pathologic conditions. Recognized changes include the following:

The amount of collagen in the heart increases with age. The excess collagen stiffens the tissue, making it less contractile.

Lipids accumulate and accelerate calcification of the heart valves. The aortic valve is typically affected more than the mitral valve.

The number of pacemaker cells in the sinoatrial (SA) node decreases with age, which may affect sinus node functioning. Fibrosis occurs throughout the conduction system although the changes in the electrocardiogram (ECG) are frequently not significant.

Resting heart rate is not affected by age, but the heart's response to exercise declines significantly. Heart rate, stroke volume, and cardiac output are all affected.

The number and function of beta-adrenergic cells decline with age, making elderly persons less responsive to beta-adrenergic agonist and antagonist drugs.

RADIOLOGIC TESTS
Echocardiography

Purpose—Echocardiography uses ultrasound to assess cardiac structures, mobility of the heart valves, and movement of myocardial walls. There are two echocardiographic techniques: M, or motion, mode uses a narrow beam of sound to view cardiac structures; two-dimensional mode transmits a wider sound beam and produces images of sound and motion.

TABLE 5-1   Blood and Urine Tests for the Cardiovascular System

TEST	NORMAL VALUES	SIGNIFICANCE IN HEART DISORDERS
Serum red blood cells (RBCs)	Men: 4.7-6.1 million/mm^3 Women: 4.2-5.4 million/mm^3	Decreased in subacute endocarditis Increased with inadequate tissue oxygenation Decreased in some congenital heart disease with right-to-left shunt
Serum white blood cells (WBCs)	5000-10,000/mm^3	Increased in acute and chronic heart inflammations and in acute MI
Erythrocyte sedimentation rate (ESR)	Men: up to 15 mm/hr Women: up to 20 mm/hr	Increased in acute MI and infectious heart disease
Prothrombin time (PT)	11-12.5 sec 100% compared to control	Indicates rapidity of blood clotting; used to monitor anticoagulant therapy with coumarin and warfarin sodium
Activated partial thromboplastin time (APPT)	30-40 sec	More sensitive than PT; used to monitor heparin therapy
International normalized ratio (INR)	2.0-3.0 for treatment of venous thrombosis, pulmonary embolism, prevention of systemic embolism with MI, atrial fibrillation	Standardization of prothrombin time (PT) assay test results for individuals on sodium warfarin (Coumadin) therapy
Blood urea nitrogen (BUN)	5-20 mg/dl	Increased with decreased cardiac output
Serum proteins	6-8 g/dl	Levels below 5 g/dl seen with edema
Cardiac isoenzymes		
Creatinine kinase (CK)	Women <2.5 U or 5-35 IU/L Men <4.3 U or 5-50 IU/L	Elevations indicate possible brain, myocardial, and skeletal muscle injury or necrosis
CK-MB	0-5% of total CK	Elevations with myocardial injury
Lactic dehydrogenase (LDH)	80-120 Wacker units or 70-207 IU/L	Elevations occur with injury to heart, liver, kidney, brain, and erythrocytes
LDH$_1$	16%-33% of total LDH	Elevation higher than LDH$_2$ with myocardial damage
LDH$_2$	28%-40% of total LDH	
LDH$_1$/LDH$_2$	<1.0	Elevation occurs with myocardial damage
Lipids		
Total lipids	40-100 mg/dl	Elevation indicates increased risk for coronary artery disease (CAD)
Cholesterol	Women: mean of 170-230 mg/dl (range increases with age) Men: mean of 140-215 mg/dl (range increases with age)	
Triglycerides	Women: mean of 90-130 mg/dl (range increases with age) Men: mean of 100-150 mg/dl (range increases with age)	
High-density lipoproteins (HDLs)	Women: mean of 55-60 mg/dl Men: mean of 45-50 mg/dl	Elevations may protect against CAD
Low-density lipoproteins (LDLs)	Women: mean of 105-150 mg/dl Men: mean of 105-145 mg/dl	Elevation indicates increased risk for CAD
HDL/LDL ratio	3:1	Elevation may protect against CAD
Electrolytes		
Sodium	136-145 mEq/L	Sodium values reflect water balance and may be decreased, indicating a water excess in patients with heart failure
Potassium	3.5-5.0 mEq/L	Effects of decreased levels include increased electrical instability, ventricular dysrhythmias, appearance of U waves on ECG, and increased risk of digitalis toxicity
Calcium	4.5-5.5 mEq/L	Manifestations of low levels include ventricular dysrhythmias, prolonged QT intervals, and cardiac arrest. Hypercalcemia shortens QT interval and causes atrioventricular (AV) block, digitalis hypersensitivity, and cardiac arrest
Magnesium	1.5-2.5 mEq/L	Cardiac manifestations of increased levels include bradycardia, peripheral vasodilation, hypotension, prolonged PR interval with widened QRS complex
Urinalysis		Helps determine effects of cardiovascular disease on renal function and existence of concurrent renal or systemic diseases Proteinuria seen in patients with malignant hypertension, CHF, or constrictive pericarditis Presence of RBCs may indicate infective endocarditis or embolic kidney disease

Procedure—A small transducer lubricated with gel to facilitate movement and conduction is placed on the patient's chest at the level of the third or fourth intercostal space, along the left sternal border. The transducer transmits high-frequency sound waves and receives them back from the patient as they are reflected from different structures.

Patient preparation and aftercare—No special preparation is necessary. The patient is told the test is painless and takes 30 to 60 minutes to complete. The patient must lie quietly, with the head of bed elevated 15 to 20 degrees during the test.

Transesophageal Echocardiography

Purpose—Transesophageal echocardiography is a semiinvasive technique using a gastroscope-like probe to pass an ultrasound transducer into the esophagus and upper stomach. Because of the proximity of the esophagus to the heart, detailed images may be obtained unobscured by the lungs and rib cage. Transesophageal echocardiography provides detailed images of the right and left atria, atrial septum, pulmonary artery and veins, and thoracic aorta. It is useful in the assessment of prosthetic valve malfunction, atrial tumor or thrombus, infective endocarditis and valvular vegetation, valvular defect, and congenital heart defect.

Procedure—A transducer affixed to the tip of a modified flexible endoscope is advanced into the esophagus and manipulated to produce images of the heart. The endoscopic device is connected to standard echocardiographic machines to provide combined two-dimensional, M-mode, pulsed Doppler, and color flow imaging.

Patient preparation and aftercare—Transesophageal echocardiography is contraindicated in patients with esophageal strictures and varices and history of dysphagia or chest wall radiation therapy because of the risk of perforation. The patient is kept NPO for 4 to 6 hours before the procedure. Dentures and other oral prosthetics must be removed. Intravenous sedation helps to reduce anxiety. Antibiotic prophylaxis for bacterial endocarditis may be ordered. Cardiac rhythm, vital signs, and SaO$_2$ are monitored throughout the procedure. The patient is given a topical anesthetic by spray or gargle. The procedure takes about 5 to 20 minutes. Vital signs and cardiac rhythm are monitored for 1 to 4 hours after the procedure, and the patient is kept NPO until sedative effects have disappeared and the gag reflex is restored.

Dobutamine Stress Echocardiography

Purpose—Dobutamine stress echocardiography is used to assess ischemic heart disease in patients who are unable to exercise because of peripheral vascular disease, chronic obstructive pulmonary disease (COPD), or neurologic or musculoskeletal disorders.

Procedure—A baseline two-dimensional echocardiogram is performed initially. An infusion of dobutamine is started at low doses and slowly increased to a maximum of 40 mg/kg/min. Continuous ECG monitoring and echocardiographic imaging are maintained during the test. The images are evaluated to determine presence of wall motion abnormalities (akinesis, dyskinesis, hyperkinesis) at rest and with stress effects induced by dobutamine.

Patient preparation and aftercare—Care is the same as for echocardiography. Dobutamine may cause transient tachycardia and hypotension. The patient may experience fatigue.

Coronary Angiography, Cardiac Catheterization, and Ventriculography

Purpose—*Coronary angiography* involves injection of radiopaque dye into the right and left epicardial coronary arteries to confirm the presence and/or degree of coronary artery stenosis, as well as the presence or absence of collateral circulation.

Cardiac catheterization describes the insertion of a catheter directly into the right and/or left ventricle to gather information about ventricular function (ejection fraction, pressures).

Ventriculography is the injection of a radiopaque dye into the left ventricle to obtain direct visualization of ventricular wall motion, mitral valve function, and status of the ventricular septum.

Procedure—After injection with a local anesthetic, a catheter is inserted via cutdown into a large vein (right side of heart studies) or artery (left side of heart studies) and threaded under fluoroscopy to the desired location. Contrast medium is injected; cineangiography films may be taken to monitor the progression of the dye. The contrast medium outlines the coronary circulation, enabling evaluation of anatomy of coronary arteries as well as stenotic segments and collateral vessels.

Patient preparation and aftercare—The procedures are explained to the patient and family. The description needs to address the procedure and anticipated sensations (flushing, nausea, chest pain, dyspnea) as well as the risks of the procedure (hemorrhage, MI, cardiovascular accident [CVA], dysrhythmia, death). The patient is NPO for at least 4 hours before the procedure. A mild sedative may be ordered. The patient and family should be informed that the procedure will last from 1 to 3 hours, during which the patient will be lying on a hard x-ray table in a cool room.

Postprocedure care may vary between institutions but will always involve frequent assessment of blood pressure, heart rate and rhythm, and peripheral circulation. Hemostasis of arterial access sites may be maintained with a pressure dressing that will be in place for at least 8 hours. The patient will be kept on bed rest, with the head of bed elevated less than 90 degrees for up to 12 hours. If bleeding occurs from arterial access sites, firm direct pressure is applied over the site and the physician is notified. Back discomfort after the procedure occurs often and should be minimized by back rubs, analgesics, and early ambulation. Research studies are looking at the safety of early ambulation after invasive studies and will impact postprocedure care in the future. Because of the nephrotoxic effects of the dye, intake and output are monitored for the first 24 hours after the procedure, as well as serum BUN and creatinine levels.

Electrophysiologic Study

Purpose—The electrophysiologic study is an invasive diagnostic procedure for the management of patients with recurrent symptomatic dysrhythmias. Internal electrodes record activity in specific areas of the cardiac conduction system, providing information about the sequence of atrial and ventricular activation, localization of conduction disturbances, and effectiveness of antidysrhythmic management. They can also deliver a stimulus to pace the heart or induce an arrhythmia. More detailed information about the heart's electrical activity can be obtained with the electrophysiologic study than with the surface ECG because of the proximity of the catheters to the cardiac conduction system.

Procedure—Before the initial electrophysiologic study the patient will be taken off antidysrhythmic medications for a period of at least 5 half-lives. The electrophysiologic study is performed under laboratory settings similar to a cardiac catheterization, using fluoroscopy to guide pacing electrodes into place. Venous access sites are generally used for catheter placement. Arterial cannulation may be required for left ventricular stimulation. The catheter is advanced until one electrode rests in the right atrium, one adjacent to the bundle of His, and one in the right ventricle. An additional electrode may be placed in the coronary sinus. Three to six intracardiac pacing catheters connected to a multichanneled electrogram may be used. A surface ECG is recorded simultaneously for comparison and evaluation.

Patient preparation and aftercare—The purpose, procedure, and risks must be explained to patient and family. The electrophysiologic study usually lasts 2 to 4 hours, during which the patient lies on an x-ray table. Back discomfort is common. The patient is NPO for at least 4 hours before the test. Intravenous access is established and maintained. The patient may be given a local anesthetic before catheter insertion and may receive a mild sedative. Patients may experience chest discomfort, dizziness, and loss of consciousness because of hypotension with prolonged episodes of dysrhythmia. Cardioversion or defibrillation may be required. Most patients will be maintained on a cardiac monitor in a telemetry unit for at least 12 to 24 hours after the procedure. Vital signs and peripheral circulation are checked frequently during the first 12 hours after the procedure. After catheters are removed, a sterile dressing is applied (pressure dressing if arterial cannulation is performed), and the patient is kept on bed rest with the head of bed elevated less than 90 degrees for at least 4

hours. Subsequent electrophysiologic studies may be required to assess the effectiveness of antidysrhythmic medications.

Myocardial Imaging Studies and Nuclear Cardiography

Purpose—Myocardial imaging shows perfusion of myocardium using radioactive tracer substances. A number of imaging studies are done. These studies help to identify appropriate candidates for coronary bypass surgery, angioplasty, and other interventions.

Procedures—In *technetium pyrophosphate scanning* a small dose of technetium pyrophosphate is injected intravenously. The radioisotope accumulates only in damaged myocardial tissue, referred to as a "hot spot."

In *thallium imaging* a small dose of ^{201}Tl is injected into the patient's antecubital vein. The imaging is done within 4 to 10 minutes, because only normal cells with intact blood supply rapidly take up this radioisotope. Necrotic or ischemic tissue will appear as "cold spots" on the scan.

Thallium imaging is most often performed with the patient at rest and during an exercise test. The exercise test may help to reveal perfusion defects that are not apparent until myocardial oxygen demands are increased. The stress test is performed as described on p. 56. After the patient reaches maximal activity level, a small dose of ^{201}Tl is injected. The patient exercises for 1 to 2 minutes and is then scanned. The patient is scanned again after 1 to 3 hours of rest to differentiate between ischemic and necrotic tissue. Changes in perfusion at rest and with exercise are called redistribution. Redistribution is the single most important predictor of future cardiac events.

For the 20% to 30% of patients unable to exercise, the cardiovascular effects of exercise may be simulated with the use of dipyridamole, adenosine, or dobutamine in conjunction with thallium imaging.

Sesta-mibi is a new nonredistributing radionuclide that binds to myocardial tissue but washes out slowly with a 6-hour half-life. This allows for more flexibility in scheduling and may be more accurate.

Positron emission tomography (*PET*) is a new noninvasive diagnostic tool that may replace thallium imaging and cardiac catheterization. PET scans differentiate between ischemic and well-perfused myocardium by demonstrating a metabolic/perfusion mismatch (elevated metabolism despite decreased blood flow). Infarcted tissue does not demonstrate this mismatch, with both metabolism and perfusion decreased. The patient, at rest, receives the first of two radioisotopes, and perfusion images are taken. Metabolism images are taken after injection with a second radioisotope, usually following a physical or chemical stress test. The PET scan looks at glucose metabolic activity. Therefore the patient's blood sugar must be within normal range.

Gated cardiac pool scanning (MUGA) analyzes ventricular function, providing information about wall motion and ejection fraction. ECG leads are attached to the patient, and the ECG is synchronized with a computer and a gamma-scintillation camera. A small amount of technetium is injected intravenously. Scanning begins after 3 to 5 minutes. The computer constructs an average cardiac cycle that represents the summation of several hundred heartbeats.

Patient preparation and aftercare—For all of the imaging studies, the patient is informed that these studies are relatively noninvasive and radiation exposure and risks are minimal. There is no specific postprocedure care, but patients may complain of fatigue. Adverse reactions to thallium, dipyridamole, adenosine, and dobutamine may include hypotension and tachycardia.

SPECIAL TESTS
Electrocardiography (EKG, ECG)

Purpose—The ECG graphically records electrical current generated by the heart. The current is measured by electrodes placed on the skin and connected to an amplifier and strip chart recorder.

Procedure—The standard 12-lead ECG has 10 electrodes attached to the arms, legs, and chest to measure current from 12 different views or leads (Figure 5-4). The electrodes are attached to lead wires that connect to the ECG machine.

Patient preparation and aftercare—The ECG is performed with the patient in a supine position with the chest exposed. Electrode sites need to be free of hair and are cleaned with alcohol swabs to decrease skin oils and improve electrode contact. Good contact between skin and electrode must be maintained. Electrode paste, gel, or saline pads may be used. The patient is asked to lie quietly during the test, which takes less than 1 minute. No specific follow-up care is necessary.

Telemetry Monitoring

Purpose—Telemetry monitoring is the continuous measurement of the cardiac activity of a patient with dysfunction that requires prompt detection and treatment. Telemetry is used for patients who need continuous monitoring but are able to ambulate.

Procedure—The patient is attached to a telemetry transmitter via lead wires (two to four wires). The

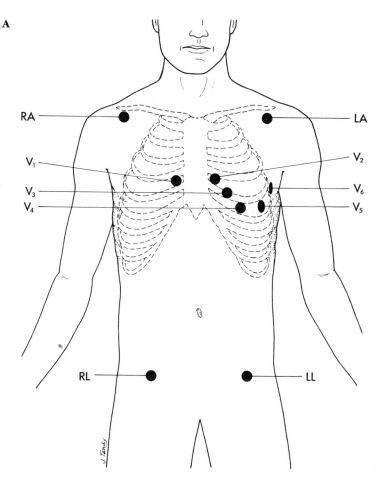

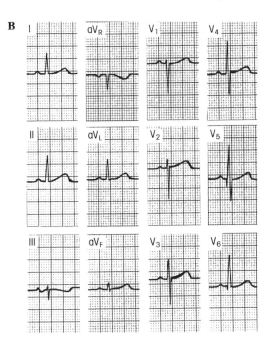

FIGURE 5-4   A, ECG leads showing placement of limb electrodes (LL, RL, RA, LA) and chest electrodes (V₁-V₆). **B,** Normal 12-lead ECG. (**A** from Flynn JB, Bruce NP: *Introduction to critical care skills,* St Louis, 1993, Mosby; **B** from Guzzetta CE, Dossey BM: *Cardiovascular nursing: bodymind tapestry,* St Louis, 1984, Mosby.)

transmitter sends ECG data to the central console of a telemetry unit.

Patient preparation and aftercare—The areas for electrode placement should be free of hair and oil. The lead wires are attached to a small transmitter that the patient carries around the neck or waist in a pouch. The patient is instructed not to leave the range of the telemetry unit and to notify the nurse if the electrodes become disconnected.

Holter Monitoring

Purpose—Holter monitoring, or ambulatory electrocardiography, allows continuous recording of the heart's electrical activity during an extended period, usually 24 hours, while the patient carries out activities of daily living (ADL). Holter monitoring allows for assessment and correlation of chest pain, dyspnea, syncope, and palpitations with cardiac events and the patient's activities.

Procedure—The patient has electrodes placed on the chest and attached to the Holter monitor, which is a small, portable ECG tape recorder, about the size of a portable radio. The monitor is worn in a holder around the chest or abdomen. After the monitoring period the device is removed and the tape is analyzed by microcomputer.

Patient preparation and aftercare—The patient is required to keep a diary of activities, medications, and symptoms during the monitoring period. The patient should be instructed to avoid bathing, showering, and participating in contact activities that may dislodge the electrodes. No specific follow-up care is required beyond informing the patient where and when to return the device.

Signal-Average Electrocardiography

Purpose—Signal-average electrocardiography is a noninvasive computerized method of analyzing standard ECGs that identifies patients at risk for ventricular tachycardia. Sustained ventricular tachycardia can be a precursor of sudden cardiac death.

Procedure—Signal-average ECG involves amplification of electrical signals from the heart that have a voltage too small to be recorded by a standard ECG. Approximately 200 identical QRS complexes are grouped and averaged, resulting in a waveform that appears smooth and continuous. Signal averaging minimizes the level of noise that contaminates the ECG signal, revealing signals of a microvolt level normally hidden in "noise" (skeletal and respiratory muscle "noise" and "noise" from electrodes).

Patient preparation and aftercare—Care is similar to that for an ECG. Cleansing and mildly abrading the skin are necessary before applying the electrodes. The patient is required to lie quietly for 10 to 20 minutes.

Stress Testing

Purpose—The stress test assesses cardiopulmonary response to an increased work load. It helps to determine the heart's functional capacity and screens for coronary artery disease (CAD).

Procedure—Electrodes are placed on the patient's chest and attached to a multilead monitoring system. Baseline blood pressure, heart rate, and respiratory rate are noted. The primary modes of exercise used include bicycle ergometry or treadmill walking. The exercise is started following patient instruction. During the test the patient's blood pressure, heart rate and rhythm, and presence of additional symptoms are assessed by a physician or nurse. The patient exercises until one of the following occurs: a predetermined heart rate is reached and maintained; signs and symptoms such as chest pain, dyspnea, fatigue, vertigo, hypotension, or ventricular dysrhythmias occur; or there are significant ECG changes.

Patient preparation and aftercare—The patient must be informed of the risks of stress testing, along with the purpose and procedure. Patient and family are assured that the procedure is performed in a controlled environment with medical and nursing care available as needed. The patient should be NPO for at least 2 hours before the test and should not eat or drink caffeine-containing foods or beverages on the day of the test. The patient should wear comfortable clothes and walking shoes. The patient is instructed to inform the physician or nurse performing the test of any symptoms (chest pain, shortness of breath, irregular heartbeat) experienced during the test.

Dipyridamole (Persantine)-Thallium Stress Testing

Purpose—The dipyridamole-thallium stress test is an alternative for patients who cannot exercise for a thallium stress test.

Procedure—An intravenous infusion of dipyridamole (Persantine) is given to dilate the coronary arteries in order to simulate the effect of exercise. Dipyridamole increases blood flow to collateral vessels, diverting it from coronary arteries and causing ischemia. Imaging is performed in the same manner as with the exercise stress test.

Patient preparation and aftercare—Care is the same as for thallium stress testing. The patient may complain of mild nausea or headache after the dipyridamole injection. The test will take about 4 hours, because imaging will again be done after a period of rest.

DISORDERS OF THE HEART

Cardiovascular diseases cause more deaths in the United States than all other diseases combined. Nearly 66 million Americans have some form of cardiovascular disease. There has, however, been a steady decline in mortality over the last decade as a result of increased knowledge regarding causes, diagnosis, treatment, and, most importantly, prevention of heart disease.

Heart diseases can be classified into two major groupings—acquired and congenital. The disorders discussed in this chapter include cardiac dysrhythmias, coronary artery disease, congestive heart failure, and inflammatory and valvular heart disease.

CARDIAC DYSRHYTHMIAS
Etiology/Epidemiology

Cardiac rhythm refers to the regular, rhythmic muscular contraction of the heart. Each mechanical contraction is initiated by an electrical wave spreading through the heart. Abnormalities of cardiac rhythm are common in individuals with and without heart disease. Any disorder of the heartbeat is termed *dysrhythmia.*

Pathophysiology

Dysrhythmias that impair cardiac output result from an alteration in the order or speed of conduction of electrical impulses. Dysrhythmias may consist of slow impulse formation, resulting in bradycardias (heart rate <60 beats/min), or rapid impulse formation, resulting in tachycardias (heart rate >100 beats/min). A delay in impulse conduction may result in AV nodal blocks or intraventricular conduction delays (bundle branch blocks). Premature, or ectopic, beats result in an irregular rhythm related to irritable cardiac cells (premature atrial, junctional, or ventricular contractions). Failure to produce an impulse may result in a pause in the conduction rhythm (sinus pause, ventricular standstill, or asystole).

The heart's electrical activity is represented in ECG tracings by P, Q, R, S, T, and U waves. Each of these waves represents a part of the cardiac cycle and is evaluated on the ECG for presence and shape. Some of the waves in combination with another represent an *interval* that is measured in fractions of a second to determine the duration of an event in the cardiac cycle (Figure 5-5).

The baseline of the ECG is known as the isoelectric line. Waves are deflections, positive (above baseline) or negative (below baseline). ECG waves are measured in amplitude (voltage) and duration (time). Amplitude is measured on the ECG by a series of horizontal lines, each 1 mm apart and representing 0.1 mV. The duration of a wave is measured by a series of vertical lines, each 1 mm apart, representing 0.04 second. The usual speed of the paper is 25 mm/sec. Every fifth line both vertically and horizontally is darker than the preceding lines, forming a large square with five smaller squares within it.

The first wave, the *P wave,* represents atrial depolarization (contraction). It begins in the sinoatrial (SA) node and then travels through the atria. The duration is normally between 0.06 and 0.12 second. The height is normally not over 3 mm. P waves are most often upright, round, and symmetric.

Following the P wave is an isoelectric line that, when combined with the P wave, constitutes the *PR interval.* The PR interval starts with the beginning of the P wave and goes to the beginning of the QRS complex. It represents the time it takes the impulse to travel from the atria to the AV node. The time interval is normally from 0.12 to 0.20 second.

The *QRS complex* represents ventricular depolarization and is composed of three waves: Q, R, and S. The Q

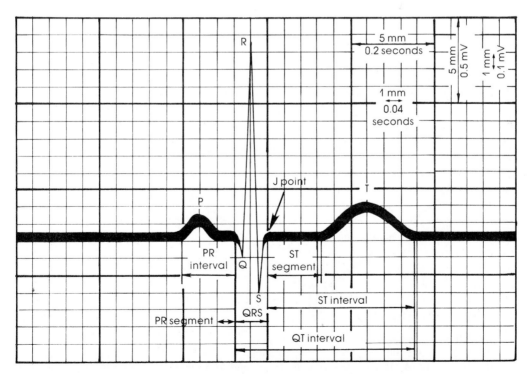

FIGURE 5-5 Deflections and intervals in a normal ECG. (From The Methodist Hospital: *Basic electrocardiography: a modular approach,* St Louis, 1986, Mosby.)

wave is the first negative deflection, the R wave is the first positive deflection, and the S wave is the second negative deflection. The impulse travels through the ventricles rapidly, and the complex normally measures between 0.06 and 0.10 second in duration.

The *ST segment* extends from termination of the QRS complex to the beginning of the T wave. It represents the time during which ventricular depolarization has occurred and repolarization may begin. Deviation of the ST segment is normal if not elevated above baseline more than 1 mm or below by 0.5 mm. Injury to the epicardium causes ST elevation; injury to the endocardium causes ST depression.

The *QT interval* follows the ST segment and is measured from the beginning of the QRS complex to the end of the T wave. It represents the time required for ventricular depolarization and repolarization to occur. The time interval is 0.34 to 0.43 second; varies with heart rate, sex, and age; and may be prolonged by antidysrhythmic medications and electrolyte disturbances.

The *T wave* represents ventricular repolarization. This represents the vulnerable period when a stimulus can produce ventricular tachycardia or fibrillation. Normally it is upright.

The *U wave* is a small, low-voltage wave that follows the T wave, occurring in the same direction as the T wave. Its etiology and clinical significance are uncertain, and it may not be seen in a normal ECG. It may be more pronounced in hypokalemia and MI.

To estimate heart rate (Figure 5-6), do the following:
- Count the number of QRS complexes in a 1-minute strip.
- Count the number of small boxes between two R waves and divide that number into 1500 (1500 small blocks in 1 minute).
- Count the number of large boxes between two R waves and divide that number into 300.
- Count the number of complexes (P waves for atrial rate, R waves for ventricular rate) in 6 seconds and multiply that number by 10 (the ECG paper is divided into 3-second intervals along the margin).

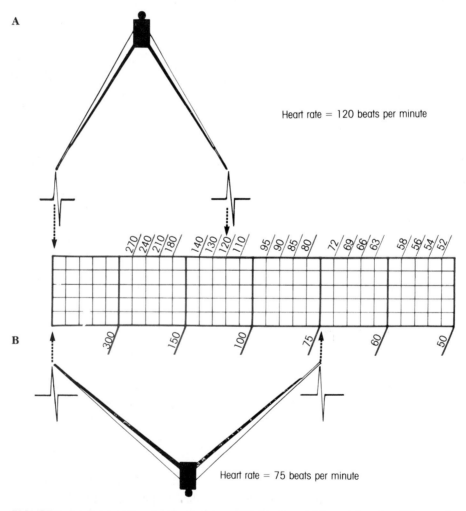

FIGURE 5-6 Determining heart rate using ECG. Locate a QRS complex that falls on a heavy black line. Count 300, 150, 100, 75, 60, 50 until a second QRS complex occurs. This will be the heart rate. **A,** Heart rate—120. **B,** Heart rate—75. (From Guzzetta CE, Dossey BM: *Cardiovascular nursing: holistic practice,* St Louis, 1992, Mosby.)

Guidelines for Interpreting an ECG Rhythm Strip

RATE

Calculate atrial and ventricular rates.
Are they fast, normal, or slow?

RR INTERVALS

Are they regular or irregular?

P WAVES

Are they present or absent?
Do they precede every QRS complex?
Are they similar in shape?

PR INTERVALS

Are they normal (0.12 to 0.20 second), short, or prolonged?
Is there a regular pattern?

QRS COMPLEXES

Are they narrow or wide?
Are they of similar shape, upright, and of regular pattern?

ST SEGMENT

Is it on the baseline, elevated, or depressed?

T WAVES

Are they upright?

QT INTERVAL

What is it?

ECTOPIC BEATS

Are they present?
Are they atrial, junctional, or ventricular?

GERONTOLOGIC PATIENT CONSIDERATIONS: ELECTROCARDIOGRAM CHANGES

P WAVE

Notching, slurring, loss of amplitude
More missing P waves (reflect fibrosis, cellular changes, or loss of atrial myocardium)

QRS COMPLEX

Greater duration of QRS interval (slowing of conduction system)
QRS complex not prolonged to 0.12 second in absence of bundle branch block
Amplitude of R and S waves decreased

BUNDLE BRANCH BLOCK

Right bundle branch block occurs more often than left
Caused by fibrocalcific changes in conduction system (rather than ischemic heart disease); prognosis dependent on cause

ST-T WAVE

ECG changes in ventricular repolarization: T wave amplitude diminishes, sometimes appearing notched, whereas ST segment flattens

BOX 5-1 Prodysrhythmia

It has long been recognized that in some individuals antidysrhythmic drugs not only aggravate existing dysrhythmias but also induce new ones. The phenomenon is called prodysrhythmia and is characterized by the development of supraventricular or ventricular dysrhythmias during therapy with antidysrhythmic drugs. This problem is particularly serious because, unlike other side effects, prodysrhythmia is often asymptomatic, unpredictable, and unrelated to the drug dosage or blood levels, yet it can be fatal. One etiologic factor is the prolongation of the QT interval, enhancing the period of vulnerability to ectopic foci. Understanding the action of antidysrhythmic drugs on the cardiac rhythm is a primary nursing responsibility when administering these medications.

For accuracy these methods should be reserved for regular rhythms. When irregular rhythms are observed, it is best to obtain the rate with a 60-second apical pulse.

Medical Management

A 12-lead ECG, along with telemetry or Holter monitoring, is used to assess the frequency and type of dysrhythmia. Stress testing, echocardiography, and electrophysiology testing may be required to determine the type, cause, and effect of the dysrhythmia.

Treatment of dysrhythmia is specific to the type of dysrhythmia, the cause, the effect it has on cardiac output, and the risk it presents to the patient. Common dysrhythmias and their treatment are listed in Table 5-2.

Noninvasive medical interventions that may be used to terminate dysrhythmias, such as supraventricular tachycardia, include carotid massage and Valsalva's maneuver.

Pharmacologic therapy for control of dysrhythmia includes drugs from one or more of the four classes of antidysrhythmic agents. They are grouped into classes on the basis of the effect they have on cardiac muscle (Table 5-3). It is important to remember that all antidysrhythmic agents can cause dysrhythmias (Box 5-1).

Temporary pacing is a nonsurgical intervention used in emergent or elective situations that require limited, short-term pacing. It provides an electrical stimulus to the right atrium, right ventricle, or both when a stimulus does not exist or when it occurs at a rate too slow for adequate cardiac output. Temporary pacemakers may also be used to provide rapid atrial pacing to overdrive atrial tachycardias. Methods of temporary pacing are external, epicardial, transthoracic, and, most commonly, transvenous.

Catheter ablation may be used to treat recurrent ventricular dysrhythmia and Wolff-Parkinson-White (WPW) syndrome that have not been adequately controlled by medical therapy. Catheter ablation is a technique whereby a catheter is positioned near the myocardial focus of the dysrhythmia. The focus is identified by

TABLE 5-2 Comparison of Selected Cardiac Rhythms

RHYTHM	DESCRIPTION	ETIOLOGY	SYMPTOMS/ CONSEQUENCES	TREATMENT
Normal sinus rhythm	Rhythm regular Heart rate 60-100 beats/min Atrial rate = ventricular rate 1 P wave preceding each QRS complex		Optimal cardiac output	None
Sinus bradycardia	P waves present Rhythm regular Heart rate <60 beats/min	Physical fitness Parasympathetic stimulation (sleep) Brain lesions Sinus dysfunction Digitalis excess	Very low rates may cause decreased cardiac output: lightheadedness, faintness, chest pain	Atropine if cardiac output decreased Pacemaker Treat underlying cause if necessary
Sinus tachycardia	P waves present followed by QRS Rhythm regular Heart rate 100-150 beats/min	Increased metabolic demands Decreased oxygen delivery, CHF, shock, hemorrhage, anemia	May produce palpitations Prolonged episodes may lead to decreased cardiac output	Treat underlying cause Occasionally sedatives
Premature atrial beats	Early P wave QRS may or may not be normal Rhythm irregular	Stress, ischemia, atrial enlargement, caffeine, nicotine	May produce palpitations Frequent episodes may decrease cardiac output Sign of chamber irritability	Sedation Quinidine May require no treatment

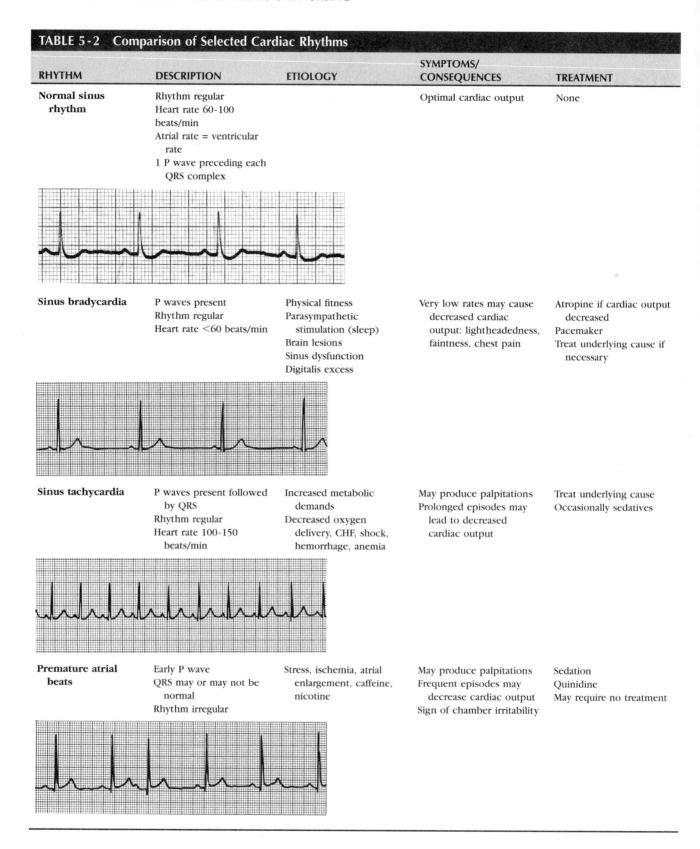

endocardial mapping. A synchronized direct current shock is delivered to cause a controlled necrosis of the area.

Cardioversion is usually an elective procedure used for hemodynamically stable ventricular or supraven-tricular tachycardias (atrial fibrillation) that are resistant to conventional medical therapies. It is the electrical reversion of a cardiac dysrhythmia to normal sinus rhythm. The electrical discharge is synchronized with the patient's QRS complex. If the patient has been

TABLE 5-2   Comparison of Selected Cardiac Rhythms—Cont'd.

RHYTHM	DESCRIPTION	ETIOLOGY	SYMPTOMS/ CONSEQUENCES	TREATMENT
Atrial flutter	Rhythm regular or irregular More than 1 P wave for every QRS Atrial rate = 250-300 beats/min f waves: sawtooth configuration	Acute and chronic heart disease; MI; valvular disease; pericarditis	Depends on rate Dizziness	Carotid massage Digoxin Quinidine Procainamide Calcium channel blocker Cardioversion

RHYTHM	DESCRIPTION	ETIOLOGY	SYMPTOMS/ CONSEQUENCES	TREATMENT
Atrial fibrillation	Rapid, irregular waves (>350/min) Ventricular rhythm irregularly irregular Ventricular rate varies, may increase to 120-150/min if untreated	Rheumatic heart disease Mitral stenosis Atrial infarction Coronary atherosclerotic heart disease Hypertensive heart disease Thyrotoxicosis	Pulse deficit Decreased cardiac output if rate is rapid Promotes thrombus formation in atria	Digitalis Quinidine Cardioversion Calcium channel blocker Beta blocker

RHYTHM	DESCRIPTION	ETIOLOGY	SYMPTOMS/ CONSEQUENCES	TREATMENT
Premature ventricular contractions (PVCs, PVBs)	Early wide bizarre QRS, not associated with a P wave Rhythm irregular	Stress, acidosis, ventricular enlargement Electrolyte imbalance Myocardial infarction Digitalis toxicity Hypoxemia, hypercapnia	Same as for premature atrial beats	Procainamide Quinidine Disopyramide (Norpace) Lidocaine Mexiletine Oxygen Sodium bicarbonate Potassium Treat CHF

Continued.

TABLE 5-2   Comparison of Selected Cardiac Rhythms—Cont'd.

RHYTHM	DESCRIPTION	ETIOLOGY	SYMPTOMS/ CONSEQUENCES	TREATMENT
Ventricular tachycardia	No P wave before QRS; QRS wide and bizarre; ventricular rate >100, usually 140-240	PVB striking during vulnerable period; hypoxemia; drug toxicity; electrolyte imbalance; bradycardia	Decreased cardiac output, hypotension, loss of consciousness, respiratory arrest	Lidocaine Procainamide Bretylium Mexiletine Cardioversion
Ventricular fibrillation	Chaotic electrical activity No recognizable QRS complex	Myocardial infarction Electrocution Freshwater drowning Drug toxicity	No cardiac output Absent pulse or respiration Cardiac arrest	Defibrillation Epinephrine Sodium bicarbonate Bretylium Cardiopulmonary resuscitation (CPR)
Ventricular standstill/ asystole	Can be distinguished from ventricular fibrillation only by ECG P waves *may* be present No QRS "Straight line"	Myocardial infarction Chronic diseases of conducting system	Same as for ventricular fibrillation	CPR Pacemaker Intracardiac epinephrine Isoproterenol

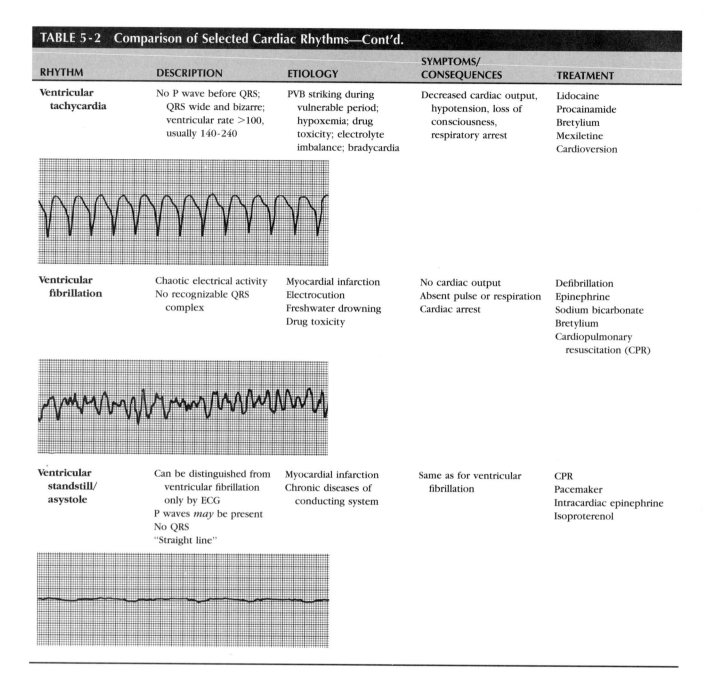

taking a digitalis preparation the drug is held, usually for 2 days, before cardioversion. Digitalis may predispose to the development of ventricular dysrhythmias. Serum potassium levels must also be within normal limits to decrease the risk of lethal dysrhythmia.

Surgical treatment for patients who experience life-threatening dysrhythmias includes *aneurysectomy,* or the surgical resection of a dyskinetic or ballooning portion of the ventricular wall. The aneurysm, usually caused by an MI, serves as a focus for dysrhythmia. *Coronary artery bypass graft* (CABG) surgery is performed if the cause of the dysrhythmia is MI secondary to coronary artery obstruction. Surgical ablation of accessory pathways (pathways that bypass the control of the AV node) of WPW may also be performed.

Permanent pacemakers are used to treat conduction disorders that are not temporary in nature. A permanent pacemaker may be single or dual chambered and consists of a pulse generator and a lead electrode system that is placed on the endocardium or epicardium. Pacemakers are programmable with a battery-operated device that adjusts mode, rate, sensitivity, and amount of energy sent to the heart with each stimulus.

The North American Society of Pacing and Electrophysiology has developed a code whereby one can differentiate a single-chamber versus a dual-chamber pacemaker and identify what chambers of the heart will be affected by the pacemaker. The first letter of the code refers to the cardiac chamber that is paced. The second letter indicates which chamber is sensed. The

TABLE 5-3   Antidysrhythmic Medications

CLASS OF DRUG	ACTION	AGENT	SIDE EFFECTS
Class 1	Depress rate of depolarization Impede flow of sodium into cell during depolarization, thus decreasing conduction velocity	Lidocaine Procainamide Quinidine Disopyramide Mexiletine Tocainide Flecainide	Hypotension Widened QRS Prolonged PR, QT intervals Bradycardia
Class 2	Depress depolarization of cardiac action potential	Propranolol	Bradycardia Hypotension
Class 3	Lengthen absolute refractory period Prolong action potential	Bretylium Amiodarone Sotalol	Bradycardia Hypotension Pulmonary fibrosis* Corneal deposits* Photophobia*
Class 4	Impede flow of calcium into cell during depolarization; depress activity of SA and AV nodes; increase AV node refractoriness	Calcium channel blockers Digoxin	Hypotension Bradycardia

*Associated with amiodarone.

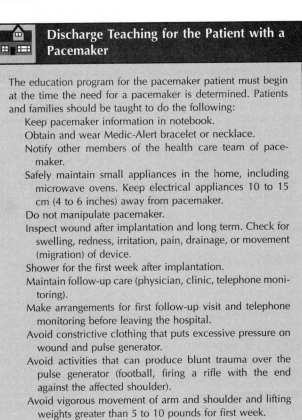

Discharge Teaching for the Patient with a Pacemaker

The education program for the pacemaker patient must begin at the time the need for a pacemaker is determined. Patients and families should be taught to do the following:

Keep pacemaker information in notebook.

Obtain and wear Medic-Alert bracelet or necklace.

Notify other members of the health care team of pacemaker.

Safely maintain small appliances in the home, including microwave ovens. Keep electrical appliances 10 to 15 cm (4 to 6 inches) away from pacemaker.

Do not manipulate pacemaker.

Inspect wound after implantation and long term. Check for swelling, redness, irritation, pain, drainage, or movement (migration) of device.

Shower for the first week after implantation.

Maintain follow-up care (physician, clinic, telephone monitoring).

Make arrangements for first follow-up visit and telephone monitoring before leaving the hospital.

Avoid constrictive clothing that puts excessive pressure on wound and pulse generator.

Avoid activities that can produce blunt trauma over the pulse generator (football, firing a rifle with the end against the affected shoulder).

Avoid vigorous movement of arm and shoulder and lifting weights greater than 5 to 10 pounds for first week.

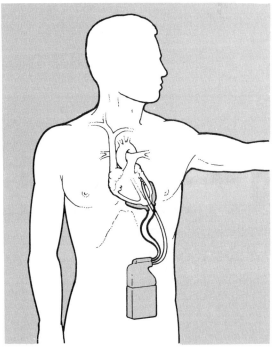

FIGURE 5-7 Internal cardioverter defibrillator (ICD). Pulse generator is implanted within a pocket created in abdominal wall. Rate-sensing electrodes and patch electrodes form a bridge between generator and heart. (From Beare PG, Myers JL: *Adult health nursing,* ed 2, St Louis, 1994, Mosby.)

third letter indicates the response to the sensed event (Table 5-4).

An *implantable cardioverter/defibrillator* (ICD) may be used for patients whose ventricular tachycardia (VT) or ventricular fibrillation (VF) is inducible during electrophysiologic studies despite antidysrhythmic therapy and for survivors of cardiac arrest whose dysrhythmia cannot be induced by electrophysiologic studies. This intervention involves the implantation of a device to detect VT or VF and to deliver a shock synchronously

for VT or asynchronously for VF if it cannot synchronize. The ICD consists of a generator, defibrillator patches, and a multilead system (Figure 5-7). It weighs about ½ pound. It is placed in one of four surgical approaches: thoracotomy, sternotomy, subxiphoid, or transvenous. The generator is usually implanted subcutaneously or submuscularly in the left parapumbilical region. The patches are attached to the inner or outer aspect of the pericardium, and the leads are placed in the epicardium. The lead system sends electrical signals from the heart to the generator, which continuously monitors the cardiac rhythm. The generator has a capacitor to store energy and deliver a shock. Most ICDs contain a power source capable of shocking the patient approximately 200 times, depending on joule setting and frequency of shocks.

The ICD is activated by sensing a rapid heart rate or a rapid heart rate and a rhythm with a wide QRS complex. The criteria used to determine defibrillator function include heart rate and probability density function (PDF). The PDF diagnoses VT or VF based on the

amount of time the QRS complex spends away from the isoelectric baseline. On ECG, wide complex VT and VF are away from the baseline a high percentage of the time as compared to sinus rhythm. When the generator receives signals that the rhythm is VT or VF it will deliver shocks to the heart or attempt to overdrive pace the rhythm back to normal sinus rhythm. The development of ICD technology is progressing quickly; thus the specific functions, placement techniques, and surgical approaches change often.

The ICD is turned on and off with a doughnut-shaped magnet. Audible tones are heard from the ICD when it is active (on) and affected by a magnetic field. The tones are synchronized with the patient's heart rate. If the tone is steady, the device has been deactivated (off). The energy discharged from the ICD can be felt to varying degrees by someone in contact with the patient. It is often described as a "buzz" and is not harmful. Because of the limited number of shocks available per device, the patient will almost always be continued on antidysrhythmic medication to limit the need for the ICD.

Complications associated with the ICD include lead fracture, migration, and dislodgement; electromechanical interference; faulty sensing and inappropriate firing; infections; fear; and anxiety. Negative changes in lifestyle associated with an ICD include less physical activity, less sexual activity, memory loss, depression, dependency, and thoughts of death.

TABLE 5-4 NBG Pacing Codes*

CODE	CHAMBERS PACED	CHAMBERS SENSED	PACEMAKER RESPONSE MODE
SINGLE CHAMBER			
AAI	A	A	Inhibited
VVI	V	V	Inhibited
VVT	V IHR/PHR	V	Triggered
A00/V00	A	None	Asynchronous
DUAL CHAMBER			
VVD	V	A and V	A triggered/V inhibited
DVI	A and A/V	V	Inhibited
DDD	A, V, and A/V	A and V	A triggered/V inhibited
D00	A/V	None	Asynchronous

From Flynn JM, Bruce NP: *Critical care skills*, St Louis, 1993, Mosby.
D, Double; *0*, none; *IHR*, intrinsic heart rate; *PHR*, pacing heart rate, *A*, atria; *V*, ventricle.

Discharge Teaching for the Patient with an ICD

Patient education is one of the most critical needs of ICD patients and families.

Patients and families should be taught to do the following:

Have realistic expectations of the ICD. The ICD does not prevent dysrhythmia; it treats dysrhythmia.

Establish a notebook containing product/device literature, patient manual.

Identify potential hazards in life-style at home, work, leisure activities, and hobbies (electrocautery, diathermy, arc welding, large transformers, running electric motors, transcutaneous electrical nerve stimulation [TENS] units, biomagnetic products, lithotripsy, and magnetic resonance imaging [MRI]).

Avoid large magnets and magnetic fields, because they may turn the device off.

Inspect incision and implant sites for signs of infection, drainage, swelling, redness, or skin warm to touch; report temperature above 38° C (100.5° F).

Protect implant site from irritation by clothing or belts, avoid scrubbing site vigorously, avoid tub baths for first week, and consider use of shower chair.

Remain on prescribed antidysrhythmics.

Carry an identification card that includes patient's physician, manufacturer's telephone number, ICD lead and model information, rate cutoff of the device, deactivation instructions, and shock sequence.

Obtain Medic-Alert bracelet or necklace.

Call physician if audible tones are heard from ICD (means the device has been exposed to a magnetic field).

Keep scheduled appointments. Anticipate seeing physician every 2 to 3 months for first year and monthly thereafter as the end of life of the ICD occurs.

Anticipate approximately 3 years of ICD battery life. Replacement usually requires only replacement of generator, not lead system.

Inform other members of health care team (dentist, surgeon, emergency personnel) of ICD.

Keep a diary of the shocks received. Notify physician of each shock to evaluate appropriate versus inappropriate shock.

In case of loss of consciousness, family should activate Emergency Medical System (EMS). In cardiac arrest family members start CPR; do not wait for ICD to fire.

Anyone touching person with ICD may sense skin tingling when device fires. It is not harmful.

Participate, if possible, in cardiac rehabilitation program.

Avoid contact sports, because they may dislodge leads.

Sit or lie down when feeling of onset of dysrhythmia occurs.

Do not drive for first 6 months after ICD placement. This allows evaluation of response to shocks and the frequency of dysrhythmia.

Participate in dysrhythmia support group.

Do not be concerned about travel restrictions. In airports only the hand-held security device contains a magnet. It must be kept 25 cm (10 inches) away from the ICD.

NURSING CARE PLAN

THE PERSON WITH DYSRHYTHMIA

■ NURSING DIAGNOSIS

Cardiac output, decreased (related to alterations in heart rate)

Expected Patient Outcome	Nursing Interventions
Patient will have a cardiac rhythm, natural or paced, that supports adequate cardiac output, as evidenced by stable blood pressure, adequate urine output, regular pulses, skin warm and dry, alert mental status.	1. Monitor patient's heart rate, rhythm, blood pressure. 2. Assess cardiac rhythm by telemetry monitoring. 3. Obtain 12-lead ECG. 4. Monitor effects and side effects of antidysrhythmic medications. 5. Monitor effect of activity on cardiac rhythm.

■ NURSING DIAGNOSIS

Activity intolerance (related to diminished cardiac output)

Expected Patient Outcome	Nursing Interventions
Patient will demonstrate cardiac tolerance of ADL.	1. Assess patient's ability to perform ADL. 2. Assess patient's activity tolerance. 3. Encourage gradual increase in activity level with shorter, more frequent activity periods. 4. Alternate activity with planned rest periods. 5. Maintain patient on telemetry monitoring, as indicated.

■ NURSING DIAGNOSIS

Tissue perfusion, altered (related to diminished cardiac output)

Expected Patient Outcome	Nursing Interventions
Patient will demonstrate improved peripheral circulation.	1. Assess adequacy of peripheral circulation (presence/absence of peripheral pulses, capillary refill, skin warm and dry). 2. Instruct patient to stop activity with occurrence of chest pain, dyspnea, palpitations, dizziness.

Continued.

NURSING MANAGEMENT

◆ ASSESSMENT

Subjective Data

Coronary artery disease
Cardiac arrest
Congestive heart failure
Congenital defects
Rheumatic fever
Cardiac medications, diuretics
Supplemental electrolyte therapy
Symptoms (palpitations, dyspnea, chest pain, weakness, dizziness, syncope)
Onset, frequency of symptoms
Precipitating factors
Exacerbating or alleviating factors
Alcohol, tobacco, other substance abuse

Objective Data

Heart rate and rhythm
Blood pressure
Peripheral circulation (pulses, capillary refill)
Apical and radial pulses, taken for 1 minute
Level of consciousness
ECG
Electrolyte levels (calcium, potassium, magnesium)
Hematocrit and hemoglobin
Arterial blood gases, SaO_2
Serum digoxin and quinidine levels
Nursing management of dysrhythmia is summarized in the "Nursing Care Plan."

NURSING CARE PLAN—CONT'D

THE PERSON WITH DYSRHYTHMIA

■ **NURSING DIAGNOSIS**
Anxiety and fear (related to life-threatening aspects of dysrhythmia)

Expected Patient Outcome	Nursing Interventions
Patient will use effective coping mechanisms to manage anxiety.	1. Assess patient's coping mechanisms. 2. Assess level of anxiety or fear. 3. Encourage patient and family to verbalize feelings, concerns about dysrhythmia. 4. Discuss with patient and family cause of dysrhythmia and treatment modalities. 5. Encourage patient and family involvement in treatment modalities (medication regimen, care of pacemaker, ICD). 6. Encourage enrollment in support group for persons with dysrhythmias and/or cardiac rehabilitation program. 7. Consider encouraging family to learn CPR. 8. Instruct patient and family in importance of maintaining regular medical follow-up.

Cardiopulmonary Resuscitation

Cardiopulmonary resuscitation (CPR) techniques are used to restore circulation and ventilation artificially during cardiopulmonary arrest. In cardiopulmonary arrest the person's heart, circulation, and respiration suddenly cease. CPR involves (1) artificial circulation by one- or two-person external cardiac massage and (2) artificial ventilation by either mouth-to-mouth, mouth-to-nose, or mouth-to-stoma technique. CPR should be initiated immediately to prevent brain damage and death. There is a window of about 4 to 6 minutes after loss of the victim's pulse and respirations before anoxic brain injury begins. CPR, however, supplies only about 20% of normal cardiac output, even when expertly administered. CPR may not be effective in reviving a victim because of the severity of heart disease. However, every attempt must be made initially to sustain the victim.

The highest priorities in CPR are the ABCs—airway, breathing, and circulation, which are the basics of resuscitation. The steps of cardiopulmonary resuscitation are outlined in Box 5-2.

Adjuncts to CPR such as endotracheal intubation and supplemental oxygen should be provided as soon as possible. If cardiac arrest occurs outside a health care facility the rescuer is to perform CPR until the victim recovers or until the rescuer is physically unable to continue.

Complications of CPR include rib fractures, fracture of the sternum, lacerations of the liver and spleen, pneumothorax, hemothorax, lung contusions, and fat emboli.

Medications commonly used during and after cardiac arrest are listed in Table 5-5. The objectives of drug therapy are to optimize cardiac function, establish spontaneous circulation, correct hypoxemia, correct acidosis, suppress sustained ventricular dysrhythmia, relieve pain, and treat congestive heart failure.

CORONARY ARTERY DISEASE
Etiology/Epidemiology

Coronary artery disease (CAD) is a general term used to describe conditions involving obstructed blood flow through the coronary arteries, the most common of which is atherosclerotic heart disease. Coronary artery disease is recognized as the leading cause of death in the Western world. Its dramatic incidence is attributed to the diet and life-style that accompany affluence and prosperity, to increased longevity, and to improved disease identification. Large-scale studies have identified factors that help define the risk of developing CAD. Common risk factors for CAD are identified in Box 5-3. Nutrition remains one of the key elements in epidemiologic studies. Despite extensive research, the exact cause of CAD remains unknown.

BOX 5-2	Steps in Cardiopulmonary Resuscitation

1. **Establish unresponsiveness.**
   a. Gently shake the person's shoulders and shout "Are you OK?"
   b. Call for help or initiate the emergency system.
   c. Position the person in a supine position on a hard, flat surface.
2. **Establish the airway.**
   a. Open the airway using the head tilt/chin lift maneuver.
   b. Look, listen, and feel for breathing for 3-5 seconds.
3. **Restore breathing.**
   a. Seal the nose, and cover the person's mouth to create a tight seal.
   b. Deliver two full breaths of 1-1½ seconds each. NOTE: **Use an airway and Ambu bag for delivering the rescue breaths as soon as possible.**
   c. Observe for rising of the chest with breaths.
   d. Allow for passive exhalation. NOTE: **If the first breath does not go in, reposition the head and try again. If it is still unsuccessful, initiate the procedure for clearing a foreign body airway obstruction (Figure 5-8).**
4. **Restore circulation.**
   a. Feel for the carotid pulse for 5-10 seconds.
   b. If no pulse is present, initiate chest compression.
      Position: Find the notch where the ribs meet the sternum. Move two fingerwidths up from the notch and place the heel of your hand along the long axis of the sternum. Place your second hand on top of the first and lace the fingers to keep them off the person's chest.
   c. Using the weight of your upper body, compress the person's sternum 1½-2 inches, delivering the pressure through the heels of your hands. Elbows are locked, and your shoulders are positioned directly over your hands.
   d. Compressions are delivered at a rate of 80-100/min. The pressure is released after each compression to allow the chest to return to its natural position. Compressions are delivered in a smooth downward thrust avoiding jerking, stabbing, or bouncing.
   e. Pause after 15 compressions and deliver two full ventilations as previously described. Continue this pattern for four full cycles and then attempt to palpate the carotid artery again. If it is still absent continue with both compressions and ventilations in the ratio described, pausing every few minutes to check for a pulse or breathing. NOTE: **If a second rescuer is present the ratio of compressions to ventilations is maintained at 5:1 with a full stop in compressions for each breath. Rescuers switch roles as needed to cope with fatigue.**

Modified from American Heart Association: *Healthcare providers' manual for basic life support,* New York, 1991, The Association.

Pathophysiology

The localized accumulation of lipids and fibrous tissue in the coronary vessels results in arterial narrowing and possible occlusion (Figure 5-9). Vascular changes gradually inhibit the ability of the arteries to dilate, thereby reducing blood flow to the myocardium. Symptoms are the result of an inadequate supply of oxygen to meet the

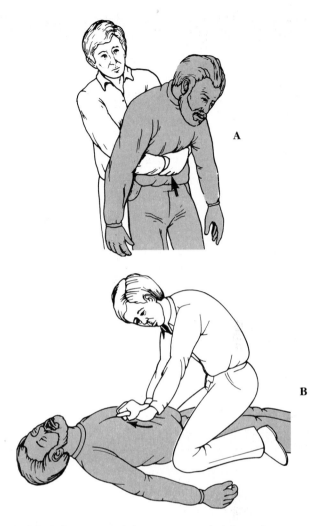

FIGURE 5-8 A, Heimlich maneuver administered to conscious (standing) victim of foreign body airway obstruction. **B,** Heimlich maneuver administered to unconscious (lying) victim of foreign body airway obstruction—astride position. (From Lewis SM, Collier IC: *Medical-surgical nursing,* St Louis, 1992, Mosby.)

demand for oxygen by the myocardium. They tend to appear only when the atherosclerotic process is well advanced, usually a greater than 75% occlusion. Myocardial ischemia results in angina, acute myocardial infarction, or sudden cardiac death.

Angina

Angina pectoris occurs when myocardial oxygen demand exceeds the supply. It is the primary manifestation of CAD and is often characterized by paroxysmal retrosternal or substernal chest pain, which may radiate into the jaw, neck, or shoulder or down the left arm. However, it may present as tightness, heaviness, aching, squeezing, indigestion, and/or pressure in the chest, throat, shoulder, or scapula. Symptoms are frequently associated with exertion, exercise, extreme cold, emotion, heavy meals, or anything that increases the work of the heart or myocardial oxygen consumption. The

TABLE 5-5 Drug Therapy in Cardiac Arrest

DRUG	INDICATIONS	ACTION
Lidocaine	PVCs, VT, VF	Depresses automaticity and conduction of ectopic beats
		Suppresses ventricular dysrhythmias
Epinephrine	Cardiac arrest, VT, VF	Increases myocardial and CNS blood flow
	Asystole	Increases heart rate
	Electromechanical dissociation	Strengthens myocardial contractility
Atropine	Sinus bradycardia	Increases heart rate
	Asystole	Enhances rate of discharge of SA node
	AV nodal block	
Dopamine	Hypotension	Increases cardiac output, renal blood flow, and blood pressure
	Shock	May cause tachydysrhythmias
Bretylium	VT and VF unresponsive to lidocaine	Raises VF threshold
		Increases action potential duration and effective refractory periods
Calcium chloride and	Hyperkalemia	Increases force of myocardial contractility
calcium gluconate	Hypocalcemia	
	Calcium channel blocker toxicity	
Dobutamine	Cardiogenic shock	Improved myocardial contractility
Isoproterenol	Bradycardia unresponsive to atropine	Increases heart rate
		Increases cardiac output
		Enhances automaticity
		Increases blood pressure
		Promotes bronchodilation
Procainamide	Ventricular ectopy when lidocaine ineffective or contraindicated	Depresses automaticity and conduction
		Prolongs refraction in atria and ventricles

BOX 5-3 Risk Factors Associated with Coronary Artery Disease

NONMODIFIABLE RISK FACTORS
1. *Age.* Mortality from CAD rapidly increases with age.
2. *Sex.* Incidence of CAD in women is very low until after menopause.
3. *Race.* Nonwhite men and women under 65 years of age have higher mortality.
4. *Family history.* A positive family history of CAD in parents or siblings under 50 years of age increases the risk.

MODIFIABLE RISK FACTORS
*1. *Hyperlipoproteinemia.* Elevated cholesterol, triglyceride, and phospholipid levels are associated with development of CAD.
*2. *Dietary patterns.* A diet chronically high in saturated fats, salt, refined sugar, and cholesterol is linked with CAD.
*3. *Hypertension.* In the presence of hyperlipidemia an elevated systolic or diastolic blood pressure often seems to accelerate atherosclerosis.
*4. *Obesity.* Overweight individuals are more prone to develop associated risk factors. The direct link to CAD is not clear.
*5. *Cigarette smoking.* Relationship is unclear but related to effects of nicotine and carbon monoxide. Risk of death is two to six times greater in heavy smokers.
6. *Diabetes.* Individuals with glucose intolerance have a greater prevalence and severity of coronary atherosclerosis.
7. *Personality and life-style.* A sedentary life-style, chronic stress, and low socioeconomic status are often associated with CAD.

*Major risk factors.

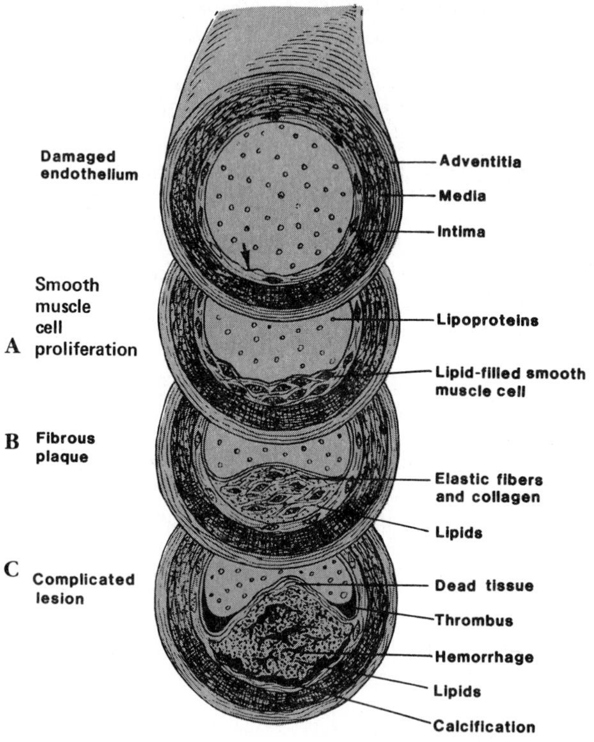

FIGURE 5-9 Stages of development in progression of atherosclerosis include, **A,** smooth muscle cell proliferation, which creates, **B,** a raised fibrous plaque and, **C,** a complicated lesion. (After Herb Smith. From Lewis SM, Collier IC: *Medical-surgical nursing,* St Louis, 1992, Mosby.)

TABLE 5-6   Drugs Used in the Management of Angina

DRUGS	ACTIONS	SIDE EFFECTS
NITRITES/NITRATES		
Nitroglycerin Isosorbide (Isordil) Nitropaste	Decrease myocardial oxygen demand by dilating peripheral vessels, decreasing peripheral resistance and systolic blood pressure Increase myocardial oxygen supply by dilating coronary arteries and intercoronary collateral vessels	Postural hypotension Burning sensation on tongue Throbbing in head, flushing Headache Tachycardia
BETA-ADRENERGIC BLOCKERS		
Propranolol (Inderal) Nadolol (Corgard) Metoprolol (Lopressor) Atenolol (Tenormin) Esmolol (Brevibloc)	Decrease myocardial oxygen demand by reducing heart rate, blood pressure, and myocardial contractility	Bradycardia (slowed heart beat) Hypotension Gastrointestinal (GI) complaints Fatigue, weakness Nightmares Depression
CALCIUM CHANNEL BLOCKERS		
Nifedipine (Procardia) Diltiazem (Cardizem) Verapamil (Calan, Isoptin)	Act at the cellular level to block movement of calcium ions, thus reducing cardiac activity and work load of heart Decrease heart rate and act as potent vasodilators Reduce coronary vasospasm	Bradycardia Hypotension Constipation Headache
ASPIRIN	Suppresses platelet aggregation that may have a role in progression of CAD by blocking a specific step in prostaglandin pathway	GI upset Allergic reaction

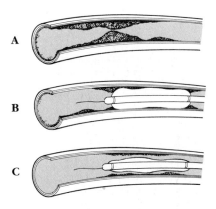

FIGURE 5-10 Percutaneous transluminal coronary angioplasty (PTCA). **A,** Plaque before PTCA. **B,** Inflation of angioplasty balloon. **C,** Plaque after PTCA. (From Beare PG, Myers JL: *Adult health nursing,* ed 2, St Louis, 1994, Mosby.)

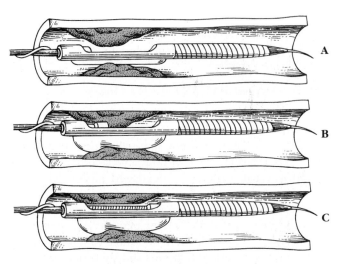

FIGURE 5-11 Directional coronary atherectomy. Variations on this procedure include use of laser tips studded with diamond chips and water blasts to pulverize or destroy plaque tissues. **A,** Bullet-shaped probe is inserted into narrowed vessel lumen. **B,** Balloon is inflated to force open side of probe against opposite vessel wall, squeezing plaque into chamber of probe. **C,** A tiny rotating cup shaves plaque that projects into chamber. Probe is rotated and repositioned as needed to shave additional plaque.

ischemia is temporary and reversible and is usually relieved by rest or vasodilation.

Diagnostic studies will include electrocardiogram, radioisotope imaging, and coronary angiography.

Medical Management

Medical management is aimed at reducing myocardial oxygen demand and increasing myocardial oxygen supply and includes the following:

Reduction or elimination of modifiable risk factors

Identification, elimination, or spacing of precipitating factors

Drug therapy with aspirin, vasodilators, beta-adrenergic blockers, and calcium channel blocking agents (Table 5-6)

Invasive and surgical management options include coronary artery bypass surgery (CABG), percutaneous coronary angioplasty, coronary atherectomy, coronary artery stents, and coronary laser angioplasty (Figures 5-10 and 5-11). These procedures do not alter the atherosclerotic process, but they do reduce angina and improve activity tolerance.

NURSING MANAGEMENT

◆ ASSESSMENT
Subjective Data

History of the disease and its treatment
Symptom pattern, severity, duration
Precipitating and relieving factors (rest, nitroglycerin)
Medications in use, understanding of drugs
Diet and exercise patterns, occupation
Knowledge of disorder, risk factor management

Objective Data

Baseline vital signs
Weight
Changes in cardiac rhythm
Associated symptoms: diaphoresis, pallor, apprehension

◆ NURSING DIAGNOSES

Nursing diagnoses for the person with angina may include, but are not limited to, the following:
Chest pain (related to temporary myocardial ischemia)
Activity intolerance (related to occurrence of chest pain with exercise or exertion)
Anxiety (related to threat of pain and change in health status)

◆ EXPECTED PATIENT OUTCOMES

Patient will have fewer attacks of pain and will have pain controlled by vasodilator drugs.
Patient will appropriately space activities to continue preferred life-style without attacks of pain.
Patient will experience decreased anxiety through better control and management of the disease.
Patient will assume informed control of life-style, will appropriately modify diet patterns and exercise/activity routines, and will be able to discuss drugs used to control symptoms and their side effects.

◆ NURSING INTERVENTIONS
Managing Chest Pain/Anginal Symptoms

Teach patient correct use of prescribed medication (Table 5-6, Discharge Teaching box, and Guidelines box).
Discuss use of nitroglycerin before planned exertion.
Emphasize need for ongoing medical care.
Instruct patient to contact physician if anginal symptom pattern changes or worsens.
Explore modifications of patient's life-style to prevent pain attacks:
Avoid physical and emotional overexertion.
Avoid overeating.
Avoid prolonged exposure to climate extremes, dress appropriately, and avoid extreme cold or hot, humid conditions.

Avoid situations that combine known precipitating factors.
Encourage activity to tolerance but avoid fatigue. Patient should stop activity immediately if pain occurs.
Patient should space activities or exercise for shorter periods and should participate in a regularly scheduled exercise regimen if available.

Decreasing Anxiety

Assess patient's and family's level of anxiety and coping mechanisms.
Assist patient and family to develop plans for cardiac risk factor reduction to enhance sense of own health management.
Plan diet for weight reduction.
Reduce salt intake.

Guidelines for Using Antianginal Drugs

SUBLINGUAL NITROGLYCERIN
Store tablets in tightly closed dark bottle; keep dry.
Sublingual administration causes burning sensation on the tongue.
Throbbing in head and flushing sensation may be felt.
Make position changes slowly after taking nitroglycerin.
Use tablets prophylactically to avoid pain if known to occur with certain activities.
Take tablet at onset of pain, and repeat every 5 minutes if pain is unrelieved. Call physician if pain is unrelieved after a total of three to four tablets.
Always carry a supply of tablets.
Replace medication every 3 to 6 months.

NITROGLYCERIN PATCHES
Apply to any nonhairy area of skin.

NITROGLYCERIN SPRAYS
Sprays are more expensive than sublingual nitroglycerin.
No evidence exists that they are more effective.

LONG-ACTING NITRATES
A 12-hour nitrate-free period is recommended to reduce the development of tolerance.

BETA BLOCKERS
Monitor pulse rate. Do not take drug if pulse rate is below 50.
Take drug with meals.
Inform physician of any history of allergy, asthma, or chronic obstructive pulmonary disease (COPD). Beta blockers may induce bronchospasm.

CALCIUM CHANNEL BLOCKERS
Take drug 1 hour before or 1 to 2 hours after meals.
Prevent constipation with use of stool softener and high-fiber foods.

ASPIRIN
Use caution when taking over-the-counter medications—avoid those that also contain aspirin.

Discharge Teaching for the Patient Following Percutaneous Transluminal Coronary Angioplasty or Atherectomy

Patient and family need to know the following:
Resumption of normal activities in 1-2 weeks.
No lifting greater than 5-10 pounds for 1-2 weeks.
Observation of insertion site for redness, swelling, soreness, drainage every day until healed; if any of these signs occur, call physician.
Return to work in 1-2 weeks, depending on occupation. Consult physician first.
If bleeding from insertion site occurs, apply firm, direct pressure with clean cloth and call physician.
Plans for cardiac risk factor reduction.
Medication regimen, which will include one aspirin every day and usually a calcium channel blocker.

Modify diet to decrease intake of cholesterol and saturated fats.
Eliminate cigarette smoking.
Maintain adequate control of hypertension if present.
Encourage patient to minimize or avoid activities that precipitate angina.
Discuss anxiety-reducing benefits of regular exercise with patient and family.
Instruct patient in relaxation and stress management techniques.

Increasing Activity Tolerance

Assess activity tolerance.
Recommend enrollment in cardiac rehabilitation program or development of a regular exercise program.
Instruct patient to stop activity with onset of anginal symptoms and to use nitroglycerin as directed.

◆ EVALUATION

Successful achievement of expected outcomes for the patient with angina is indicated by the following:
Ability to space daily activities to maintain life-style without occurrence of pain
Report of less anxiety as a result of improved disease control
Management of antianginal drugs to keep free of pain
Ability to describe effects of drugs, appropriate diet and activity, and signs and symptoms that indicate need to contact physician
Ability to describe plan for cardiac risk factor reduction (smoking cessation; exercise program; stress management; modified salt, fat, and cholesterol diet; control of hypertension and diabetes)

MYOCARDIAL INFARCTION
Etiology/Epidemiology

Myocardial infarction (MI) is caused by a sudden blockage, most often secondary to thrombosis, of one of the branches of a coronary artery that interferes with the blood supply to a portion of the myocardium, producing ischemic death

of tissue over a period of hours. The location and size of the infarct determine the consequences in terms of contractility and myocardial function. The mortality from MI remains high (30% to 40%), with most deaths occurring before the patient reaches the hospital.

Pathophysiology

Ischemic injury evolves over a period of hours. Ischemia depresses cardiac function and triggers autonomic nervous system responses that worsen the imbalance between oxygen supply and demand. When oxygen supply is severely decreased myocardial cellular damage begins subendocardially and slowly extends to the epicardium. Necrosis of the affected area occurs within approximately 6 hours. Once necrosis has occurred the healing process takes 2 to 3 months. Prolonged ischemia and necrosis produce irreversible cellular damage to the cardiac muscle, and contractile function in the area is permanently lost. MI may be complicated by the development of dysrhythmias, congestive failure, pericarditis, or cardiogenic shock (see Box 5-6).

The two general types of MI are transmural (Q wave infarction), which involves the full thickness of the myocardium, and subendocardial (non-Q wave or incomplete infarction), which involves only a partial thickness of the ventricular wall.

Medical Management

The diagnosis is based on the following symptoms and diagnostic study results:
Severe crushing chest pain unrelieved by rest or nitroglycerin, accompanied by diaphoresis, nausea, anxiety, feeling of impending doom.
ECG changes—may include Q waves, elevated ST segments, T wave abnormalities
Serum enzymes—creatine kinase (CK-MB) and lactic dehydrogenase (LDH) released into bloodstream from death of tissue (Figure 5-12)

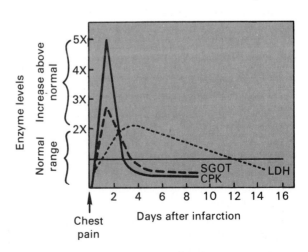

FIGURE 5-12 Heart muscle enzyme levels in blood after MI. (From Lewis SM, Collier IC: *Medical-surgical nursing,* St Louis, 1993, Mosby.)

BOX 5-4	Use of Thrombolytics in Treatment of MI

PURPOSE

Used to restore blood flow and preserve injured myocardial tissue to limit area of infarction

ACTION

Thrombolytics accelerate the natural fibrinolytic process by activating plasminogen, thereby lysing the clot

AGENTS USED

Streptokinase—activates all circulating plasminogen, creating a systemic lysis state

Tissue plasminogen activator (t-PA)—activates only fibrin-bound plasminogen and is more clot specific, causes less systemic risk and is associated with greater effectiveness in reperfusion

CONCERNS

Must be given within 4-6 hours of onset of MI

Contraindicated in presence of bleeding disorders, severe hypertension, or history of CVA

Used cautiously if at all in patients of advanced age with recent history of trauma, surgery, GI bleed

All patients at risk for bleeding and/or reocclusion

Heparin used in conjunction with thrombolytic therapy to prevent reocclusion secondary to new thrombus formation

BOX 5-5	Cardiac Rehabilitation

Cardiac rehabilitation is a comprehensive program to help the cardiac patient achieve and maintain optimal health and well-being. The rehabilitation process begins in the hospital, with phase 1, and continues indefinitely, with phases 2 and 3. Risk factor reduction, cardiovascular fitness, and psychologic well-being are goals. The components of rehabilitation are activity progression, medical therapy, education, and counseling. A team approach is optimal, involving physicians, nurses, exercise physiologists/physical therapists, nutritionists, counselors, and vocational counselors.

BOX 5-6	Cardiogenic Shock

DEFINITION

Inadequate tissue perfusion of cardiac origin, most commonly caused by MI with severe left ventricular failure. Mortality is 80%-90%.

PATHOLOGIC SEQUENCE

1. Cardiac function and output are insufficient to perfuse body cells.
2. Vital organs do not receive nutrients and/or discharge cellular waste, producing metabolic acidosis.
3. Progressive damage occurs in vital organs from prolonged ischemia.
4. Decreased coronary artery perfusion causes progressive ischemia and infarction.

SIGNS AND SYMPTOMS

Hyperventilation—shallow respirations

Falling blood pressure—tachycardia, weak pulse

Decreasing urine output, oliguria (less than 20 ml/hr)

Cool clammy skin, pallor

Restlessness, decreasing level of consciousness, mental confusion, lethargy

Metabolic acidosis

MEDICAL AND NURSING CARE

Monitor arterial lines and pulmonary artery catheters

Drug therapy:
    Vasopressors and cardiotonics
    Dopamine and norepinephrine

Intraaortic balloon pump

Careful fluid replacement

Supplemental oxygen

Support and reassurance to patient and family

Medical management is directed toward limiting infarct size, improving oxygenation, relieving pain, and preventing complications. Specifics include the following:

Reperfusion efforts with thrombolytic agents (Box 5-4)

Oxygen, nitrates, beta-adrenergic blockers, and rest to reestablish a balance in myocardial supply and demand

Intravenous morphine sulfate for chest pain

Aspirin (chewed, not enteric coated) to decrease platelet adhesion and thrombosis

Cardiac monitoring for early recognition of dysrhythmia

Heparin therapy

Percutaneous transluminal coronary angioplasty

Coronary artery bypass surgery (Box 5-8)

Staged cardiac rehabilitation begins as soon as the patient is stable (Box 5-5).

NURSING MANAGEMENT

◆ ASSESSMENT (ACUTE PHASE)

Subjective Data

Character of pain and accompanying symptoms (there may be none in elderly persons)

History of onset, treatment attempted, prior CAD history

Dyspnea

Objective Data

Vital signs (signs of shock), increased pulse, decreased blood pressure

Diaphoresis (perspiration), skin temperature

Skin color, cyanosis

Dysrhythmias

Intense anxiety and apprehension

Presence of nausea/vomiting

Nursing management of the person with an MI is summarized in the nursing care plans.

NURSING CARE PLAN

PERSON WITH MYOCARDIAL INFARCTION—ACUTE PHASE

■ NURSING DIAGNOSIS
Chest pain (related to myocardial ischemia)

Expected Patient Outcome	Nursing Interventions
Patient's pain will be relieved.	1. Assess degree of pain and effectiveness of interventions.
	2. Give prescribed medication as needed (thrombolytics, nitrates, morphine, beta-adrenergic blockers, aspirin, heparin).
	3. Stay with patient and offer reassurance.
	4. Administer prescribed oxygen by nasal cannula.
	5. Monitor vital signs and cardiac rhythm.
	6. Obtain serial cardiac isoenzymes and 12-lead ECGs.
	7. Maintain quiet, calm environment.

■ NURSING DIAGNOSIS
Cardiac output decreased (related to loss of myocardial contractility, dysrhythmia)

Expected Patient Outcomes	Nursing Interventions
Patient's vital signs will be stable. Patient will not exhibit dysrhythmia.	1. Monitor vital signs for signs of shock.
	2. Use measures to decrease anxiety.
	3. Provide absolute rest.
	4. Assist with all ADL.
	5. Teach patient to avoid Valsalva maneuvers.
	6. Monitor cardiac rhythm.
	7. Maintain intravenous access.
	8. Monitor I & O.
	9. Place patient in semi-Fowler's position.

■ NURSING DIAGNOSIS
Anxiety (related to intense pain and fear of death)

Expected Patient Outcome	Nursing Interventions
Patient will not experience disabling anxiety.	1. Assess anxiety level and coping mechanisms.
	2. Give family members opportunities to discuss their concerns, and keep them informed of patient's progress.
	3. Provide a calm, unhurried environment.
	4. Be sure patient understands that the function of the continuous ECG is to monitor, not to keep the heart beating.
	5. Give prescribed tranquilizers or sedatives as needed.
	6. Promote rest.

NURSING CARE PLAN

MYOCARDIAL INFARCTION—REHABILITATIVE PHASE

■ NURSING DIAGNOSIS
Activity intolerance (related to myocardial ischemia, fatigue)

Expected Patient Outcome	Nursing Interventions
Patient will tolerate progression of activities.	1. Maintain bed rest with bathroom privileges for 4-24 hours. 2. Assess for signs and symptoms of activity intolerance (weakness, dyspnea, chest pain, diaphoresis, dysrhythmia, orthostatic hypotension). 3. Progress activity gradually. 4. Alternate activity and rest periods. 5. Encourage patient to recognize activity limitations.

■ NURSING DIAGNOSIS
Activity intolerance (related to decreased myocardial function)

Expected Patient Outcome	Nursing Interventions

Patient will have sufficient energy to gradually resume self-care activities.	1. Space activities with rest.
	2. Encourage a gradual increase in self-care activities 12-24 hours after symptoms are controlled and vital signs are stable.
	3. Begin rehabilitation teaching early, so patient has sense of expected recovery.
	4. Encourage and supervise an increased activity schedule (Box 5-7):
	  a. Assess orthostatic heart rate and blood pressure before beginning activity.
	  b. Encourage out of bed to chair, with progression to ambulation in room and then hall.
	  c. Have patient increase ambulation time (1 minute to 5 minutes) gradually.
	  d. Encourage patient to ambulate two to six times per day.
	  e. Instruct patient to stop activity with onset of symptoms of activity intolerance.
	5. Reinforce plans for home activity program and/or enrollment in cardiac rehabilitation phase 2 program.

CONGESTIVE HEART FAILURE
Etiology/Epidemiology

Congestive heart failure (CHF) represents a state in which the heart is no longer able to pump an adequate supply of blood to meet the demands of the body (Box 5-9). The failure may be acute or chronic. The chronic form develops gradually and generally produces milder symptoms. Congestive heart failure is caused by two types of conditions:

1. Conditions resulting in direct heart damage, such as MI
2. Conditions that produce ventricular overload
   a. Preload—Amount of blood in ventricle at end of diastole is increased as in fluid overload or valvular and septal defects.
   b. Afterload—Force that the ventricle must exert to eject blood into the circulatory system is increased as with valvular stenosis or pulmonary or systemic hypertension.

NURSING CARE PLAN

MYOCARDIAL INFARCTION—REHABILITATIVE PHASE

■ NURSING DIAGNOSIS
Sexual dysfunction, high risk (related to fears of recurrent MI)

Expected Patient Outcome	Nursing Interventions
Patient will gradually resume preillness pattern of sexuality.	1. Give patient opportunities to explore concerns about own sexuality and resumption of sexual activity (usually after 6 weeks). 2. Correct misunderstandings about effect of coitus after infarction. 3. Encourage patient and partner to identify coital positions that are less stressful to patient. 4. Suggest that coitus be delayed until 3 hours after a heavy meal or excessive alcohol intake. 5. Teach patient symptoms occurring during coitus that need to be reported to physician.

■ NURSING DIAGNOSIS
Ineffective individual and family coping, high risk (related to life-style changes required by the MI)

Expected Patient Outcome	Nursing Interventions
Patient and family will receive ongoing support and education and be encouraged to discuss their feelings and fears.	1. Provide patient and family with teaching and reteaching as needed. 2. Clarify misconceptions and misunderstandings. 3. Discuss return to employment and leisure patterns. 4. Refer for counseling follow-up if appropriate. 5. Patient and family will be able to describe plans for cardiac risk factor reduction.

Congestive heart failure is a major community health problem in the United States, affecting 3 million persons. Factors contributing to the increasing incidence include the increased number of elderly persons in the population and the decreased mortality from CAD. Risk factors for CHF include hypertension, diabetes, cigarette smoking, obesity, poor total cholesterol/HDL cholesterol ratio, and proteinuria. CHF is associated with a very high mortality.

Pathophysiology

The overt symptoms of CHF appear as the heart's compensatory mechanisms are first set in motion and then exhausted. Symptoms include the following:

Tachycardia—Heart rate increases to increase cardiac output, but diastole is shortened and inadequate filling time is present.

Ventricular dilation—Myocardial fibers stretch to provide more forceful contractions.

Myocardial hypertrophy—Increased muscle mass causes more efficient contraction. Muscle mass can outgrow the blood supply and cause hypoxia.

As the mechanisms of cardiac compensation become inadequate, additional homeostatic mechanisms are triggered:

Sympathetic stimulation with release of norepinephrine causes general vasoconstriction.

Glomerular filtration is reduced, and aldosterone secretion causes retention of sodium and water.

Hepatic congestion decreases clearance of aldosterone and antidiuretic hormone (ADH), worsening the fluid overload.

CHF may be classified in a variety of ways. The mechanisms of left and right ventricular failure are described in Box 5-9. Excess fluid retention by the body results in venous stasis, an increase in venous pressure, and congestion in either the pulmonary system or systemic venous circulation.

CRITICAL PATHWAY   **Coronary Artery Bypass Graft Without Complications**

DRG #: 107; expected LOS: 9

	Day of Admission Day 1	To ICU After Surgery Day 2	Day 3	Transfer Out of ICU Day 4
Diagnostic Tests	CBC, UA, SMA/18*, PT/PTT, T & X, ABGs, chest x-ray, ECG	CBC, SMA/6†, Mg++, PT/PTT, ABGs, ECG, chest x-ray	CBC, SMA/6,† PT/PTT, ABGs, ECG, chest x-ray after removal of PCT	CBC, SMA/6†, PT/PTT
Medications	Home medications, no aspirin	IVs (filling pressure maintained), IV antibiotic, KCl replacement, IV analgesic, nitroglycerin	IVs, IV analgesic, IV antibiotic, aspirin 5 gr daily, stool softener	IV to saline lock, IV or PO analgesic, IV antibiotic, aspirin 5 gr daily, iron tab daily, stool softener
Treatments	Weight and height, VS q 8 hr, I & O q 8 hr, elastic leg stockings, pHisoHex shower	Monitor I & O q 2 hr (including nasogastric, Foley, chest tube), VS q 1 hr; intubated on ventilator with O₂; thigh-high elastic leg stockings on unaffected leg; weight	Monitor I & O q 4 hr (nasogastric, Foley, PCT removed), VS q 4 hr; nasal O₂; after extubation inspiratory spirometer; thigh-high elastic leg stockings on unaffected leg; weight	Telemetry, I & O q 8 hr, VS q 6 hr; dressings changed chest and leg; inspiratory spirometer, elastic leg stockings, weight
Diet	As at home	NPO	Clear liquids to full liquids, fluid restriction	Diet as tolerated, low sodium, fat, and cholesterol; fluid restriction
Activity	Up as tolerated	Bed rest, head of bed elevated 30 degrees; T q 1 hr	Bed rest, dangle and up in chair with assistance × 2; T, C, & DB q 2 hr	Bed rest, up in chair × 3, brief walk in hall with assistance; T, C, & DB q 2 hr
Consultations	Respiratory therapist, perioperative nurse, primary nurse, anesthesiologist			Cardiac rehabilitation (dietary, exercise therapist, counselor on stress reduction)

NOTE: Acknowledge that patients recover at varying rates; therefore specified daily actions should be based solely on patient need.
ABGs, Arterial blood gases; *CBC,* complete blood cell count; *T, C, & DB,* turn, cough, and deep breathe; *PCT,* pleural chest tube; *PT,* prothrombin time; *PTT,* partial thromboplastin time; *SMA,* sequential multiple analysis; *T & X,* type and crossmatch; *UA,* urinalysis; *VS,* vital signs.

BOX 5-7   **Common Activities Categorized by Energy Expenditure**

VERY LIGHT ACTIVITY

Eating, dressing, bathing
Driving, walking ≤2 mph
Cooking
Bowling
Golfing (cart use)

LIGHT ACTIVITY

Use of commode or bedpan
Housework
Stair climbing (one flight)
Sexual activity
Fitness walking ≤4 mph
Gardening
Dancing
Cycling <8 mph
Lawn mowing (power-mower)

MODERATE ACTIVITY

Jogging
Snow shoveling
Tennis
Skiing
Swimming
Skating
Basketball

HEAVY ACTIVITY

Handball
Jump rope
Cross country skiing
Lifting >75 lb
Carrying loads upstairs
Wet snow shoveling

Modified from Beare PG, Myers JL: *Principles and practice of adult health nursing,* ed 2, St Louis, 1994, Mosby.

BOX 5-8   **Coronary Artery Bypass Graft (CABG) Surgery**

The most common type of cardiac surgery over the past 2 decades has been coronary artery bypass graft (CABG). In this procedure a blood vessel (internal mammary artery or saphenous vein) is anastomosed to a coronary artery distal to the point of occlusion and to the ascending aorta, thus bypassing the area of vessel obstruction and reestablishing effective coronary artery perfusion (Figure 5-13).

The purpose of CABG is to relieve angina, prevent MI, and preserve myocardial function. Determining the best candidate for CABG is somewhat controversial. There is consensus that life expectancy is increased when CABG is performed on patients with left main coronary artery disease or severe three-vessel disease. Of concern, however, are research studies that indicate lower return to work rates and, in general, less productivity among post-CABG patients than post-MI patients.

The mortality for CABG is 1% to 2%, with 90% of patients demonstrating improved cardiac function and 60% of patients demonstrating elimination of anginal symptoms. The benefits of CABG surgery last for approximately 5 to 10 years, longer with use of the internal mammary artery. It is important that patients and families be informed about the continued need for cardiac risk factor reduction efforts. CABG treats the manifestations of coronary artery disease; it is not a curative intervention (see Critical Pathway).

CRITICAL PATHWAY   Coronary Artery Bypass Graft Without Complications

DRG #: 107; expected LOS: 9

Day 5	Day 6	Day 7	Day 8	Day of Discharge Day 9
	CBC, SMA/6†	ECG, chest x-ray after removal of pacing wire		
IV saline lock, PO analgesic, IV antibiotic, aspirin 5 gr daily, iron tab daily, stool softener	IV saline lock, PO analgesic; discontinue antibiotic; aspirin 5 gr daily, iron tab daily, stool softener	Discontinue saline lock; PO analgesic; aspirin 5 gr daily, iron tab daily, stool softener	PO analgesic, aspirin 5 gr daily, iron tab daily, stool softener	PO analgesic, aspirin 5 gr daily, iron tab daily, stool softener
Telemetry, I & O q 8 hr, VS q 6 hr; discontinue all dressings; inspiratory spirometer; elastic leg stockings, weight	Telemetry, I & O q 8 hr, VS q 6 hr, elastic leg stockings, weight	Discontinue pacing wire (VS q 30 min after removal × 4); discontinue telemetry; I & O q 8 hr, VS q 6 hrs, elastic leg stockings	Discontinue I & O; VS q 8 hr, elastic leg stockings, weight	Staples removed, VS q 8 hr, elastic leg stockings
Regular diet, low sodium, fat, and cholesterol; fluid restriction	Regular diet, low sodium, fat, and cholesterol; fluid restriction	Regular diet, low sodium, fat, and cholesterol	Regular diet, low sodium, fat, and cholesterol	Regular diet, low sodium, fat, and cholesterol
Up walking in room × 4, walk in hallway with assistance × 1; T, C, & DB q 2 hr	Up walking in room × 4, walk in hallway with assistance × 2; T, C, & DB q 2 hr	Up walking in room × 4, walk in hallway with assistance × 3; C & DB q 2 hr	Up walking in room × 4, walk in hallway × 4; C & DB q 2 hr	Up walking ad lib

*Serum calcium, phosphorus, triglycerides, uric acid, creatinine, BUN, total bilirubin, alkaline phosphate, aspartate aminotransferase (AST) (formerly serum glutamic-oxaloacetic transaminase [SGOT]), alanine aminotransferase (ALT) (formerly serum glutamate pyruvate transaminase [SGPT]), lactic dehydrogenase (LDH), total protein, albumin, sodium, potassium, chloride, total CO_2, glucose.
†Serum sodium, potassium, chloride, total CO_2, glucose, BUN.

Medical Management

Primary goals of treatment are aimed at decreasing oxygen requirements, optimizing cardiac output, removing excess fluid, and restoring the balance between the supply of and demand for blood by body tissue. Major approaches include the following:

Providing supplemental oxygen, usually by nasal cannula

Reducing body's need for oxygen

Restricting sodium and fluid intake

Administering medications

Inotropes to increase contractility (digoxin, dopamine, dobutamine, milrinone, amrinone)

Vasodilators to increase cardiac output (nitrates, hydralazine, calcium channel blockers)

ACE -inhibitors to decrease afterload, increase cardiac output (captopril, enalapril)

Beta-adrenergic blocking agents to decrease sympathetic stimulation, decrease dysrhythmias (metoprolol, atenolol)

Using an intraaortic balloon pump

Using a ventricular assist device

Doing a cardiac transplantation

 Hemodynamic Monitoring

Hemodynamic monitoring is the measurement of hemodynamic status. Hemodynamic status is an index of the pressure and the flow within the pulmonary and systemic circulations. Patients with heart failure, fluid overload, shock, pulmonary hypertension, and other such problems have altered hemodynamic status. Invasive hemodynamic monitoring requires cardiac catheterization and arterial pressure monitoring. The Swan-Ganz catheter made bedside catheterization feasible and revolutionized hemodynamic evaluation. The cardiac indices measured include central venous pressure (CVP), pulmonary artery pressure (PAP), pulmonary artery wedge pressure (PAWP), and cardiac output (CO) (Figure 5-14). Bedside monitoring may also include systemic intraarterial pressure measurement. The critical care nurse must be able to operate hemodynamic monitoring equipment and assess and interpret trends in values.

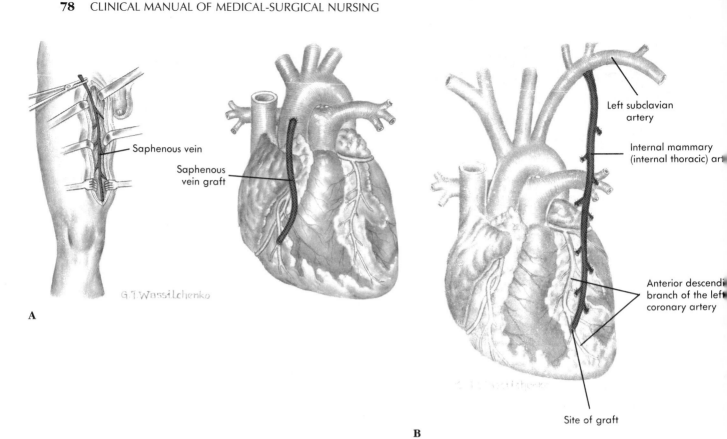

FIGURE 5-13 **A,** Saphenous vein graft. **B,** Internal mammary artery graft. (From Thelan LA et al: *Critical care nursing,* ed 2, St Louis, 1994, Mosby.)

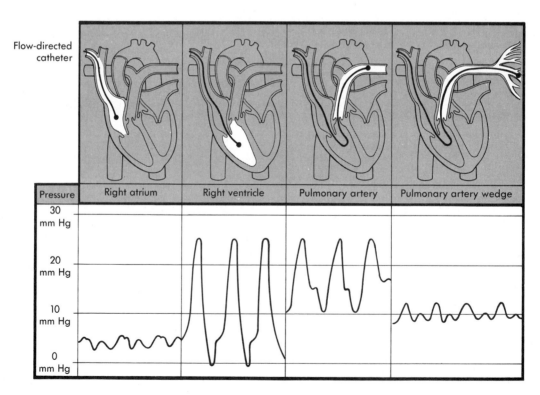

FIGURE 5-14 Pulmonary artery catheter insertion with corresponding waveforms. (From Thelan LA et al: *Textbook of critical care nursing: diagnosis and management,* ed 2, St Louis, 1994, Mosby.)

Congestive Heart Failure*

LEFT-SIDED FAILURE

Left ventricle cannot pump all the blood coming from the lungs. The symptoms are primarily the result of lung congestion.

  Blood backs up into pulmonary bed.
  Increased hydrostatic pressure causes fluid to accumulate in the pulmonary tissues.
  Blood flow is decreased to brain, kidneys, and systemic cells.

Symptoms

  Severe dyspnea, orthopnea, rales, cough productive of frothy, blood-tinged sputum
  Severe anxiety, restlessness, confusion
  Severe weakness, fatigue
  Oliguria

RIGHT-SIDED FAILURE

Right ventricle cannot pump all the blood coming from the right atria; right atria cannot accept all the blood coming from the systemic circulation. Rarely seen alone—usually occurs with left-sided failure.

  Blood backs up into systemic circulation.
  Increased hydrostatic pressure causes peripheral and dependent pitting edema. Fluid may weep from edematous tissues.
  Venous congestion in kidneys, liver, and GI tract.

Symptoms

  Peripheral and dependent edema—pitting type
  Distended neck veins
  Anorexia, nausea, bloating

----

*Although CHF may initially manifest as failure of one side of the heart, the inability to reverse these effects will ultimately lead to failure of the unaffected side, because the heart is one organ.

NURSING MANAGEMENT

◆ ASSESSMENT

Subjective Data

  History and development of symptoms, history of heart disease
  Dyspnea, orthopnea, paroxysmal nocturnal dyspnea
  Recent abrupt weight gain
  Ankle swelling
  Increasing fatigue, loss of appetite, dizziness
  Exercise intolerance

Objective Data

  Tachypnea, use of accessory muscles
  Edema: site, degree
  Abdominal distention
  Neck vein distention
  Baseline vital signs

  Baseline weight, daily weights
  Presence of adventitious breath sounds
  Level of consciousness

The nursing management of the patient with CHF is summarized in the "Nursing Care Plan" and the "Critical Pathway."

CARDIAC TRANSPLANTATION

During the past decade, cardiac transplantation has become a therapeutic option for patients with end-stage cardiovascular disease. Survival rates are 80% to 90% at 1 year, 70% at 5 years, and 50% at 10 years. Success of cardiac transplantation is attributed to advances in immunosuppressive drugs, antimicrobial agents, methods to detect rejection, and organ procurement and preservation. The primary indication for a transplant is cardiomyopathy, end-stage coronary artery disease, and congenital heart disease. The limiting factor is the lack of available donor organs. The median waiting time for a heart has increased to over 200 days. Approximately 2% of those individuals awaiting donor hearts actually receive them. Chapter 18 contains an overview of the management of transplantation.

INFLAMMATORY HEART DISEASE

Bacterial, viral, and fungal disorders, as well as inflammatory reactions, may produce inflammatory heart disease. Any layer of the heart muscle may be involved. The process may be acute and life threatening or mild and relatively asymptomatic. It may cause no residual damage or trigger serious problems in later years. A description of the major forms of inflammatory heart disease is presented in Table 5-7. Infective endocarditis is described in the text as a model.

Infective Endocarditis: Acute Endocarditis, Subacute Bacterial Endocarditis

Etiology/epidemiology

Infective endocarditis is an infection of the endocardium, usually involving the heart valves. Acute endocarditis often develops on normal valves, has a rapid onset, and can cause death within days or weeks even with treatment. Subacute endocarditis develops more slowly, usually on previously damaged valves, and responds well to treatment. The disease may also be classified according to causative organism. Viridans (alpha) streptococci, staphylococci, and enterococci are the major infective agents.

Pathophysiology

Patients who experience intrusive procedures, mainline drugs, or have cardiac anomalies and faulty valves that increase blood turbulence are at high risk for endocarditis. The infecting organisms are carried in the bloodstream and deposited on heart valves or other portions of the endocardium. The organisms bombard the valves

NURSING CARE PLAN

THE PERSON WITH CONGESTIVE HEART FAILURE

■ NURSING DIAGNOSIS
Cardiac output, decreased (related to ventricular dysfunction)

Expected Patient Outcome	Nursing Interventions
Patient will demonstrate an improvement in cardiac output.	1. Monitor respirations q 4 hr for increased effort and rate, and pulse for tachycardia or for rate <60. 2. Monitor heart sounds q 4 hr for presence of S_3 or gallop rhythm. 3. Give prescribed inotropes, vasodilators. Monitor patient's response. 4. Teach patient to avoid Valsalva maneuver. 5. Monitor cardiac rhythm (dysrhythmias may occur because of ventricular dysfunction, effects of medicines). 6. Monitor electrolyte levels.

■ NURSING DIAGNOSIS
Fluid volume excess (related to impaired cardiac pump, retention of sodium and water)

Expected Patient Outcomes	Nursing Interventions
Patient will gradually excrete excess fluid. Patient will maintain stable weight.	1. Assess extremities for edema (site, degree of pitting) and coolness of skin q 4 hr. 2. Maintain an accurate intake and output. 3. Weigh daily. 4. Give prescribed diuretics. 5. Give sodium-restricted diet as prescribed. 6. Assess need for fluid restriction. 7. Provide mouth care. 8. Report weight gain of 2-3 pounds over 1-2 days. 9. Monitor BUN, creatinine levels (most diuretics only effective with adequate renal function).

■ NURSING DIAGNOSIS
Activity intolerance (related to dyspnea, fatigue)

Expected Patient Outcomes	Nursing Interventions
Patient will gradually resume self-care activities without excessive fatigue. Patient will demonstrate cardiac tolerance to increased activity.	1. Plan rest periods. Space activity and rest. 2. Encourage gradually increasing activity within prescribed restrictions; monitor for intolerance. 3. Assist with ADL as necessary; encourage self-care as tolerated. 4. Provide small frequent feedings. Prevent constipation. 5. Advise patient on energy conservation techniques. 6. Encourage patient to avoid fatigue and stress.

NURSING CARE PLAN—CONT'D

THE PERSON WITH CONGESTIVE HEART FAILURE

■ NURSING DIAGNOSIS
Gas exchange, impaired (related to ventilation-perfusion imbalance)

Expected Patient Outcomes	Nursing Interventions
The exchange of O_2 and CO_2 in the lungs will improve. Patient will not need supplemental oxygen.	1. Assess for evidence of hypoxia. 2. Monitor for adventitious breath sounds q 4 hr. 3. Assess neck vein distention q 4 hr (presence, degree). 4. Provide oxygen by nasal cannula or face mask at 2 to 6 L/min as prescribed during early period. 5. Place patient in well-supported high Fowler's or semi-Fowler's position; elevate feet if sitting in chair.

■ NURSING DIAGNOSIS
Skin integrity, high risk for impaired (related to tissue edema)

Expected Patient Outcome	Nursing Interventions
Patient's skin remains intact.	1. Keep patient's legs elevated when sitting in chair. 2. Encourage frequent position changes when lying in bed. 3. Keep skin soft and supple with special attention to sacrum and heels. 4. Use additional measures, as necessary, to protect skin from pressure. Avoid abrasion or shearing force. 5. Assess skin integrity every day (legs, sacrum, heels).

■ NURSING DIAGNOSIS
Anxiety (related to severe dyspnea)

Expected Patient Outcome	Nursing Interventions
Patient will use effective coping mechanisms to manage anxiety.	1. Give patient opportunities to explore feelings about effect of illness on life-style. 2. Assist patient to identify personal strengths. 3. Give medications to reduce anxiety, if prescribed. 4. Teach measures to control heart failure and reduce stress.

and become embedded. The hallmark of the disease is the platelet-fibrin-bacteria mass termed a *vegetation* that develops and then scars and perforates the valve leaflets. The growths may also break off as emboli.

Medical management
Medical management includes intravenous antibiotic therapy specific to cultured organism (usually a penicillin). Therapy is continued even after symptom cessation to eliminate all microorganisms from the vegetations and prevent complications. Heart action is reduced and

supported as needed. Diagnostic studies may include blood cultures, echocardiogram, transesophageal echocardiogram, and cardiac catheterization.

NURSING MANAGEMENT

◆ ASSESSMENT
Subjective Data

History of heart, valvular, or rheumatic disease
Recent history of intrusive procedure, such as dental work, minor surgery, Foley catheters, or cystoscopy

CRITICAL PATHWAY	**Congestive Heart Failure Without Complications**

DGR #: 127; expected LOS: 6

	Day of Admission Day 1	Day 2	Day 3
Diagnostic Tests	CBC, UA, SMA/18,* ABGs, PT/PTT, chest x-ray, ECG	SMA/6,† PT/PTT, echocardiogram	SMA/6†, PT/PTT, chest x-ray, ABGs
Medications	IV @ TKO rate; digitalis, diuretic, low-dosage anticoagulant, vasodilator, bronchodilator, antidysrhythmic; Rx for rest/anxiety	IV @ TKO rate; digitalis, diuretic, low-dosage anticoagulant, vasodilator, bronchodilator, antidysrhythmic; Rx for rest; stool softener	IV @ TKO rate; digitalis, diuretic, low-dosage anticoagulant, vasodilator, bronchodilator, antidysrhythmic; Rx for rest; stool softener
Treatments	I & O q 8 hr; weight; O$_2$; VS q 4 hr; cardiac monitor; assess cardiopulmonary system q 4 hr; assess skin and give special care q 2 hr; elastic leg stockings	I & O q 8 hr; weight; O$_2$; VS q 4 hr; cardiac monitor; assess cardiopulmonary system q 4 hr; assess skin and give special care q 2 hr; elastic leg stockings	I & O q 8 hr; weight; O$_2$; VS q 6 hr; cardiac monitor; assess cardiopulmonary system q 6 hr; assess skin and give special care q 6 hr; elastic leg stockings
Diet	Full liquids, low sodium; restrict fluids	Soft, low sodium; provide 6 small meals/day	Soft, low sodium; provide 6 small meals/day
Activity	Bed rest, head of bed elevated 30 degrees	Bed rest, head of bed elevated 30 degrees; to BR with assistance	Up in chair with assistance × 4; head of bed elevated 30 degrees while in bed
Consultations	Cardiology	Home health, dietary	

NOTE: Acknowledge that patients recover at varying rates; therefore specified daily actions should be based solely on patient need.
ABGs, Arterial blood gases; *BR,* bathroom; *CBC,* complete blood cell count; *PT,* prothrombin time; *PTT,* partial thromboplastin time; *SMA,* sequential multiple analysis; *TKO,* to keep open; *UA,* urinalysis; *VS,* vital signs.

Guidelines for Administration of Digitalis

ADMINISTERING DIGITALIS

Take apical pulse before administering digitalis preparations; withhold medication and notify physician if pulse is below 60 or above 120.

Monitor serum potassium blood levels. Hypokalemia potentiates the effects of digoxin and the heart becomes more excitable. Hypokalemia is the most common cause of digitalis toxicity.

Give potassium supplements (if prescribed) and instruct patient in potassium-rich food sources.

MONITORING PATIENT FOR DIGITALIS TOXICITY

Cardiovascular Effects

Bradycardia
Tachycardia
Bigeminy (double beats)
Ectopic beats
Pulse deficit (difference between apical and radial pulse)

Gastrointestinal Effects

Anorexia
Nausea and vomiting
Abdominal pain
Diarrhea

Neurologic Effects

Headache
Double, blurred, or colored vision
Drowsiness, confusion
Restlessness, irritability
Muscle weakness

Guidelines for Administration of Intravenous Inotropes*

Use an infusion pump. The infusion rate determines the drug's action so it must be carefully controlled to achieve the desired effect.

Continually monitor the patient's heart rate and rhythm, blood pressure, and urine output.

Do not add an alkaline solution such as sodium bicarbonate to the solution or infusion line, because it will inactivate the drug.

Weigh the patient every day; dosages are determined based on patient's weight (milligrams per kilogram per hour).

———
*Dopamine, dobutamine, milrinone, amrinone.

History of IV drug abuse
Malaise, fatigue, joint pain
Anorexia

Objective Data

Presence of fever (low grade or high grade)
Dyspnea
Edema
Weight loss
New murmur over cardiac valves or change in quality of existing murmur
Anemia and petechiae (conjunctive, mouth, nails)
Osler's nodes (finger and toe pads)

CRITICAL PATHWAY   Congestive Heart Failure Without Complications

DGR #: 127; expected LOS: 6

Day 4	Day 5	Day of Discharge Day 6
ECG	SMA/6†, PT/PTT, chest x-ray, ABGs	PT/PTT
IV saline lock; adjust drugs for home use; Rx for rest; stool softener	IV saline lock; adjust drugs for home use; Rx for rest; stool softener	Discontinue IV saline lock; adjust drugs for home use
I & O q 8 hr; weight; O$_2$; VS q 8 hr; cardiac monitor; assess cardiopulmonary system q 8 hr; assess skin and give special care q 8 hr; elastic leg stockings	I & O q 8 hr; weight; discontinue O$_2$; VS q 8 hr; discontinue cardiac monitor; assess cardiopulmonary system q 8 hr; elastic leg stockings	Weight; discontinue I & O; VS q 8 hr; assess cardiopulmonary system q 8 hr; elastic leg stockings
Soft, low sodium; provide 6 small meals/day	Soft, low sodium; provide 6 small meals/day	Soft, low sodium; provide 6 small meals/day
Up walking in hallway with assistance × 2, up in chair × 4; head of bed elevated 30 degrees while in bed	Up walking in hallway with assistance × 2, up in chair × 4; HOB elevated 30 degrees while in bed	Up walking in hallway

*Serum calcium, phosphorus, triglycerides, uric acid, creatinine, BUN, total bilirubin, alkaline phosphate, aspartate aminotransferase (AST) (formerly serum glutamic-oxaloacetic transaminase [SGOT]), alanine aminotransferase (ALT) (formerly serum glutamate pyruvate transaminase [SGPT]), lactic dehydrogenase (LDH), total protein, albumin, sodium, potassium, chloride, total CO$_2$, glucose.
†Serum sodium, potassium, chloride, total CO$_2$, glucose, BUN.

TABLE 5-7   Pericarditis, Myocarditis, and Rheumatic Heart Disease

DISORDER	ETIOLOGY	SIGNS AND SYMPTOMS	MEDICAL MANAGEMENT
Pericarditis	Inflammation of the sac that contains the heart, as a result of trauma, neoplasm, systemic disease, or infection—fluid accumulates in the pericardial space (acute); fibrous thickening of pericardial layers occurs; follows both an acute and a chronic course	Severe chest pain, aggravated by deep breathing; pain is precordial, radiates to left shoulder, and is relieved by sitting up and leaning forward Pericardial friction rub Fever; increased WBCs Signs of CHF (chronic) Cardiac tamponade (acute): excess fluid impairs diastolic filling and cardiac output	Treatment of underlying condition or organism if known Pericardiocentesis if large effusion or tamponade Fenestration or pericardectomy for severe cases Symptomatic treatment for pain and fever
Myocarditis	Inflammation of heart muscle—may occur alone or with systemic illnesses, especially infectious ones; may develop secondary to endocarditis or pericarditis	May be nonspecific, such as fever, fatigue, dyspnea, flulike symptoms Signs of CHF Pericardial pain, arrhythmia	Identification and treatment of underlying condition Supportive CHF therapy, digoxin General comfort measures Possible use of immunosuppressives
Rheumatic heart disease	Inflammatory disease involving all three heart layers—residual damage through scarring and deformity of heart valves occurs in 10%; seen in conjunction with beta-hemolytic streptococcal infections; autoimmune response causes antibody formation	Joint pain, recurrent heart murmur, friction rub Follows upper respiratory infection by 1-4 wk May advance to signs of arrhythmias, CHF	Parenteral antibiotics Antiinflammatory drugs Comfort measures Symptom management Prophylactic antibiotic use for years

◆ NURSING DIAGNOSES

Nursing diagnoses for the patient with infective endocarditis may include, but are not limited to, the following:

Activity intolerance (related to systemic illness and decreased tissue oxygenation)

Cardiac output, decreased (related to failing valvular function)

Infection, high risk for (related to valvular dysfunction, invasive procedures)

Tissue perfusion, decreased (related to decreased cardiac output)

◆ EXPECTED PATIENT OUTCOMES

Patient's energy level will gradually increase until patient can resume normal activity pattern.

Patient's cardiac function will return to normal with effective antibiotic therapy.

Patient will gradually resume normal activity without incidence of pain or dyspnea.

Patient practices preventive behaviors to minimize future episodes of endocarditis.

◆ NURSING INTERVENTIONS

Enhancing Cardiac Output

Monitor vital signs frequently.

Be alert for complications, such as signs of CHF or emboli.

Assess heart and lung sounds frequently.

Provide supplemental oxygen as needed.

Monitor I & O.

Promoting Tissue Perfusion

Provide for adequate rest, but strict bed rest is not necessary. Gradually increase activity as cardiac status improves.

Assess orthostatic heart rate and blood pressure.

Assess peripheral circulation (pulses, capillary refill).

Instruct patient to rest with onset of dyspnea, chest pain, syncope.

Progressing Activity Tolerance

Assess activity tolerance.

Gradually increase activity level.

Provide comfort measures for fever and joint aches.

Encourage well-balanced diet.

Assist patient to find adequate diversionary activities.

Treating and Preventing Infection

Assess temperature patterns.

Administer prescribed intravenous antibiotics.

Teach patient role of antibiotics in controlling the disease. Prolonged antibiotic treatment is essential.

Teach patient importance of scrupulous oral hygiene and regular dental care.

Teach patient to follow healthy heart diet, eating foods that contain cholesterol, saturated fat, and sodium in moderation.

Teach patient about need for prophylactic antibiotics in the future, especially before dental work. Strict adherence is essential.

◆ EVALUATION

Successful achievement of expected outcomes for the patient with infective endocarditis is indicated by the following:

Resumption of normal activities and no unusual fatigue

Discusses origins of disease, purposes and goals of treatment regimen, and measures to follow to prevent recurrence

Cardiac function returns to preillness levels or patient is scheduled for surgical replacement of damaged heart valves

NOTE: The major features of pericarditis, myocarditis, and rheumatic heart disease are summarized in Table 5-7.

VALVULAR HEART DISEASE
Etiology/Epidemiology

Valvular heart disease may occur congenitally or as a sequela of the inflammatory disorders previously discussed. Rheumatic heart disease is one of the most common precipitating disorders. Diseased or impaired heart valves may become stenosed and obstruct the normal flow of blood through the heart or become insufficient and cause regurgitation and backflow of blood. Initially the heart compensates through gradual myocardial hypertrophy, but as the condition worsens CHF eventually develops and may necessitate valve replacement or repair.

Pathophysiology

Initially the heart is able to compensate for the diseased valves through myocardial hypertrophy. Effective medical treatment may extend the compensatory period by years. If the condition worsens, CHF will develop. Table 5-8 describes the specific forms of valvular dysfunction.

Medical Management

Initial treatment is conservative and is aimed at reducing circulatory congestion and decreasing the cardiac work load. Surgical repair or replacement is typically delayed until the symptoms are significantly impairing the patient's ADL. Types of valve repair are listed in Box 5-10.

NURSING MANAGEMENT

◆ ASSESSMENT (PREOPERATIVE)
Subjective Data

History and course of disease

Current medical treatment

    Diet and activity

    Medications

Knowledge and attitude about proposed surgery

TABLE 5-8   Valvular Heart Disorders

ETIOLOGY	SIGNS AND SYMPTOMS	MEDICAL MANAGEMENT
MITRAL INSUFFICIENCY		
Papillary muscle dysfunction allows valve to flap in direction of atria during systole. Caused by rheumatic heart disease, congenital factors, bacterial endocarditis. Primarily affects males.	Fatigue and weakness Right-sided heart failure Frequently accompanied by atrial fibrillation Blowing, high-pitched systolic murmur Third heart sound	Restricted activity Low-sodium diet Diuretics Cardiac glycosides to augment left ventricular output Surgical valve repair or replacement when symptoms are advanced
MITRAL STENOSIS		
Valve leaflets become thickened and calcified and eventually fuse, resulting in progressively narrowed and immobile valve. Caused by rheumatic heart disease, congenital factors. Two thirds of patients are female.	Fatigue Dyspnea Pulmonary hypertension Right-sided failure Atrial fibrillation with pooled blood in atria, causing thrombus Low-pitched, rumbling presystolic murmur Snapping, loud first heart sound May be asymptomatic for 20 or more years	Low-sodium diet Diuretics Cardioversion or drug treatment for atrial fibrillation Surgical valve repair or replacement when activity is significantly impaired
AORTIC INSUFFICIENCY		
Deforming of valve leaflets causes them to close improperly, allowing blood to backflow. Caused by rheumatic heart disease, congenital factors. Primarily affects males.	Symptoms rare until left ventricular failure is imminent Palpitations, exertional dyspnea Angina at rest or with exertion Soft blowing aortic diastolic murmur Widened pulse pressure	Cardiac glycosides Low-sodium diet Diuretics Nitroglycerin Surgical valve replacement usually necessary
AORTIC STENOSIS		
Aortic valve becomes stenosed, obstructing left ventricular outflow during systole. Caused by congenital valvular problem (most common cause), rheumatic heart disease, atherosclerosis in elderly persons. Eighty percent of patients are male.	Exertional dyspnea Angina Exertional syncope (loss of consciousness) Harsh, rough midsystolic murmur Systolic thrill over aortic area	Rest Cardiac glycosides Diuretics Low-sodium diet Nitroglycerin if angina is present Surgical valve replacement as severity of symptoms worsens
TRICUSPID INSUFFICIENCY		
Rare disorder since normal valve leaflets are very small and play less of a role in valve closure. Impaired valve allows backflow of blood into right atrium. Caused by rheumatic heart disease (rare), congenital factors. Primarily affects females.	Symptoms of right-sided heart failure Hepatomegaly, jugular vein distention	Cardiac glycosides Low-sodium diet Diuretics Surgical valve repair or replacement
TRICUSPID STENOSIS		
Rare disorder in which shortening and fusion of commissures cause orifice to narrow and block blood returning to heart. Caused by rheumatic heart disease. Usually occurs with mitral or aortic stenosis. Primarily affects females.	Symptoms of right-sided heart failure Hepatomegaly, jugular vein distention	Cardiac glycosides Low-sodium diet Diuretics Surgical valve repair or replacement

Patient's complaints:
  Fatigue
  Dyspnea on exertion, orthopnea, or paroxysmal nocturnal dyspnea
  Angina
  Palpitations or syncope (fainting with drop in blood pressure)

Objective Data

Activity and energy level
Respiratory rate and quality—breath sounds
Baseline vital signs
Presence of abnormal heart sounds
Presence of edema, pitting or nonpitting
Prominent neck veins

BOX 5-10	Types of Valve Repair
Annuloplasty	Repair of ring or annulus of incompetent or diseased valve
Valvuloplasty	Repair of valve, suturing of torn leaflets
Commissurotomy	Dilation of valve; repair of a leaflet or commissure, fibrous bond or ring
Percutaneous balloon valvuloplasty	Dilation of valve by balloon; nonsurgical procedure

Peripheral oxygenation—nail beds, skin tone, temperature, pulses, and capillary refill

Heart rate, cardiac rhythm

◆ NURSING DIAGNOSES

Nursing diagnoses for the patient with valvular disorder may include, but are not limited to, the following:

Activity intolerance (related to insufficient cardiac output)

Breathing pattern, ineffective (related to fluid accumulation in lung spaces)

Cardiac output, decreased (related to failing valves and cardiac pumping mechanism)

Anxiety (related to seriousness of open heart surgery and uncertainty of prognosis)

Fluid volume excess (related to retained extracellular fluids)

Sleep pattern disturbance (related to dyspnea in recumbent position)

◆ EXPECTED PATIENT OUTCOMES

Patient will modify activities as needed to adjust to fluctuating energy levels.

Patient will experience optimum oxygen and carbon dioxide exchange in lungs.

Patient will steadily improve cardiac output after surgery.

Patient will experience manageable levels of anxiety over anticipated surgical procedure, using effective coping mechanisms.

Patient will have normal fluid volume as cardiac function improves.

Patient will reestablish a pattern of restful sleep.

◆ NURSING INTERVENTIONS

Patient care during the extended period of medical management is similar to that received by the patient with CHF and focuses on patient teaching for adherence to diet and medication protocols, strategies for balancing activity and rest, and preparing for cardiac surgery.

◆ NURSING DIAGNOSES

Nursing diagnoses for the patient following cardiac surgery may include, but are not limited to, the following:

Cardiac output, decreased (related to cardiopulmonary bypass, low cardiac output syndrome, vasodilation, bleeding)

Gas exchange, impaired (related to hypoventilation)

Pain (related to surgery)

Activity intolerance (related to pain, fear, invasive lines)

Thought processes, altered (related to postpericardiotomy delirium, medication effects)

Infection, potential for (related to surgery, invasive lines)

Fear (related to cardiovascular surgery, invasive procedures, pain)

◆ EXPECTED PATIENT OUTCOMES

Patient will demonstrate hemodynamic stability with adequate cardiac output and tissue perfusion.

Patient will demonstrate adequate gas exchange (arterial blood gases within normal limits or at patient's baseline).

Patient will indicate discomfort within tolerable limits.

Patient will progress activity to resumption of self-care.

Patient will be alert, oriented, and able to participate in postoperative regimen.

Patient will exhibit no evidence of infection (healing incisions, afebrile, clear lung sounds).

Patient will demonstrate psychosocial and physical comfort.

◆ NURSING INTERVENTIONS

Nursing interventions for the patient having cardiac surgery are given below.

Preoperative

See Guidelines box on p. 87 for preoperative teaching plan.

Preoperative care is similar to that for other major surgeries indicated in the text.

Postoperative

Enhancing cardiac output

Monitor vital signs, cardiac rhythm, intake and output.

Maintain hemodynamic monitoring as needed.

Maintain adequate oxygenation to reduce myocardial irritability.

Warm patient to 36° C using heating blanket, lights.

Auscultate heart and lung sounds.

Promoting adequate gas exchange

Assess respiratory rate, lung sounds.

Maintain turning, coughing, and deep breathing schedule. Suction as necessary.

Provide supplemental oxygen.

Increase activity as early as possible.

Guidelines for Preoperative Teaching for the Person Undergoing Cardiac Surgery

1. General information
   a. Places of care during hospitalization
      (1) CCU or ICU after surgery
      (2) Return to general patient care division in 2-3 days
   b. Visiting hours and location of waiting rooms
2. Description of surgery
   a. Simple explanation of anatomy of heart and effect of the patient's cardiovascular disorder (e.g., incompetent valve, obstructed coronary artery)
   b. Explanation of surgical procedure
   c. Definition of unfamiliar terms: bypass, extracorporeal
   d. Length of time in surgery: 2-4 hours
   e. Length of time until able to see family (usually 1½-2 hours after surgery)
3. Preparation for surgery
   a. Shower or bath night before surgery with special antimicrobial soap
   b. Surgical shave: shaving of entire chest and abdomen neck to groin and left midaxillary line to right
   c. Legs shaved if saphenous vein grafts will be used
   d. Preoperative medication
4. Explanation of monitors
   a. Round patches on chest connected to a cardiac monitor that records patient's heartbeats
   b. Monitor makes beeping sound all the time
5. Explanation of lines
   a. Intravenous routes for fluid and medications
   b. Central venous line in neck or chest to monitor fluid status
   c. Pulmonary artery catheter in chest or neck to measure pulmonary pressures and monitor fluid status
   d. Plastic connector line to obtain blood samples without a needle stick

6. Explanation of drainage tubes
   a. Indwelling urinary catheter
   b. Chest tube: bloody drainage expected
7. Explanation of breathing tube
   a. Tube in windpipe connected to machine called ventilator
   b. Unable to speak with tube in place but can mouth words and communicate in writing
   c. Tube removed when patient is fully awake and stable
   d. Secretions in lungs or tube removed by nurse using a suction catheter
   e. Food and oral fluids not permitted until breathing tube is removed
8. Explanation and demonstration of activities and exercises
   a. Purpose of activity is to promote circulation, keep lungs clear, and prevent infection
   b. Activity includes:
      (1) Turning from side to side in bed
      (2) Sitting on edge of bed
      (3) Sitting in chair the night of or the morning after surgery
   c. Range-of-motion exercises
   d. Deep breathing using sustained maximal inspiration
   e. Tubes and lines will restrict movement somewhat, but nurse will assist patient
9. Relief of pain
   a. Some pain will be experienced, but it will not be excruciating (different pain than original angina if this was present)
   b. Frequent pain medication will be given to help relieve the pain, but patient should always tell nurse when pain is present

---

Administer analgesics before turning, deep breathing exercises.

Provide pillow for splinting.

Promoting comfort

Assess level of discomfort.

Provide analgesics as needed; consider patient-controlled analgesia.

Progressing activity

Encourage patient to begin progressive activity and ambulation (dangle and to chair on postoperative day 1, ambulate in room on postoperative day 2, ambulate in hall on postoperative day 3).

Encourage enrollment in cardiac rehabilitation program; development of home walking/exercise program.

Maintaining orientation

Assess level of consciousness, mental status.

Reorient as necessary.

Minimize patient stay in ICU.

Provide concise explanations of procedures.

Encourage family to visit.

Maintain day and night environments.

Assess medication regimen; administer mild sedation as needed.

Provide for uninterrupted sleep.

Minimizing risk of infection

Maintain sterile technique with dressing changes.

Do careful hand washing.

Assess incision, intravenous site.

Reducing fear/enhancing self-care

Teach relaxation techniques; provide diversional activities.

Encourage patient involvement in planning and carrying out care regimens.

Encourage enrollment in cardiac rehabilitation program.

Reinforce the importance of regular medical follow-up.

For patients with mechanical prosthetic valves, instruct patient in importance of long-term anticoagulation with warfarin sodium (Coumadin).

◆ EVALUATION

Successful achievement of expected outcomes for the patient undergoing cardiac surgery is indicated by the following:

Patient is without systemic signs of cardiac failure.

Patient has effective respiratory pattern; lungs are clear to auscultation.

Patient's incisions heal without complications.

Patient maintains a normal fluid balance.

Patient is knowledgeable about postdischarge diet and activity patterns; can state purpose and side effects of all medications.

Patient can state signs that indicate need for immediate medical follow-up.

Patient returns to normal occupational and recreational patterns and has increased activity tolerance.

SELECTED REFERENCES

Afridi I et al: Dobutamine stress echocardiography, *Am Heart J* 127:1510-1515, 1994.

Arteago WJ, Drew BJ: Device therapy for ventricular tachycardia or ventricular fibrillation: the implantable cardioverter/defibrillator and antitachycardia pacing, *Crit Care Nurse Q* 14(2):60-71, 1991.

Beare PG, Myers JL: *Adult health nursing,* St Louis, 1994, Mosby.

Braun A: When arrest is imminent, *RN,* pp 22-29, March 1994.

Brown KK: Boosting the failing heart with inotropic drugs, *Nursing,* pp 34-39, April 1993.

Cliff DL, Blazewicz PA: Radiofrequency catheter ablation. I, *Dimen Crit Care* 12(6):313-318, 1993.

Drew BJ: Bedside electrocardiographic monitoring, *Heart Lung* 20(6):10-23, 1991.

Drew BJ, Sparacino PSA: Bedside electrographic monitoring, *Heart Lung* 20(6):597-607, 1991.

Feagins C, Daniel D: Management of CHF in the home setting, *Home Health Care Practice* 4(1):31-37, 1991.

Flynn JB, Bruce NP: *Critical care skills,* St Louis, 1993, Mosby.

Funk M: Epidemiology of heart failure, *Crit Care Nurs Clin North Am* 5(4):569-573, 1993.

Hochrein MA, Sohl L: Heart smart: a guide to cardiac tests, *Am J Nurs,* pp 22-25, Dec 1992.

Marrie TJ: Infective endocarditis: a serious and changing disease, *Crit Care Nurse* 7(2):31-46, 1987.

Matrisciana L: Unstable angina, *Crit Care Nurse,* pp 30-39, Dec 1992.

Schactman M, Grune JS: Signal-averaged electrocardiography: a new technique for determining which patients may be at risk for sudden cardiac death, *Focus Crit Care* 18(3):202-210, 1991.

Schoenbaum MP, Drew BJ: Proarrhythmia: mechanisms, evaluation, and treatment, *Crit Care Nurs Q* 14(2):10-18, 1991.

Scrima DA: Infective endocarditis: nursing considerations, *Crit Care Nurse* 7(2):47-56, 1987.

Teplitz L: Classification of cardiac pacemakers: the Pacemaker Code, *J Cardiovasc Nurs* 5(3):1-8, 1992.

Verdeber A et al: Preparation for cardiac catheterization, *J Cardiovasc Nurs* 7(1):75-77, 1992.

Weikart CJ: New eye into the heart, *RN,* pp 36-39, Oct 1993.

Zimmaro DM: Catheter ablation of ventricular tachycardia and related nursing interventions, *Crit Care Nurse* 7(4):20-29, 1987.

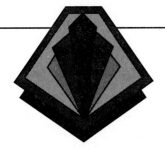

Disorders of the Vascular System

♦ ASSESSMENT

SUBJECTIVE DATA

Demographic data
  Age, sex, ethnic background
  Menopausal status
  Occupation
    Physical stresses of job
      Prolonged standing, sitting, lifting
  Smoking history, pack years
Health history
  Family or personal history of:
    Coronary artery disease (CAD), hypertension, hyperlipidemia
    Cerebrovascular disease or stroke
    Diabetes mellitus
    Renal disease
    Bleeding disorders, thrombotic disease
  Current drug use
    Prescription and over the counter (OTC)
    Oral contraceptive use in females, estrogen replacement therapy
Diet history
  Usual dietary pattern
    Special diet if any
  Height and weight balance
  Cholesterol level if known
  Use of alcohol
Activity level/fitness
  Exercise pattern
    Frequency, duration, intensity
Current health problem
  Onset, duration, severity
    Self-treatment measures attempted, success
  Edema
  Extremity pain
    Feeling of heaviness in legs
    Cramping pain with exercise
  Fatigue
  Paresthesia, numbness

OBJECTIVE DATA

Skin and extremities
  Color, temperature, texture of skin
    Pallor or cyanosis
    Capillary refill
  Edema
    Unilateral, bilateral, severity
  Hair distribution
  Peripheral pulses
    Presence and symmetry (Figure 6-2)
Blood pressure

✍ DIAGNOSTIC TESTS

LABORATORY TESTS

Laboratory tests do not play a primary role in the evaluation of the vascular system, but a number of tests will be utilized in conjunction with a general workup of the overall cardiovascular system. Some of the most common tests include cholesterol and various lipid studies and blood coagulation studies such as prothrombin time and partial thromboplastin time. Normal values are presented in Chapters 5 and 7.

RADIOGRAPHIC TESTS

Venography

Purpose—Venography is used to assess the condition of the deep veins of the leg after injection of a

GERONTOLOGIC PATIENT CONSIDERATIONS: PHYSIOLOGIC CHANGES IN THE VASCULAR SYSTEM

A number of changes occur in the vascular system with advancing age. These are most significant when the body is under stress from trauma or illness. Some of the major changes include the following:
  Thickening and increased stiffness of the aorta and large arteries
    Increased thickness of the intimal wall from fibrosis
    Thinning and calcification of the medial wall
  Increased vascular resistance
    Increased systolic blood pressure
  Atherosclerosis
    Accumulation of plaque within the intimal wall
  Venous valve insufficiency

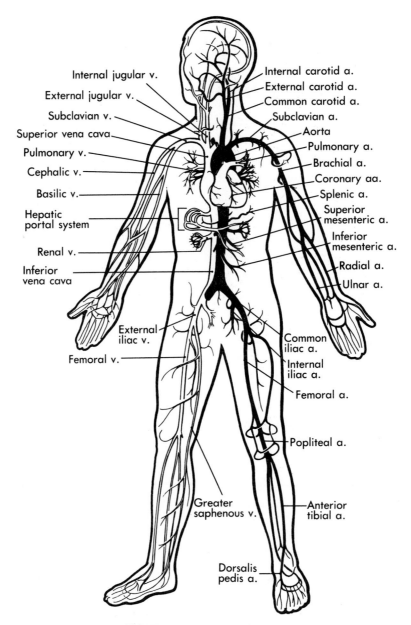

FIGURE 6-1 Vascular system.

contrast medium. It is used primarily to confirm or rule out the presence of a thrombosis. The test is not used for routine screening because of the relatively high radiation exposure.

Procedure—The patient is positioned on a tilt table, and an intravenous (IV) line is inserted into the dorsum of the foot. Contrast medium is injected, and its distribution through the leg is followed fluoroscopically. The test takes about 30 to 45 minutes.

Patient preparation and aftercare—The patient is restricted to clear liquids for 4 hours before the test and assessed carefully for any allergy to iodine, shellfish, or contrast media. The patient is informed that injection of the dye causes a burning sensation and some discomfort is present in the leg during the test. The peripheral pulses are monitored after the test, and the injection site is assessed for hematoma, inflammation, or bleeding. No other posttest care is required.

Impedance Plethysmography

Purpose—Impedance plethysmography is a reliable noninvasive test used to measure venous flow in the extremities and detect the presence of deep vein thrombosis, particularly in the proximal deep veins of the leg.

Procedure—The patient is placed in a supine position, electrodes are attached to the calf, and a pressure cuff is wrapped around the thigh about 2 inches above the knee. The cuff is inflated to impede venous return without interfering with arterial flow. Tracings are made of the increase in venous volume following inflation and the corresponding decrease following deflation. This is done several times. If veins are obstructed they are unable to respond when additional pressure is applied. The test takes about 30 to 45 minutes.

Patient preparation and aftercare—No special care is indicated except routine patient teaching regarding this little known test.

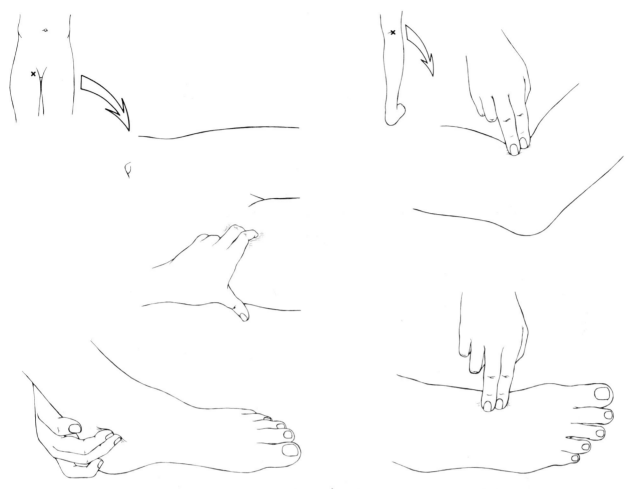

FIGURE 6-2 Palpating peripheral pulses. (From Potter PA: *Pocket guide to health assessment,* ed 3, St Louis, 1994, Mosby.)

Doppler Ultrasonography

Purpose—Doppler ultrasonography, a noninvasive test, evaluates the blood flow in the major veins and arteries of the extremities and provides a safe, inexpensive alternative to arteriography and venography. It assists in the diagnosis of thromboses, peripheral arterial disease, and the patency of bypass grafts (Figure 6-3).

Procedure—The patient is placed supine, and the transducer is placed at various points along the path of the test vessels. The waveforms are recorded for analysis. Segmental limb blood pressure is obtained via cuff compression to localize arterial occlusive disease. The test takes about 20 minutes. An ankle brachial index (AB index) may also be computed.

Patient preparation and aftercare—No special care is required except patient teaching and reassurance that the test is painless.

NOTE: Ultrasonography can also be used to evaluate the abdominal aorta for the presence of aneurysm.

Arteriography

Purpose—Arteriography is an invasive test that utilizes a contrast medium to visualize the arterial sys-

tem, assess blood flow, and detect obstruction or abnormality.

Procedure—The patient is placed supine. A catheter is inserted into the femoral or brachial artery with the patient under local anesthesia and is threaded to the desired location. Dye is inserted into the catheter to visualize the vessels and blood flow, and x-ray films are taken. The test takes about 1 to 2 hours.

Patient preparation and aftercare—Careful teaching is the foundation of pretest care. Infusion of the dye typically causes a transient flushing or burning sensation. The patient is carefully assessed for allergy to iodine, shellfish, or contrast dyes. The patient is instructed to fast the night before the test. After the test the insertion site is carefully monitored for signs of bleeding or hematoma, and vital signs, peripheral pulses, and sensation are evaluated hourly for 4 to 8 hours. The patient is instructed to lie flat in bed with the affected leg straight for about 6 hours. The patient is encouraged to drink a liberal amount of fluids to assist in the excretion of the dye.

NOTE: Digital subtraction angiography may be employed to improve the quality of the images. Fluoro-

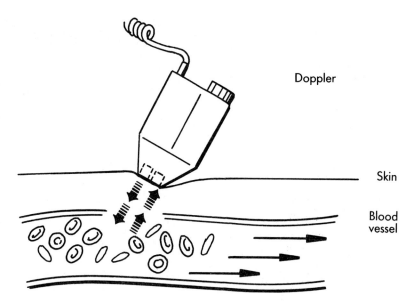

FIGURE 6-3 Doppler effect showing RBCs reflecting sound.

scopic images are enhanced by computer, and the masking effects of adjacent bone or tissue are minimized.

ARTERIAL DISORDERS
ARTERIAL OCCLUSIVE DISEASE
Etiology/Epidemiology

The symptoms of arterial disease are the result of disturbances in the delivery of blood and oxygen to the tissues. The severity of the symptoms clearly reflects the degree of circulatory impairment. Several specific disorders are related in various ways to the development of arteriosclerosis and atherosclerosis in the periphery.

Arteriosclerosis obliterans is used as the prototypical disease. Table 6-1 summarizes other problems.

Arteriosclerosis obliterans is the most common cause of arterial occlusive disease in individuals over 30 years of age. It causes segmental arteriosclerotic narrowing or obstruction within the intima of the artery. It primarily affects the lower extremity, and the iliac and popliteal arteries are involved most frequently. Plaque typically develops at the points of bifurcation or narrowing. The disease affects more men than women, and clinical symptoms appear between the ages of 50 and 70 years in most cases. Identified risk factors include cigarette smoking (chronic vasoconstrictive effect of nicotine), obesity, hypertension and hyperlipidemia, and diabetes mellitus.

TABLE 6-1 Peripheral Arterial Disorders		
ETIOLOGY	**SIGNS AND SYMPTOMS**	**MEDICAL MANAGEMENT**
THROMBOANGIITIS OBLITERANS (BUERGER'S DISEASE)		
Obstructive inflammatory process in small arteries and veins	Pain: intermittent claudication, pain at rest, or general aching; cold sensitivity	Stopping smoking (may be enough to reverse symptoms)
Strongly associated with cigarette smoking	Numbness and tingling	Sympathectomy if unresponsive to conservative measures
Appears in males aged 20-40 yr and slightly more often in Semitic and Oriental persons	Superficial thrombophlebitis	May require amputation of affected digits
		Preventive measures
RAYNAUD'S PHENOMENON OR DISEASE		
Epidoses of arterial spasm—most often in hands	Cold, numbness, and pain in one or more fingers or toes	Avoiding cold
May appear alone or secondary to another disease process	Bilateral process, affects both hands	Stopping smoking
Occurs primarily in women aged 20-40 yr	Fingers appear white or mottled	Calcium antagonists or muscle relaxants
	Cold aggravates spasms	Sympathectomy if unresponsive to conservative measures
	Intense redness and throbbing follow spasms	May require amputation of affected digits
ARTERIAL EMBOLISM		
Blood clots floating in arterial blood usually originate in heart and tend to lodge in bifurcation of an artery, severely impairing blood flow	Symptoms depend on size and location	Bed rest and anticoagulants or fibrinolytics
	Abrupt onset of severe pain and burning, loss of distal pulses, and a cold, pale, numb extremity	Surgery—embolectomy or endarterectomy within 6-10 hr

Pathophysiology

Arteriosclerosis obliterans occurs when there is segmented arteriosclerotic narrowing or obstruction of the intimal and medial layers of the artery. The primary lesion is plaque formation that causes partial or complete occlusion. Calcification of the medial layer with loss of elasticity further weakens the arterial walls and predisposes to aneurysm and thrombus formation. The pathology can progress to ulceration, necrosis, and gangrene.

Symptoms appear when the vessels can no longer provide enough blood to supply oxygen and nutrients and remove metabolic wastes from the tissues. Symptoms develop gradually. Intermittent claudication, an aching pain or cramping that occurs while walking, is the primary symptom. The pain is usually relieved after 1 to 2 minutes of rest. The muscles of the calf are affected most frequently, although the pain may occur in the lower back, buttocks, thigh, or foot. Pain that occurs at rest indicates severe disease and may be described as a burning pain. It frequently occurs at night. The affected extremity is also typically cold and numb and experiences paresthesias.

Medical Management

A presumptive diagnosis is established from the pattern of the patient's symptoms. Other tests may include noninvasive ultrasonography with pressure and volume determinations and angiography if indicated. Medical management is directed at maintaining or improving peripheral circulation and preventing occlusion. It includes a variety of medications and general life-style modifications. Drug therapy may include antilipidemics, vasodilators, and agents such as dipyridamole (Persantine) and pentoxifylline (Trental) that inhibit platelet adhesion and improve capillary blood flow by increasing red blood cell (RBC) flexibility. Surgical management is used for the patient who does not respond to more conservative management and for individuals who develop an acute obstruction. Options include bypass grafting, endarterectomy, and endovascular procedures such as balloon or laser angioplasty (Box 6-1). Amputation may be required if complications such as infection and gangrene occur.

NURSING MANAGEMENT

◆ ASSESSMENT
Subjective Data

History of disease and its treatment
    History of CAD or hypertension
Presence of aching pain in the calf, lower back, buttocks, thigh, or foot
    Relationship to exercise
    Effect of rest
    Severity and duration
Night pain

BOX 6-1 | Surgical Options for Arterial Vascular Disease

BYPASS GRAFTS

The procedure involves the bypass of an obstructed segment using the saphenous vein or a synthetic material. Autogenous grafts are more successful. The bypass may involve the aorta or a more distal vessel. Small artery bypasses are experimental (see Guidelines box on p. 93).

ENDARTERECTOMY

The procedure involves the stripping and removal of plaque using a specially designed catheter. Extremely hardened vessels may not survive the attempt at plaque removal.

ENDOVASCULAR SURGERY

Balloon and Laser Angioplasty

The procedure can be used as primary treatment or as an adjunct to surgery. The balloon inflation compresses and ruptures the plaque. It is often used to improve iliac artery flow as part of a more extensive surgical procedure.

Atherectomy

The procedure uses a special catheter to strip away the atherosclerotic plaque, and its use is still experimental.

Numbness, paresthesias in feet or legs
Usual diet, life-style, occupation, and exercise routines
Smoking history

Objective Data

Presence, strength, and equality of peripheral pulses
Prolonged or absent capillary refill
Skin
    Temperature, color, hair growth pattern
    Thickened nails
    Presence of ulcers or skin breakdown
Obesity
Color change in feet with elevation and dangling
Results of Doppler ultrasonography

◆ NURSING DIAGNOSES

Nursing diagnoses for the person with arteriosclerosis obliterans may include, but are not limited, to the following:
    Tissue perfusion, altered (peripheral; related to arterial obstruction)
    Injury, high risk for (related to decreased sensory perception in extremities)
    Activity intolerance (related to intermittent claudication with exercise)

◆ EXPECTED PATIENT OUTCOMES

Patient will experience increased perfusion to the extremities.
Patient will be free of tissue injury related to trauma, heat, cold, or pressure.
Patient will be able to engage in daily activities without the onset of claudication pain.

◆ NURSING INTERVENTIONS

Supporting Peripheral Tissue Perfusion

Maintain a warm environmental temperature.
  Avoid chilling and exposure to the cold.
  Avoid the use of any direct heat to the extremities.
  Layer clothes for warmth; wear socks.
Avoid elevating the legs; maintain slight dependency.
Avoid sitting or standing in one position for too long.
  Arrange frequent rest periods when traveling.
  Avoid crossing the legs when sitting.
  Ensure that chairs do not impair the circulation.
Avoid constrictive clothing, such as garters, girdles, tight waistbands, socks with tight banding.
Reinforce the importance of *not smoking*.
Administer vasodilator or other medication as ordered.

Preventing Injury

Wear comfortable protective shoes at all times.
Trim nails carefully straight across, soaking feet first.
Seek professional assistance for care of corns, calluses, or ingrown toenails.
  Avoid trauma to the extremities.
  Refrain from massaging the legs.
  Cleanse feet daily and lubricate with moisturizing lotion. Avoid use of rubbing alcohol or oversoftening.
  Use clean cotton socks and change daily.
  Do not go barefoot.
Assess the condition of the feet daily, using a mirror if necessary.
Check water temperature carefully before immersing feet.

Promoting Pain-free Activity

Help patient develop an exercise plan that carefully balances rest and activity. *Moderate* regular exercise improves arterial circulation by stimulating the development of collateral circulation.
Exercise only to the point of pain and then rest. NOTE: Excess exercise puts additional metabolic demand on the circulation. Walking is ideal exercise.
Add Buerger-Allen exercises if physician approves:
  Lie flat with legs elevated for 2 to 3 minutes.
  Sit for 2 to 3 minutes with legs relaxed and slightly dependent.
  Flex, extend, evert, and invert the feet. Hold each position for 30 seconds.
  Lie flat for 5 minutes with legs covered for warmth.
Help patient reduce body weight if indicated.
Reinforce principles of a low-cholesterol, low-saturated fat diet.

◆ EVALUATION

Successful achievement of expected outcomes for the patient with arteriosclerosis obliterans is indicated by the following:

Guidelines for Nursing Care for Bypass Graft Surgery

PREOPERATIVE

Monitor affected limb for changes in color, temperature, sensation.
Assess peripheral pulses by palpation or with Doppler probe.
Place cradle on bed to protect limb from pressure.

POSTOPERATIVE

Monitor peripheral pulses, color, temperature, and sensation in affected limb hourly.
  Use Doppler if pulses are difficult to palpate.
  Report any sudden changes or deterioration.
Monitor incision for redness or drainage.
Reposition patient every 2 hours.
Maintain cradle to prevent pressure on extremities.
Avoid sharp or prolonged flexion in region of the graft.
Encourage progressive activity and monitor patient response.

Incorporation of life-style modifications into activities of daily living; absence of smoking
Intact skin without evidence of injury or infection
A balance of activity and rest that allows the patient to remain free of claudication

ANEURYSM

Etiology/Epidemiology

An aneurysm is a localized or diffuse enlargement of an artery at some point along its course. Aneurysms typically occur when the vessel wall becomes weakened by trauma, congenital disease, infection, or atherosclerosis. They can occur virtually anywhere, but the most common site is along the course of the aorta, particularly in the abdomen. There has been an increased incidence of aneurysm noted in recent years, possibly related to the ongoing aging of the population. Risk factors again include cigarette smoking and hypertension.

GERONTOLOGIC PATIENT CONSIDERATIONS FOR ARTERIAL OCCLUSIVE DISEASE

Arteriosclerosis obliterans is primarily a problem of the elderly, particularly in association with insulin-dependent diabetes mellitus (IDDM) or non–insulin dependent diabetes mellitus (NIDDM). The disease is often fairly advanced on diagnosis, and the risk factors such as smoking, diet, and obesity often represent the patterns of half a century or more. Decreased immune function also increases the risk of concurrent infection from minor trauma or irritation. It is important for the nurse to take the time to involve the patient in all home management strategies, modifying recommendations as needed to increase acceptability. Major life-style changes are often unrealistic. Stress is placed on adherence to effective management of diabetes and hypertension, which worsen the incidence of complications such as infection, gangrene, and amputation.

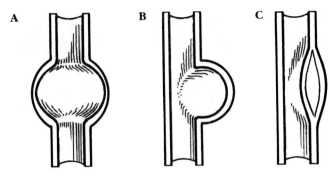

FIGURE 6-4 Types of aneurysms. **A,** Fusiform. **B,** Saccular. **C,** Dissecting.

Pathophysiology

A series of pathophysiologic changes cause weakness of the arterial wall, resulting in dilation and potential rupture. The intimal wall is destroyed, and the tunica media is damaged, with a marked loss of elastin. Once the process begins there is a tendency toward progressive dilatation and degeneration, with a risk of rupture. There are three major types of aneurysms (Figure 6-4):

saccular Involving only part of the artery's circumference. They take the form of a sac or pouch attached to the side of the vessel.
fusiform A spindle-shaped defect involving the entire circumference of the arterial wall.
dissecting Produced when there is hemorrhage into a vessel wall that splits and dissects the wall, causing it to widen. They are usually caused by a degenerative defect.

The symptoms depend on the size, type, and location of the aneurysm. Compression of adjacent structures may create abdominal, flank, or back pain. Many aneurysms are essentially asymptomatic and picked up as part of an unrelated diagnostic process.

Medical Management

Ultrasonography is useful in determining the size and location of the aneurysm. Computed tomography (CT) scanning may be used to obtain cross-sectional images of the aorta. Angiography may also be employed. The diagnostic process may be initiated by the detection of a pulsating mass in the abdomen.

Small, asymptomatic aneurysms are usually managed medically with careful follow-up and control of hypertension. Aneurysms over 6.0 cm are usually treated surgically, because the risk of rupture increases steadily. Replacement of the diseased segment with a Teflon or Dacron graft is standard although surgical approaches vary depending on the size and location of the aneurysm.

NURSING MANAGEMENT

Patients undergoing aneurysm surgery receive standard but meticulous postoperative care. Special attention is focused on monitoring the adequacy of urine output and peripheral perfusion, which serve as indicators of graft patency. Urine output should be at least 50 ml/hr, and the patient's extremities should remain warm to the touch. The incidence of pale, mottled skin with cold numb extremities is a serious complication. Initial management may take place in an intensive care unit. A critical pathway for a patient undergoing abdominal aortic aneurysm repair is included on p. 96.

HYPERTENSION
Etiology/Epidemiology

Hypertension is defined as a consistent elevation of blood pressure above 140/90 mm Hg or a consistent elevation of diastolic pressure above 90 mm Hg on an average of two or more readings.

Hypertension is commonly classified into two types: primary and secondary. The cause of primary or essential hypertension, which accounts for 90% of all cases, is basically unknown. Secondary hypertension results from a known cause such as glomerulonephritis, Cushing's disease, or renal stenosis.

Hypertension affects over 58 million people, and the incidence increases with age. Hypertension occurs more often in men and is nearly twice as prevalent among African-Americans as among Whites. The disease also tends to be more severe in the African-American population. It is also theorized that millions more have hypertension that is neither diagnosed nor treated.

Pathophysiology

Blood pressure is determined by the following:
Volume of blood flow and strength, rate, and rhythm of the heart
Peripheral vascular resistance as determined by the diameter of blood vessels and the viscosity of the blood
Increased peripheral resistance from narrowing of the arterioles is the single most common characteristic of hypertension. This peripheral resistance is influenced by renal regulation of the renin angiotensin network and by stimulation of the sympathetic system and release of catecholamines.

Figure 6-5 illustrates the sites of blood pressure regulation. These are the targets of pharmacologic control discussed under "Medical Management."

With prolonged hypertension, the elastic tissue of arterioles is replaced by fibrous collagen tissue, making the arteriole walls less distensible. As resistance increases, so does the ventricular workload, leading to possible congestive heart failure. The process of atherosclerosis also appears to be accelerated. Inadequate blood supply to the coronary arteries can lead to angina and myocardial infarction. Permanent damage may occur in the kidneys and cerebral vessels.

Hypertension is typically asymptomatic. When symptoms are present they usually indicate the presence of advanced disease. Early morning headache, blurred vision, and spontaneous epistaxis are possible.

CRITICAL PATHWAY   **Abdominal Aortic Aneurysm (AAA) Below Level of Kidney**

DRG #: 108, Expected LOS: 7 to 10 Days

	Day of Admission Day 1	Day of Surgery (to ICU from OR) Day 2	Day 3	Day 4	Transfer Out of ICU Day 5
Diagnostic Tests	CBC, UA, SMA/18* PT/PTT, T & X, chest and abdominal x-ray films, CT chest and abdomen, ECG	CBC, SMA/6,† ABGs	CBC, SMA/6†		CBC, SMA/6†
Medications	IVs, IV antibiotics, IM/PO analgesic; antihypertensive medications as necessary; other medications for chronic health problems as necessary	IVs, IV antibiotics, IV analgesic; antihypertensive medications as necessary; other medications for chronic health problems as necessary	IVs, IV antibiotics, IV analgesic; antihypertensive medications as necessary; other medications for chronic health problems as necessary	IVs, IV antibiotics, IV/IM analgesic; antihypertensive medications as necessary; other medications for chronic health problems as necessary	IV rate decreased, PO intake becomes adequate; IV antibiotic; IV/IM analgesic; antihypertensive medications as necessary; other medications for chronic health problems as necessary
Treatments	I&O q 8 hr; VS q 4 hr; CSS	I & O (including Foley and NG) q hr × 12, then q 2 hr × 12; VS and assess pulmonary and neurocirculatory systems to legs q hr × 12, then q 2 hr × 12; monitor hemodynamic parameters and check dressing q hr; CSS; intubated on ventilator with O₂ (extubate when appropriate)	I & O q 4 hr including NG and Foley; VS and assess pulmonary and neurocirculatory systems to legs q 2 hr; monitor hemodynamic parameters and check dressing q 2 hr; CSS	I & O q 8 hr including NG and Foley; VS and assess pulmonary and neurocirculatory systems to legs q 4 hr; disc central lines; assess BS q 2 hr; remove dressing; CSS	I & O q 8 hr; discontinue NG and Foley; VS and assess pulmonary and neurocirculatory systems to legs q 6 hr; assess BS q 2 hr; CSS
Diet	Clear liquids if no nausea, NPO p MN	NPO	NPO	NPO	Begin clear liquids if no nausea and BS present
Activity	Bed rest, DB q 2 hr; keep HOB <30 degrees	Bed rest; keep bed flat without sharp flexion of hip/knee; DB q 2 hr	Bed rest; keep bed flat without sharp flexion of hip/knee; T & DB q 2 hr	Bed rest; keep HOB <30 degrees; up walking in room with help × 4; T & DB q 2 hr	Bed rest; keep HOB <30 degrees; up walking in room with help × 4; T & DB q 2 hr
Consultations	RT, perioperative nurse, primary nurse, other specialists as needed for other medical problems; anesthesiologist	RT	RT	RT	Social service

NOTE: Acknowledge that patients recover at varying rates; therefore specified daily actions should be based solely on patient need.
ABGs, arterial blood gas values; *BS,* Bowel sounds; *CBC,* complete blood cell count; *CSS,* compression support stocking; *CT,* computed tomography; *DB,* deep breathe; *HOB,* head of bed; *IM,* intramuscular; *I & O,* intake and output; *NG,* nasogastric tube; *NPO,* nothing by mouth, *p MN,* after midnight; *PO,* by mouth; *PT,* prothrombin time; *PTT,* partial thromboplastin time; *RT,* respiratory therapist; *SMA,* sequential multiple analysis; *T & DB,* turn and deep breathe; *TKO,* to keep open; *T & X,* type and crossmatch; *UA,* urinalysis.
*Serum calcium, phosphorus, triglycerides, uric acid, creatinine, BUN, total bilirubin, alkaline phosphate, aspartate aminotransferase (AST) (formerly serum glutamic oxaloacetic transaminase [SGOT], alanine aminotransferase (ALT) (formerly serum glutamatic pyruvate transaminase [SGPT]), lactic dehydrogenase (LDH), total protein, albumin, sodium, potassium, chloride, total CO₂, glucose.
†Serum sodium, potassium, chloride, total CO₂, glucose, BUN.

	CRITICAL PATHWAY	Abdominal Aortic Aneurysm (AAA) Below Level of Kidney

DRG #: 108, Expected LOS: 7 to 10 Days

	Day 6	Day 7	Day 8	Day 9	Day of Discharge Day 10
		CBC, SMA/6†	CBC, SMA/18*		
	IV rate decreased as PO intake becomes adequate; IV antibiotics; IM/PO analgesic; antihypertensive medications as necessary; other medications for chronic health problems as necessary	IV @ TKO rate; IV antibiotics; IM/PO analgesic; antihypertensive medications as necessary; other medications for chronic health problems as necessary	IV to saline lock; PO analgesic; antihypertensive medications as necessary; other medications for chronic health problems as necessary	Discontinue saline lock; PO analgesic; antihypertensive medications as necessary; other medications for chronic health problems as necessary	PO analgesic; adjust medications for home use
	I & O q 8 hr; VS and assess pulmonary and neurocirculatory systems to legs q 6 hr; assess BS q 2 hr; CSS	I & O q 8 hr; VS and assess pulmonary and neurocirculatory systems to legs q 6 hrs; assess BS q 2 hr; CSS	I & O q 8 hr; VS and assess pulmonary and neurocirculatory systems to legs q 8 hr; CSS	Discontinue I & O; VS and assess pulmonary and neurocirculatory systems to legs q 8 hr; CSS	VS and assess pulmonary and neurocirculatory systems to legs q 8 hr; CSS
	Clear liquids; advance to full liquids or soft diet	Full liquids or soft diet	Regular diet	Regular diet	Regular diet
	Up walking in room with help × 6; T & DB q 2 hr	Up walking in hallway with help × 2; up ad lib in room	Up walking in hallway with help × 6; up ad lib in room	Up walking in hallway with help × 6; up ad lib	Up ad lib

BOX 6-2	Malignant Hypertension

Malignant hypertension is a severe, rapidly progressive rise in blood pressure that damages the small arterioles of the major organ systems. Inflammation of the arterioles of the eye is a classic finding. Malignant hypertension primarily affects African-American males under 40 years of age. Unless medical treatment is successful, the disease is rapidly fatal.

Medical Management

Hypertension is typically diagnosed simply on the presence of a consistent blood pressure elevation. Further diagnostic studies are not usually warranted unless the patient does not respond to therapy as expected. Other diagnostic data could include electrolytes, urinalysis, electrocardiogram (ECG), and an intravenous pyelogram (IVP) to evaluate potential renal involvement.

Medical management of hypertension is directed at control of the disease and prevention of associated

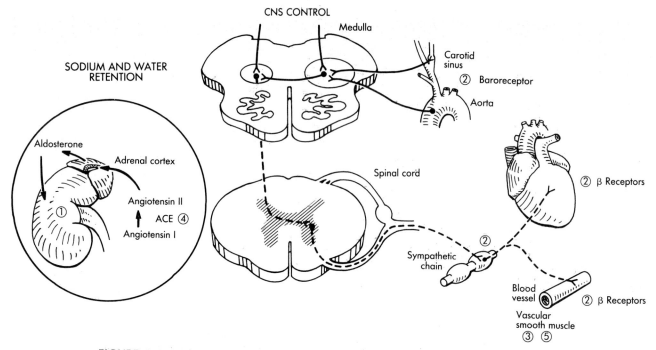

FIGURE 6-5 Sites of blood pressure regulation and action of antihypertensive drugs. *1*, Diuretics. *2*, Adrenergic inhibitors. *3*, Vasodilators. *4*, ACE inhibitors. *5*, Calcium antagonists.

Guidelines for Use of Antihypertensive Medications

1. Use a diuretic, beta blocker, calcium channel antagonist, or angiotensin converting enzyme (ACE) inhibitor.
2. If ineffective after 1-3 months, increase dosage of drug, add a second drug of a different class, or substitute a second drug.
3. Add a third drug of a different class or substitute a second drug.
4. Add a fourth drug of a different class or substitute a third drug.
5. Evaluate further and refer if indicated.

diseases and complications. Nonpharmacologic strategies include risk factor reduction through weight loss, regular aerobic exercise, stress management, reduction of dietary sodium, and smoking cessation. These strategies are frequently employed first and are often successful at initial control, although drug therapy is usually necessary eventually. A wide range of drugs exists. Some of the commonly prescribed drugs are described in Table 6-2. The current recommendations for the prescription of various antihypertensive agents are summarized in the Guidelines box above.

NURSING MANAGEMENT

♦ ASSESSMENT
Subjective Data

Knowledge of hypertension and its treatment
Presence of risk factors
    Obesity
    Smoking and alcohol use
    Sedentary life-style
    Positive family history
Usual dietary and activity patterns
Occupation and life-style
Symptoms, if any

Objective Data

Vital signs
Weight
Increased cholesterol or lipid levels

♦ NURSING DIAGNOSES

Nursing diagnoses for the person with hypertension may include, but are not limited to, the following:
    Knowledge deficit (related to disease, treatment, side effects of medications, nonpharmacologic management)
    Noncompliance, high risk for (related to side effects of medications, absence of clinical symptoms, cost of therapy)

♦ EXPECTED PATIENT OUTCOMES

Patient will be knowledgeable about hypertension and its pharmacologic and nonpharmacologic management.
Patient will adhere to prescribed regimen and successfully manage treatment-related side effects.

♦ NURSING INTERVENTIONS
Teaching about Hypertension Management

Reduce risk factors.
Help patient reduce weight and maintain desired weight.
Teach patient principles of modified fat and sodium diets.

TABLE 6-2   Antihypertensive Medications*

DRUG	ACTION†	SIDE EFFECTS†
DIURETICS		
Thiazide/Thiazide-like Diuretics		
Bendroflumethiazide (Naturetin) Benzthiazide (Aquatag, Exna) Chlorothiazide (Diuril) Chlorthalidone (Hygroton) Cyclothiazide (Fluidil) Hydrochlorothiazide (Esidrix, Hydrodiuril) Hydroflumethiazide (Saluron) Indapamide (Lozol) Methyclothiazide (Enduron) Metolazone (Zaroxolyn) Polythiazide (Renese) Quinethazone (Hydromox) Trichlormethiazide (Diurese, Metahydrin)	Block sodium reabsorption in cortical portion of ascending tubule; water excreted with sodium, producing decreased blood volume; NOTE: thiazides ineffective in renal failure	Increased levels of BUN, uric acid, blood glucose, calcium, cholesterol, and triglycerides Decreased potassium Possible postural hypotension in summer from sodium loss Gastrointestinal (GI) upset, dry mouth, thirst, weakness, muscle aches, fatigue, tachycardia Sexual dysfunction May cause increased blood levels of lithium
Loop Diuretics		
Bumetanide (Bumex) Ethacrynic acid (Edecrin) Furosemide (Lasix)	Block sodium and water reabsorption in medullary portion of ascending tubule; cause rapid volume depletion	Decreased potassium Thirst, skin rash, postural hypotension, nausea, vomiting
Potassium-sparing Diuretics		
Amiloride (Midamor) Spironolactone (Aldactone) Triamterene (Dyrenium)	Inhibit aldosterone; sodium excreted in exchange for potassium	Drowsiness, confusion Increased potassium levels Diarrhea Gynecomastia with Aldactone
ADRENERGIC INHIBITORS		
Beta-Adrenergic Blockers		
Acebutolol (Sectral) Atenolol (Tenormin) Betaxolol (Kerlone) Carteolol (Cartrol) Metoprolol (Lopressor) Nadolol (Corgard) Penbutolol (Levatol) Pindolol (Visken) Propranolol (Inderal) Timolol (Blocadren)	Block beta-adrenergic receptors of sympathetic nervous system, decreasing heart rate and blood pressure; NOTE: beta blockers should not be used in patients with asthma, COPD, CHF, and heart block; use with caution in diabetes and peripheral vascular disease	Bronchospasm Bradycardia, fatigue, insomnia Sexual dysfunction Peripheral vascular insufficiency Increased triglycerides
Centrally Acting Alpha Blockers		
Clonidine (Catapres) Guanabenz (Wytensin) Guanfacine (Tenex) Methyldopa (Aldomet)	Activate central receptors that suppress vasomotor and cardiac centers, causing decrease in peripheral resistance; NOTE: rebound hypertension may occur with abrupt discontinuation of drug (except with Aldomet)	Drowsiness, sedation Dry mouth Fatigue Sexual dysfunction Orthostatic hypotension Positive Coombs' test with Aldomet
Peripheral-Acting Adrenergic Antagonists		
Guanadrel (Hylorel) Guanethidine (Ismelin) Rauwolfia serpentina (Raudixin) Reserpine (Serpasil)	Deplete catecholamines in peripheral sympathetic postganglionic fibers Block norepinephrine release from adrenergic nerve endings	Orthostatic hypotension Lethargy, depression Sexual dysfunction Nasal congestion (with Raudixin and Serpasil)
Alpha₁-Adrenergic Blockers		
Doxazosin mesylate (Cardura) Prazosin (Minipress) Terazosin (Vasocard, Hytrin)	Block synaptic receptors that regulate vasomotor tone; reduce peripheral resistance by dilating arterioles and venules	"First dose" syncope, orthostatic hypotension, weakness, palpitations, decreased low-density lipoproteins
Combined Alpha- and Beta-Adrenergic Blockers		
Labetalol (Normodyne, Trandate)	Same as for beta blockers	Bronchospasm, orthostatic hypotension, peripheral vascular insufficiency

TABLE 6-2 Antihypertensive Medications—Cont'd

DRUG	ACTION[†]	SIDE EFFECTS[†]
VASODILATORS		
Hydralazine (Apresoline) Minoxidil (Loniten)	Dilate peripheral blood vessels by directly relaxing vascular smooth muscle; NOTE: usually used in combination with other antihypertensives, because they increase sodium and fluid retention and can cause reflex cardiac stimulation	Headache, dizziness Tachycardia, palpitations, fatigue, edema
ACE INHIBITORS		
Benazepril (Lotensin) Captopril (Capoten), captopril/HCTZ (Capozide) Enalapril (Vasotec), enalapril/HCTZ (Vaseretic) Fosinopril (Monopril) Lisinopril (Prinivil, Zestril), lisinopril/HCTZ (Prinzide, Zestoretic) Ramipril (Altace) Quinapril (Accupril)	Inhibit conversion of angiotensin to angiotensin II, thus blocking release of aldosterone, thereby reducing sodium and water retention	"First dose" hypotension, headache, dizziness, fatigue Increased potassium Cough, skin reactions
CALCIUM ANTAGONISTS		
Amlodipine besylate (Norvasc) Diltiazem (Cardizem) Diltiazem XR (Dilacor) Felodipine (Plendil) Isradipine (DynaCirc) Nifedipine (Procardia), nifedipine XR (Adalat) Nitrendipine Verapamil (Calan, Isoptin) Verapamil SR	Inhibit influx of calcium into muscle cells; act on vascular smooth muscles (primary arteries) to reduce spasms and promote vasodilation	Dizziness, fatigue, nausea, headache, edema

*In addition to this large group of drugs there are also numerous combination agents that contain two or more drugs.
[†]Primary actions and most common side effects are included and are related to entire drug category; consult a drug reference or drug package insert for more specific information.
COPD, Chronic obstructive pulmonary disease; *CHF,* congestive heart failure.

Help patient explore and reduce factors contributing to personal and occupational stress. Patient should do the following:
Balance rest, recreation, and activity.
Plan regular exercise patterns.
Use relaxation techniques.
Help patient reduce or stop smoking.
Help patient master the treatment plan.
Teach patient about prescribed medications. Provide written materials.
Monitor lying, sitting, and standing blood pressures.
Teach patient to accurately monitor own blood pressure.

Fostering Adherence

Teach patient how to manage side effects of medications. Patient should do the following:
Take diuretics early in the day.
Maintain adequate intake of potassium in diet.
Recognize symptoms of hypovolemia.
Prevent or control orthostatic hypotension by avoiding alcohol use and hot baths and making position changes slowly.
Sit immediately if faintness is felt.
Avoid prolonged periods of standing.

Be alert for symptoms of depression or impotence.
Encourage patient to report changes in sexual functioning (libido, erection, or decreased ejaculation), because changes in drug regimen are possible. Sexual problems are common with alpha and beta blockers.
Explore adjustment of drugs or doses with physician.
Support patient's adjustment to long-term management of the disease. Explore obstacles to compliance.

◆ EVALUATION

Successful achievement of expected outcomes for the patient with hypertension is indicated by the following:
Correct description of hypertension, disease management, and reduction of risk factors
Adherence to prescribed regimen and effective control of drug side effects

VENOUS DISORDERS

Venous problems develop when there is an alteration in the transport of blood from the capillary beds back to the heart. Valves may malfunction, or muscle and connective tissue can make the veins less distensible.

DEEP VEIN THROMBOSIS/ THROMBOPHLEBITIS
Etiology/Epidemiology

Thrombophlebitis and deep vein thrombosis (DVT) are common venous disorders characterized by vein inflammation and/or clot formation. Venous stasis, vessel wall injury, and hypercoagulability of the blood are the primary etiologic factors. Stasis can be caused by both incompetent valves and immobility. The presence of thrombosis may be accompanied by or trigger phlebitis in the affected vessel. Thrombophlebitis occurs primarily in the greater or lesser saphenous veins of the lower extremities.

DVT is a common problem in hospitalized persons, causing between 50,00 and 100,000 deaths annually from pulmonary emboli. Both DVT and thrombophlebitis occur more commonly in women and elderly persons. Other risk factors are as follows:

Major abdominal, pelvic, or orthopedic surgery
Oral contraceptive use
Obesity
Pregnancy
Heart disease
Advanced cancer
Coagulation disorders

Pathophysiology

A thrombosis forms as a result of the accumulation of platelets, fibrin, and white and red blood cells that attach at one end to the vein wall. The other end of the thrombus floats freely in the lumen and can break off and migrate as an embolism. The accumulation tends to occur at the bifurcations of deep veins in the leg, particularly the smaller calf veins.

The symptoms depend on the location and size of the thrombus and the adequacy of the collateral circulation. It is estimated that more than 50% of DVTs are asymptomatic. When symptoms develop they include calf pain, edema, and increased calf circumference. Thrombi in the iliac or femoral veins may cause acute pain and pronounced leg swelling. The severity of the symptoms reflects in part the degree of inflammation that is triggered in the vessel by the thrombus. Superficial thrombophlebitis may cause a vessel to feel hard and thready.

Medical Management

DVT is diagnosed through the use of Doppler ultrasonography, impedance plethysmography, and possible venography. Anticoagulation with heparin is the foundation of care for DVT. This prevents the extension of the thrombus and inhibits any new thrombus formation. Heparin therapy is followed by long-term oral anticoagulation, usually with sodium warfarin (Coumadin) (Table 6-3). If the thrombus is causing acute obstruction, thrombolysis with a fibrinolytic agent such as streptokinase or tissue plasminogen activator may be attempted. Bed rest is usually maintained for about 5 to 7 days to allow time for the thrombus to adhere firmly to the wall of the vein.

TABLE 6-3 Anticoagulants		
ACTION	**DOSAGE**	**SIDE EFFECTS**
HEPARIN		
Forms complex with antithrombin III, which inhibits thrombin action	Intravenous: Bolus 5000-10,0000 U	Hemorrhage, spontaneous bleeding, epistaxis, bleeding gums, hematoma, GI bleeding with black tarry stools
Intravenous route produces immediate action; duration is 2 hr	Continuous drip: 20,000-30,000 U/day at 0.5 U/kg/min in 5% dextrose or normal saline	
Subcutaneous route used for maintenance and prophylaxis	Subcutaneous: 5000 U 2 hr before surgery and every 8-12 hr thereafter	
	NOTE: dosage adjusted to maintain APTT at 1.5-2 times laboratory control	
	Normal APTT = 33-45 sec	
	Prolonged APTT = 60-100 sec	
	Acute arterial embolism: 100,000 U	
	Deep vein thrombosis: bolus 5000-10,000 U (1000 U/hr)	
WARFARIN SODIUM (COUMADIN, PANWARFIN)		
Inhibits vitamin K—dependent clotting factor synthesis (factors II, VII, IX, and X)	Oral: 10-15 mg/day until prothrombin time within therapeutic range	Same as for heparin
Depresses prothrombin activity	Then 2-10 mg/day	
Peaks in 36-72 hr	NOTE: dosage adjusted to maintain PT at 2.0-2.5 times laboratory control	
Duration is 2-5 days	Normal PT = 11-12 sec	
	Prolonged PT = 17-19 sec	

APTT, Activated partial thromboplastin time; *PT,* prothrombin time.

NURSING MANAGEMENT

◆ ASSESSMENT

Subjective Data

History of:
  Immobility: long car trip, bed rest
  Surgery: abdominal, pelvic, orthopedic
  Minor trauma to the leg
Pain in calf muscle or thigh during rest or exercise
  Tenderness to palpation
  Pain with dorsiflexion of foot (Homan's sign)

Objective Data

Unilateral edema in ankle, calf, or thigh
Difference in calf circumference of 1.2 cm or more
Redness or heat in affected leg
Positive Doppler or other venous study

◆ NURSING DIAGNOSES

Nursing diagnoses for the person with a deep vein thrombosis may include, but are not limited to, the following:
  Pain (related to inflammation and venous stasis in leg)
  Risk of bleeding (related to anticoagulant therapy)
  Home maintenance management, risk of impaired (related to inadequate knowledge about long-term management of anticoagulant therapy and prevention of future episodes)

◆ EXPECTED PATIENT OUTCOMES

Patient's pain will decrease.
Patient will not experience bleeding while receiving anticoagulant therapy.
Patient will manage home care effectively and take measures to prevent the recurrence of DVT.

◆ NURSING INTERVENTIONS

Relieving Pain

Medicate with analgesics as needed. *Do not administer any products containing aspirin, and teach the patient the importance of checking all OTC products for aspirin content.*
Administer nonsteroidal antiinflammatory drugs (NSAIDs) as ordered to reduce edema.
Maintain patient on bed rest or activity restriction as prescribed with affected leg elevated.
Apply warm, moist heat or cold packs as ordered.

Preventing Bleeding

Administer anticoagulants and/or fibrinolytics as ordered and check for signs of bleeding.
Administer heparin IV or deep subcutaneously with a fine-gauge needle, using a 90-degree angle into lower abdomen.
  Do not aspirate or massage site.
Hold all venipuncture sites firmly for 3 to 5 minutes.

Avoid rectal temperature and intramuscular injections.
Monitor patient's partial thromboplastin time (PTT).
Have protamine sulfate available to reverse effects of heparin.
Hematest urine, emesis, and stools.
Examine skin for petechiae or ecchymoses.
Measure calf or thigh circumference daily.
Assess adequacy of peripheral circulation.
Observe for signs of pulmonary embolism, such as sudden sharp chest pain or dyspnea.

Teaching for Effective Home Management

Apply TED stockings. Measure leg carefully for correct fit. Teach patient proper use for home care—put on before getting out of bed in morning.
Teach patient general principles of leg and foot care.
  Elevate legs above the heart at intervals throughout the day.
  Perform ankle flexion and extension exercises frequently when standing or sitting.
  Engage in regular aerobic exercise.
Teach patient to use soft toothbrushes and avoid use of straight razors.
Teach patient to avoid products containing aspirin.
Teach patient to avoid constricting clothing around the knee or calf.
Teach patient to wear support hose/TED stockings, particularly during periods of enforced immobility such as long car or plane trips.

◆ EVALUATION

Successful achievement of expected outcomes for the patient with deep vein thrombosis is indicated by the following:
  Absence of leg pain
  No evidence of bleeding
  Correct description of life-style modifications required for safe, long-term anticoagulation

VARICOSE VEINS
Etiology/Epidemiology

Varicose veins are abnormally dilated veins with incompetent valves. They affect up to 20% of the population

---

BOX 6-3   The Greenfield Filter

The Greenfield filter (Figure 6-6) is a small device that can be inserted percutaneously through the jugular or the femoral vein. It is typically positioned in the inferior vena cava just below the renal veins. It is effective in preventing clots from traveling to the lungs, and the design of the filter is successful in preventing its migration within the vena cava. The filter is left in place for life, and the patient typically continues to receive low-dose oral anticoagulant therapy.

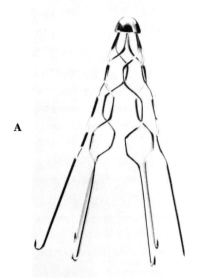

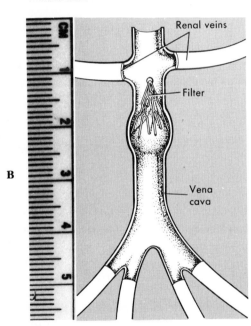

FIGURE 6-6   A, Greenfield vena cava filter. **B,** Greenfield filter is placed in inferior vena cava just below renal veins. (**A** from Davis JH et al: *Clinical surgery,* St Louis, 1987, Mosby. **B** from Beare PG, Myers JL: *Principles and practice of adult health nursing,* ed 2, St Louis, 1994, Mosby.)

and occur most often in the lower extremities and lower trunk, usually in the great and small saphenous veins. The highest incidence is in women between 30 and 50 years of age. Congenitally defective valves, prolonged standing, and systemic conditions that interfere with venous return such as pregnancy or ascites all contribute to the development of varicosities.

Spider veins, venous stars, or telangiectasias are not varicose veins. They are small dilated cutaneous veins that appear as a blemish. They do not typically require surgical intervention.

BOX 6-4	Pulmonary Embolism

Pulmonary embolism remains a major cause of mortality for hospitalized patients. The resulting pathologic condition is complex. Blockage of the pulmonary arterioles can prevent oxygen from reaching the circulation, and the patient becomes profoundly hypoxemic. Failure of surfactant production causes the alveoli to collapse, and pulmonary hypertension develops rapidly and severely with a subsequent decline in cardiac output.

SYMPTOMS

There are no warning signs. Symptoms relate to the size of the clot and overall health of the tissue. Common symptoms include the following:

Sudden, severe dyspnea, tachypnea, and chest pain
Restlessness and anxiety
Tachycardia
Cough and hemoptysis
Cyanosis

TREATMENT

Treatment revolves around anticoagulation and supportive care to sustain cardiopulmonary function. Death results in 10% of cases within 1 hour. Treatment measures include the following:

IV heparin
Oxygen therapy, intubation if necessary
Correction of dysrhythmia
Pain relief
Treatment of shock

Pathophysiology

The primary pathologic factor is weakening of the vein wall. The vein wall weakens from a deficiency of elastin or collagen and cannot withstand normal pressures. The vessel dilates with pooling of blood, and the valves become stretched and incompetent. A primary disease process usually has a slow onset and affects the superficial veins. A secondary process affects the deep veins, often from injury or DVT. Classic symptoms of varicose veins include dull aching or heaviness, fatigue, and edema.

Medical Management

Most varicose veins can be managed conservatively with life-style modifications and the use of support stockings. Surgical intervention with ligation and stripping is indicated for more complex cases. Incisions are made at the ankle, knee, and groin to strip the involved vein. The limb is completely wrapped postsurgically in compression dressings.

NURSING MANAGEMENT

Nursing care following surgery involves the standard postoperative measures. The affected leg is kept elevated when lying or sitting to promote venous return. Pain management is essential before attempts at ambulation. Teaching for long-term management involves

BOX
6-5 **Leg Ulcers**

Most leg ulcers result from chronic venous insufficiency. Persons with diabetes are at particular risk because of their corresponding deficits in sensory awareness. Arterial insufficiency can also result in ulceration from inadequate exchange of oxygen and other nutrients. The lesions are open and necrotic and are rapidly complicated by bacterial invasion.

Most venous ulcers are located on the medial aspect of the ankle and are moderately painful. Edema and changes in pigmentation in the area are common. Arterial ulcers tend to develop on the heel, toes, and dorsum of the foot. They are more painful and often present with a pale or mottled appearance.

TREATMENT

Necrotic tissue is debrided, and the ulcer is treated with wet to dry dressings, chemical agents, or hydrophilic coverings. An Unna boot, created from gauze impregnated with substances that harden around the leg, may be applied to a small new ulcer. The boot is changed weekly during the healing process. Whirlpool therapy is also helpful in some situations. Topical and systemic antibiotics are also typically administered. Healing time is often prolonged, and future breakdown in the area is common.

BOX
6-6 **Common Causes of Shock**

HYPOVOLEMIC SHOCK

Excessive blood loss from trauma, GI bleeding, surgery, or coagulation disorders
Loss of body fluids other than blood—vomiting and diarrhea, ketoacidosis
Movement of fluids from the vascular to the interstitial compartment or peritoneal cavity, as in burns or complete bowel obstruction

CARDIOGENIC SHOCK

Myocardial infarction
Pulmonary embolism
Cardiac tamponade
Dysrhythmia

NEUROGENIC/VASOGENIC SHOCK

Spinal cord injury
Anaphylactic response to drugs, toxins, dyes
Gram-negative sepsis, particularly involving the urinary tract and prostate

---

ongoing use of elastic stockings for activities that will require prolonged standing. Moderate active exercise is recommended daily. The patient is also encouraged to elevate the legs at intervals throughout the day if possible to facilitate venous return and to monitor the development of local edema. The affected limb should be protected from trauma if possible, because local infection is an ongoing concern.

SHOCK
ETIOLOGY/EPIDEMIOLOGY

Shock is a life-threatening condition involving virtually all body systems that is characterized by inadequate perfusion at the cellular level. With the level of patient acuity that defines tertiary-care institutions today, virtually any patient can be considered at risk for shock. Any condition in which the level of tissue perfusion is inadequate to meet the cells' needs for oxygen and nutrients can result in shock. A common classification system for shock is as follows:

cardiogenic Related to inability of the heart to pump sufficient blood to perfuse the body. Myocardial infarction is the most common cause (see Chapter 5).
hypovolemic Related to an inadequate volume within the vascular compartment. It is the most common form of shock and will serve as the model for discussion.
neurogenic/vasogenic Related to massive dilation of the blood vessels caused by interference with the sympathetic nervous system, as occurs with spinal cord injury (see Chapter 13); release of vasoactive substances during an

allergic response or anaphylaxis; (see Chapter 17); or release of endotoxins from gram-negative organisms, which triggers release of numerous vasoactive substances in sepsis.

Common causes of each type of shock are summarized in Box 6-6. A description of the various stages of shock is presented in Box 6-7.

PATHOPHYSIOLOGY

In the early stages of shock the body's compensatory mechanisms are able to sustain adequate blood flow to the tissues. The mechanisms primarily involved in compensation include the sympathetic nervous system, which stimulates the heart and causes peripheral vasoconstriction; and the endocrine system, which initiates the fight-or-flight response with increased secretion of glucocorticoids, antidiuretic hormone (ADH), and renin/aldosterone to conserve body fluids.

As shock progresses, however, blood flow to all body tissues becomes impaired. Anaerobic metabolism takes over, and adenosine triphosphate production is severely impaired. Acid metabolites accumulate and cause dilation at the arteriole end of the capillaries. Fluid shifts to the interstitium and decreases blood volume. Decreased flow to the kidney results in oliguria and anuria, with accumulation of metabolic wastes. Ischemia of the abdominal organs causes release of a myocardial depressant factor from the pancreas, which compromises cardiac contractility. Beyond a certain point the cycle of shock becomes irreversible. At this point the patient is vulnerable to tubular necrosis and renal failure, paralytic ileus and stress ulcers, falling cardiac output and dysrhythmias, adult respiratory distress system (ARDS),

BOX 6-7 Stages of Shock

INITIAL STAGE
Inadequate oxygen delivery initiates the early cellular changes as evidenced by increased levels of blood lactates.

COMPENSATORY STAGE
Decreased cardiac output triggers multiple nervous, hormonal, and chemical mechanisms to maintain perfusion to the vital organs. These include classic features such as tachycardia, tachypnea, increased force of contraction of the ventricles, peripheral vasoconstriction, fluid retention, and shunting of the blood to the vital organs.

PROGRESSIVE STAGE
The compensatory mechanisms are no longer able to maintain vital organ perfusion. Organ function begins to deteriorate. Classic symptoms include a falling blood pressure, tachycardia with or without dysrhythmia, weak or absent peripheral pulses, urine volume of less than 20 ml/hr, cold mottled skin, and decreased responsiveness progressing to coma.

REFRACTORY STAGE
The shock state is so advanced that death from multiple organ failure is imminent.

BOX 6-8 Signs and Symptoms of Shock

EARLY SHOCK
Tachycardia, tachypnea
Blood pressure normal or slightly lowered, decreased pulse pressure
Decreased urine output, increased specific gravity, thirst
Alert, restless, nonspecific anxiety

PROGRESSIVE SHOCK
Tachycardia
Decreased blood pressure
Rapid shallow respirations
Oliguria or anuria
Cool clammy skin
Decreased bowel sounds, ileus
Petechiae, spontaneous bleeding
Lethargy, coma

GERONTOLOGIC PATIENT CONSIDERATIONS FOR SEPTIC SHOCK

Almost half of all cases of septic shock develop in persons over 65 years of age. Organ function is impaired from chronic illnesses, and poor nutrition can worsen overall immune system functioning. The gram-negative bacilli, such as *Escherichia coli, Klebsiella, Enterobacter, Serratia,* and *Pseudomonas,* account for about 50% of all cases of septic shock. These organisms contain a lipoprotein called an endotoxin that is responsible for the multiple adverse effects throughout the body. The multiple chemical mediators include histamine, prostaglandins, kinins, interleukins, and endorphins. Elderly patients are more likely to come into contact with these bacilli from catheterization, intrusive procedures, and residence in long-term care facilities.

Volume replacement in elderly persons must be undertaken with caution. The elderly person is often unable to tolerate rapid infusion and can experience heart failure. Drug metabolism and excretion are also typically impaired, and drug dosages may need to be adjusted.

Commonly employed drugs in shock states include the following:
Mixed alpha- and beta-adrenergics—dopamine, dobutamine, epinephrine, amrinone
Beta-adrenergics—isoproteronol
Vasodilators—nitroprusside, nitroglycerin
Vasopressors—norepinephrine, phentolamine, and phenylephrine

Supportive measure in shock may include oxygen therapy and intubation for mechanical ventilation; blood product transfusion; and correction of acidosis.

NURSING MANAGEMENT

◆ ASSESSMENT
Subjective Data
History of surgery, trauma, infection
Level of consciousness—presence of confusion
Sense of anxiety or restlessness
Nausea or thirst

Objective Data
Vital signs—lying and sitting if possible
Central venous pressure, other hemodynamic monitoring as available
Respiratory rate, depth, pattern; breath sounds
Blood gases
Intake and output, urine specific gravity
Bowel sounds
Skin temperature, moisture
  Cool, pale, and moist in hypovolemic shock
  Warm, dry, and pink in neurogenic shock

sepsis, and disseminated intravascular coagulation (DIC). The classic symptoms are summarized in Box 6-8.

MEDICAL MANAGEMENT

Medical management is determined by the stage of shock and the patient's unique condition. Strategies include fluid replacement with crystalloid, colloid, and blood solutions; vasoactive drugs to sustain blood pressure; antibiotics; and supplemental oxygen. An intraaortic balloon may be inserted to support the action of a failing left ventricle.

◆ NURSING DIAGNOSES

Nursing diagnoses for the person in shock may include, but are not limited to, the following:

Fluid volume deficit (related to fluid shifts or direct losses)

Cardiac output, decreased (related to damage to the heart muscle and effects of waste products and depressant factors)

Gas exchange, impaired (related to decreased lung compliance and interstitial edema)

Infection or bleeding, risk of (related to suppressed immune system functioning and excess gastric acid production)

Anxiety (related to seriousness of condition and uncertainty of outcomes)

◆ EXPECTED PATIENT OUTCOMES

Patient will maintain an acceptable balance of intake and output.

Patient will maintain cardiac output within normal range.

Patient will maintain a satisfactory exchange of oxygen and carbon dioxide.

Patient will not experience infection or bleeding.

Patient will report decreased anxiety.

◆ NURSING INTERVENTIONS

Restoring Fluid Balance

Administer IV fluids as ordered.

Administer blood products if ordered.

Measure and record intake and output hourly.

Auscultate bowel sounds.

Keep patient NPO if ileus is present.

Provide ice chips for thirst and comfort.

Provide mouth care.

Supporting Cardiac Output

Monitor and record vital signs, right atrial pressure, pulmonary artery pressure, and cardiac output hourly or as ordered.

Administer vasoactive drugs as ordered:

Always use IV pump to control flow.

Monitor vital signs continuously every 5 to 15 minutes.

Maintain patency of infusions—drugs are very irritating to tissue.

Follow hemodynamic parameters if available.

Place patient flat in bed with legs slightly elevated.

Change positions frequently.

Keep patient at absolute rest. Maintain a neutral environmental temperature to conserve energy.

Supporting Gas Exchange

Administer prescribed supplemental oxygen.

NOTE: Patient will need to be intubated if symptoms of ARDS develop.

Encourage deep breathing—actively prevent complications related to immobility.

Assess level of consciousness every hour.

Assess skin color and temperature.

Monitor oxygen saturation and Po_2 regularly.

Preventing Injury

Protect patient from injury if restless or confused.

Maintain strict aseptic technique for inserting all monitoring lines, suctioning, and so forth. Monitor carefully for signs of infection.

Monitor frequently for petechiae or signs of bleeding.

Administer antacids or histamine H_2 receptor blockers as ordered to prevent stress ulceration.

Relieving Anxiety

Support and reassure patient and family frequently. Assist to remain quiet and relaxed if possible.

Explain all equipment and monitoring lines.

Describe treatments before use.

Make time for the family to be present at the bedside if possible.

Keep the family informed of the patient's progress.

Make appropriate use of touch.

Arrange for support from minister or chaplain if desired.

◆ EVALUATION

Successful achievement of expected outcomes for the patient in shock is indicated by the following:

A balanced intake and output; urine output of 30 to 50 ml/hr

Stable blood pressure without drug support

Oxygen saturation >94; Po_2 >90

Absence of infection or bleeding

Verbalization of decreased anxiety; presence of family or other support persons at the bedside

SELECTED REFERENCES

Anderson K: Thrombolytic therapy for treatment of acute peripheral arterial occlusion, *J Vasc Nurs* 10(3):20-24, 1992.

Blank CA, Irwin GH: Peripheral vascular disorders, *Nurs Clin North Am* 25(4):777-794, 1990.

Bright LD, Georgi S: Peripheral vascular disease: is it arterial or venous? *Am J Nurs* 92:34-47, 1992.

Davis E: The diagnostic puzzle and management challenge of Raynaud's syndrome, *Nurse Pract* 18:18-25, 1993.

Eliopoulos C: PVD: protecting patients from complications, *Nurs 91*, pp 32-34, 1991.

Emma LA: Chronic arterial occlusive disease, *J Cardiovasc Nurs* 7:14-24, 1992.

Fellows E, Jocz AM: Getting the upper hand on lower extremity arterial disease, *Nurs 91*, pp 34-42, 1991.

Harris KA: Graft infections, *J Vasc Nurs* 10(1):13-17, 1992.

Herzog J: Deep vein thrombosis in the rehabilitation client: diagnostic tools, prevention, and treatment modalities, *Rehabil Nurs* 18:8-11, 1993.

Hill MN, Cunningham SG: The latest words for high blood pressure, *Am J Nurs* 89:504-509, 1989.

Johannsen JM: Update: guidelines for treating hypertension, *Am J Nurs* 93 42-49, 1993.

LaQuaglia JD, Appleton DL: Vascular disease and postoperative nursing management, *Crit Care Nurse* 5:34-42, 1990.

Lovell MB, Harris KA: Abdominal aortic aneurysms, *J Vasc Nurs* 9:2-6, 1991.

Lovell MB et al: The management of chronic venous disease, *J Vasc Nurs* 11(2):43-47, 1993.

Nunnelee JD, Kurgan A: Interruption of the inferior vena cava for venous thromboembolic disease, *J Vasc Nurs* 11(3):80-82, 1993.

Payne JS: Alternative for revascularization: peripheral atherectomy devices, *J Vasc Nurs* 10(3):2-8, 1992.

Rice V: Shock, a clinical syndrome: an update. I. An overview of shock. II. The stages of shock. III. Therapeutic management. IV. Nursing care of the shock patient, *Crit Care Nurse* 11(4):20-27, 11(5):74-82, 11(6):34-39, 11(7):28-40, 1991.

Rice V, editor: Shock, *Crit Care Nurs Clin North Am* 2(2):143-342, 1990.

Rudolphi D: Limb loss in the elderly peripheral vascular disease patient, *J Vasc Nurs* 10(3):8-13, 1992.

Siedlecki B: Peripheral vascular disease, *Can Nurse* 88:26-28, 1992.

Trottier DI, Kochar MS: Hypertension and high cholesterol: a dangerous synergy, *Am J Nurs* 92:40-43, 1992.

Young JR et al: *Peripheral vascular diseases,* St Louis, 1991, Mosby.

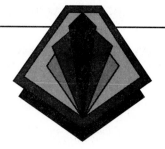

C H A P T E R   7

Disorders of the Blood and Blood-Forming Organs

◆ ASSESSMENT

SUBJECTIVE DATA

Health history
    Family history of inherited hematologic disorders
        Sickle cell trait, anemia; thalassemia
        Hemophilia
    Work-related exposure to toxins
    Medications in use:
        prescription and over the counter (OTC)
        Use of aspirin
        Use of anticoagulants
        Antibiotic use, particularly chloramphenicol
        Use of prescription tranquilizers or sedatives
    Treatment for tuberculosis, such as isoniazid, PASA, streptomycin
    Exposure to or use of cytotoxic agents
    History of frequent nosebleeds; prolonged bleeding after injury or extraction
    Diet history
        Use of vitamin and mineral supplements
Current health problem
    Chronic fatigue, activity intolerance
    Dyspnea on exertion, palpitations
    Dizziness or faintness, vertigo
    Fever or night sweats, frequent infection
    Increased or excess menstrual flow
    Easy bruising
    Presence of paresthesias
    Anorexia, sore tongue, dysphagia
        Weight loss

OBJECTIVE DATA

Skin
    Petechiae, ecchymoses, and/or purpura
    Jaundice (skin and sclerae)
    Pallor (skin, mucous membranes, conjunctivae)
    Changes in skin texture
        Dry skin and hair, brittle nails, concave nails
    Lesions or draining areas (surface skin and on mucous membranes)
    Atrophy of tongue papilla; smooth, red appearance
    Cracks at the corners of the mouth

Lymph node enlargement
    Pain or tenderness
Liver or spleen enlargement
Joint or bone pain, particularly along ribs or sternum
Nervous system
    Cranial nerve function
    Sensory function, paresthesias

✍ LABORATORY TESTS

Blood Tests

Blood tests form the cornerstone of evaluation of persons with suspected problems involving the blood and blood-forming organs. Blood tests are also used to monitor the response to therapy. Table 7-1 summarizes the basic blood tests used to evaluate the hematologic system, which are also described below:

1. Hemoglobin: measures the amount of Hb in the circulation
2. Hematocrit: represents the ratio of red blood cells (RBCs) to total blood volume

GERONTOLOGIC PATIENT CONSIDERATIONS: PHYSIOLOGIC CHANGES IN HEMATOLOGIC FUNCTION

Findings from animal studies suggest that changes associated with the aging process have little clinical significance. The cellularity of the marrow decreases, but the actual counts exhibit minimal change.
    Minimal changes in leukocyte count and differential
        Less response to the stimulus of infection
    Hemoglobin (Hb) decreases after middle age, more strongly in men than women
    Iron absorption unimpaired
    Serum iron and iron binding capacity decrease
    Low serum levels of B_{12} and folic acid but no evidence of corresponding anemia in most people
    (**NOTE:** Nutritional anemias are common in elderly persons, but their presence appears to be more related to dietary inadequacies than to physiologic changes and blood cell production.)
    No change in platelet number or function
    Slight increase in some clotting factors

TABLE 7-1 Common Laboratory Tests Used to Evaluate the Hematologic System

TEST	NORMAL VALUES	SIGNIFICANCE OF ABNORMAL FINDINGS
TESTS OF THE HEMATOLOGIC SYSTEM		
RBC count	3.6-5.0 million/mm³ (women)	*Decreased levels* indicate possible anemia or hemorrhage.
	4.2-5.5 million/mm³ (men)	*Elevations* indicate possible chronic anoxia.
Hemoglobin (Hb)	12-15 g/dl (women)	Same as for RBC count.
	14-16.5 g/dl (men)	
Hematocrit (Hct)	37%-45% (women)	Same as for RBC count.
	42%-50% (men)	
Mean corpuscular volume (MCV)	80-95 μm³	*Elevations* indicate possible macrocytic RBCs.
		Decreased levels indicate possible microcytic RBCs.
Mean corpuscular hemoglobin (MCH)	27-31 pg	*Elevations* are associated with macrocytic anemia.
		Decreased levels are associated with microcytic anemia.
Mean corpuscular hemoglobin concentration (MCHC)	32-36 g/dl (32%-36%)	*Decreased levels* indicate possible hypochromic cells.
		Elevations are associated with spherocytosis.
White blood cell (WBC) count	4,500-11,000/mm³	*Elevations* indicate possible infection.
		Decreased levels indicate possible bone marrow failure.
Reticulocyte count	0.5%-2% of total RBC count	*Elevations* indicate possible polycythemia vera.
		Decreased levels indicate possible inadequate RBC production.
Iron (Fe)	60-90 μg/dL	*Decreased levels* indicate possible iron deficiency anemia.
Platelet count	150,000-350,000/mm³	*Elevations* indicate possible hemorrhage, polycythemia vera, or malignancy.
		Decreased levels indicate possible bone marrow failure, hypersplenism, or accelerated consumption of platelets.
Coagulation Tests		
Prothrombin time (PT)	11-12.5 sec (85-100%)	*Elevations* indicate possible deficiency of factors V and VII.
Partial thromboplastin time (PTT)	30-40 sec	*Elevations* indicate possible deficiency of factors II, V, VIII, IX, XI, or XII.
Bleeding time	1-9 min	*Elevations* indicate possible thrombocytopenia, marrow infiltration, or inadequate platelet function.

3. Red blood cell indices
   a. Mean corpuscular volume (MCV): estimates the average size of the RBC
   b. Mean corpuscular hemoglobin (MCH): measures the content of hemoglobin in the RBC
   c. Mean corpuscular hemoglobin concentration (MCHC): measures the entire blood volume of hemoglobin rather than just a single cell
4. Reticulocyte count: measures the number of immature RBCs in the circulation; serves as a measure of bone marrow function
5. Coombs' test: detects antibodies against RBCs and is crucial in blood typing
6. Prothrombin time (PT): evaluates the intactness of the extrinsic coagulation cascade (factors V and VII)
7. Partial thromboplastin time (PTT): evaluates the intactness of the intrinsic coagulation cascade (factors II, V, VIII, IX, XI, XII)

Biopsies
Bone marrow aspiration and biopsy

Purpose—Bone marrow aspiration and biopsy are used to obtain a sample of marrow for histologic and hematologic examination to support the diagnosis of blood disorders (Figure 7-1). Aspiration permits retrieval

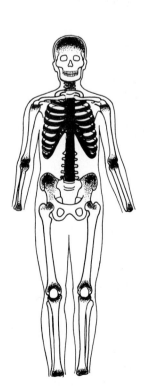

FIGURE 7-1 Sites of active bone marrow hematopoiesis.

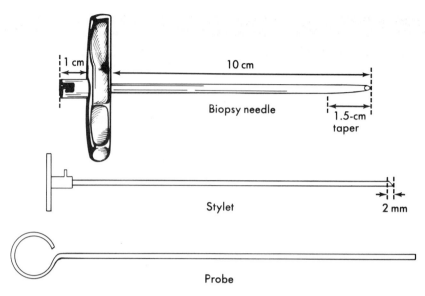

FIGURE 7-2 Bone marrow biopsy needle showing shape and size.

of a fluid sample, whereas actual biopsy removes a core of bone marrow.

Procedure—The skin over the biopsy site is cleansed, and a local anesthetic is injected. The biopsy needle (Figure 7-2) is inserted and carefully advanced into the cortex of the bone. A tissue plug is removed, and a pressure dressing is applied. The test takes about 15 minutes.

Patient preparation and aftercare—No special preparation is needed except careful patient teaching about the nature of the procedure and the importance of remaining completely still. A consent form is usually required. The patient is informed that a local anesthetic is used, but that a sudden sharp pain will still be experienced when the marrow is aspirated. After the biopsy the puncture site is carefully checked for bleeding and inflammation.

DISORDERS OF THE RED BLOOD CELLS
ANEMIA

The development of the various component blood cells is illustrated in Figure 7-3. Anemia is a broad category of disorders involving a deficiency of RBCs as reflected in

BOX 7-1	Classifying Anemias by Red Cell Morphology

-cytic: suffix refers to the size of the cell
-chromic: suffix refers to the amount of Hb

NORMOCYTIC NORMOCHROMIC ANEMIA

- Normal cell size and hemoglobin content
- Caused by acute blood loss and most hemolytic processes

MICROCYTIC NORMOCHROMIC ANEMIA

- Small cell size but normal hemoglobin content
- Caused by infection, tumor, and chronic illness

MACROCYTIC NORMOCHROMIC ANEMIA

- Large irregular cell size with normal hemoglobin content
- Caused by nutritional deficiencies such as folic acid or vitamin B_{12}

MICROCYTIC HYPOCHROMIC ANEMIA

- Small cell size and decreased hemoglobin content
- Caused by nutritional deficiency of iron or chronic blood loss, such as from the gastrointestinal (GI) tract or menses

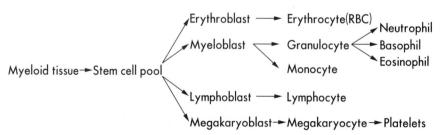

FIGURE 7-3 Formation of blood cells from myeloid tissue. (From Yasko J: *Guidelines for cancer care: symptom management,* Reston, VA, 1983, Reston Publishing.)

TABLE 7-2   The Anemias Classified by Common Causes

ETIOLOGY	SIGNS AND SYMPTOMS	MEDICAL MANAGEMENT
BLOOD LOSS		
Acute		
Hemorrhage (trauma, GI bleeding)	Physiologic signs of shock	Stop source of bleeding; restore losses with IV fluid, whole blood, or packed cell transfusions. Treat shock.
Chronic		
Slow GI loss (malignancy, peptic ulcers) Vaginal bleeding (menstrual disorders) Hemorrhoids	Patient may remain asymptomatic with RBC and Hb at significantly depressed levels, then have chronic fatigue, weakness, tachycardia, exertional dyspnea, pallor of skin and mucous membranes	Stop source of blood loss. Promote proper nutrition; give supplemental iron.
IMPAIRED PRODUCTION		
Aplastic Anemia (Depression or Cessation of *All* Blood-forming Elements)		
Bone marrow depression from drugs, chemicals, virus, radiation; unidentified causes in 50% of cases Special attention to: Chloramphenicol Anticonvulsants Sulfonamides Butazolidine	Symptoms as with chronic blood loss; problem often also affects white cells and platelets	Remove causative agent if possible. Provide supportive care until bone marrow regeneration is possible: transfusions of RBCs, platelets; laminar air flow to protect from infection. Perform bone marrow transplant if suitable donor available.
INCREASED DESTRUCTION OF RBCs (HEMOLYSIS)		
Congenital		
Sickle cell disease (hemoglobinopathy)		
Hereditary abnormality in hemoglobin protein that occurs primarily in African-American population; hemoglobin S variant tends to sickle in shape in presence of low oxygen tension, slowing circulation and increasing cellular hypoxia and infarcts; RBC life span shortened	General symptoms of anemia plus painful episodes of vasoocclusive crisis (see p. 114)	No specific therapy. Treat symptoms with analgesics, oxygen, IV hydration. Provide supportive care during exacerbations. Provide genetic counseling for carriers.
Thalassemia		
Inherited disorder of decreased synthesis of hemoglobin and malformation of RBCs that increases their hemolysis; occurs primarily in Orientals or persons of Mediterranean heritage	Thalassemia minor—usually asymptomatic or symptoms of mild anemia Thalassemia major—severe anemia, enlarged spleen, jaundice, growth failure	No therapy usually needed. Transfusions for severe form to maintain patient in relatively symptom-free state; usually fatal in young adulthood.
Enzyme deficiency of G-6-PD (glucose-6-phosphate dehydrogenase)		
Inherited deficiency of enzyme in pathways that metabolize glucose and generate ATP, leading to premature RBC destruction	General symptoms of anemia are produced through acute hemolysis occurring when cells are exposed to oxidant drugs such as aspirin or sulfonamides, usually in response to infection	Diagnose condition and remove the drug stimulus.
Acquired Hemolytic		
Most often drug-induced or autoimmune; antibodies are produced that cause premature destruction of the RBCs	General symptoms of anemia reflecting severity of disorder	Attempt to suppress antigen-antibody reactions through administration of corticosteroids. Beneficial in about 50% of cases.

hemoglobin level, hematocrit, and RBC count. The anemias can be classified in a variety of ways. The two major classifications are by red cell morphology or by etiology. The morphology classification is demonstrated in Box 7-1, and Table 7-2 classifies the anemias by etiologic group.

Iron Deficiency Anemia
Etiology/epidemiology

Iron deficiency is the most common form of anemia. The basic disorder involves an inadequate supply of iron to meet the needs for developing RBCs. The body first depletes its iron stores in the bone marrow, spleen, liver,

TABLE 7-2 The Anemias Classified by Common Causes—Continued

ETIOLOGY	SIGNS AND SYMPTOMS	MEDICAL MANAGEMENT
NUTRITIONAL DEFICIENCY		
Iron Deficiency		
Deficiency of iron leads to synthesis of RBCs with a decreased amount of hemoglobin; eventually leads to decreased number of cells	Few overt clinical signs in early stages, then gradual development of fatigue and exertional dyspnea, plus: Brittle concave nails Shiny, bright red, smooth tongue Cracks in corner of mouth	Determine cause and correct. Provide adequate balanced diet (rarely a major factor). Administer ferrous sulfate orally or parenterally if GI absorption is insufficient.
Megaloblastic Anemia		
Vitamin B₁₂ deficiency (pernicious anemia)		
Insufficient amount of B_{12} absorbed from intestine (B_{12} is essential for synthesis of RBCs); malabsorption syndrome and loss of intrinsic factor following gastric surgery are possible causes	General signs of anemia plus: Peripheral neuropathy Ataxia	Administer vitamin B_{12} parenterally weekly or monthly.
Folic acid deficiency		
Often occurs with chronic alcoholism, or malabsorption syndromes (folic acid is essential for synthesis of RBCs)	General signs of anemia plus symptoms of underlying disease	Administer oral folic acid and a well-balanced diet. Treat underlying disorder.

and muscle before turning to the hemoglobin pool. The anemia results from chronic blood loss, increased body demand as during pregnancy, adolescence, or infection; or from dietary inadequacy related to malnutrition, malabsorption, or inadequate intake. It is a worldwide problem but occurs most often in women, children, and elderly persons.

Pathophysiology

Iron is an essential component of the hemoglobin molecule, and its deficiency leads to the production of fewer RBCs and cells with a decreased hemoglobin content. The anemia typically develops gradually, and the individual may adapt successfully to the changes and exhibit few overt symptoms. The anemia interferes with the transport of oxygen to the tissues and leads to tissue hypoxia. The body compensates by increasing both the rate of circulation and respiration. Fatigue, mild tachycardia, and exertional dyspnea are the most characteristic symptoms of mild disease. Severe deficiency may cause the nails to become brittle and concave (spoon shaped) with longitudinal ridges. The papillae of the tongue atrophy and create a smooth red appearance. The corners of the mouth may crack and become red and painful.

Medical management

Iron deficiency anemia creates a microcytic hypochromic form of anemia. The diagnosis is confirmed by the presence of a low serum iron or ferritin and an elevated serum iron-binding capacity. The primary treatment is to increase the amount of iron in the diet. Oral iron supplement is usually given in the form of ferrous sulfate. Blood transfusion with packed red blood cells

may occasionally be needed (see Guidelines box on p. 114). Table 7-3 presents various types of blood components that may be administered.

NURSING MANAGEMENT

Patient teaching for successful self-care is the major nursing consideration. Poor diet is rarely the sole cause of iron deficiency anemia, but it often is a contributory cause. The nurse assists the patient to analyze the diet for adequacy of iron intake and instructs the patient on iron-rich sources such as red meats, organ meats, whole wheat products, egg yolks, spinach, kidney beans, carrots, and raisins. An adequate intake should provide about 10 to 15 mg of iron daily.

The nurse also instructs the patient about iron supplement use. The pills should be taken after meals with a vitamin C source such as orange juice to promote iron absorption. Iron is initially irritating to the GI tract and may cause nausea. Either diarrhea or constipation can occur, and the stools will be black. A stool softener may be needed. If the individual cannot absorb sufficient iron orally, parenteral iron therapy, administered via deep Z track injection, may be used.

Sickle Cell Anemia
Etiology/epidemiology

Sickle cell anemia is the most common genetic disorder in the United States. It predominates in the African-American population, where it is estimated that 1 in 12 persons is a carrier and 1 in 65 develops the anemia. The disease is transmitted as a homozygous recessive disorder and creates a chronic hemolytic anemia. A heterozygous state creates a usually asymptomatic con-

TABLE 7-3 Types of Blood Components

BLOOD COMPONENT	DESCRIPTION	USAGE	COMMENTS
RED BLOOD CELLS (RBCs)			
Packed RBCs (PRBCs)	RBCs separated from plasma and platelets	Anemia Moderate blood loss	Decreased risk of fluid overload as compared to whole blood
Autologous PRBCs	Same as packed RBCs	Elective surgery for which blood replacement is expected	Units may be stored for up to 35 days
Washed RBCs	RBCs washed with sterile isotonic saline before transfusion	Previous allergic reactions to transfusions	Increased removal of immunoglobulins and protein
Frozen RBCs	RBCs frozen in a glycerol solution; cells washed after thawing to remove the glycerol	Storage of rare type of blood Storage of autologous blood for future use	Relatively free of leukocytes and microemboli Expensive
Leukocyte-poor RBCs	RBCs from which most leukocytes have been removed	Previous sensitivity to leukocyte antigens from prior transfusions or from pregnancy	Fewer RBCs than packed RBCs; washed leukocyte-poor RBC units have more RBCs than nonwashed
Neocytes	RBC units with high number of reticulocytes (young RBCs)	Transfusion-dependent anemias	Fewer problems with iron overload Expensive
OTHER CELLULAR COMPONENTS			
Platelets			
Random donor packs	Platelets separated from RBCs by centrifuge; given in 50 ml of plasma	Thrombocytopenia DIC	Plasma base is rich in coagulation factors Platelet preparations can also be packed, washed, or made leukocyte-poor
Pheresis packs	Platelets from an HLA-matched donor, separated by pheresis	Allosensitized persons with thrombocytopenia	Requires specialized techniques
Granulocytes	Granular leukocytes separated by pheresis	Granulocytopenia from malignancy or chemotherapy	Allergen sensitization may occur with chills and fever
PLASMA COMPONENTS			
Fresh frozen plasma (FFP)	Freezing of plasma within 4 hr of collection	Clotting deficiencies Liver disease Hemophilia Defibrination	Preserves factors V, VII, VIII, IX, and X and prothrombin Minimizes hepatitis risk Administered through a filter
Factor concentrates VIII and IX	Prepared from large donor pools Heated to inactivate HIV	VIII: hemophilia A IX: hemophilia B	Increased risk of hepatitis (VIII, IX) and thromboembolism (IX) Given in small volumes
Cryoprecipitate	Precipitated material obtained from FFP when thawed	Hemophilia A Infection of burns Hypofibrinogenemia Uremic bleeding	Contains factors VIII and XIII and fibrinogen

Serum albumin
  Normal serum albumin (NSA)
  Plasma protein fraction (PPF)
	Albumin chemically processed from pooled plasma	Hypovolemic shock
		Hypoalbuminemia
		Burns
		Hemorrhagic shock
			No risk of hepatitis
			Does not require ABO compatibility
			Lacks clotting factors
			Hypotension may occur if PPF is given faster than 10 ml/min

Immune serum globulin	Obtained from plasma of preselected donors with specific antibodies	Hypogammaglobulinemia Prophylaxis for hepatitis A	Given intramuscularly

dition called the sickle cell trait. The basic abnormality involves the substitution of a single amino acid within the beta polypeptide chain of the globin portion of hemoglobin.

Pathophysiology

The rearrangement of the structure of the polypeptide chain of hemoglobin dramatically alters the properties of the hemoglobin molecule. Hemoglobin S is formed instead of the normal hemoglobin A. The variant has a normal oxygen-carrying capacity; however, when oxygen tension decreases, the molecule polymerizes, causing distortion and realignment of the RBC into a sickle shape. The sickle cell causes an increased blood viscosity, decreases circulation time, worsens cell hypoxia, and promotes further sickling. The rigid sickled cells

Guidelines for Nursing Care During Blood Transfusions

BEFORE TRANSFUSION

Take baseline set of vital signs.

Keep blood refrigerated in the blood bank until ready for use.

Use two nurses to check blood bag data and ensure positive identification. Verify data with patient ID band before starting blood.

Prime tubing with normal saline solution—IV should have 18-gauge needle.

Note: Never hang blood products with glucose solutions, because they induce RBC hemolysis and clumping.

Tell patient to immediately report signs of reactions (Box 7-2).

DURING TRANSFUSION

Stay with patient during first 15 minutes of transfusion to observe for reaction. Run blood slowly during first 15 minutes. Compare serial vital signs.

Administer remainder of unit in less than 4 hours. If whole blood is used, watch for signs of fluid overload.

Monitor vital signs at regular intervals throughout transfusion.

Monitor for signs of delayed transfusion reactions.

If a reaction of any kind occurs:

Stop the transfusion immediately.

Administer the normal saline IV.

Notify physician.

Treat symptomatically as prescribed with antihistamine or other drug.

Collect the first available urine specimen.

Send urine specimen, unused blood and tubing, and all laboratory tags to blood bank for immediate analysis.

Continue to closely monitor the patient.

Collect follow-up blood work as ordered.

BOX 7-2 | **Signs and Symptoms of Transfusion Reactions**

ACUTE HEMOLYTIC REACTIONS (USUALLY OCCUR IMMEDIATELY)

Burning sensation along the vein

Flushed face, abrupt fever and chills

Chest pain, labored breathing

Headache, backache, flank pain

ALLERGIC REACTIONS (USUALLY OCCUR WITHIN 1½ HOURS)

Hives and itching

Facial edema

Dyspnea, wheezing, anaphylaxis

Note: Transfusion may be continued under close supervision if the reaction is mild.

PYOGENIC REACTIONS (USUALLY OCCUR WITHIN 1½ HOURS)

Chills and fever

Headache and tachycardia

Palpitations or abdominal pain

---

tend to plug the capillary network and can lead to local infarction and worsening tissue hypoxia. The central nervous system, liver, spleen, eyes, kidneys, bones, and joints are all potential sites for infarction. The affected cells also have a much shortened life span of 7 to 20 days versus a normal 120.

An acute episode is generally characterized by localized, migratory, or generalized pain. It is usually accompanied by fever and often leads to vasoocclusive crises in occluded blood vessels. Frequency and severity of episodes vary markedly from one or two per year to one or two per month. Dehydration, infection, stress, and abrupt weather changes have all been known to precipitate an acute episode, which may last from 1 to 10 days. The disease can be fatal by middle adulthood, but increasing numbers of patients with sickle cell disease are living healthy, normal life spans. The risk of frequent infection increases over time as the patient has less and less infection-fighting reserve from the spleen.

Medical management

No specific therapy is available to treat sickle cell disease. Supportive care during exacerbations or crises usually consists of analgesics, oxygen, and adequate hydration. Transfusion therapy may be indicated to replace lost RBCs and improve oxygen tension in the tissues. Adequate pain management during crises is critical to prevent the development of patterns of drug-seeking behavior from inadequate management of pain.

NURSING MANAGEMENT

◆ ASSESSMENT
Subjective Data

Pain
    Location, duration, severity
    Local, migratory, generalized
    Knowledge of successful management strategies from prior experience
Fatigue
    Severity, impact on life-style and activities of daily living (ADL)

Objective Data

Low-grade fever
Presence of signs of crisis
    Acute abdominal pain
    Priapism
    Neurologic deficits
Evidence of chronic problems
    Leg ulcers
    Ocular problems
    Renal insufficiency

The remainder of the nursing management for the person with a sickle cell disease crisis is presented in the nursing care plan.

NURSING CARE PLAN

THE PERSON EXPERIENCING A SICKLE CELL DISEASE CRISIS

■ **NURSING DIAGNOSIS**

Pain (related to imbalance in oxygen supply and demand)

Expected Patient Outcomes	Nursing Interventions
Patient will experience reduced pain and report that existing pain is managed effectively.	1. Perform good pain assessment. 2. Give prescribed analgesics as needed, and evaluate effectiveness of medication. 3. Explore the use of patient-controlled analgesia for pain control. 4. Identify measures patient has found helpful and include these measures in the care. 5. Support joints gently when assisting patient to do range of motion (ROM) exercises. 6. Use moist heat or massage, if helpful. 7. Use other pain-relieving measures; person with frequent crises may benefit from learning special techniques such as biofeedback or self-hypnosis. 8. Assist patient in avoiding habituation and dependence on narcotics if possible.

■ **NURSING DIAGNOSIS**

Tissue perfusion, altered peripheral (related to blockage in small arterioles and capillaries)

Expected Patient Outcomes	Nursing Interventions
Patient will not develop thrombosis, skin ulcerations, or retinal infarction.	1. Administer prescribed IV fluids; because large amounts may be given, monitor patient for fluid overload (5 to 8 L). 2. Encourage oral fluids, if permitted. 3. Teach patient to drink 4 to 6 L of fluid daily and more during hot weather. 4. Monitor for signs of thrombosis (pain in chest or abdomen, headache, decreased vision, oliguria or low urinary specific gravity). 5. Assess legs, especially medial malleoli, for signs of skin breakdown; use measures to prevent skin dryness or injury from trauma. 6. Provide prescribed oxygen. 7. Reduce activity to lower body's metabolic needs.

Continued.

ERYTHROCYTOSIS

The term *erythrocytosis* refers to an abnormal increase in the number of RBCs. It is frequently a secondary response to hypoxia or chronic cardiac or pulmonary disease. The primary form of the disease is polycythemia vera, which is a bone marrow dysfunction of unknown etiology. Leukocytosis and thrombocytosis often occur as well. Problems related to increased blood volume and viscosity frequently develop as the disease worsens.

The standard treatment for polycythemia vera is periodic phlebotomy designed to maintain a normal hemoglobin and hematocrit. In fulminant cases the patient may be treated with an alkylating agent or

NURSING CARE PLAN—CONT'D

THE PERSON EXPERIENCING A SICKLE CELL DISEASE CRISIS

■ **NURSING DIAGNOSIS**

Activity intolerance (related to pain and decreased tissue oxygenation)

Expected Patient Outcome	Nursing Interventions
Patient will have sufficient energy to remain independent in the activities of daily living.	1. Space daily activities and encourage frequent rest periods. 2. Assist with activities of daily living as needed. 3. Assist with gentle ROM exercise each shift. 4. Assess for incidence and severity of dyspnea. Encourage use of oxygen if ordered.

■ **NURSING DIAGNOSIS**

Coping, risk of ineffective individual (related to disease exacerbations)

Expected Patient Outcome	Nursing Interventions
Patient will utilize positive coping strategies to deal with illness-related problems.	1. Provide opportunities for patient to discuss feelings about inability to fulfill expected roles. 2. Assist patient to identify personal strengths. 3. Identify and support all positive coping strategies. 4. Suggest joining a support group or obtaining counseling to minimize dependency behaviors.

■ **NURSING DIAGNOSIS**

Knowledge deficit (related to disease origins and treatment and genetic implications)

Expected Patient Outcome	Nursing Interventions

Patient/family understand the nature of the disorder and its treatment and receive appropriate genetic testing and counseling.	1. Assess patient's knowledge of sickle cell anemia and correct misunderstandings.
	 2. Teach patient the basis of sickle cell disease and genetic effects.
	 3. Provide resources for family planning and genetic counseling.
	 4. Teach patient to avoid situations that cause crises.
	    a. Infection, dehydration, and overexertion
	    b. Smoking and alcohol use
	 5. Reinforce importance of folic acid supplement to support RBC formation.
	 6. Teach patient to drink 4 to 6 quarts of fluid daily.
	 7. Discuss genetic counseling and contraceptive methods if patient is concerned about transmitting disease.

radioactive phosphorus to suppress the bone marrow. Patients are monitored carefully for the development of other bone marrow problems such as leukemia, which develop at a markedly increased rate. Close medical follow-up is important.

DISORDERS OF HEMOSTASIS AND COAGULATION

The normal functioning of the hemostatic network requires the complex interplay of numerous elements

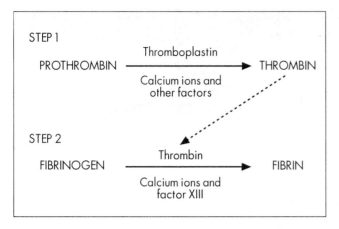

FIGURE 7-4   Basic steps in coagulation process.

BOX 7-3	Disorders Associated with Platelets and Coagulation	
PLATELETS		
Thrombocytopenia	Decreased number of platelets	
Thrombocytosis	Increased number of platelets	
Bleeding syndromes	Disorders of platelet function	
COAGULATION		
Congenital		
Hemophilia A	Decrease of factor VIII	
Hemophilia B	Decrease of factor IX	
von Willebrand's disease	Decrease of factor VIII and defective platelet aggregation	
Acquired		
Vitamin K deficiency	Decrease of factors II, VII, IX, and X	
Disseminated intravascular coagulation	Stimulates first the clotting process, then the fibrinolytic process	

and factors. An abbreviated overview of the process of clot formation is presented in Figure 7-4. Each element is independently produced and regulated and is vulnerable to a variety of disorders. Box 7-3 summarizes potential disorders associated with platelets and coagulation.

THROMBOCYTOPENIA
Etiology/Epidemiology

Thrombocytopenia exists by definition when the number of platelets falls below the normal level of 150,000 to 400,000/mm^3. The condition may reflect increased platelet destruction, decreased survival, or decreased production. It is a common adverse effect of cancer treatment with chemotherapy or radiation. A primary rare form, idiopathic thrombocytopenia purpura (ITP), affects young adults as a result of the production of an autoantibody to a platelet antigen.

Pathophysiology

Platelets are the body's first barrier to blood loss from blood vessel injury. They aggregate and adhere to the site of vessel injury and can effectively plug small leaks. They also release thromboplastin as the first step of the clotting cascade. A decrease in circulating platelets interferes with effective hemostasis and leaves the patient vulnerable to excessive and spontaneous bleeding. Patients often exhibit petechiae, purpura, and ecchymoses on the skin. Petechiae occur only in platelet disorders. Epistaxis, menorrhagia, and gingival bleeding are also common. The threat of serious bleeding always exists.

Medical Management

The diagnosis is established by the examination of complete laboratory studies of all blood elements. Bleeding and coagulation tests will be carefully analyzed. A bone marrow biopsy may be taken to search for megakaryocytes—platelet precursors.

Treatment of thrombocytopenia rests on the isolation and removal of the cause of platelet depression if possible. ITP is treated with corticosteroids to decrease antibody production and splenectomy to remove the organ principally involved in platelet destruction. Plasmapheresis is being used on an experimental basis. Transfusions of platelets may be given if the patient is experiencing active bleeding. A normal platelet life span is only 10 days, and transfused platelets survive only 2 to 3 days; therefore transfusions must be repeated every few days during an acute period. Transfusion is not particularly helpful in ITP, because the transfused platelets are rapidly destroyed by the circulating antibodies. Platelets may be obtained from random or HLA-matched donors. Random donors are much easier to obtain but may eventually lead to antibody formation, which decreases effectiveness.

NURSING MANAGEMENT

Nursing care focuses on the patient's risk of injury from bleeding. Spontaneous hemorrhage is potentially life threatening when the platelet count is below 20,000/mm^3. The nurse assesses and documents the presence and severity of all petechiae and bruises. The following bleeding precautions are instituted:

Testing urine, stool, and any secretions for blood
Avoiding rectal temperatures
No intramuscular (IM) injections
Applying pressure to all venipuncture sites for at least 5 minutes
Teaching the patient the importance of:
    Soft gentle mouth care
    Avoiding use of straight razors
    Avoiding any contact sports
    Assessing the home for risks of falls
    Avoiding the use of any product containing aspirin
    Avoiding anal sex

HEMOPHILIA

Etiology/Epidemiology

Hemophilia is a hereditary coagulation disorder. Both hemophilia A (factor VIII) and hemophilia B (factor IX) are sex-linked recessive disorders that affect males almost exclusively.

Pathophysiology

Patients with hemophilia have lifelong histories of bleeding, both spontaneous and trauma related. Disease complications are a direct result of the bleeding tendency and include (1) joint deformities from repeated bleeds and (2) bleeding into soft tissue areas such as the brain and retroperitoneum.

Medical Management

Treatment consists of replacement of the deficient clotting factors if bleeding episodes do not respond to local treatment such as pressure and ice application. Transfusions of cryoprecipitate or concentrates of other deficient factors are given. Concentrated factors restore blood levels without volume overload. Desmopressin acetate (DDAVP) has been shown to increase the levels of factor VIII in persons with mild hemophilia A. Ambulatory and home administration programs have dramatically increased the quality of life in persons with hemophilia. The transmission of HIV has been a major concern, since the factors have traditionally been prepared from pools of donors. More rigorous screening of donors and treatment of the factors with heat to kill the virus have largely corrected this serious concern for hemophiliacs.

NURSING MANAGEMENT

Most adults with hemophilia are extremely knowledgeable about their disease and its management. The nurse assesses the patient's knowledge base and reinforces it as needed. The patient is reminded about the importance of wearing Medic-Alert identification and informing all health care providers about the disorder. Positive coping strategies are reinforced, and the patient is encouraged to make the kind of life-style adaptations that will allow for safe and complete participation in occupational and social activities. Genetic counseling is an important consideration. Referral to the National Hemophilia Foundation can represent another source of support for the patient and family.

DISSEMINATED INTRAVASCULAR COAGULATION

Etiology/Epidemiology

Disseminated intravascular coagulation (DIC) is a complicated and potentially fatal disruption of the body's hemostatic mechanisms that occurs in response to a variety of primary diseases or injury. It involves an imbalance between the processes of coagulation and

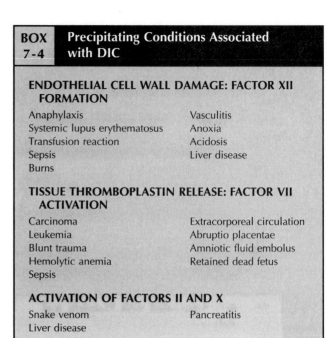

BOX 7-4 Precipitating Conditions Associated with DIC

ENDOTHELIAL CELL WALL DAMAGE: FACTOR XII FORMATION

Anaphylaxis	Vasculitis
Systemic lupus erythematosus	Anoxia
Transfusion reaction	Acidosis
Sepsis	Liver disease
Burns	

TISSUE THROMBOPLASTIN RELEASE: FACTOR VII ACTIVATION

Carcinoma	Extracorporeal circulation
Leukemia	Abruptio placentae
Blunt trauma	Amniotic fluid embolus
Hemolytic anemia	Retained dead fetus
Sepsis	

ACTIVATION OF FACTORS II AND X

Snake venom	Pancreatitis
Liver disease	

anticoagulation and is characterized by initial clotting followed by hemorrhage. DIC can be triggered directly or indirectly by conditions that stimulate or activate clotting factors or cause the release of tissue thromboplastin. Conditions known to trigger DIC are summarized in Box 7-4.

Pathophysiology

Once the clotting process is initiated, the body's response is generalized and occurs throughout the vascular system. This creates a state of hypercoagulability. The fibrinolytic processes are then stimulated and act to dissolve the widespread clots. This depletes the clotting factors and rapidly creates a state of hypocoagulability. The next step is usually widespread hemorrhage. Early signs include bleeding into the mucous membranes and tissues; oral, vaginal, or rectal bleeding; and laboratory values showing a prolonged prothrombin time and partial thromboplastin time.

Medical Management

The focus of medical management in DIC is the control of the underlying primary disease process. Concurrent efforts are made to control the bleeding and restore the balance of clotting factors. This is accomplished primarily through the administration of blood products such as platelets, cryoprecipitate, fresh frozen plasma, and fresh whole blood. Heparin has been administered in the attempt to inhibit the underlying microthrombosis, but its use is extremely controversial since it may also significantly increase the bleeding.

NURSING MANAGEMENT

The patient with DIC is cared for in a critical care area, and nursing care is based on constant body system assessment. All actual and potential bleeding sites are monitored, and careful records are made of all drainage and blood loss. Medications are administered orally or intravenously, and the patient is handled with great care to prevent injury. Fluid balance is a critical element, and the nurse balances the rapid replacement of lost blood and fluid with accurate recording of all losses. Frequent vital signs, urine output, and level of consciousness are assessed to monitor for hypovolemic shock and the development of other complications related to the bleeding.

The patient with DIC is critically ill, and the often visible bleeding creates a very frightening situation for the family. The nurse supports the patient and family throughout the crisis, keeping them informed of all changes in the patient's condition, and involves them at the bedside where feasible.

DISORDERS OF THE WHITE BLOOD CELLS

The white blood cells (WBCs) provide the humoral and cellular response to infection. Any disorder involving the WBCs leaves the individual susceptible to infection.

Disorders of immune function are described in Chapter 17. The leukemias are the primary disorders involving the WBCs.

LEUKEMIAS

The leukemias are malignant disorders of the bone marrow and lymph nodes that are characterized by uncontrolled proliferation of the WBCs and their precursors. The leukemias are classified as acute or chronic and are further subdivided according to cell type. The major forms of leukemia are presented in Table 7-4. Acute leukemias have a rapid onset and lead quickly to death, usually from overwhelming infection, if not adequately treated. The chronic leukemias develop more insidiously and may persist for years. The etiology of the leukemias remains unknown, although predisposing variables have been identified, including chronic exposure to chemicals, drugs, or radiation and a few specific chromosomal aberrations.

Acute Myelogenous Leukemia
Etiology/epidemiology

Acute myelogenous leukemia (AML) can occur at any age but is most common in adolescence and late middle

TABLE 7-4 Leukemias			
PEAK AGE	**PROGNOSIS**	**SYMPTOMS**	**MEDICAL MANAGEMENT**
ACUTE LEUKEMIAS			
Acute Lymphocytic Leukemia (ALL)			
2-4 yr (80% are children)	Good response to treatment; over 50% of patients under 15 achieve 5-yr survival	Fever, respiratory infections, anemia, bleeding mucous membranes, lymphadenopathy, fatigue and weakness, tendency to infection	Combined chemotherapy Drugs: Vincristine Prednisone 6-Mercaptopurine Methotrexate
Acute Myelogenous Leukemia (AML)			
12-20 yr, after 55 yr	High mortality from infection and hemorrhage; an initial remission is possible in 50%-75%, but 5-yr survival is poor	Same symptoms as ALL but less lymphadenopathy	Chemotherapy: Cystosine arabinoside Thioguanine Adriamycin Daunorubicin Bone marrow transplant
CHRONIC LEUKEMIAS			
Chronic Lymphocytic Leukemia (CLL)			
50-70 yr but can occur at any age; three times more common in men	Most patients do quite well; survive 10 or more yr with disease	Insidious onset; weakness, fatigue, massive lymphadenopathy, pruritic vesicular skin lesions, anemia, thrombocytopenia	Chemotherapy: Alkylating agents—chlorambucil and glucocorticoids Treated only when patient is symptomatic
Chronic Myelogenous Leukemia (CML)			
30-50 yr	Death usually occurs in less than 5 yr from infection and hemorrhage	Weakness, fatigue, anorexia, weight loss, splenomegaly, anemia, thrombocytopenia, fever; can have fulminant stage	Chemotherapy with same agents used with AML; also vincristine, busulfan, hydroxyurea Bone marrow transplant

age. It arises from a single myeloid stem cell and is characterized by the development of immature myeloblasts in the bone marrow. It carries an extremely high mortality from infection and hemorrhage, although an initial remission is common with aggressive therapy. The 5-year survival rate is poor.

Pathophysiology

Large numbers of abnormal WBCs accumulate in the bone marrow and then spread to the other hematopoietic organs, causing enlargement. The proliferation of one cell type interferes with the production of other blood components. The abnormal or immature WBCs are unable to perform their function and dramatically increase the individual's susceptibility to infection. The potential symptoms include infection, fatigue and malaise, anemia, bruising and bleeding, and lymphadenopathy.

Medical management

Medical management utilizes aggressive chemotherapy in an attempt to achieve disease remission. The treatment is arduous and commonly involves a combination of drugs such as cytosine arabinoside, 6-thioguanine, and doxorubicin. The patient needs prolonged supportive care with blood component replacement and antibiotic therapy during this time. Prophylactic treatment of the central nervous system with intrathecal chemotherapy is critical to prevent the sequestering of leukemic cells behind the blood-brain barrier. Bone marrow transplant with HLA-matched bone marrow is being used with increasing frequency.

NURSING MANAGEMENT

◆ ASSESSMENT
Subjective Data

History and duration of symptoms
History of prior treatment, if any
Patient's complaint of fatigue and weakness
History of frequent infection
Possible weight loss or anorexia
Family's response to symptoms and diagnosis
Medications in current use

Objective Data

Fever
Presence of anemia, thrombocytopenia
Bruising, petechiae
Lymphadenopathy
Bleeding or ulceration of mucous membranes
General systems assessment

◆ NURSING DIAGNOSES

Nursing diagnoses for the person with acute myelogenous leukemia may include, but are not limited to, the following:

Injury and infection, risk of (related to the disease symptoms and side effects of the treatment regimen)
Nutrition altered: less than body requirements (related to anorexia and GI side effects of chemotherapy)
Activity intolerance (related to severe fatigue and weakness)
Coping, ineffective individual or family (related to the treatment regimen and prognosis of the disease)
Knowledge deficit (related to the management of the side effects of chemotherapy)

◆ EXPECTED PATIENT OUTCOMES

Patient will be protected from bleeding and infection during chemotherapy.
Patient will maintain an adequate nutrient intake to meet minimal body requirements.
Patient will maintain sufficient energy to remain independent in the activities of daily living.
Patient and family will receive support and honestly share their feelings and fears about the disease.
Patient will be knowledgeable about treatment regimen, expected side effects, and their management.

◆ NURSING INTERVENTIONS
Preventing Bleeding and Infection

Administer combined chemotherapy, if covered by hospital policy. Ensure patency of vascular access (see Chapter 1 for specific interventions for IV administration of chemotherapy).
Administer blood and blood products as ordered.
Institute bleeding precautions.
  See discussion under thrombocytopenia.
  Monitor for signs of bleeding.
  Promptly report the incidence of petechiae, ecchymoses, and gingival bleeding.
Protect patient against nosocomial infection.
  Promote scrupulous hygiene, particularly oral.
  Insist on rigorous handwashing by staff.
  Prep skin thoroughly before skin puncture.
  Monitor for early signs of infection.
  Establish protective isolation if indicated: laminar airflow rooms may be needed to preserve life in severely leukopenic patients.
  Examine the mouth every 4 hours for signs of stomatitis.
  Assist the patient with frequent gentle mouth care.

Promoting Adequate Nutrition

Employ nursing measures to counter anorexia and nausea (see Chapter 1 for specific nutrition interventions for chemotherapy).

Conserving Energy

Assist patient to space activity to conserve energy.

Assist patient with activities of daily living as needed.

Encourage patient to remain involved with normal daily activities but to avoid overexertion.

Teach patient and family the importance of adequate rest at intervals throughout the day.

Supporting Effective Coping

Provide emotional support to patient and family. Ensure adequate time for questions; encourage expression of fears and concerns.

Include family in all aspects of care.

Explore community agencies that can provide patient and family with support and specific assistance, such as the American Cancer Society and the Leukemia Society.

Teaching for Effective Self-care

Teach patient and family about treatment regimen including the following:

Purposes of combination drug therapy

Expected side effects of drugs

Management of side effects

Purpose of isolation

Measures to prevent infection or bleeding

Symptoms indicating complications

Symptoms of infection or clotting problems

Importance of scheduled follow-up

◆ EVALUATION

Successful achievement of expected outcomes for the patient with acute myelogenous leukemia is indicated by the following:

Absence of bleeding or infection

Intake of balanced nutrients and stable body weight

Sufficient energy for self-care and involvement in family or social activities

Open communication between patient and family concerning disease, treatment, and prognosis; involvement with support activities

Correct description of:

Disease and treatment regimen

Side effects of all medications

Diet adjustments

Measures to prevent bleeding and infection

Symptoms of complications needing medical evaluation

DISORDERS OF THE LYMPH SYSTEM

The chief functions of the lymph nodes and lymph system are to assist in phagocytosis of cellular debris and to provide an immune response to antigens received from the structures drained by the lymph nodes. Lymph nodes are not normally palpable but enlarge in the presence of a wide variety of infectious processes. Infectious mononucleosis is the best known primary disorder and is summarized in Box 7-5. Most of the other disorders of the lymph system are malignant.

LYMPHOMA

The category of lymphoma includes a variety of malignant disorders in which the lymph tissue is infiltrated with malignant cells and the affected nodes enlarge. The disease then spreads to lymph tissue of other nodes such as the liver or spleen. Lymphomas usually follow a pattern of exacerbation and remission.

Lymphomas are generally categorized into two major groupings. *Hodgkin's disease* is a potentially curable disease characterized by the presence of Reed-Sternberg cells in affected lymph nodes. *Non-Hodgkin's lymphoma* is the term used for a broad spectrum of lymphoid malignancies that have different histologic features and prognosis. Table 7-5 compares the major features of the two categories.

TABLE 7-5   Malignant Disorders of the Lymph System

ETIOLOGY	SIGNS AND SYMPTOMS	MEDICAL MANAGEMENT
Hodgkin's disease		
Unknown, viruses possibly implicated Affects primarily young adults	Lymph node enlargement (firm, nontender, painless), fever, weight loss, night sweats, pruritus (itching), fatigue and weakness, presence of Reed-Sternberg cells, enlarged liver and spleen	Radiotherapy for early stages; combination chemotherapy for middle and late stages MOPP regimen most commonly used: nitrogen mustard, vincristine, procarbazine, and prednisone
Non-Hodgkin's lymphoma		
Unknown, viruses implicated Affects 50 to 70 year olds	Nontender "bulky" lymphadenopathy, moderate hepatomegaly and splenomegaly; patient may experience unexplained weight loss, fever, night sweats	Radiotherapy for initial treatment for localized disease Combination chemotherapy is mainstay of treatment for diffuse disease; variety of drug combinations employed

BOX 7-5	Infectious Mononucleosis

Infectious mononucleosis is an acute self-limiting disease caused by the Epstein-Barr virus. It is more common in young persons and is usually a benign disease with a good prognosis. The symptoms are variable:

Malaise—usual early complaint

Flulike symptoms—fever, sore throat, generalized aches, enlarged lymph nodes

Moderate spleen enlargement

MEDICAL AND NURSING CARE

Promote rest and comfort.

Avoid stress and strain.

Prepare patient for persistent fatigue.

Most persons recover spontaneously within a few weeks.

Hodgkin's Disease

Etiology/epidemiology

Hodgkin's disease primarily affects young adults in late adolescence or the 20s. Its etiology is unknown. The four different histologic varieties of the disease are each associated with a different outcome. The diagnosis and treatment are rigorous, but prolonged remission and even cure are possible in many cases. The best indicator of prognosis is the stage of the disease at the time of diagnosis.

Pathophysiology

Presence of the Reed-Sternberg cell is the pathologic hallmark of Hodgkin's disease. General clinical symptoms associated with Hodgkin's disease include fatigue, weakness, anorexia, fever, night sweats, and general pruritus. The lymph nodes are generally enlarged, as are the liver and spleen. A mediastinal mass may be present.

Medical management

Diagnosis and staging of Hodgkin's disease are complex. A lymphangiogram is performed to evaluate the intraabdominal lymph nodes. A bone marrow biopsy is frequently performed to search for disease involvement. A staging laparotomy may be performed to assess the extent of the disease and take tissue for biopsy. Radiation therapy is employed for early stage disease (I and II) and effects a cure in 80% to 90% of patients. Combination chemotherapy is usually added at stage III, with the drugs administered for 2 weeks of each month over a 6-month period. Remission is achieved in approximately 80% of cases.

NURSING MANAGEMENT

♦ ASSESSMENT

Subjective Data

History, duration, and severity of symptoms

Knowledge of disorder

Prior treatment and response if appropriate

Patient's complaints of the following:

Fever

Weakness

Anorexia

Night sweats

General pruritus (itching)

Effect of fatigue on self-care capabilities

Objective Data

Nontender, enlarged lymph nodes

Weight loss

Fever

Nutritional status

Enlarged liver and spleen

Positive lymph node biopsy or lymphangiogram

Condition of skin

♦ NURSING DIAGNOSES

Nursing diagnoses for the person with Hodgkin's disease may include, but are not limited to, the following:

Activity intolerance (related to systemic fatigue and fever)

Skin integrity, high risk for impaired (related to pruritus, fever, and night sweats)

Knowledge deficit (related to treatment regimen and side effects of chemotherapy)

♦ EXPECTED PATIENT OUTCOMES

Patient will maintain sufficient energy to be independent in self-care.

Patient will maintain an intact skin.

Patient will be knowledgeable of the treatment regimen and the management of the side effects of drugs.

♦ NURSING INTERVENTIONS

Conserving Energy

Monitor activity tolerance and assess for dyspnea with exertion.

Assist patient to deal with the side effects of chemotherapy and radiation (see Chapter 1 for specific interventions).

Help patient to arrange activities to conserve energy.

Encourage patient to remain active in self-care to the degree possible.

Maintaining an Intact Skin

Provide comfort measures appropriate to symptoms.

Keep bedding and linen fresh and dry.

Offer baths and skin care.

Administer antipyretic and antipruritic medication as prescribed.

Plan with patient to adjust diet to ensure adequate nutritional intake and fluids.

Teaching for Self-Care

Teach patient about treatment regimen and measures to control side effects.

Explain importance of detailed diagnostic workup.

Assist patient to schedule treatments for minimal disruption of normal life-style.

Provide teaching about the effects of broad field radiation and chemotherapy on reproductive capacities.

Males are frequently sterile and should consider sperm banking.

Females usually regain fertility in time; may have ovaries relocated outside radiation treatment zone.

Provide ongoing support to patient and family.

◆ EVALUATION

Successful achievement of expected outcomes for the patient with Hodgkin's disease is indicated by the following:

Sufficient energy to maintain independence in self-care and involvement in usual daily activities

An intact skin, effective control of pruritus

Correct description of:

Disease

Treatment regimen

Management of treatment side effects

Symptoms indicating complications and need for medical evaluation

Non-Hodgkin's Lymphoma
Etiology/epidemiology

Non-Hodgkin's lymphoma is a broad category of malignancies that includes disease processes with variable pathologic manifestations, courses, and responses to therapy. Their cause is unknown although the role of viruses is under investigation. The cancer typically affects persons in their 50s and 60s.

Pathophysiology

The various forms of lymphoma can be grouped by prognosis or histologic type. One broad grouping includes lymphocytic, histiocytic, or mixed cell types. Patients typically have nontender, peripheral lymphadenopathy and enlargement of the liver and spleen. Unexplained fever, night sweats, and weight loss are also common.

Medical management

Diagnosis is made from examination of the lymph node tissue. Treatment decisions are based on the tissue histology, so an accurate diagnosis is critical. The disease is also staged in a manner similar to Hodgkin's

disease. There are numerous possible treatment regimens. Radiotherapy is generally the first step when the disease is localized. Chemotherapy is extensively used when the disease is generalized. Most protocols use combination chemotherapy.

NURSING MANAGEMENT

The nursing management is similar to that presented under Hodgkin's disease. The nurse supports the patient during the rigorous diagnosis and staging process and then assists the patient to cope with the side effects of treatment. Outcomes are not as positive as with Hodgkin's disease, but many patients are able to achieve significant intervals of remission.

SELECTED REFERENCES

Armitage JO: Treatment of non-Hodgkin's lymphoma, *N Engl J Med* 328(14):1023-1030, 1993.

Brain MC, Carbonne PP: *Current therapy in hematology-oncology,* ed 4, St Louis, 1991, Mosby.

Brandt BA: A nursing protocol for the client with neutropenia, *Oncol Nurs Forum* 17(1, suppl):9-15, 1990.

Callery MF, Culbana MB, Francis CK: Building a safe community blood supply, *Am J Nurs* 91(6):51-52, 1991.

Callery MF, Culbana MB, Francis CK: Choosing blood components and equipment, *Am J Nurs* 91(6):42-48, 1991.

Callery MF, Culbana MB, Francis CK: Preventing and managing transfusion reactions, *Am J Nurs* 91(6):48-50, 1991.

Canellos G et al: Chemotherapy of advanced Hodgkin's disease with MOPP, ABVD, or MOPP alternating with ABVD, *N Engl J Med* 327(21):1478-1484, 1992.

Doheny MO, Sedlak C, Broome B, Murphy L: Caring for the orthopaedic patient with sickle cell disease, *Orthop Nurs* 11(1):41-48, 1992.

Froberg J: The anemias: causes and courses of action, *RN* 52(1):24-29, 1989.

Harmening DM: *Clinical hematology and fundamentals of hemostasis,* ed 2, Philadelphia, 1992, FA Davis Co.

Harovas J, Anthony, HH: Managing transfusion reactions, *RN* 56(12):32-36, 1993.

Johnson J: Prevention and management of neutropenia in the cancer patient, *Oncol Nurs Forum* 17(1, suppl):3-6, 1990.

Lakhani AK: Current management of acute leukemias, *Nurs '88 (Lond)* 3:755-758, 1988.

London F: Nursing diagnoses and caring for patients with sickle cell disease, *Adv Clin Care* 5(5):12-16, 1990.

Martinelli A: Sickle cell disease: etiology, symptoms, patient care, *AORN J* 53:716-724, 1991.

Piomelli S: Sickle cell diseases in the 1990s: the need for active and preventative intervention, *Semin Hematol* 28(3):227-232, 1991.

Rostad ME: Management of myelosuppression in the patient with cancer, *Oncol Nurs Forum* 17(1, suppl):4-8, 1990.

Simonson GM: Caring for patients with acute myelocytic leukemia, *Am J Nurs* 88:304-309, 1988.

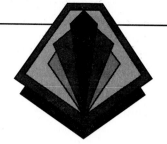

Disorders of the Respiratory System

◆ ASSESSMENT

SUBJECTIVE DATA

Health history
  Past history of respiratory system illnesses, surgery, or trauma
    Childhood illnesses, for example, asthma, croup, ear infections, tonsillitis
    Adult illnesses, for example, pneumonia, sinusitis, chronic obstructive pulmonary disease (COPD)
    Surgical procedures, for example, tonsillectomy, myringotomy
    History of rib fracture or other chest trauma
  Immunization history, for example, influenza and pneumococcal vaccine
  Results of tuberculin testing
    Date of last test, reaction
  Environmental exposure to respiratory irritants
    Home, for example, wood-burning stove, kerosene heaters
    Occupational exposure, for example, chemicals, fumes, pollutants
  Recent travel plans and area of residence: rural versus urban
Family history
  Allergies and hay fever
  Asthma
  Emphysema
  Genetic disorders, for example, cystic fibrosis
Smoking history
  Use of cigarettes, cigars, pipe, marijuana
    Extent and duration of smoking; pack years
    Efforts to quit if any and methods used
  Exposure to passive smoke at home or work
    Extent and duration of exposure
Allergy history/hay fever
  Nature and severity of respiratory symptoms
  Standard treatment and effectiveness
Medication history
  Current and past use of prescription and over the counter (OTC) medications affecting the respiratory system
    Antihistamines, decongestants, cough preparations, nasal sprays, bronchodilator
    Use of inhalers or nebulizers

Current problem
  Dyspnea,* or shortness of breath
    Onset, perceived severity, duration
    Precipitating and relieving factors
    Effect on activities of daily living (ADL), work and leisure time activities, and sexuality
  Paroxysmal nocturnal dyspnea or orthopnea
    Presence and severity
    Effect on sleep patterns
    Methods of treatment
  Cough
    Duration and severity, pattern of incidence, for example, morning versus nighttime or constant
    Productive or nonproductive
      Consistency, quantity, color, and odor of sputum
      Treatment methods used if any; effectiveness
  Presence of chest pain
    Location, severity, relationship to breathing

OBJECTIVE DATA

Inspection
  Nose and sinuses
    Size, shape, and symmetry; presence of visible deformity or tumor
    Presence of nasal flaring
    Condition of mucous membranes, presence of septal deviation or perforation, polyps
  Neck and throat
    Symmetry
    Presence of postnasal discharge, inflammation, tonsillar enlargement or discharge
    Tracheal alignment, swelling, bruising
  Lungs and thorax
    Chest configuration and symmetry; anteroposterior (AP) to lateral diameter
    Skin color, condition
    Presence of spinal deformities, for example, kyphosis, lordosis, scoliosis

---

*NOTE: Dyspnea is a subjective symptom that cannot be objectively evaluated and may not correlate well with observable or measurable parameters.

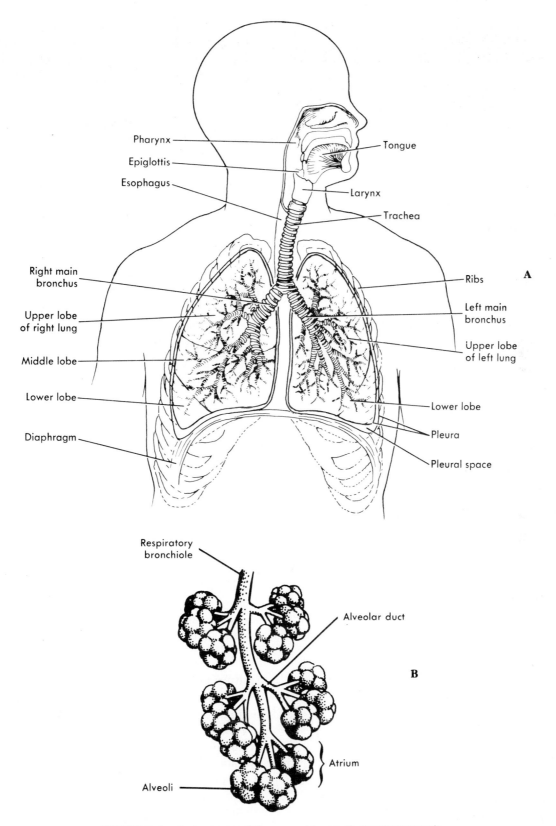

FIGURE 8-1 **A,** Anatomy of thorax and lungs. **B,** Respiratory unit.

Symmetry of chest movement with inspiration
   Presence of splinting
Use of accessory muscles in breathing; pursed lip
   or diaphragmatic breathing; presence of rib
   retractions

Rate, rhythm, and depth of respiration
Palpation
   Nose and paranasal sinuses for tenderness and swelling
   Neck for size, shape, consistency, mobility of lymph
      nodes

BOX 8-1 Adventitious Breath Sounds

RALES

Crackling, discontinuous sounds frequently described as the sound of hair being rolled between the fingers near the ear

Caused by air passing through moisture in alveoli or bronchiole; associated with infection and atelectasis; more commonly heard on inspiration

RHONCHI

Continuous musical or coarse rattling sounds that typically change following coughing or suctioning

Caused by fluid, secretions, or obstruction within larger airways; associated with infection, tumor, and chronic lung disease; more prominent on expiration

WHEEZES

Squeaky, musical sounds that can usually be heard without a stethoscope

Caused by air rushing through narrowed small airways; associated with bronchospasm and secretions; heard during both inspiration and expiration

GERONTOLOGIC PATIENT CONSIDERATIONS: PHYSIOLOGIC CHANGES IN THE RESPIRATORY SYSTEM

The effects of aging leave the older adult more vulnerable to problems involving the respiratory tract, and when problems develop they are frequently more difficult to manage. In general, the connective tissue becomes weaker and less elastic. This affects respiratory function in several ways:

Increased rigidity of the rib cage

Increased anteroposterior (AP) diameter

50% increase in residual volume between early adulthood and 70 years of age

Parallel decrease in vital capacity (FEV_1 decreases about 30 ml/yr)

Alveoli less elastic and fibrotic tissue increases with fewer functional capillaries

pO_2 decreases about 4 mm Hg each decade

O_2 saturation reduced gradually to approximately 94%

pCO_2 unchanged

In addition, the loss of skeletal muscle strength weakens effective coughing. The reduction in body fluid can cause drier mucous membranes and thickened mucus. The gradual decline in immunocompetence leaves the elderly individual increasingly vulnerable to infections of all types.

Chest

  Vocal and tactile fremitus

  Masses, swelling, areas of tenderness

  Presence and location of any crepitus (subcutaneous emphysema or a crackling sensation)

Percussion

  Used to assess for pulmonary resonance, organ boundaries, and diaphragmatic excursion

Auscultation

  Breath sounds, normal and adventitious

  Location, intensity, pitch, and duration

  Normal vesicular breath sounds

    Low pitched, soft, breezy; expiration heard as a puff (heard primarily over outer aspects of lungs)

  Normal bronchovesicular breath sounds

    Harsher, moderate in pitch and intensity (heard primarily over the thorax near the main-stem bronchi)

  Normal bronchial breath sounds

    Fairly loud, coarse, with a blowing hollow quality (heard primarily over the trachea)

  Adventitious breath sounds

    Superimposed over normal lung sounds

    Rales, rhonchi, wheezes (Box 8-1)

✍ DIAGNOSTIC TESTS

LABORATORY TESTS
Blood and Urine Tests

Many tests are used to evaluate the status and functioning of the respiratory system. Major tests include complete blood counts (CBCs), arterial blood gases, and other measures of oxygenation. These have been described in Chapter 7.

Cultures
Throat culture

Purpose—Throat cultures are used primarily to isolate and identify pathogens, particularly group A beta-hemolytic streptococci, and allow for prompt intervention.

Procedure—The tonsillar areas are swabbed from side to side with a cotton-tipped applicator, including any inflamed or purulent areas. Care is taken to avoid touching the tongue, cheeks, or teeth. The swab is immediately placed in a culture tube and transported.

Patient preparation and aftercare—No special preparation is needed beyond instruction in how to cooperate in the specimen collection. The swab frequently induces a brief gagging sensation. No aftercare is required.

Sputum culture

Purpose—Sputum culture is performed to isolate and identify the cause of pulmonary infection.

Procedure—Most specimens are collected by expectoration, which may require ultrasonic nebulization, hydration, postural drainage, or chest physiotherapy to accomplish effectively. Tracheal suctioning may be used in other situations. The specimen is collected in a sterile container that is placed in a leak-proof bag before transport.

Patient preparation and aftercare—The patient should be well hydrated before specimen collection and instructed in the proper technique for deep breathing and forceful coughing. Mouth care should not be performed before the collection but is offered at its conclusion.

Fluid Analysis (Sweat Test)

Purpose—The sweat test quantitatively measures electrolyte concentrations in the sweat and is primarily used to confirm or rule out cystic fibrosis. Elevated levels of sodium and chloride confirm the diagnosis of cystic fibrosis.

Procedure—Electrodes are placed on the patient's right forearm. A gauze pad is placed under each electrode and secured in place. The pads are saturated with pilocarpine solution on the positive electrode and saline solution on the negative electrode. A small adhesive bandage is applied, and a slight electrical current is passed through the area at 15- to 20-second intervals for about 5 minutes. The pads are then discarded, and the skin is cleansed. Clean dry gauze pads are then applied to the region where the pilocarpine was administered and sealed with waterproof tape. The pad is left in place for about 30 to 40 minutes and then is removed and analyzed for sweat content.

Patient preparation and aftercare—The test is explained in language the child can understand, and the patient is informed that the electrodes may cause a tingling sensation but they will not hurt. No special aftercare is required after the area has been washed with soap and water and examined for redness. The patient is monitored throughout the test for any complaints of burning that could indicate dislodgement of the electrodes.

RADIOLOGIC TESTS
Chest Radiography

Purpose—Chest radiography is used to detect pulmonary disorders and the location and size of lesions and to help assess pulmonary function.

Procedure—The patient is positioned standing or sitting in front of the machine, and x-ray films can be taken from the anterior, posterior, and lateral positions.

Patient preparation and aftercare—No special preparation is required beyond patient teaching. The patient must be able to hold his or her breath and remain very still during the film exposure. All jewelry is removed, and tubes and equipment should be cleared from the x-ray portal if possible. No aftercare is needed.

NOTE: Radiography may also be performed to assist in visualizing the sinuses. Radiopaque substances may be instilled to improve visualization of the trachea and bronchi under fluoroscopy.

Thoracic Computed Tomography

Purpose—Computed tomography (CT) of the thorax provides a three-dimensional image of the chest that is one of the most accurate diagnostic tests. It is used to locate suspected neoplasms, evaluate lymph nodes, and differentiate calcified lesions from tumors.

Procedure—The patient is placed in a supine position, and the machine scans the chest from numerous different angles, which the computer then uses to create three-dimensional images of the area. A contrast medium may be injected to enhance the images.

Patient preparation and aftercare—Patient teaching about the test is the primary preparation. The test requires about one-half hour, and the hard table may cause moderate discomfort. If contrast medium is planned the patient is instructed to fast for about 4 hours before the test and is carefully assessed for allergies to dye, iodine, or shellfish. No specific aftercare is required.

Pulmonary Angiography

Purpose—Pulmonary angiography is used most commonly to confirm the presence of pulmonary emboli when scans prove to be nondiagnostic. It can also be used to evaluate the pulmonary circulation before surgery.

Procedure—The patient is placed in a supine position, local anesthetic is administered, and a catheter is inserted into the femoral or antecubital vein. The catheter is advanced into the right side of the heart and on into the pulmonary artery, where dye is injected that outlines the pulmonary circulation. The test takes about 1 hour.

Patient preparation and aftercare—The patient is NPO for about 8 hours before the test, and patient teaching concerning the test is provided. The patient is carefully assessed for any history of allergy to contrast media, iodine, or shellfish. The patient is informed that the introduction of the dye frequently induces a flushed feeling, a salty taste, and transient nausea and may cause an urge to cough. A pressure dressing is applied over the insertion site at the conclusion of the test, and the patient is typically kept on bed rest for about 6 hours. Vital signs are monitored, and the insertion site is checked frequently for bleeding. No further restrictions are required.

SPECIAL TESTS
Pulmonary Function Tests

Purpose—Pulmonary function tests are a series of tests that evaluate ventilatory function through spirometric measurements and are used to evaluate pulmonary dysfunction, assess the effectiveness of a treatment regimen, and measure the progression of pulmonary disease.

Procedure—The tests begin with having the patient breathe normally into the spirometer to adjust to the mouthpiece and nose clip. The patient is then serially coaxed through a series of analyses that seek to determine maximal lung volumes during various phases of respiration (Table 8-1 and Figure 8-2).

Patient preparation and aftercare—The patient is instructed about the nature of the tests and reassured that they are not painful, although they may be fatiguing to a dyspneic patient. The patient should not eat heavily before the test, should not smoke for at least 4 to 6 hours, and should empty the bladder and wear loose

TABLE 8-1 Pulmonary Function Tests	
MEASUREMENT	**IMPLICATIONS OF RESULTS**
Tidal volume (Vt): amount of air inhaled or exhaled during normal breathing	Decreased Vt could indicate restrictive disease and requires further testing.
Minute volume (MV): total amount of air expired per minute	Normal MV may be present even with severe disease. Increased MV occurs with hypoxemia, acidosis, and increased CO_2 levels.
Inspiratory reserve volume (IRV): amount of air inspired *after* a normal inspiration	An abnormal IRV can accompany many pulmonary pathologic conditions but by itself is not diagnostic.
Expiratory reserve volume (ERV): amount of air expired *after* a normal exhalation	ERV varies in normal persons but is typically decreased in obese persons.
Residual volume (RV): amount of air remaining in lungs *after* a forced exhalation	An RV greater than 35% of total lung capacity may indicate obstructive lung disease.
Vital capacity (VC): total volume of air that can be inspired and expired	Decreased VC may indicate decreased respiratory effort, decreased thoracic expansion, or limited movement of diaphragm.
Total lung capacity (TLC): total volume of lungs when fully expanded	A low TLC indicates restrictive disease, whereas a high TLC indicates overdistended lungs from obstructive disease.
Forced expiratory volume (FEV): volume of air expired in first, second, or third second of forced exhalation; usually expressed as FEV_1	A decreased FEV_1 with an increase in FEV_2 and FEV_3 may accompany obstructive disease.

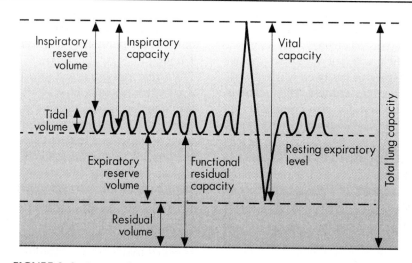

FIGURE 8-2 Lung volumes and capacities illustrated by spirography tracing.

comfortable clothing. Clarification should be sought concerning the administration of medications such as analgesics and bronchodilators before the test. The patient should be allowed to rest following the test and then resume a normal routine.

Lung Perfusion Scan

Purpose—A lung perfusion scan is used to assess the arterial perfusion of the lungs, usually to detect the presence of pulmonary emboli.

Procedure—A radiopharmaceutical is injected intravenously with the patient first in a supine position and then lying prone. Following uptake of the drug, a series of films are taken in a variety of chest views, which can be projected onto a screen. Normal lungs exhibit a uniform high uptake of the substance, whereas areas of low uptake indicate poor perfusion. The test takes about 15 to 30 minutes.

Patient preparation and aftercare—No special preparation is required beyond teaching concerning the

test and reassurance that the amount of radioactivity is minimal and not harmful. The injection site is carefully monitored following the test, but no specific posttest care is required.

Lung Ventilation Scan

Purpose—A lung ventilation scan uses air mixed with radioactive gas to identify the areas of the lung that are ventilated during respiration. It is used primarily to help diagnose pulmonary emboli and is frequently combined with a lung perfusion scan.

Procedure—The patient inhales air mixed with a small amount of radioactive gas through a mask. Its distribution throughout the lungs is then monitored on a nuclear scan. Normal findings show even distribution throughout the lungs, whereas unequal distribution indicates poor ventilation or airway obstruction in the outlined areas. The test takes about 15 to 30 minutes.

Patient preparation and aftercare—No special preparation is indicated except for careful instruction about the test and reassurance about its safety. No posttest care is required.

Thoracentesis (Pleural Fluid Analysis)

Purpose—Thoracentesis involves the puncture of the chest wall to obtain a specimen of pleural fluid or to relieve the pressure of accumulated fluid buildup.

Procedure—The patient is positioned either leaning forward supported by pillows on an overbed table or on the side with the head of the bed elevated about 30 to 45 degrees to widen the intercostal interspaces. The skin is prepared, a local anesthetic is injected, and the thoracentesis needle is inserted above the rib over the fluid accumulation. Fluid is aspirated into a container. A small pressure bandage is applied to the site at the conclusion of the test. Pleural biopsy may also be performed at the conclusion of the thoracentesis to aid in the evaluation.

Patient preparation and aftercare—The patient is instructed about the test and encouraged not to cough, move, or deep breathe if possible during the test to minimize the risk of injury. The patient is monitored carefully during and after the test for the development of pneumothorax or respiratory distress. The site is monitored for any sign of bleeding or infection after the test, and the patient is encouraged to rest on the affected side for at least 1 hour to help seal the puncture site. Vital signs are monitored frequently for 4 hours.

NOTE: Although the chest is normally a negative pressure environment, a substantial fluid accumulation can be accompanied by a rise in pressure and the risk of fluid spraying during the aspiration. The need for protective eyewear and/or face shields should be considered.

Lung Biopsy

Purpose—Specimens of pulmonary tissue are excised to establish a diagnosis of diffuse pulmonary disease when other less invasive tests are inconclusive and to obtain specimens for evaluating lung lesions.

Procedure—The procedure can be performed closed through needle biopsy or as part of a bronchoscopy or by the open method in the operating room. The procedure for closed biopsy is similar to that described for a thoracentesis (see above), with the biopsy needle inserted through an intercostal space with the patient under local anesthetic. A small pressure dressing is applied following the test.

Patient preparation and aftercare—Patient teaching is provided, and the patient is instructed to fast before the test. The patient should be informed that despite the anesthetic, he or she is likely to feel a sharp brief pain as the biopsy needle touches the lung. This is important, because the patient should remain still and not breathe deeply during the test. Vital signs are monitored frequently following the test, and the patient is assessed for any difficulty in breathing. The patient is

usually encouraged to rest in bed on the affected side for about 30 minutes to help seal the puncture site, which is then monitored for any signs of infection or drainage.

ENDOSCOPY
Bronchoscopy

Purpose—The test involves direct visualization of the larynx, trachea, and bronchi to examine for possible tumor or obstruction, to help locate a bleeding site, and to obtain specimens to aid in the diagnosis of infectious or degenerative processes.

Procedure—The patient is positioned on a bed or in a chair. A local anesthetic is applied to the throat, and a bronchoscope is inserted through the mouth or nose. Additional anesthetic is introduced to facilitate the movement of the scope through the larynx. The structure of the airways is analyzed, and bronchial brushes or biopsy forceps may be used to obtain tissue specimens. The procedure takes about 45 to 60 minutes.

Patient preparation and aftercare—Teaching about the procedure is a critical aspect of patient preparation. The patient fasts for about 6 to 12 hours before the test. Sedatives are frequently administered, but the patient should be aware that he or she will be awake during the test and that the introduction of the bronchoscope does cause discomfort and a gagging sensation despite the anesthetic. Breathing through the nose helps relieve perceived breathlessness.

Posttest care involves monitoring vital signs with particular attention to any hoarseness, difficulty in swallowing, dyspnea, stridor, or the development of subcutaneous emphysema around the face or neck. A semi-Fowler's position is used, and the patient is encouraged to avoid coughing or clearing the throat if possible and to spit out saliva rather than swallow it until the gag reflex is fully restored. Food and fluid are also restricted until the gag reflex returns, which may take 1 to 2 hours. Clear liquids or ice chips should be used initially to assess for intact swallowing. Temporary sore throat and hoarseness are expected and should clear within 1 to 2 days. Blood-tinged sputum is expected after the test, but any frank hemoptysis should be reported immediately.

Mediastinoscopy

Purpose—The mediastinum is the cavity behind the sternum that separates the lungs. Mediastinoscopy allows for visualization of these structures directly and permits palpation and biopsy of lymph nodes. It is useful in the detection and staging of lung cancer.

Procedure—The test is performed with the patient under general anesthesia. The patient is intubated, and a small incision is made in the suprasternal region. A channel is created for palpation of the lymph nodes, and the mediastinoscope is inserted. Tissue specimens are collected. The test takes about 1 hour.

Patient preparation and aftercare—Patient teaching about the test is performed, and the patient is instructed to fast after midnight before the test. Vital signs are carefully monitored after the test, and the site is checked for bleeding and/or drainage. The patient is monitored for signs of infection, subcutaneous emphysema, or diminished breath sounds on the affected side. Temporary chest pain at the incision site and sore throat are common and may require mild analgesics.

Direct Laryngoscopy

Purpose—Direct visualization of the larynx is performed to see areas that are inaccessible through the indirect approach and is used to detect lesions, strictures, or foreign bodies; to remove benign lesions; and to aid in the accurate diagnosis of laryngeal cancer. Indirect laryngoscopy, which is a less invasive office procedure, is performed more commonly.

Procedure—After the administration of a general or local anesthetic, the laryngoscope is inserted through the patient's mouth. The larynx is examined, and minor surgery may be performed.

Patient preparation and aftercare—Patient teaching is essential, particularly if a local anesthetic is to be used. The patient fasts for 6 to 8 hours before the test. A sedative is administered as well as medication to reduce secretions. The patient is placed in a semi-Fowler's position after the test, and vital signs are monitored frequently. An ice collar may be administered to reduce edema, and the patient is encouraged to avoid coughing or clearing the throat and to expectorate saliva into an emesis basin initially to monitor for bleeding. Food and fluid are restricted until the gag reflex returns, and the patient is carefully monitored for any sign of airway obstruction, such as stridor, dyspnea, or subcutaneous emphysema. Hoarseness, voice loss, and sore throat are common, and lozenges and gargles may be comforting once the gag reflex returns.

INFECTIONS OF THE RESPIRATORY SYSTEM

INFECTIONS OF THE NOSE AND SINUSES

Acute rhinitis and sinusitis are extremely common viral health problems that affect almost everyone at some time and are usually treated effectively by the patient with the use of a variety of OTC preparations such as decongestants and antihistamines. Allergic problems are also extremely common and affect millions of persons on a seasonal basis.

All forms of rhinitis and sinusitis cause sneezing, nasal discharge, nasal obstruction, and headache. Symptoms of acute inflammation (malaise, anorexia, body aches) may not be present to any significant degree. The problems are usually self-limiting and resolve within 1 week, but patients can at any time acquire a bacterial secondary infection that can progress into a much more serious illness. Acute bacterial sinusitis is extremely painful and may require hospitalization for effective management. Drainage of obstructed sinuses may be necessary in severe situations.

There is no specific treatment, so interventions are directed at improving comfort by successfully suppressing the symptoms. Decongestants are recommended for rhinitis, whereas sinusitis often responds well to the use of antihistamines. Nursing care focuses on patient comfort and teaching about preventing spread of the infection, attributed primarily to hand-to-hand contact.

INFECTIONS OF THE PHARYNX AND LARYNX

Acute *pharyngitis* is the most common throat inflammation. It may be caused by numerous viruses as well as streptococci, staphylococci, and other bacteria. Viruses account for over 70% of the cases. Classic symptoms include dryness and pain in the throat and a red appearance. Other symptoms of upper respiratory infection may also be present. Unless a bacterial origin can be determined, the treatment is usually symptomatic in nature with a focus on patient comfort. If antibiotics are indicated, the patient is instructed to complete the entire prescription.

Acute *tonsillitis* involves inflammation of the tonsils and their crypts. It is frequently caused by *Streptococcus* and may follow a respiratory tract infection when the patient's resistance is already low. The onset is rapid and usually involves sore throat, fever, muscle aches, and malaise. The peritonsillar tissue is red and swollen and may produce a yellowish exudate. Treatment involves general comfort measures and the administration of antibiotics if the infection is bacterial. Tonsillectomy may be recommended if the person experiences repeated episodes of infection. Care of the patient following tonsillectomy is presented in the Guidelines box.

Acute *laryngitis* is an inflammation of the mucous membrane that lines the vocal cords accompanied by edema. It usually occurs with or following another respiratory infection. Symptoms vary from slight scratchiness to absolute voice loss. Pain and cough may also be present. Treatment is symptomatic and primarily involves voice rest and general comfort measures.

ACUTE BRONCHITIS
Etiology/Epidemiology

Acute bronchitis is an inflammation of the bronchi and usually the trachea that develops typically as an extension of an upper respiratory infection. Although it is most common in persons with chronic pulmonary disease, it also occurs in communicable forms in persons without an underlying lung pathologic condition. Acute bronchitis is usually viral in origin but can result from either primary or secondary bacterial infection. It can also be triggered by environmental pollution and the inhalation of noxious fumes or chemicals.

Guidelines for Nursing Care of the Person with Tonsillectomy

PREOPERATIVE CARE

Teach patient about the surgical procedure and type of anesthesia planned.
Teach patient about diet and analgesia after surgery.

POSTOPERATIVE CARE

Position patient on side until fully awake and alert.
Use Fowler's position once patient is awake.
Provide adequate analgesia. Avoid use of aspirin.
Apply ice collar if prescribed.
Observe for bleeding:
　Teach patient not to cough or attempt to clear throat for 1-2 weeks.
　Observe patient for frequent swallowing.
　Prevent vomiting if possible; observe for blood.
Offer ice-cold fluids and soft bland diet when patient is stable:
　Avoid use of straw, because it creates throat suction.
　Suggest patient use large swallows since they hurt less.
　Cold items are better tolerated.
　Avoid irritating foods until healing is complete.
Keep fluid intake high, at least 2-3 L.
Patient should avoid rigorous activity and exercise during first 3-5 days but can resume normal activity.
Teach patient to expect worsening of pain between days 4 and 8 when the membrane separates over the incision.

Pathophysiology

The inflammatory process causes an increased blood flow to the affected area with an increase in secretions. Productive cough, low-grade fever, and malaise are typical symptoms. Crackles and wheezes are heard on auscultation. The infection lasts anywhere from 1 to 4 weeks and can deteriorate into acute pneumonia in severe cases.

Medical Management

Treatment is largely symptomatic and revolves around control of fever, management of cough and secretions, rest, and ensuring an adequate fluid intake. A patient with a chronic, nonproductive cough may be given codeine for suppression, particularly at night. Amantadine (Symmetrel) may be given to high-risk patients to shorten the course of the illness, but antibiotics are not administered unless there is clear evidence of bacterial involvement. A bronchodilator may be prescribed if there is significant wheezing or prolongation of peak flow.

NURSING MANAGEMENT

Nursing care is also supportive. The patient is instructed or assisted to cough effectively to clear the airway. Persistent coughing produces significant discomfort, and the patient should be assisted to splint the affected area appropriately. Fluids are encouraged to thin the secretions, and the patient is encouraged not to take OTC antihistamines or decongestants unless truly indi-

cated, since these preparations tend to dry the secretions and make them more difficult to expectorate. An episode of bronchitis may represent an opening to work with a patient on smoking cessation if appropriate.

PNEUMONIA
Etiology/Epidemiology

Pneumonia involves acute inflammation of the lung tissue that can result from inhalation of an infectious agent, transport of organisms via the bloodstream, aspiration, or inhalation of noxious fumes or chemicals. It is the leading cause of infectious disease death in the United States. Over 3 million cases are diagnosed each year. The disease is classified according to the causative organism and is further subdivided according to organisms that are typically acquired in the community versus those acquired in the hospital (Box 8-2).

Community-acquired pneumonias can affect otherwise healthy individuals but more commonly affect individuals with preexisting chronic illnesses or disease states, elderly persons, and immunocompromised persons. The causative agents, severity, and typical symptoms vary substantially among various groups. The atypical pneumonias, which include those caused by viruses, do not present with the classic clinical picture and may not be readily diagnosed in their early stages.

BOX 8-2 Causes of Community- and Hospital-Acquired Pneumonias

COMMUNITY ACQUIRED

Streptococcus pneumoniae: 30%-70%
　Most common in young adults
Haemophilus influenzae: 8%-20%
　Mortality high in bacteremic patients
Atypical pneumonias
　Mycoplasma pneumoniae: 2%-15%
　　Primarily affect adolescents and young adults
　Chlamydia pneumoniae: 2%-6%
　　Occurs primarily in overcrowded and communal sleeping areas
　Legionella pneumophilia: 2%-8%
　　Virulent, with high mortality
　Viruses: 5%-15%
Aspiration pneumonias: 5%-15%
　Involve anaerobic organisms of upper airway

HOSPITAL ACQUIRED

Gram-negative bacteria: 75%-85%
　Pseudomonas aeruginosa alone causes 20%-30%
　Enterobacteriaceae (*Proteus, Klebsiella, Escherichia*): 20%-50%
Staphylococcus aureus: 10%-20%
　Associated with impaired host defense and presence of invasive lines or catheters
Aspiration pneumonias: 2%-20%
　Involve anaerobic organisms of upper airway and pharynx
　Suppression of gastric pH can lead to stomach colonization by bacteria and subsequent migration to airway

> **BOX 8-3** **Risk Factors for Nosocomial Pneumonia**
>
> Age >60 years
> Prolonged hospitalization
> Serious underlying disease state or recent surgery
> Malnutrition or prolonged immobility
> Endotracheal intubation, tracheostomy, or mechanical ventilation
> Invasive lines or monitoring devices
> Depressed alertness, aspiration
> High-dose histamine H_2 blocker use

Hospital-acquired infections are typically caused by different organisms and carry an associated mortality of as much as 30% to 50% because of the presence of coexisting diseases and the high proportion of gram-negative, antibiotic-resistant organisms. Risk factors for the development of nosocomial pneumonia are summarized in Box 8-3.

Pathophysiology

Pneumonia results in inflammation of the lung tissue. The inflammatory process may cause a variety of responses depending on the specific pathogen and the physical status of the individual. Classic pneumonia causes inflammatory exudate to fill the alveolar air spaces, producing lung consolidation that blocks effective gas exchange in the affected alveoli. Excess mucous production, bronchospasm, increased capillary permeability, and pleural inflammation can all occur. Hypoxemia, respiratory acidosis, and bacteremia may occur in virulent cases.

Classic symptoms of pneumonia are as follows:
Abrupt onset
High fever (39° to 40° C with shaking chills)
Pleuritic chest pain with restricted chest movement
Productive cough with purulent, green, or rusty sputum
Tachypnea, inspiratory rales, and dullness to percussion

This pattern is not present in all cases, however. The onset may be more insidious and be accompanied by a lower-grade fever, fatigue, and malaise. This is common with the viral and atypical pneumonias. Some organisms trigger more gastrointestinal (GI) than respiratory symptoms with headache, nausea, and vomiting. Aspiration pneumonias often present with an insidious onset followed by a rapid downhill progression into bacteremia and shock. Organisms that spread to the lungs via the blood rarely trigger significant pulmonary symptoms and instead present with general septicemia.

Medical Management

The diagnosis of pneumonia is confirmed by chest x-ray and obtaining sputum smears and cultures. The white blood cell (WBC) count will be markedly elevated (15,000 to 25,000/mm^3) in the presence of bacterial infection. Initial treatment usually involves a broad-spectrum antibiotic, which is then modified based on the data from culture and sensitivity. Most patients can be safely treated at home. In more severe cases, usually involving elderly persons, hospitalization allows for initial treatment with parenteral antibiotics for 2 to 3 days. The response to appropriate therapy is usually prompt. Hospital-acquired pneumonia requires extremely aggressive treatment because of its associated mortality.

Supplemental oxygen may be needed for patients who are markedly hypoxemic. Supportive care is offered to deal with fever, fatigue, and airway clearance. Strict isolation is rarely required except for staphylococcal pneumonia, and scrupulous hand washing is usually sufficient protection.

NURSING MANAGEMENT

◆ ASSESSMENT
Subjective Data

History and duration of symptoms
History of recent upper respiratory tract infection
Location and degree of chest pain or discomfort
Patient's complaints of the following:
  Fatigue
  Anorexia
  Dyspnea
  Fever and chills

Objective Data

Fever, tachycardia, tachypnea
Decreased breath sounds, inspiratory rales, cyanosis
Dullness to percussion
Productive cough: rusty, purulent, or green sputum
Use of accessory muscles, nasal flaring
Chest splinting
Positive chest x-ray
WBCs >15,000/mm^3

The remainder of the nursing management of the patient with bacterial pneumonia is presented in the "Nursing Care Plan." A "Critical Pathway" for pneumonia is also included.

> **GERONTOLOGIC PATIENT CONSIDERATIONS FOR PNEUMONIA**
>
> Pneumonia is the most frequent cause of death from infection in persons over 65 years of age, and it is the third leading cause of death from any cause in persons over 85 years. The incidence and mortality are both higher in elders with a history of COPD or other chronic illness. Pneumonia is of particular concern during the late fall and winter months when it typically follows infection with a virus. Outreach and teaching concerning the importance of pneumonia vaccine and annual flu shots in this population are essential.

NURSING CARE PLAN

THE PERSON WITH BACTERIAL PNEUMONIA

■ NURSING DIAGNOSIS
Airway clearance, ineffective (related to increased mucous production, inflammation, and alveolar consolidation)

Expected Patient Outcome	Nursing Interventions
Patient's lungs will become progressively clear to auscultation.	1. Collect adequate sputum specimens before administration of antibiotics.
	2. Administer medications as prescribed: antibiotics, expectorants, antitussives.
	3. Ensure adequate room humidity.
	4. Encourage patient to cough and deep breathe effectively.
	5. Encourage deep breathing every 1-2 hours.
	6. Utilize chest physical therapy if patient cannot clear airway by coughing.
	7. Suction airway if patient is unable to effectively clear secretions. Administer nebulizer treatment or bronchodilators as ordered.

■ NURSING DIAGNOSIS
Breathing pattern, ineffective (related to restricted chest movement and splinting)

Expected Patient Outcome	Nursing Interventions
Patient will return to a normal breathing pattern, fully inflating all lung segments.	1. Position patient in semi-Fowler's position to facilitate breathing. Do not position on affected side. Encourage frequent position changes.
	2. Administer oxygen if prescribed by mask or nasal cannula.
	3. Utilize incentive spirometer to encourage effective inhalation.
	4. Assess adequacy of ventilatory effort. Observe for cyanosis, use of accessory muscles.
	5. Monitor arterial blood gases.

■ NURSING DIAGNOSIS
Pain (related to pleural irritation)

Expected Patient Outcome	Nursing Interventions
Patient will experience minimal chest pain.	1. Assist patient to assume position of comfort.
	2. Administer mild analgesics if chest pain is severe.
	3. Splint chest while coughing.
	4. Provide comfort measures: linen, bathing for elevated temperature, mouth care if cough is productive.
	5. Ensure adequate fluids to keep secretions thin.

Continued.

NURSING CARE PLAN—CONT'D

THE PERSON WITH BACTERIAL PNEUMONIA

■ NURSING DIAGNOSIS
Activity intolerance (related to hypoxemia and overwhelming fatigue)

Expected Patient Outcome	Nursing Interventions
Patient will have sufficient energy to return to normal pattern of activities.	1. Encourage adequate rest. 2. Assist patient with activities of daily living as needed. 3. Encourage patient to restrict activity level until disease resolves to prevent relapse.

■ NURSING DIAGNOSIS
Fluid volume deficit, risk of (related to fever and anorexia)

Expected Patient Outcome	Nursing Interventions
Patient will receive sufficient fluids orally and intravenously to compensate for losses and maintain a normal fluid balance.	1. Administer parenteral fluids as ordered. 2. Offer fluids orally as tolerated. Record intake and output accurately. Ensure adequate fluids. 3. Offer small frequent meals high in protein and carbohydrates.

■ NURSING DIAGNOSIS
Impaired home maintenance management, risk of (related to insufficient knowledge about follow-up care and prevention of reinfection)

Expected Patient Outcome	Nursing Interventions

Patient will correctly describe measures to follow after discharge and ways to prevent future reinfection.	1. Prevent spread of disease:
	    Use scrupulous hand-washing procedures.
	    Teach patient about coughing and tissue disposal.
	    Complete full course of antibiotic therapy.
	2. Teach patient importance of frequent thorough cleansing of any vaporizers used in the home.
	3. Teach patient about available immunizations:
	    Annual flu vaccine
	    Pneumonia vaccine every 3-5 years
	4. Encourage patient to maintain adequate nutrition and avoid overfatigue during the recovery period. Four to six weeks of restricted activity is generally needed.
	5. Encourage elderly patients to seek prompt treatment for respiratory infections.

TUBERCULOSIS
Etiology/Epidemiology

Tuberculosis (TB) is an infectious disease caused by *Mycobacterium tuberculosis*, a gram-positive, acid-fast bacillus. The disease was the leading cause of death in the United States in 1900 and remained a major health problem until the introduction of effective drug therapy in the late 1940s and 1950s. Although TB is considered to be both preventable and controllable, it is once again a significant health problem in the United States. The last 20 years have witnessed a massive tide of immigration from Asia where the disease remains endemic and the emergence of HIV infection, which leaves the individual vulnerable to infection by the organism. The

CRITICAL PATHWAY   Pneumonia Without Complications

DRG #: 090; expected LOS: 6

	Day of Admission Day 1	Day 2	Day 3	Day 4	Day 5	Day of Discharge Day 6
Diagnostic Tests	CBC, UA, SMA/18,* chest x-ray, sputum and blood for C & S, ABGs, ECG >40 yr, ?theophylline level	Electrolytes, ABGs, chest x-ray	Check C & S results		Chest x-ray, CBC, electrolytes	
Medications	IVs, IV antibiotics, review/continue home Rxs	IV to saline lock, IV antibiotics, review/continue home Rxs	IV saline lock, IV antibiotics, review/continue home Rxs	IV saline lock, IV antibiotics, review/continue home Rxs	IV saline lock, PO antibiotics, adjust drugs for home use	Discontinue saline lock, PO antibiotics, adjust drugs for home use
Treatments	I & O q 8 hr, VS q 4 hr, weight, O$_2$, respiratory assessment q 4 hr, skin assessment and special care q 4 hr	I & O q 8 hr, VS q 8 hr, respiratory assessment q 4 hr, skin assessment and special care q 4 hr	I & O q 8 hr. VS q 6 gr, weight, O$_2$ PRN. respiratory assessment q 6 hr, skin assessment and special care q 4 hr	I & O q 8 hr. VS q 6 hr, respiratory assessment q 6 hr	Discontinue I & O, VS q 8 hr, weight, respiratory assessment q 8 hr	VS q 8 hr, respiratory assessment q 8 hr
Diet	Clear liquids	Advance diet as tolerated, force fluids	Regular diet, force fluids	Regular diet, force fluids	Regular diet, force fluids	Regular diet, force fluids
Activity	Bed rest with bathroom privileges, head of bed elevated 30 degrees, T, C, & DB q 1 hr	Up in chair and walk with assistance, T, C, & DB q 1 hr, head of bed elevated 30 degrees	Up in room and walk with assistance × 2, T, C, & DB q 2 hr	Up in room and walk with assistance × 4, T, C, & DB q 2 hr	Up ad lib	Up ad lib
Consultations	Respiratory therapy	Social service, skilled nursing unit &/or home health				

*Serum calcium, phosphorus, triglycerides, uric acid, creatinine, BUN, total bilirubin, alkaline phosphate, aspartate aminotransferase (AST; formerly serum glutamic oxaloacetic transaminase [SGOT]), alanine aminotransferase (ALT; formerly serum glutamic oxaloacetic transaminase [SGPT]), lactic dehydrogenase (LDH), total protein, albumin, sodium, potassium, chloride, total CO$_2$, glucose.

BOX 8-4	Multidrug-Resistant Tuberculosis

It is estimated that nearly 10% of TB cases were resistant to isoniazid (INH) and/or rifampin in 1993. Resistance to *both* drugs has been reported in 13 states. New York City had an incidence of multidrug-resistant tuberculosis 52 times that of the rest of the United States. Asians and non-Hispanic blacks are at highest risk. Persons with multidrug-resistant tuberculosis are treated with a four-drug protocol in the attempt to prevent further drug resistance. Preventing infection in others is a major concern, especially in institutional care settings.

recent development of drug-resistant forms of the bacillus is creating pockets of extremely high risk among disadvantaged and substance-abusing populations in major cities that may pose a critical risk to the majority population in the years to come (Box 8-4). This ancient disease has once again taken a place on center stage in public health discussions. Sixteen states plus the District of Columbia again showed increases in their TB case rate during 1993.

TB statistics vary by race, age, and ethnicity. TB has traditionally been seen in minority and immigrant populations, with most new cases occurring in elderly persons. Recently the new case incidence has shifted dramatically toward the 25- to 44-year age-group, which is now showing an expected parallel increase in rates among children under 15 years of age who are presumed to have household contact. Outreach and detection efforts are shifting once again toward the schools and toward the largely urban-based population of HIV-positive individuals who are at high risk for infection and active disease.

Pathophysiology

Tuberculosis is spread by the inhalation of tubercle-laden droplets. When a person with no previous exposure to TB inhales a sufficient number of tubercle bacilli into the alveoli, a TB infection occurs. Inflammation occurs within the alveoli, and natural body defenses attempt to counteract the infection. The body's reaction depends on the susceptibility of the individual, the size of the dose, and the virulence of the organism. NOTE: Most individuals infected by the organism do not develop active disease but demonstrate only positive skin testing and x-ray evidence of calcified nodes or cavities. If the initial immune response is not adequate, clinical disease will then occur.

TB infection is unique in that a person who has been infected with the bacillus harbors the organism for the remainder of life in a so-called dormant or resting state. If a person comes under intense physical or emotional stress or experiences a decline in immune function, the bacilli can become active and begin to multiply. It is estimated, however, that fewer than 1 out of 10 persons with a positive skin test ever develops active disease. TB can affect other areas of the body beside the lungs, and this aspect of the disease assumes significant proportions in the HIV-positive population. The lymph nodes, GI tract, kidneys, and skeletal system all can be affected.

Medical Management

The diagnosis is carefully established through a combination of skin testing, x-ray examinations, and culture of the sputum. Most persons with TB do not have positive smears, and a full culture is required. Because the tubercle bacillus grows slowly, the full culture may take 3 to 6 weeks.

The foundation of treatment is drug therapy, with at least four drugs initially to prevent the further development of resistant organisms. Drug susceptibility testing should be performed as soon as the organism can be successfully cultured. The drug regimen can be modified as needed once susceptibility results are available. INH and rifampin are the cornerstones of treatment, supplemented with pyrazinamide (PZA), ethambutol, and streptomycin as needed. Drug therapy is summarized in Table 8-2. Four-drug treatment is indicated for 2 months followed by at least 6 months of therapy with

TABLE 8-2 Drugs Used to Treat Tuberculosis

DRUG	DOSAGE	SIDE EFFECTS
FIRST-LINE DRUGS		
Isoniazid (INH)	5-10 mg/kg/day	Peripheral neuritis, hepatic toxicity, hypersensitivity (skin rash, fever, arthralgia)
Ethambutol (EMB)	15-25 mg/kg/day	Optic neuritis, peripheral neuritis, skin rash, GI upset
Rifampin	10-20 mg/kg/day	Hepatitis, fever, GI upset, peripheral neuropathy
Streptomycin	15-20 mg/kg/day	Auditory toxicity, nephrotoxicity
SECOND-LINE DRUGS		
Para-aminosalicylic acid (PAS)	150 mg/kg/day	GI upset, hypersensitivity, hepatotoxicity
Ethionamide	750-1000 mg/day	GI upset, hepatotoxicity
Kanamycin	0.5-1 g/day	Auditory toxicity, nephrotoxicity
Capreomycin	1 g/day	Auditory toxicity, nephrotoxicity
Pyrazinamide (PZA)	15-30 mg/kg/day	Hyperuricemia, hepatotoxicity
Cycloserine	750 mg/day	Psychosis, personality change, skin rash

BOX 8-5 — Directly Observed Therapy Programs

Nonadherence to TB drug therapy can lead to prolonged infectiousness and increased transmission of TB in the local community. It is also a major factor in the development of drug-resistant organisms. Directly observed therapy requires a setting where the patient goes to receive medication two or three times per week. Clinics, shelters, drug treatment centers, schools, and jails are all possible sites. The medication is then administered under the direct observation of a designated responsible person who is not necessarily a health care provider. Community nurses in the inner city are providing direct outreach services in some settings to take the medication directly to the target population. Legislation is in place in some settings that allows TB patients to be taken into custody for treatment if they fail to comply with the requirements of direct observation.

INH and rifampin if the organism is resistant. Patients who are HIV positive are treated for at least 9 months. Since nonadherence to the drug regimen is a major factor in the development of resistant organisms, many communities are developing directly observed therapy programs (Box 8-5). Immunization with bacille Calmette Guérin (BCG) vaccine, which has long been practiced around the world, is again being considered in the United States in light of the increased threat of TB to the population at large (see Home Care box).

Adequate rest and optimal nutrition are the other components of basic care. Management is also directed at preventing the spread of the disease. Basic hygiene precautions for coughing and sputum disposal are important, but strict isolation at home is not necessary. Family and social contacts are skin tested, and high-risk individuals may receive preventive drug therapy.

Home Care for TB Prevention

Prophylactic chemotherapy with INH is recommended for persons with recent skin test conversions, persons who are close contacts of individuals diagnosed with infectious TB, and persons with medical conditions that increase their risk of TB, such as HIV-positive status. Patients are monitored closely during therapy, particularly individuals over 35 years who are at greater risk for drug-related hepatitis. Therapy is continued for 6 months.

BCG vaccine is used worldwide as a TB vaccine but has never achieved widespread acceptance in the United States because of controversy about its safety and effectiveness. It is used only in persons who have a negative response to a TB skin test. Recent students indicate that the vaccine significantly reduces the risk of active TB and death with an overall protective effect of 50%. With this level of success, the vaccine is again being considered for infants and children who have continuing exposure to persons with resistant organisms or in communities where the infection rate exceeds 1% per year. It is also being considered for use in institutional settings. Broader recommendations may emerge in the future.

NURSING MANAGEMENT

◆ ASSESSMENT
Subjective Data

History and progression of symptoms
History of TB exposure
Family composition—members at risk
Patient's complaints of the following:
   Fatigue and malaise
   Anorexia and weight loss
   Afternoon or night sweats
Patient's perceptions of or attitudes toward the diagnosis of tuberculosis

Objective Data

Vital signs; presence of low-grade fever, particularly in the afternoon
Productive cough, character of sputum (may be blood streaked)
Decreasing weight
Positive skin test (see Guidelines box), chest x-ray

◆ NURSING DIAGNOSES

Nursing diagnoses for the person with tuberculosis may include, but are not limited to, the following:
   Activity intolerance (related to fatigue generated by inflammatory response)

Guidelines for Administering a PPD Skin Test

1. Choose an injection site on the inner aspect of the forearm that is free of hair, lesions, and tatoos.
2. Wipe the site with alcohol and pat dry.
3. Pull the skin taut, and position the 25- or 27-gauge ½- to ⅝-inch needle at a 10- to 15-degree angle.
4. Smoothly insert the needle, bevel up, until the bevel is fully inserted. *The needle tip should still be visible under the skin.* If it is not, the needle is inserted too deeply.
5. Slowly inject 0.1 ml of the PPD solution into the dermis. You should feel slight resistance, and a raised whitish wheal will appear under the skin.
6. Wipe the injection site with gauze, circle the site with a pen for easy identification, and cover with an adhesive bandage.

READING THE TEST
1. Read at 48-72 hours.
2. Measure the induration with a flexible metric ruler:
   a. Indurations of 5 mm or more: immunocompromised patients; persons with chest x-rays that confirm old healed TB; persons with close contact with someone with infectious TB
   b. Indurations of 10 mm or more: immigrants from indigenous TB areas; medically underserved, low-income populations; health care workers caring for high-risk patients; residents of long-term care facilities such as nursing homes, shelters, or jails
   c. Indurations of 15 mm or more: a positive reaction for anyone

Airway clearance, ineffective (related to excess mucus production)

Knowledge deficit (related to tuberculosis, its treatment, and prevention of its spread)

◆ EXPECTED PATIENT OUTCOMES

Patient will experience increased energy and be able to resume normal ADL.

Patient will experience decreased sputum production and maintain a clear airway.

Patient will be knowledgeable about the tuberculosis disease process, need for long-term therapy, and measures to prevent spread of the disease.

◆ NURSING INTERVENTIONS

Conserving Energy

Encourage patient to allow for adequate rest until energy level improves.

Space and limit activities.

Assist patient with ADL as required.

Explore ways to modify food patterns to meet nutritional needs within the constraints of persistent anorexia.

Employ appropriate nursing measures to increase patient's comfort level: linen changes, tepid baths.

Promoting Airway Clearance

Establish degree of respiratory isolation indicated (Box 8-6).

Teach patient rationale for restrictions.

Teach patient importance of covering mouth when coughing or sneezing.

BOX 8-6	Inpatient Precautions for Patients with TB

1. Patient is placed in a private room with the hallway door kept closed.
2. Negative airflow should be present in the room to prevent room air from moving out into the hallway.
3. Room air is exchanged at least six times per hour with fresh air from the outside.
4. High-energy particulate air filters can be installed over ventilation ducts, and ultraviolet lights may be used to disinfect the room air.
5. Personnel caring for the patient should use disposable particulate respirators that fit snugly over the nose and mouth.
6. Patients who need to leave the room for tests should wear particulate respirators with a one-way valve.
7. Precautions are maintained until the patient has three negative smears for TB and is considered noninfectious.
8. All health care workers should know their tuberculin status and be tested at least yearly.
9. Health care workers who convert to a positive tuberculin test should be examined for active disease and offered INH preventive therapy.

Teach patient proper technique for disposal of contaminated tissues and importance of good hand washing.

Follow strict hand-washing precautions.

Encourage the patient to maintain a high fluid intake.

Teaching for Effective Self-Care

Administer medications as prescribed (see Table 8-2). Teach patient about expected side effects, especially GI disturbances.

Patient should take supplemental vitamin B_6 while taking first-line drugs.

Tell patient taking rifampin that it turns body secretions orangy red.

Teach patient importance of taking all medications for as long as prescribed (may be 9 to 24 months).

Stress importance of routine follow-up to monitor for toxic effects of medications.

Encourage patient and family to verbalize feelings and concerns about diagnosis of tuberculosis.

Reinforce the importance of completing the full course of therapy to prevent the incidence of resistant organisms.

Teach family importance of ongoing screening for family members exposed to tuberculosis.

Teach patient facts about possibility of future recurrence and importance of being alert to symptoms.

◆ EVALUATION

Successful achievement of expected outcomes for the patient with tuberculosis is indicated by the following:

Resumption of usual daily pattern of activity without fatigue

Minimal cough and sputum production; clear airway

Correct statements about medication side effects and their management; expressed commitment to long-term care and follow-up

FUNGAL INFECTIONS OF THE LUNG

The three major fungal infections of the lungs (histoplasmosis, coccidioidomycosis, and blastomycosis) are classified as deep mycoses, because there is involve-

---

GERONTOLOGIC PATIENT CONSIDERATIONS FOR TUBERCULOSIS

Elderly persons are at significantly high risk of developing active TB. General immunocompetence declines steadily with age, and elders may also be affected by inadequate nutrition and a variety of chronic illnesses that also impair their ability to maintain adequate immune surveillance. Many of these cases will involve reactivation of organisms that had been encountered and walled off earlier in the person's life, but primary first-encounter tuberculosis also occurs with greater frequency in this population.

TABLE 8-3 Fungal Infections of the Lung

DESCRIPTION	COMMON SYMPTOMS	TREATMENT
HISTOPLASMOSIS		
Most common systemic mycotic disease in United States; occurs from inhalation of spores of *Histoplasma capsulatum* from soil contaminated with infected excreta from fowl and bats	Severe infections: acute onset with fever, chest pain, dyspnea, prostration, weight loss, widespread pulmonary infiltrates, hepatomegaly, and splenomegaly; no symptoms in mild cases	Drug(s) of choice: amphotericin B (Fungizone intravenous) and ketoconazole (Nizoral); 75% of patients cured; without treatment patient with disseminated disease will die
COCCIDIOIDOMYCOSIS (VALLEY FEVER, SAN JOAQUIN VALLEY FEVER)		
Endemic to well-defined areas in southwestern United States, Mexico, and South America; occurs from inhalation of spores of *Coccidioides immitis* from contaminated soil; growth enhanced by rainfall and inhibited by sunlight	Asymptomatic upper respiratory tract infection in about 60% of those who inhaled spores; 40% have symptoms ranging from flulike illness to frank pneumonia	Amphotericin B IV Therapy required for only 10% of those with symptoms; remainder have spontaneous remission
BLASTOMYCOSIS		
Most prevalent in the United States and Canadian valley areas Believed to be caused by inhalation of *Blastomyces dermatitidis* from soil contaminated with spores carried on air currents and inhaled by humans and animals	Skin lesions that appear as small papular or pustular lesions on exposed parts of the body such as hands and face Peripheral development of lesions; may become raised and do not itch	Amphotericin B IV; mandatory in immunocomprised patients Ketoconazole orally

ment of the parasite in deeper tissues and internal organs of the body. These disorders are summarized in Table 8-3.

OCCUPATIONAL LUNG DISEASES

Many pulmonary diseases are believed to be caused by substances that are inhaled in the workplace. However, disorders such as asthma, bronchitis, and emphysema are almost impossible to directly attribute to occupational risk, since their incidence is indirectly related to some very diverse variables. Even so, it is estimated that millions of Americans experience job-related pulmonary disorders and the risk of developing a work-related disorder is dramatically increased by a smoking history. Some of the more common forms are summarized in Table 8-4.

OBSTRUCTIVE PROBLEMS OF THE UPPER AIRWAY

Partial obstruction of the airway results from several common problems, including deviated septum, nasal polyps, and enlarged tonsils and adenoids. Most of these disorders lead to some difficulty with breathing and may manifest as noisy breathing, snoring, postnasal drip, or loss of the sense of smell. Nasal trauma is also quite common and may result in abrupt displacement of the bones. Cosmetic problems are another common complaint of persons who seek medical care. The management is typically surgical in nature and may involve

Guidelines for Nursing Care of the Patient After Nasal Surgery

PREOPERATIVE TEACHING

Teach the patient concerning the following:
  Procedure and type of anesthesia to be used (general or local)
  Necessity for mouth breathing after surgery because of nasal packing
  Appearance: significant swelling and bruising expected

POSTOPERATIVE CARE

Monitor vital signs regularly.
Monitor for signs of bleeding:
  Observe for excessive swallowing and hematemesis.
  Assess bleeding through nasal drip pad.
Change drip pad under nose as needed.
Place patient in mid-Fowler's position—apply ice over nose for 24 hours.
Encourage fluid intake.
Provide oral mouth care frequently.
Provide adequate analgesia and relief for nausea if indicated.
Maintain or provide adequate room humidity. Utilize cool mist via collar.
Inform patient that first stools may be tarry from swallowing blood.
Avoid constipation and vigorous coughing if possible during healing.

tonsillectomy/adenoidectomy, septoplasty, rhinoplasty, or polypectomy. Tonsillectomy was presented in the Guidelines box on p. 131, and the general care for patients undergoing nasal surgery is presented in the Guidelines box above.

TABLE 8-4 Major Occupational Lung Diseases

DISEASE	DESCRIPTION	COMMON SYMPTOMS/COURSE
ASBESTOS-RELATED LUNG DISEASE		
	One of the most dangerous occupational hazards; can cause both fibrosis and cancer in asbestos workers	After fibrosis begins, cough, sputum, weight loss, increasing breathlessness; most die within 15 yr of first symptoms
	20%-25% of deaths of workers with heavy exposure are from lung cancer; cancer related to degree of asbestos and to *cigarette smoking, which enhances carcinogenic properties of asbestos*	
	Mesothelioma (cancer of pleura) accounts for 7%-10% of deaths of asbestos workers; inoperable and always fatal; can occur after very little exposure	
PNEUMOCONIOSES		
Coal worker's pneumoconiosis (CWP; "black lung disease")	150,000 coal miners in United States at risk	Simple CWP: dust accumulation in lungs; over years dust piles up, and respiratory bronchioles are dilated (called focal emphysema); no symptoms; no respiratory difficulty
	10%-30% of all coal miners develop simple form of disease, more prevalent in miners of anthracite or hard coal	
Complicated CWP or progressive massive fibrosis (PMF)	3% of persons with simple CWP develop complicated form: more often occurs in miners with heavy deposits of coal dust in lungs	Fibrosis develops in some dust-laden areas; fibrosis spreads and fibrotic areas coalesce; eventually most of lung is stiffened and useless
		PMF shortens life span; may die from respiratory failure, cor pulmonale, or superimposed infection
Acute silicosis	1 million people in United States run risk of developing silicosis	Inflammatory reaction within alveoli, diffuse fibrosis
	Rapidly progressive disease, leading to severe disability and death within 5 yr of diagnosis	Early symptoms: difficulty in breathing, weight loss, fever, cough
Chronic silicosis	Inhaled silica dust; commonest form seen in miners, foundry workers, and others who inhaled relatively low concentrations of dust for 10-20 yr	Dust accumulated in tissue → breathlessness with exercise
Complicated silicosis	20%-30% of persons with chronic silicosis develop this	Progressive massive fibrosis (PMF) throughout lungs → decreased lung function and cor pulmonale
		Breathlessness, weakness, chest pain, productive cough with sputum, respiratory cripple, dies of heart failure
Allergic alveolitis (farmer's lung)	Hypersensitivity disease caused by fine organic dust inhaled into smallest airways; cause of farmer's lung is moldy hay; other dusts can cause allergic alveolitis	Alveoli inflamed inundated by WBCs, sometimes filled with fluid
		Chronic form develops over time; eventually, fibrosis occurs
		Symptoms begin some hours after exposure to offending dust and include fatigue, shortness of breath, dry cough, fever, and chills; recovery may take 6 wk, and patient may suffer residual lung damage
Byssinosis (brown lung)	Occupational disease occurs in textile workers; mainly in cotton workers but also afflicts workers in flax and hemp industries	Chronic bronchitis and emphysema develop in time
		Symptoms of asthma and allergy persist as long as there is exposure to cotton antigen
		Strong relationship between amount of dust inhaled and symptoms
MIXED-DUST PNEUMOCONIOSES		
	Many workers exposed to a mixture of dusts	Individual dusts usually deposit in patterns that can be recognized on x-ray film; mixed dusts result in different patterns
	Not known whether mixed dusts in lungs are additive (1 + 1 = 2) or potentiating (1 + 1 = 5)	Amount of fibrosis present depends on amount of silica inhaled

---

BOX 8-7   **Acute Airway Obstruction: Laryngeal Edema**

Acute laryngeal edema is a medical emergency that can be caused by anaphylaxis or massive edema following inflammation, trauma, intubation, or surgery to the throat. The airway narrows acutely and obstructs normal ventilation. Emergency management involves the administration of corticosteroids and/or epinephrine and may necessitate intubation or the formation of a tracheostomy. Respiratory arrest occurs rapidly if the patency of the airway is not promptly restored.

CANCER OF THE RESPIRATORY SYSTEM
CANCER OF THE LARYNX
Etiology/Epidemiology

Squamous cell carcinoma of the larynx is a relatively rare cancer that has been steadily increasing in frequency in recent years. Approximately 12,500 cases are diagnosed each year. The disease occurs five times more commonly in men than in women and typically affects individuals over 60 years of age. Risk factors include heavy smoking and extensive alcohol use. Links have also been found with chronic laryngitis and voice abuse.

Pathophysiology

The disease can arise from any part of the laryngeal mucous membrane. It is slow growing when confined to the true vocal cords because of the limited lymphatic supply. It becomes much more aggressive when found elsewhere in the laryngeal area. Tumor growth prevents the free vibration of the vocal cords and creates the classic early sign of progressive persistent hoarseness. As the disease advances it can cause dysphagia, a feeling of obstruction in the throat, or pain in the region of the Adam's apple.

Medical Management

The diagnosis is usually confirmed by fiberoptic laryngoscopy, possibly supplemented by biopsy. Treatment options for early disease include radiation and surgery. Laser excision or partial laryngectomy is a common approach. When the tumor is more advanced, more aggressive surgical excision is indicated and usually is combined with postoperative radiation and possibly chemotherapy in the attempt to preserve laryngeal function. Extensive tumors necessitate complete laryngectomy, usually coupled with some degree of radical neck dissection (Box 8-8 and Figure 8-3).

NURSING MANAGEMENT

◆ ASSESSMENT (PREOPERATIVE)
Subjective Data

History and severity of symptoms
Patient's history of smoking, alcohol use, or voice abuse

BOX 8-8   **Options for Surgical Treatment of Laryngeal Cancer**

VERTICAL PARTIAL LARYNGECTOMY

One half of the larynx is removed. The voice is hoarse but adequate for communication, and there are minimal problems with swallowing.

SUBTOTAL LARYNGECTOMY

Removal of more than one half of the larynx or a portion of the second vocal cord. Voice is increasingly compromised, and the individual has significant problems with swallowing.

SUPRAGLOTTIC LARYNGECTOMY

This procedure is used to remove larger supraglottic tumors and excises the top of the larynx horizontally, leaving the true vocal cords intact. Voice quality remains intact, but the patient has significant swallowing impairment that creates a high risk for aspiration.

TOTAL LARYNGECTOMY

The procedure involves the removal of the epiglottis, thyroid cartilage, hyoid bone, cricoid cartilage, and three or four rings of the trachea in addition to the entire larynx. The pharyngeal tracheal opening is closed, as is the anterior wall of the hypopharynx, and the remaining trachea is brought out to the neck and sutured, creating a permanent tracheostomy. The voice is lost, and the sense of smell is severely compromised.

Patient's knowledge of surgical procedure and outcomes
Patient's response to potential loss of vocal function
Assessment of past coping mechanisms
Occupation and leisure activities

Objective Data

General health status, especially respiratory system
Degree of hoarseness
Difficulty with swallowing, pain

◆ NURSING DIAGNOSES

Nursing diagnoses for the person with laryngeal cancer undergoing laryngectomy may include, but are not limited to, the following:

Airway clearance, ineffective (related to edema around surgical area and increased volume of secretions)
Communication, impaired verbal (related to loss of vocal mechanism)
Infection and nonhealing of surgical wounds, risk of
Altered nutrition, risk of: less than body requirements (related to initial NPO status and impaired swallowing)
Impaired home maintenance management, risk of (related to inadequate knowledge about laryngectomy stoma care)

◆ EXPECTED PATIENT OUTCOMES

Patient will maintain a clear airway through appropriate use of positioning and suctioning.
Patient will effectively communicate needs to nursing staff.

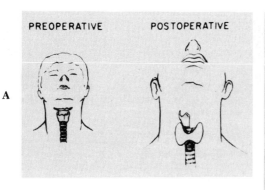

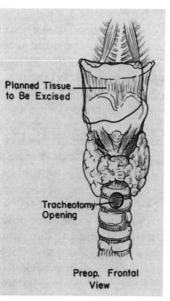

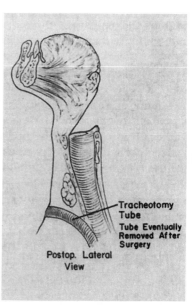

FIGURE 8-3 **A,** Hemilaryngectomy (vertical partial laryngectomy). **B,** Supraglottic (horizontal partial) laryngectomy. (From DeWeese DD et al: *Otolaryngology: head and neck surgery,* ed 7, St Louis, 1988, Mosby.)

Patient's incisions will heal without infection.

Patient will ingest a normal diet orally without evidence of aspiration and will maintain a stable body weight.

Patient will demonstrate mastery of all skills needed for home stoma care and correctly describe symptoms needing medical evaluation.

◆ NURSING INTERVENTIONS

Preoperative Teaching

Prepare patient for surgery and postoperative care.
Explain the following:

Presence and appearance of stoma and nature of neck breathing

Hemovac or other wound drainage if planned

Technique of suctioning and equipment

Devices to deliver humidity

Presence of nasogastric tube for tube feeding

Encourage patient and family to ask questions and discuss fears and concerns about surgery and rehabilitation.

Discuss loss of normal speech.

Discuss with patient the communication device to be used after the operation, such as magic slate, chalkboard, or pad and pencil.

Present options of speech rehabilitation:

Assess patient for readiness for visit from a rehabilitated patient.

Facilitating Airway Clearance

Position the patient with the head of bed elevated 30 to 45 degrees.

Maintain the neck in a slightly flexed position to minimize tension on the suture lines and instruct the patient to support the head during movement and position changes.

Suction tracheostomy frequently to keep the airway clear (see box on tracheostomy care).

NOTE: Suctioning may be needed very frequently during the first few postoperative hours.

Keep the cuff inflated for the first 16 to 24 hours or as ordered to minimize the risk of aspiration. Suction the airway thoroughly when the cuff is deflated.

NOTE: A cuffed tube is not needed after total laryngectomy surgery, since the entire upper airway has been removed and aspiration is not physically possible.

Auscultate the lungs before and after each episode of suctioning.

Maintain humidity to the stoma.

Administer cool mist therapy via T-tube or cervical mask.

Encourage deep breathing and perform chest physiotherapy as needed.

Promoting Effective Communication of Needs

Ensure that call bell remains within easy reach. Answer promptly.

Utilize yes and no questions to minimize frustration and effort required of patient.

Provide patient with the agreed upon communication device at the bedside.

Avoid using the patient's writing arm for IV tubing.

Preventing Infection and Promoting Wound Healing

Monitor the surgical site frequently. Dressings are not usually used after surgery.

Note and record color, temperature, capillary refill, and induration of all skin flaps.

Assess suture line for color, approximation of edges, edema, and presence and character of drainage.

Keep the incision lines free of crusting and exudate. Cleanse with saline or half-strength hydrogen peroxide as ordered and apply antibiotic ointment.

Monitor for signs of wound dehiscence or the development of fistulas, particularly if the patient has received radiation therapy.

Cleanse and inspect all drainage tubes. Monitor and record all wound drainage. Initial drainage will be bloody to serosanguineous in nature. The amount of drainage should decrease steadily in the first postoperative days.

Supporting Adequate Nutrition

Initiate nasogastric tube feedings, and assess tolerance.

Assess bowel sounds, and record frequency and character of stools.

Ensure adequate fluid intake; monitor intake and output, and assess patient for indications of dehydration.

Weigh patient daily.

Provide frequent mouth care, and keep mucous membranes moist.

Assess swallowing ability, and assist occupational therapy in swallowing retraining efforts.

Begin oral feedings cautiously with clear water; keep head of bed elevated.

Provide support and reassurance for total laryngectomy patient that aspiration can not occur.

Assess partial laryngectomy patients for signs of aspiration. A sensation of choking is common.

Explain the loss of smell sensation to the patient, and assist with nasal hygiene as needed.

Teaching for Effective Home Management

Teach patient self-care of tube if permanent stoma has not been created (suctioning is rarely needed after discharge). See Home Care box.

Help patient plan for life-style modifications that will be necessary after discharge:

Prevent water and foreign objects from entering stoma.

Adjust hygiene routines—take precautions when bathing or showering and when shaving (avoid use of talc).

Make clothing adjustments such as scarf or collar of porous material to cover stoma.

Make recreational adjustments—swimming and water sports are contraindicated.

Refer patient and family for community support services:

Services of the American Cancer Society

Home Care after Laryngectomy

HUMIDITY

Use a cool mist humidifier whenever possible and especially at night. Be sure to follow product recommendations concerning care and cleaning.

Cover the stoma during the day with a dampened gauze cover, and remoisten as needed throughout the day.

Instill 3-5 ml of normal saline into the tube if mucous plugs become a problem.

Drink at least 8-10 glasses of fluid daily.

PRECAUTIONS

Keep stoma covered when outdoors to protect the airway from dust, pollen, or other substances.

Tub baths are fine. If a shower is preferred use a hand-held shower head or acquire a stoma shower guard.

The stoma can be washed daily with warm water and soap, taking care to prevent introduction of soap or water into the airway.

Use particular caution when washing the hair.

Cover the stoma during shaving. Avoid use of talc or baby powder.

Carry a Medic-Alert tag or bracelet that identifies you as a neck breather.

OTHER

Pay special attention to mouth care. Dryness contributes to bad breath and tooth decay.

Adjust routines to keep nasal passages free of secretions.

Discuss sexuality issues with partner. The loss of normal airflow can be extremely upsetting to the partner who may be afraid to verbalize feelings.

Location of nearest Lost Chord or New Voice club, and the International Association for Laryngectomies

Support and visitation from family and friends

Arrange for follow-up services from speech pathology department. Options for rehabilitation are described in Box 8-9.

Support all positive coping behaviors. Reinforce a positive body image.

♦ EVALUATION

Successful achievement of expected outcomes for the patient with laryngectomy surgery is indicated by the following:

Airway clear to auscultation; thin scant sputum

Ability to communicate needs effectively; referrals for speech rehabilitation

Incisions healed without breakdown or infection

Stable body weight, ability to swallow a soft diet without choking or aspiration

Demonstration of all aspects of stoma management; correct listing of precautions to be followed during daily activities; positive expressions concerning physical self

BOX 8-9 Speech Rehabilitation after Laryngectomy

ESOPHAGEAL SPEECH

Speech is produced by voluntarily expelling swallowed air. This used to be the primary patient option, but the increasing use of postoperative radiotherapy causes fibrotic tissue formation that impairs this method. Many patients were also unable to learn to eructate frequently and on demand.

TRACHEOESOPHAGEAL SPEECH

A tracheoesophageal puncture is made to create a tracheoesophageal fistula large enough to permit the insertion of a valve prosthesis. The prosthesis is a hollow silicone tube that is open at the tracheal end and closed with a valve at the pharyngeal end. The patient covers the opening with a finger or opens and closes a special valve to divert air from the lungs. When the patient talks, air pressure opens the valve and permits air to enter the esophageal area (Figure 8-4).

ELECTROLARYNX

Several mechanical devices can be used externally to produce speech sound. These speech aids, which function as vibrators or artificial larynxes, have improved dramatically in the quality of the voice product and now provide for pitch inflection, but they are still clearly electronic in nature. Most contain a battery-powered device that is placed against the side of the neck. This method can be easily mastered by any patient.

LUNG CANCER

Etiology/Epidemiology

Lung cancer is the leading cause of cancer death in both men and women. The disease may be either a primary tumor in the lung or a metastatic process from a primary site elsewhere in the body. Metastasis from the colon is extremely common. Approximately 172,000 new cases were diagnosed in 1993, with over 153,000 deaths. Less than 15% of individuals are expected to survive for 5 or more years after diagnosis. The incidence statistics have increased dramatically over the last 50 years, primarily related to levels of cigarette smoking, industrial exposure, and environmental pollution. The longer the duration of the smoking history, the greater the risk. Most individuals are over 50 years of age at the time of diagnosis. The actual mortality risk of any particular case of lung cancer depends on the type of cancer cell involved and the location and size of the tumor at the time of diagnosis. Early detection remains a severe problem in disease management, because there are few early symptoms.

Pathophysiology

Adenocarcinomas are the most common form of lung cancer, followed closely by squamous cell tumors. Each represents about 40% of the total. Small cell (oat cell) tumors represent an additional and extremely deadly 15% to 20%. Histologic analysis is essential. Specimens are obtained by bronchoscopy, sputum collection, and excision of the lesion.

TABLE 8-5 Major Types of Lung Surgery

PROCEDURE	DESCRIPTION
Pneumonectomy	Entire lung removed; phrenic nerve crushed to allow diaphragm to rise and partially fill space; drainage tubes not used
Lobectomy	One lobe of a lung removed; remaining tissue must be capable of overexpanding to fill up space; two chest tubes used for postoperative drainage
Segmental resection	One or more lung segments removed; procedure attempts to preserve maximum amount of functional lung tissue; two chest tubes used for postoperative drainage; air leaks may delay reexpansion
Wedge resection	Well-circumscribed diseased portion removed without regard for segmental planes; two chest tubes used for postoperative drainage

Most lung tumors arise in the bronchi. The patient may be asymptomatic or simply have a cough. As the tumor grows, hemoptysis, shortness of breath, and unilateral wheezing are common. When tumors grow peripherally, they may perforate the pleural space and create extrapulmonary symptoms such as pleural effusion or pain and friction rub. The incidence of weight loss and debility usually indicates the presence of metastases.

Medical Management

Medical management is complicated by the difficulty in early diagnosis of the disease. Specific treatment depends on the tumor histology and disease staging. Treatment options include surgery with either local resection or wide excision, radiation, and chemotherapy, which may be used as primary, adjuvant, or palliative therapy. Table 8-5 describes the basic types of lung surgery.

The nursing management that follows is targeted to the care of the patient undergoing thoracic surgery.

NURSING MANAGEMENT

◆ ASSESSMENT
Subjective Data

Patient's complaints of the following:
  Cough and dyspnea, pain with breathing
  Hemoptysis
  Fever and chills
  Fatigue and weight loss
  Smoking history: amount, duration, type
  Occupational exposure to carcinogens
  Understanding of diagnosis and proposed treatment

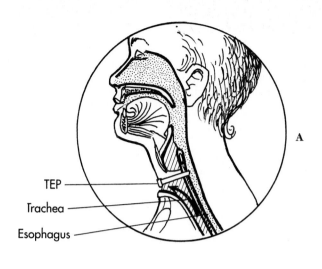

TEP

Trachea

Esophagus

A

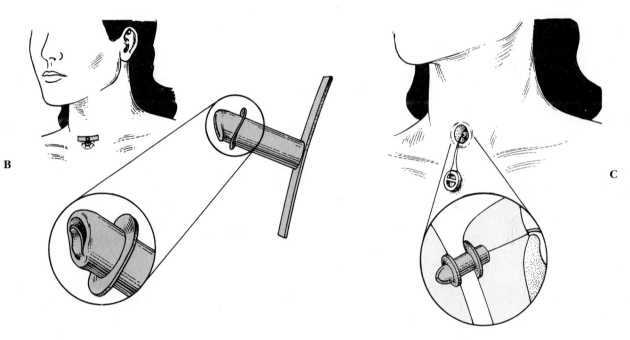

B

C

FIGURE 8-4   Options for Tracheoesophageal Voice Prostheses (TEPs). **A,** Placement of voice prosthesis in relation to trachea and esophagus. **B,** Trapdoor prosthesis. **C,** Voice button.

Objective Data

Visible shortness of breath
Unilateral wheezing
Cough productive of blood-tinged sputum
Positive chest x-ray, CT, or bronchoscopy findings

◆ NURSING DIAGNOSES

Nursing diagnoses for the person undergoing surgery for lung cancer may include, but are not limited to, the following:

Pain (related to incisional tissue damage)

Breathing pattern, ineffective (related to postoperative pain and the presence of chest drainage tubes)
Knowledge deficit (related to surgical treatment of lung cancer)

◆ EXPECTED PATIENT OUTCOMES

Patient will report only manageable incisional pain.
Patient will maintain an effective breathing pattern and a clear airway.
Patient and family will be knowledgeable concerning all aspects of surgical care.

BOX 8-10	Water Seal Chest Drainage

PURPOSE

To remove fluid and air from the intrapleural space to allow for lung reexpansion

TUBE PLACEMENT

One or two tubes may be used

Anterior chest above affected area; used primarily to remove air from the pleural space

Posterior chest below affected area; used primarily to drain serosanguineous fluid that results from surgery

WATER SEAL CHEST DRAINAGE EQUIPMENT

One-, two-, or three-bottle systems or self-contained disposable units (Pleur-Evac) (Figure 8-5)

One-bottle system: provides for gravity drainage of the chest; air and fluid are forced out on inspiration

Two-bottle system: allows for either the addition of suction to aid in chest reexpansion or a separate bottle for drainage collection

Three-bottle system: has separate bottles for water seal, drainage collection, and suction

Pleur-Evac: provides for three-bottle setup in one unit

Water seal established by placing the tip of the tube under water; allows fluid and air to drain from the pleural space but prevents air from reentering the pleural space; lung reexpansion and preservation of negative pressure in the chest supported

---

◆ NURSING INTERVENTIONS

Preoperative Teaching

Teach patient concerning the following:

Diagnostic tests and proposed surgical procedure

Equipment to be used in postoperative care

Correct technique for abdominal breathing and effective coughing

Range of motion exercises for the arm and shoulder

Method of pain control planned for postoperative period

Controlling Postoperative Pain

Administer analgesics as ordered.

Explore the use of patient-controlled analgesia (PCA) if approved.

Ensure adequate pain relief to support effective coughing and deep breathing.

Assist the patient to splint the chest wall during movement and pulmonary hygiene.

Supporting an Effective Breathing Pattern

Maintain patient in a semi-Fowler's position once hemodynamic stability is achieved.

Turn patients with all procedures except pneumonectomies with operative side uppermost to promote lung reexpansion.

Patients with pneumonectomies are positioned on their backs or tilted toward their operative side in

	Guidelines for Nursing Management of Chest Tubes

GENERAL

Check all connections to ensure that they are taped securely.

Fasten tubing to bed to prevent dependent loops.

Ensure that side rails and bed will not come down on top of bottle.

Monitor patient's status regularly—answer all questions about equipment and precautions.

Encourage patient to cough and deep breathe.

Ambulation may be encouraged with water seal drainage.

MONITORING THE WATER SEAL SYSTEM

Check frequently to be sure water is oscillating in water seal.

Tip of chest tube should be 1-2 cm below the water level.

Water level rises during inspiration and falls on expiration.

If water is not moving, check system for obstruction, such as patient lying on tubes.

Water will cease oscillating when lung is fully reexpanded.

Monitor for bubbling in the water seal bottle/chamber, which indicates the continuing presence of an air leak in the lung.

If suction is in use, check regularly to ensure that it is at the prescribed level.

Monitor for bubbling in the suction bottle/chamber, which should be gentle and continuous.

Milk or strip chest tubes only if specifically ordered. This procedure is controversial, since it significantly increases negative pressure in the chest. Gentle squeezing should successfully maintain tube patency.

Keep two hemostats at bedside to clamp chest tube if bottle is accidentally broken. **Note:** Clamping is never done except in emergency or with direct order. It can cause tension pneumothorax. If emergency occurs, reconnect tubes with new sterile setup as quickly as possible.

Never lift chest tube bottles above level of the chest, which would allow fluid to be pulled into the chest.

Mark level in drainage bottle regularly—check every hour while drainage is heavy.

---

their initial care to protect the intact lung from fluid drainage.

Provide supplemental oxygen at 4 to 6 L/min.

Initiate coughing and deep breathing exercises every hour.

Splint chest wall firmly during pulmonary care.

Promote deep abdominal breathing.

Monitor for patency of the water seal drainage system (Box 8-10, Guidelines box, and Figure 8-5).

Monitor for excess drainage and the presence of subcutaneous emphysema.

Report the development of subcutaneous emphysema following pneumonectomy immediately. It could indicate the presence of an air leak in the bronchial stump.

Report the presence of blood on the dressings.

Auscultate lungs and monitor vital signs frequently.

Ensure adequate room humidity.

Maintain an adequate fluid intake to keep secretions thin.

Encourage early and frequent ambulation to tolerance.

Initiate arm and shoulder exercises.

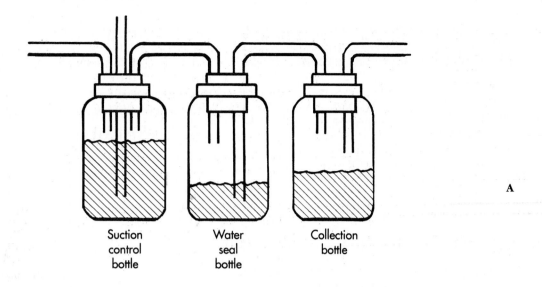

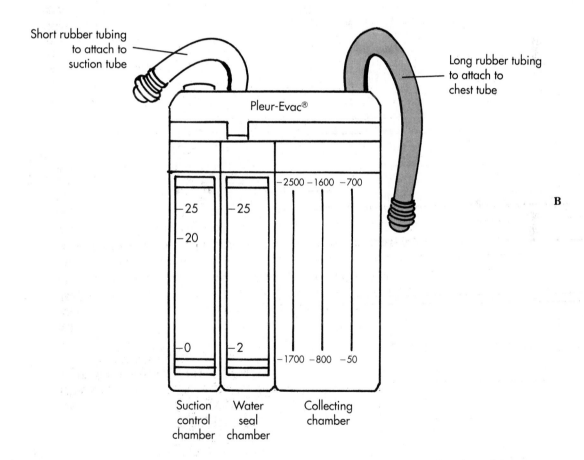

FIGURE 8-5 Options for water seal chest drainage. **A,** Three-bottle system. **B,** Disposable Pleur-Evac.

♦ EVALUATION

Successful achievement of expected outcomes for the patient with lung cancer undergoing surgery is indicated by the following:

Absence of reported incisional pain

Lungs clear to auscultation, normal breathing pattern

Correct description of postsurgical care and home care management

NOTE: Modifications in postoperative care for the patient undergoing pneumonectomy are summarized in the Guidelines box.

Guidelines for Nursing Care Following Pneumonectomy

Chest tubes are not necessary. There is no lung tissue left to reexpand on the operative side.

Patient is positioned on the operative side or back. The patient is *not* positioned on the good side to prevent the drainage of fluid from the surgical side.

Serous drainage collects in the operative space and, over time, congeals and helps to support the mediastinum and remaining thoracic structures in correct position. Patients are initially monitored closely for signs of mediastinal shift (tracheal displacement, dyspnea, distention of the neck veins).

Fluids are carefully monitored for 2-4 days to allow the remaining lung to adjust to the increase in blood flow. Rales are typically audible over the base of the remaining lung.

Activity tolerance is carefully monitored. Decreased vital capacity compromises the patient's ability to engage in activity without severe dyspnea. Heart rate and subjective dyspnea are carefully monitored.

Standard pulmonary hygiene measures are implemented with the remaining functioning lung.

CHEST TRAUMA

Injuries to the chest may affect the bony chest cage, pleurae and lungs, diaphragm, and/or the heart and major blood vessels. Chest injuries are broadly classified as being either blunt or penetrating in nature. Motor vehicle accidents in which the driver is not wearing a seat belt restraint are the leading cause of blunt injury. Violent injury from gunshots or stabbings is the most common cause of penetrating chest injury. Initial treatment is typically begun in the emergency room and supplemented by more definitive surgery or monitoring. The associated nursing care is determined by the nature and extent of the injuries but shares many common features with the care described for patients undergoing thoracic surgery for other causes. Common forms of chest trauma are described in Table 8-6.

ADULT RESPIRATORY DISTRESS SYNDROME

Adult respiratory distress syndrome (ARDS) is the name given to a life-threatening syndrome of acute hypoxemic respiratory failure that is associated with shock, trauma, sepsis, disseminated intravascular coagulation (DIC), emboli, and other critical illnesses. It is characterized by severe dyspnea, hypoxemia, and diffuse pulmonary infiltrations. The pathophysiologic alterations of ARDS are typically initiated by a massive event that may not initially involve the respiratory system. The capillary walls become extremely permeable, allowing fluid, protein, and cells to leak into the interstitial and eventually the alveolar lung spaces. Ventilation and perfusion are both impaired, which induces severe hypoxemia. The normal cells that line the alveoli are destroyed and replaced by cells that cannot produce surfactant (hyaline membrane), which increases surface tension and results in widespread atelectasis and increased pressure to ventilate. The pathophysiologic sequence is outlined in Figure 8-6.

Patients with ARDS are critically ill. They are treated with high concentrations of oxygen and mechanical ventilation support and frequently require the addition of positive end-expiratory pressure (PEEP) to support successful ventilation. Other interventions are similar to those described for the patient in respiratory failure (see p. 163).

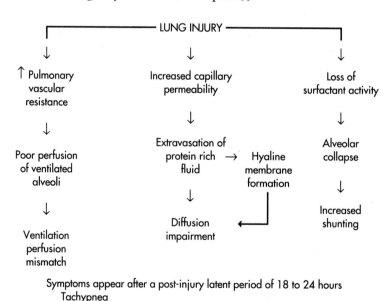

FIGURE 8-6 Pathophysiology of adult respiratory distress syndrome.

TABLE 8-6 Chest Trauma

INJURY	MANAGEMENT
BLUNT INJURIES	
Rib Fractures	
Most common type of chest trauma; usually involves third to tenth ribs; caused by blows or crushing injury	Unless rib fragments penetrate pleura, treatment is conservative, with tight strapping of affected side; nursing care focuses on pain management, support of airway, and assisting patient to adapt self-care skills
Flail Chest	
When ribs or sternum are fractured in more than one place and a portion of chest wall separates from chest cage; chest wall becomes unstable on affected side; insufficient bony support to maintain bellows function of lungs; breathing pattern becomes paradoxical (affected segment pulls inward on inspiration and is forced out on expiration)	Internal stabilization of affected segment; patient intubated on volume-controlled ventilator to stabilize ventilation until bony union occurs; nursing care focuses on airway management, pain control, and prevention of complications
PENETRATING INJURIES	
Pneumothorax	
Chest wall injury allows air to enter pleural space between lung and chest wall; exposure to atmospheric pressure causes lung collapse; condition also known to occur spontaneously or in response to blunt injury; *tension pneumothorax* occurs when air enters pleural space on inspiration but cannot leave on expiration; accumulating air rapidly increases pressure in chest cavity and can result in compression of heart and great vessels or shift of mediastinal contents toward unaffected side	Insertion of chest tube with water seal drainage to effectively reinflate collapsed lung; *tension pneumothorax* is true emergency and may require needle aspiration of accumulated air; nursing care involves maintenance of drainage system and support of effective breathing pattern
Hemothorax	
Blood leaks into pleural space and collapses affected lung; usually occurs in conjunction with pneumothorax	Drainage and reexpansion of affected lung with chest tubes and water seal drainage; related nursing care similar to pneumothorax
Pulmonary Contusion	
Usually results from sudden compression of thorax; blood extravasates into pulmonary tissue; usually self-limiting but can advance rapidly to severe pulmonary edema	Depends on severity of injury; patient may simply require close monitoring or intubation with mechanical ventilation; nursing care focuses on pain management and close monitoring of pulmonary status
Cardiac Tamponade	
Injury causes blood to accumulate in pericardial sac, gradually compressing heart and interfering with effective function	Emergency pericardiocentesis to remove blood and pressure, followed by surgical repair as needed; nursing care involves close monitoring of all vital signs

PULMONARY EMBOLUS

Etiology/Epidemiology

A pulmonary embolus involves the lodging of a clot or other foreign matter within a pulmonary arterial vessel. If the embolus involves a medium-sized artery, an area of infarction occurs in the affected lung. Any condition that predisposes to the development of deep vein thrombosis can result in pulmonary embolus if the clot does not securely adhere to the vessel and the initiating site.

Pathophysiology

An embolus obstructs the blood flow and causes local tissue hypoxia. Associated pulmonary vessels vasoconstrict in response to the hypoxia, creating a ventilation-perfusion mismatch that leads to arterial hypoxemia. A major embolic episode causes abrupt pain, severe dyspnea, coughing, and hemoptysis that can progress rapidly to shock. Emboli in smaller vessels typically produce milder symptoms.

Medical Management

The diagnosis is not always easy to confirm in milder forms. Definitive diagnosis is established by pulmonary angiography. Anticoagulant therapy with heparin is the cornerstone of treatment. Thrombolytic therapy to promote dissolution of the embolus is undergoing research trials. It cannot be used postsurgically, however, because of the significant risk of bleeding. In nonresponsive cases, surgical extraction of the embolus may also be attempted.

NURSING MANAGEMENT

The associated nursing care is largely collaborative and supportive. The nurse maintains meticulous monitoring of all vital functions and assesses for the associated side effects of anticoagulant or thrombolytic therapy. Pulmonary hygiene is maintained hourly. Patient teaching and support are critical interventions during this highly anxious time. After the initial treatment period the nurse instructs the patient in long-term anticoagulant therapy with warfarin sodium (Coumadin) and how to reduce the risk factors for deep vein thrombosis (DVT) in the future (see Chapter 4). The importance of ongoing medical follow-up is emphasized.

CHRONIC OBSTRUCTIVE PULMONARY DISEASE

The category of diseases traditionally labeled chronic obstructive pulmonary disease has been broadened to include other diseases of airflow limitation such as cystic fibrosis, tracheal stenosis, and bronchiolitis. Actual obstruction is therefore not always the only or even the major pathophysiologic component. The term *COPD,* however, is traditionally used to describe a variable combination of asthma, chronic bronchitis, and pulmonary emphysema and remains in widespread use. COPD is a major health problem in the United States, and its associated morbidity and mortality continue to rise. It affects approximately 20 million people, and the associated mortality is one of the fastest growing among all disease processes. The diseases are more common among men, typically appear in middle to late middle age, and are strongly related to cigarette smoking, environmental pollution, chronic infection, and hypersensitivity.

The discussion that follows describes the unique pathophysiologic base of each of the three primary disorders. Most patients exhibit variable mixes of the predominant disease types. The nursing management of chronic bronchitis and emphysema overlaps in most respects and is presented as a unit. Asthma is presented separately.

CHRONIC BRONCHITIS
Etiology/Epidemiology

Chronic bronchitis is defined clinically by its symptoms: hypersecretion of mucus and recurrent or chronic productive cough for at least 3 months per year for at least 2 years. The physiologic signs include hypertrophy and hypersecretion of the bronchial mucous glands caused by inhalation of chemical or physical irritants or by bacterial and viral infections. Cigarette smoking is by far the most common irritant.

Pathophysiology

Two pathologic changes typify chronic bronchitis: hypertrophy in the mucus-secreting glands and chronic inflammatory changes in the small airways. The excessive mucus and impaired ciliary movement increase susceptibility to infection. Increased airway resistance results from tissue changes in the bronchial walls, and the excessive mucus frequently triggers bronchospasm. As the disease progresses, altered O_2 and CO_2 exchange occurs, typically resulting in progressively severe hypoxemia, hypercapnia, and respiratory acidosis.

The earliest symptom of chronic bronchitis is a productive cough, especially on awakening. Compromises in pulmonary function often go unrecognized until they become severe. The individual simply gradually modifies and restricts his or her usual activities to remain within limitations and relatively asymptomatic. An acute respiratory infection usually precipitates the exacerbation of symptoms to a level demanding attention. As the disease progresses, the symptoms increase from episodic to constant in nature, with visible dyspnea the most characteristic feature.

EMPHYSEMA
Etiology/Epidemiology

Emphysema is a disorder characterized by increased lung compliance, decreased diffusing capacity in the lung, and increased airway resistance. It is defined pathologically by destructive changes in the alveolar walls and enlargement of the air spaces that are distal to the terminal bronchiole. The cause remains unknown but appears to involve destruction of the connective tissue of the lung by proteases that may be facilitated by the effects of cigarette smoke. The typical patient is a man between 50 and 60 years old with a long history of cigarette smoking.

Pathophysiology

Two major forms of emphysema can be distinguished by their morphologic features. Centrilobular emphysema is the most common form and involves distention and damage of selective respiratory bronchioles. Openings form in the bronchiole walls that gradually enlarge to form a single distended space. The upper lung segments are primarily affected. In panlobular disease the disease involvement is more uniform and primarily involves destruction of the alveoli. It is more severe in the lower lung segments and appears in individuals without a history of chronic bronchitis or impaired lung functioning.

Characteristic physiologic abnormalities associated with emphysema include (1) increased lung compliance from a loss of elastic recoil (The lungs are permanently overdistended.), (2) increased airway resistance from the narrowing or collapse of the small airways (particularly striking during expiration when air becomes trapped in the distal airspaces), (3) altered oxygen and carbon dioxide exchange from destruction of the bronchiole walls, which decreases the available surface area for gaseous diffusion.

The earliest symptom of emphysema is dyspnea on exertion, which gradually progresses to continuous dys-

BOX 8-11	Clinical Manifestations of Chronic Bronchitis and Emphysema

CHRONIC BRONCHITIS

Early Symptom

Productive morning cough

Later Symptoms

Noticeable shortness of breath
Use of accessory muscles for breathing
Edema, bloated appearance, distended neck veins

Complications of Advanced Disease

Right-sided congestive heart failure
Cor pulmonale
Respiratory failure

Blood Gas Values

Low resting pO_2
Elevated pCO_2

EMPHYSEMA

Early Symptom

Dyspnea on exertion

Later Symptoms

Severe dyspnea
Use of accessory muscles for breathing
Increased (AP) chest diameter

Complications of Advanced Disease

Severe hypercapnia
Cor pulmonale
Respiratory failure

Blood Gas Values

Normal pO_2 at rest; falls with activity
Normal pCO_2 until disease well advanced

BOX 8-12	Drug Therapy in COPD

BRONCHODILATOR

Sympathomimetic agents (adrenergic agents; administered by metered-dose inhaler)
   Albuterol (Proventil)
   Metaproterenol (Alupent, Metaprel)
   Terbutaline (Brethaire)
Xanthine compound
   Theophylline (Theodur); evening administration appears to reduce overnight decline in FEV_1

CORTICOSTEROIDS

Use controversial and not effective in all patients; used primarily when patients show inadequate response to other traditional therapy
   Methylprednisolone (Solu-Medrol)
   Prednisone

ANTICHOLINERGIC AGENT (ADMINISTERED BY INHALER)

Ipratropium (Atrovent)

ANTIBIOTICS

Prophylactic administration not recommended
Commonly prescribed agents:
   Ampicillin
   Amoxicillin
   Tetracycline
   Trimethoprim-sulfamethoxazole
   Ciproflaxin

pnea. Sputum production is scant or absent. Air trapping gradually increases the individual's AP chest diameter. Pursed lip breathing and the use of accessory muscles for breathing are classic indicators. The diagnosis is confirmed from pulmonary function tests that show a decrease in airflow and an increase in residual volumes. The major clinical manifestations of bronchitis and emphysema are presented in Box 8-11.

Medical Management

The management of bronchitis and emphysema overlaps in many ways, and therapy is individualized on the basis of the patient's symptoms, blood gases, and pulmonary function studies. Treatment options include adequate nutrition and hydration, avoidance of environmental irritants, relaxation and breathing retraining, respiratory therapy with oxygen or aerosols, and drug therapy. Options for drug management include the use of bronchodilators, antibiotics, and corticosteroids (Box 8-12).

A critical pathway for a patient with COPD follows the Nursing Management section.

NURSING MANAGEMENT

◆ ASSESSMENT
Subjective Data

History and severity of disease symptoms
Medications and treatments in use
Smoking history
Family history and occupational exposures
History of upper respiratory infections
Knowledge of disease process
Patient's and family's response to progressive disability
Patient's complaints of the following:
   Shortness of breath
   Sleep disturbances
   Chronic cough
   Anorexia
   Fatigue
Perception of general health and fitness

Objective Data

Pulmonary inspection and auscultation
Forward leaning posture
Use of pursed lip breathing, prolonged exhalation
Shortness of breath at rest or with speech or exercise
Use of accessory muscles in respiration

Diminished chest excursion

Increased AP chest diameter

Decreased breath sounds—crackles and rhonchi

Presence and degree of cyanosis

Productive cough—amount and appearance of sputum

Vital signs—presence of tachycardia and tachypnea

Signs of right-sided congestive heart failure, edema

Normal or decreased lung volumes

Blood gases—hypoxemia, hypercapnia, respiratory acidosis

◆ NURSING DIAGNOSES

Nursing diagnoses for the person with COPD may include, but are not limited to, the following:

Gas exchange, impaired (related to destructive changes in the alveolar membrane)

Breathing pattern, ineffective (related to airway changes and fatigue)

Airway clearance, ineffective (related to excessive mucous production and decreased expiratory force)

Impaired home maintenance management, risk of (related to insufficient knowledge about COPD management and measures to improve general health)

◆ EXPECTED PATIENT OUTCOMES

Patient will demonstrate improved ventilation and oxygenation.

Patient will utilize an effective breathing pattern.

Patient will adequately clear the airway with appropriate use of medications and coughing and deep breathing exercises.

Patient will be knowledgeable about the disease process and its treatment and will incorporate health-promoting measures into daily life-style.

◆ NURSING INTERVENTIONS

Promoting Gas Exchange

Monitor blood gases for signs of hypoxemia, hypercapnia, or respiratory acidosis/alkalosis:

Headache and irritability

Confusion

Increasing somnolence

Tachycardia

Administer and teach patient proper use of aerosol therapy (see Guidelines box on p. 153).

Teach safe use of humidifiers and nebulizers.

Teach proper use of hand-held inhalers.

Administer oxygen as prescribed (given when patients are unable to maintain a pO_2 greater than 55 mm Hg or for patients who cannot complete ADL without severe dyspnea): 1 to 2 L of O_2 by nasal prongs or cannula.

Encourage patient to use O_2 continuously for best results, particularly for meals and at night.

NOTE: Only low-flow oxygen is used (1 to 2 L). Low blood oxygen serves as the primary stimulus for breathing in patients with chronically elevated pCO_2 levels. Raising the pO_2 level significantly with supplemental oxygen would eliminate the stimulus to breathe and induce respiratory failure.

Encourage the use of pursed lip breathing to help lower CO_2 levels and improve oxygenation.

Improving Breathing Pattern Efficiency

Assist patient to adjust breathing pattern by doing the following:

Use pursed lips breathing to prolong exhalation and stabilize airway.

Practice diaphragmatic or abdominal breathing.

Exhale with activity.

Assume leaning-forward posture for rest.

Assist patient to consciously slow breathing rate, inhaling over 5 seconds and exhaling over 10 seconds.

Teach patient progressive relaxation exercises.

Assist patient with muscle reconditioning as tolerated.

Promoting Airway Clearance

Administer medications as prescribed.

Teach patient about expected side effects and their management.

Reinforce principles of effective deep breathing and "huff" coughing.

Ensure an adequate daily fluid intake.

Teach patient and family how to perform postural drainage and chest physiotherapy (Box 8-13).

Promoting Effective Home Management

Teach patient about disease progression management.

Assist patient and family members to give up smoking.

Discuss modification of life-style and home environment to reduce exposure to pollutants.

Teach patient measures to avoid infection. Minimize contacts with crowds and young children.

Patient should contact physician promptly if changes occur in the color or amount of the sputum.

Patient should receive an annual flu vaccine and be immunized against pneumonia.

Avoid extremes of hot and cold. Ensure adequate humidity in winter.

Teach patient importance of balanced, nutritious diet and maintaining normal weight.

Use small, frequent feedings if anorexic.

Ensure protein adequacy but limit the amount of carbohydrates, because they produce CO_2 in the body.

Ensure adequate fluid intake.

Reinforce the importance of maintaining or increasing activity level. Explore the availability of a structured rehabilitation program.

Avoid bed rest at all costs.

Guidelines for Use of Hand-held Nebulizers and Metered-dose Inhalers

Solutions of bronchodilator should be diluted in water or saline. This decreases particle size and facilitates deposit of the solution deeper in the smaller airways.

The use of spacers increases the safety and effectiveness of inhaler use (Figure 8-7). They require less coordination of breathing with the administration of the dose.

Note: All aerosol devices are excellent sites for bacterial growth, and proper cleaning is essential to safe use.

METERED-DOSE INHALERS

1. Assess pulse rate before use of the bronchodilator and again after administration to assess response to the medication. Notify the physician if the pulse is greater than 20% faster or stays elevated for more than a few minutes.
2. Shake the canister to mix the medication and propellant.
3. Take a full breath and exhale.
4. Place the mouthpiece into the mouth beyond the teeth. Close the lips tightly around the mouthpiece.
5. Inhale slowly and deeply and depress the canister once during inhalation. **Note:** If using a spacer the patient releases the medication into the spacer and then inhales the drug directly from the device. No coordination of breathing with administration is required. Up to 80% more medication is delivered to the lungs rather than the oropharynx.
6. Hold the breath for 5-10 seconds.
7. Exhale slowly through pursed lips.
8. Gargle with tap water and blow the nose to remove any residual medication.
9. Equipment care:
   a. Clean the metered-dose inhaler mouthpiece daily with mild soap and water, rinse with warm tap water, and allow to air dry.
   b. Soak the mouthpiece once each week for 20 minutes in 1 pint of water mixed with 2 ounces of vinegar.
   c. Protect the canister from extreme temperatures. If the metered-dose inhaler is carried in a purse or bag, keep it in a clean plastic bag.

HAND-HELD NEBULIZERS

1. Exhale fully.
2. Position nebulizer in mouth *without* sealing lips around it.
3. Take a deep breath through mouth while squeezing the bulb of the nebulizer *once*.
4. Hold breath for 3-4 seconds at full inspiration.
5. Exhale slowly through pursed lips.
6. Usually one inhalation is sufficient. Several inhalations of a bronchodilator may cause medication overdosage and result in side effects (e.g., tachycardia, palpitation, and nervousness).

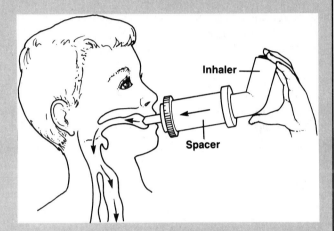

FIGURE 8-7   Patient using inhaler with spacer attached to allow for better dispersal of medication.

♦ EVALUATION

Successful achievement of expected outcomes for the patient with COPD is indicated by the following:

Blood gases maintained within acceptable levels

An effective breathing pattern with a respiratory rate no greater than 24 to 28/min

A clear airway after coughing

Ability to successfully expectorate thin mucus

Correct description of disease components and management

Maintenance of a smoke-free home

A stable body weight

Correct description of measures to avoid infection

ASTHMA

Etiology/Epidemiology

Although asthma is frequently considered to be a disease of childhood, the disorder affects over 10 million persons and over two thirds of them are adults. Both

TABLE 8-7	Asthma Syndromes Classified by Precipitating Factor and Response Pattern	
ASTHMA SYNDROMES	**CHARACTERISTICS**
Atopic asthma	Childhood onset, allergic rhinitis, allergic dermopathy, identifiable environmental precipitating events
Exercise-induced asthma	Airway constriction after exercise
Aspirin-hypersensitivity triad	Presence of nasal polyps, urticaria, and asthma after aspirin ingestion
Bronchospasm associated with nonbacterial upper respiratory tract infections	As described by patient
Industrial asthma	Bronchoconstriction associated with certain industrial precipitating factors

BOX 8-13 Chest Physiotherapy—Clapping and Vibration

PURPOSE

To combine the force of gravity with natural ciliary activity of the small bronchial airways to move secretions upward toward the main bronchi and the trachea.

Usually combined with postural drainage (see Figure 8-8 for positions).

PROCEDURE

Help patient assume appropriate position for lung segment to be drained.

Clap over area with cupped hands for approximately 1 minute to loosen secretions and stimulate coughing.

At conclusion of clapping, instruct patient to breathe deeply; apply vibrating pressure during the expiratory phase.

Have patient cough effectively to clear the airway.

Repeat as needed, and include all appropriate positions.

GENERAL INFORMATION

Modify desired positions as needed to increase patient tolerance.

Clapping is not done over bare skin—provide cloth barrier.

Time treatments for maximal benefit:
Soon after arising
At bedtime
More often as prescribed and tolerated
Complete procedure at least 1 hour before meals

Provide rest and mouth care after procedures.

Auscultate lungs before and after treatment to assess effectiveness.

Humidity and bronchodilators may be given 15-20 minutes before treatment.

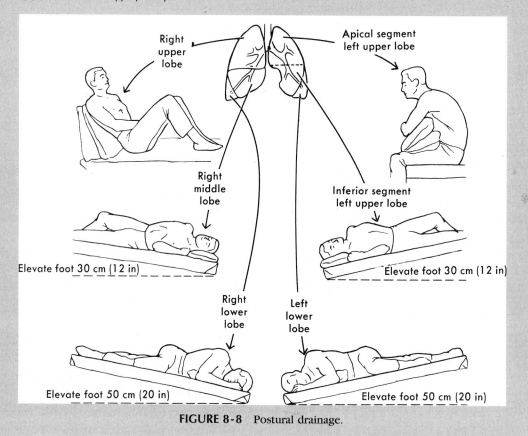

FIGURE 8-8 Postural drainage.

morbidity and mortality associated with the disorder are on the rise. Asthma is characterized by an increased responsiveness of the trachea and bronchi to various stimuli that result in narrowing of the airway.

The underlying basis of asthma involves either genetic or immunologic factors, and a wide variety of precipitating factors for the disease have been identified, including environmental factors, exercise, infection, and stress. Most cases of asthma involve a mix of both intrinsic and extrinsic factors. Several of the distinct asthma syndromes are described in Table 8-7.

Pathophysiology

An asthma attack is the result of several physiologic alterations. Antigen-antibody reactions are at the heart of immunologic asthma. They trigger the release of chemical mediators such as histamine that produce three major reactions in the airway:

1. Constriction of smooth muscles in the large and small airways, which results in bronchospasm
2. Increased capillary permeability, which produces mucosal edema
3. Increased production and secretion by the mucous glands

CRITICAL PATHWAY Chronic Obstructive Pulmonary Disease Without Intubation

DRG #: 088; *Expected LOS: 6*

	Day of Admission Day 1	Day 2	Day 3	Day 4	Day 5	Day of Discharge Day 6
Diagnostic Tests	CBC, UA, SMA/18,* ABGs, sputum C & S, ECG, Pulmonary function tests, Chest x-ray	SMA/6,† ABGs	Chest x-ray	SMA/6,† ABGs	Chest x-ray, ECG	
Medications	IV at TKO, digitalis, antibiotic, diuretic, bronchodilator, aerosol Tx, Rx for rest	IV at TKO, digitalis, antibiotic, diuretic, bronchodilator, aerosol Tx, stool softener, Rx for rest	IV to saline lock, digitalis, antibiotic, diuretic, bronchodilator, stool softener, Rx for rest	IV saline lock, adjust drugs for home use, stool softener, Rx for rest	IV saline lock, adjust drugs for home use, stool softener, Rx for rest	Discontinue IV saline lock, adjust drugs for home use
Treatments	I & O q 8 hr, weight, O$_2$, VS q 4 hr, cardiac monitor, assess cardiopulmonary systems and level of consciousness (LOC) q 4 hr, elastic leg stockings	I & O q 8 hr, weight, O$_2$, VS q 4 hr, cardiac monitor, assess cardiopulmonary systems and LOC q 4 hr, elastic leg stockings	I & O q 6 hr, weight, O$_2$, VS q 6 hr, cardiac monitor, assess cardiopulmonary systems and LOC q 6 hr, elastic leg stockings	I & O q 8 hr, weight, O$_2$, VS q 8 hr, discontinue cardiac monitor, assess cardiopulmonary systems and LOC q 8 hr, elastic leg stockings	I & O q 8 hr, weight, discontinue O$_2$ unless chronic use, VS q 8 hr, assess cardiopulmonary systems and LOC q 8 hr, elastic leg stockings	Weight, discontinue I & O, VS q 8 hr, assess cardiopulmonary systems and LOC q 8 hr, elastic leg stockings
Diet	Full liquids, low sodium	Advance diet to soft diet, provide 6 small meals/day, high protein and calorie, low sodium	Soft diet, provide 6 small meals/day, high protein and calorie, low sodium	Soft diet, provide 6 small meals/day, high protein and calorie, low sodium	Soft diet, provide 6 small meals/day, high protein and calorie, low sodium	Soft, low sodium, provide 6 small meals/day, high protein and calorie
Activity	Bed rest, head of bed elevated 30 degrees	Bed rest, head of bed elevated 30 degrees, up to bathroom with assistance	Head of bed elevated 30 degrees while in bed, up in chair × 4 with help	Head of bed elevated 30 degrees, up in hallway × 4 with help and in chair × 4	Up in hallway × 6 with help and chair as desired	Up walking in hallway as desired
Consultations	Respiratory therapy, pulmonary medicine	Home health, dietary, respiratory rehab	Respiratory rehab team	Respiratory rehab	Respiratory rehab	

*Serum calcium, phosphorus, triglycerides, uric acid, creatinine, BUN, total bilirubin, alkaline phosphate, aspartate aminotransferase (AST; formerly serum glutamic oxaloacetic transaminase [SGOT]), alanine aminotransferase (ALT; formerly serum glutamic oxaloacetic transaminase [SGPT]), lactic dehydrogenase (LDH), total protein, albumin, sodium, potassium chloride, total CO$_2$, glucose.
†Serum sodium, potassium, chloride, total CO$_2$, glucose, BUN.

> ### Guidelines for Teaching Patients the Safe Use of Methylxanthines
>
> Individual responses to theophylline vary, and blood levels need to be monitored at intervals. Therapeutic levels are 10-20 µg/ml.
>
> Cigarette and marijuana smoking significantly increases the plasma clearance of theophylline, necessitating higher doses to achieve a therapeutic effect.
>
> Numerous medications interact with theophylline and alter its absorption rate. Physicians need to be made aware of *all* medications taken by a patient.
>
> Chronic liver disease, infection, and congestive heart failure all decrease plasma clearance of the drug. Initial doses need to be monitored carefully, especially in elderly patients.
>
> There are a wide variety of theophylline preparations. Patients should follow product directions carefully for their correct use in regard to the ingestion of food. Food delays absorption. Most GI symptoms can be successfully controlled by administering the drug with a full glass of water.

The net result is an airway that is acutely narrowed by spasm. Airway resistance is increased, and the lungs become hyperinflated because of air trapping with a resulting increase in lung compliance. The work of breathing is substantially increased, and the muscles can become rapidly exhausted. Hyperventilation can trigger an initial respiratory alkalosis. Ventilation-perfusion mismatch can trigger hypoxemia. With exhaustion the respiratory rate falls and severe respiratory acidosis and hypoxemia can occur that can result in death if not reversed.

Visible symptoms vary with the severity of the attack. The airway is essentially asymptomatic between attacks and exhibits no structural damage. Mild attacks are characterized by dyspnea and wheezing following exercise, laughing, singing, or excitement. The attack can usually be promptly controlled with medication. Acute attacks are characterized by severe respiratory distress, both expiratory and inspiratory wheezing, severe apprehension, and diaphoresis. When treatment is successful the attack ends with the individual coughing up large quantities of thick mucus.

Medical Management

The treatment plan attempts to provide symptomatic relief from attacks, control specific causative factors, and promote optimum health. The chief aim of drug therapy is to provide the patient immediate and ongoing bronchial relaxation. Drug therapy is the key component and focuses on the use of short-acting bronchodilators such as epinephrine; long-acting agents such as ephedrine, terbutaline, and theophylline; and antiinflammatory agents such as corticosteroids and cromolyn (Guidelines box). Oxygen therapy is also used as needed during acute attacks.

NURSING MANAGEMENT

◆ ASSESSMENT
Subjective Data

History of disease and its treatment
History of onset of attack
Factors that precipitate attack
    Allergy history
Medications in use and patient's knowledge of them and their correct usage
Other self-care methods used to control symptoms
Patient's complaints of the following:
    Shortness of breath
    Severe anxiety
    Feeling of suffocation

Objective Data

Presence of inspiratory and expiratory wheezing, prolonged expiration, diffuse rhonchi
Productive or nonproductive cough
Presence and severity of dyspnea, tachycardia, and tachypnea
Apparent respiratory distress
    Use of accessory muscles to breathe
    Forward positioning to breathe
Transient cyanosis, diaphoresis
Blood gases—early changes are mild hypoxemia and respiratory alkalosis; late effects are severe hypoxemia and acidosis

The remainder of the nursing care for the person with asthma is presented in the "Nursing Care Plan."

CYSTIC FIBROSIS
Etiology/Epidemiology

Cystic fibrosis (CF) is an autosomal recessive disease that is the most lethal genetic disorder affecting whites. The disease affects the exocrine glands of various systems, creating obstruction of the gland ducts and passageways. A couple who are both carriers has a one in four chance of the disease affecting their offspring with each pregnancy. CF has traditionally been considered to be a pediatric disorder, but the improvement in disease treatment has created a steadily increasing adult population with the disorder. At present, about 25% of all patients with CF are adults, and reaching adulthood is now considered to be a reasonable expectation for infants and children with the disease. Average life expectancy is about 24 years.

Pathophysiology

Cystic fibrosis is an obstructive disease of the exocrine glands and may involve any or all of the pulmonary, pancreatic/hepatic, GI, and reproductive systems. Although the specific defect is not well defined, the

NURSING CARE PLAN

THE PERSON WITH ASTHMA

■ NURSING DIAGNOSIS
Gas exchange, impaired (related to bronchospasm and ventilation-perfusion imbalance)

Expected Patient Outcomes	Nursing Interventions
Patient will experience improved gas exchange in the lungs as evidenced by the following: Arterial blood pH within normal limits pO_2 above 80 mm Hg	1. Position patient in high Fowler's position. 2. Monitor vital signs and respiratory status regularly. a. Auscultate lungs. b. Observe for cyanosis. 3. Administer bronchodilators as ordered. a. Monitor IV rates carefully. b. Monitor patient for medication's side effects: tachycardia, palpitations, sweating. 4. Administer humidified oxygen as ordered. 5. Establish calm environment; reassure patient. Do not leave patient alone. 6. Encourage relaxation and controlled breathing. a. Encourage patient to inhale through the nose and exhale through pursed lips.

■ NURSING DIAGNOSIS
Airway clearance, ineffective (related to excess mucus production in lungs)

Expected Patient Outcome	Nursing Interventions
Patient will utilize effective coughing to maintain a clear airway.	1. Encourage fluids by mouth. 2. Ensure adequate environmental humidity. 3. Assist patient to cough effectively. Administer chest physiotherapy if coughing is ineffective. 4. Promote comfort measures for diaphoretic patient.

Continued.

exocrine gland secretions display a variety of abnormalities:

Decreased water content

Altered electrolyte concentration

Abnormal organic components

The damage to the respiratory system is typically most profound. The changes in the airways predispose the patient to recurrent infection, inflammation, edema, and smooth muscle restriction. Blood vessels can erode over time and predispose to bleeding. Death typically results from pulmonary complications and respiratory failure. Digestion is affected in about 80% to 90% of all patients, with pancreatic insufficiency the primary problem. Intestinal obstruction and glucose intolerance are also related to the pancreatic problems.

The three primary clinical symptoms associated with CF include recurrent respiratory infections, malnutrition, and excessive salt losses. In infancy the diagnosis is established by exclusion as the child is checked for otherwise unexplained symptoms such as meconium ileus or failure to thrive. Respiratory problems predominate when the disease is diagnosed in later childhood and adolescence, and infertility may be the only complaint in the rare situation when the presence of CF is confirmed in adulthood. Classic clinical manifestations of CF are summarized in Box 8-14.

Medical Management

The diagnosis of CF is confirmed by a positive sweat test with a chloride level greater than 60 mEq/L with x-ray

NURSING CARE PLAN—CONT'D

THE PERSON WITH ASTHMA

■ NURSING DIAGNOSIS

Impaired home maintenance management, risk of (related to insufficient knowledge of the disease process, precipitating factors, and treatment regimen)

Expected Patient Outcome	Nursing Interventions
Patient will be knowledgeable concerning disease and proposed treatment plan.	1. Teach patient about medications and their safe use. Teach patient to use inhaled bronchodilators before planned exercise.
	2. Teach patient safe use and care of all equipment such as inhalers and nebulizers.
	3. Encourage patient to keep a symptom diary to help identify possible precipitating factors, symptom patterns, and effectiveness of treatment modalities.
	4. Teach patient to avoid potential allergens and precipitating factors if possible, such as smoking, exertion, cold air, and dust.
	5. Teach patient to seek prompt treatment of upper respiratory tract infections.
	6. Teach patient breathing exercises and use of chest physiotherapy if appropriate.
	7. Teach patient to maintain optimum nutrition, adequate rest, and sufficient fluids.
	8. Teach patient relaxation and stress management techniques.

BOX 8-14	Classic Clinical Manifestations of Cystic Fibrosis

RESPIRATORY

Chronic productive cough
Recurrent bronchitis or pneumonia
Pulmonary crackles and rhonchi, wheezing
Shortness of breath, dyspnea on exertion

GASTROINTESTINAL

Frequent bulky, greasy stools
Weight loss, low weight/height percentile
Cramps and abdominal pain

GLUCOSE METABOLISM

Polyuria, polydipsia, polyphagia
Hyperglycemia without ketoacidosis

---

evidence of COPD or evidence of pancreatic insufficiency. Medical management is multifaceted, with primary emphasis on the prevention of respiratory obstruction and infection. Measures include regular chest physiotherapy with percussion and postural drainage; the administration of humidification and mucolytic agents; the administration of the new drug dornase-alfa (Pulmozyme) by nebulizer, which has been shown in research trials to improve lung function and reduce the risk of pulmonary infection. Infections are treated aggressively when they occur, with culture-specific antibiotics. Hospitalization is frequently required to supply the needed aggressive infection management.

GI and growth problems are managed by the administration of supplemental fat-soluble vitamins and pancreatic enzyme supplementation, which is individualized to the needs of the specific patient to keep fatty stools to under three per day. The occurrence of pulmonary infection usually entails a significant loss as far as body weight and general nutrition are concerned. The dietitian is consulted for options for meeting the patient's ongoing accelerated nutritional needs. Aggressive intervention with tube feedings, gastrostomy, or total parenteral nutrition (TPN) may be necessary if the patient is unable to meet nutritional needs orally.

NURSING MANAGEMENT

◆ ASSESSMENT
Subjective Data

Patient's understanding of the disease and its treatment

Adherence to home regimens, for example, postural drainage, chest percussion, aerosol therapy, nutritional supplements

Shortness of breath, dyspnea on exertion

Fatigue, ability to complete ADL, usual activities

24-hour diet intake; degree of anorexia, abdominal discomfort

Weight fluctuations over last 2 to 4 weeks

Frequency and appearance of stools

Medications in current use: pattern of use, side effects, and their management

Patient and family structure, support mechanisms, and usual coping patterns

Objective Data

Presence of wheezing, crackles, rhonchi

Finger clubbing, presence of cyanosis

Severity of cough; sputum quantity, character

Fever, presence of tachycardia, tachypnea

Blood gases, results of pulmonary function studies

Body weight

Stool color, appearance, frequency

Blood and urine glucose levels

◆ NURSING DIAGNOSES

Nursing diagnoses for the person with CF admitted for a respiratory infection may include, but are not limited to, the following:

Airway clearance, ineffective (related to copious thick secretions)

Activity intolerance (related to decreased oxygenation, infection, and inadequate nutrition)

Nutrition, altered: less than body requirements (related to anorexia, increased need)

Impaired home maintenance, risk of (related to complex disease regimen, fatal disease prognosis)

◆ EXPECTED PATIENT OUTCOMES

Patient will successfully cough up mucus and have clear breath sounds in all lobes.

Patient will regain sufficient energy to maintain independence in self-care activities and engage in preferred life-style.

Patient will stabilize weight and slowly regain weight to within 10% to 20% of ideal weight. Serum albumin levels will be within normal limits.

Patient and family will manage disease regimen effectively, talk openly about the present and the future, and sustain optimism.

BOX 8-15	Options for Intubation

NASAL ENDOTRACHEAL

Tube is comfortable for the patient and easily anchored. It can kink and obstruct the airway, however, and predisposes the patient to nasal and/or sinus infection.

ORAL ENDOTRACHEAL

Route permits use of a larger-diameter tube and is less traumatic to insert. However, it is very uncomfortable for the patient, is difficult to anchor securely, makes oral hygiene difficult, and predisposes the patient to mouth sores. A bite block is required to lower the risk of obstruction.

COMPLICATIONS OF INTUBATION

Tissue trauma (tracheal or laryngeal damage or necrosis)
Tube displacement
Nosocomial infection and aspiration
Early conversion to a tracheostomy is frequently recommended to prevent injury and increase patient comfort, facilitate oral hygiene and effective suctioning, and secure the airway. The disadvantages include cost and the risk of bleeding or dislodgement. Various tracheostomy options are shown in Box 8-16.

◆ NURSING INTERVENTIONS
Facilitating Airway Clearance

Maintain bronchial hygiene regimen every 2 to 4 hours:
    Postural drainage
    Chest percussion/clapping
    Assessment of breath sounds before and after each treatment

Assist patient to cough effectively and safely dispose of tissues.

Encourage slow rhythmic breathing.
    Teach patient controlled breathing: inhaling through the nose and exhaling through the mouth.

Ensure adequate room humidity.

Encourage patient to increase fluid intake to 3 to 4 L/24 hr.
    Supplement with IV fluids if needed, particularly if fever is present.

Utilize high Fowler's position.

Monitor blood gases and O_2 saturation.
    Administer supplemental oxygen as ordered.

Reducing Fatigue

Assess activity tolerance frequently.

Plan for frequent rest periods, especially after each respiratory treatment.

Monitor pulse, perceived dyspnea with activity.

Encourage patient to use supplemental oxygen if ordered.

Encourage patient to remain involved in self-care activities. Provide assistance as needed.

BOX 8-16 · Tracheostomy Tubes

Tracheostomy tubes are constructed of semiflexible plastic, rigid plastic, or metal and may be cuffed, uncuffed, or fenestrated. Tubes are available with and without inner cannulas, which may or may not be disposable. Periodically cleaning and replacing an inner cannula preserves the patency of the tube, minimizes the risk of airway plugging, and reduces the patient's work of breathing. The choice of tube is based on the patient's condition and the physician's preference. All tracheostomy tubes consist of a main shaft and a neck plate, or flange.

UNCUFFED TUBES

Uncuffed tubes may be plastic or metal. They permit the free flow of air around the tube and reduce the risk of tracheal damage. They may be single lumen or have an inner removable cannula. The risk of aspiration exists, however, and some form of adaptor is usually needed for mechanical ventilation. Metal tubes that can be cleaned and reused are more cost effective for long-term airway maintenance. They do not have an adaptor at the neck plate, however, and must be replaced with a plastic tube if emergency resuscitation is required.

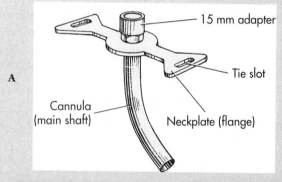

CUFFED TUBES

Most cuffed tubes are disposable plastic. They provide for low pressure in the airway with high volume in the cuff. The low pressure within the cuff is evenly distributed against the tracheal wall and reduces the chance of tracheal injury. The cuff is bonded to the tube and cannot accidentally dislodge in the trachea. It does not require interval deflation. Cuffed tubes have an inflation line leading to the cuff and a pilot balloon that inflates when the cuff contains air. The balloon itself, however, does not tell how much air is in the cuff.

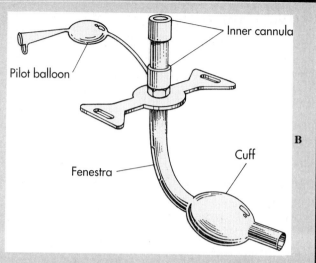

FENESTRATED TUBES

Fenestrated tubes allow the flexibility of mechanical ventilation with the cuff inflated and the inner cannula in place and speech through the upper airway with the cuff deflated and the external opening capped. An opening on the upper surface of the outer cannula allows inspired air to pass through the tube and over the vocal cords. They are also very useful in the gradual process of weaning patients from mechanical ventilation. The inner cannula *must* be in place before suctioning to prevent the catheter from passing through one of the openings and injuring the trachea.

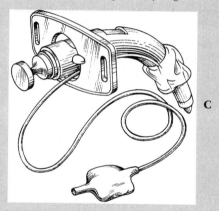

FIGURE 8-9 Tracheostomy tubes. **A,** Uncuffed tube. **B,** Cuffed tube. **C,** Fenestrated tube.

Promoting Adequate Nutrition

Perform ongoing nutritional assessment.
  Keep calorie counts, food diaries.
  Monitor serum albumin levels.
Record daily weight.
Provide small frequent feedings.
Work with patient to establish satisfactory plan for meeting needs for supplemental calories and nutrition.

Administer vitamins and pancreatic enzymes with each meal and snack.
Monitor frequency, volume, and consistency of stools.
Involve family and dietitian in all meal planning.
Monitor blood glucose levels as ordered.

Promoting Effective Home Management

Encourage patient and family to verbalize feelings, fears, and frustrations.

Guidelines for Tracheostomy Care and Suctioning

GENERAL CARE

Provide constant airway humidification.
Change all respiratory equipment every 24 hours.
Provide frequent mouth care.
Establish communication and minimize sensory deprivation.

TRACHEOSTOMY SUCTIONING

Explain the procedure to patient.
Wash hands before the procedure.
Auscultate lungs before the procedure.
Suction *only* if indicated by assessment findings, that is, presence of wheezing or rhonchi. Suctioning can cause hypoxemia, arrhythmias, and damage to the tracheal mucosa and should never be performed routinely.
Coordinate suctioning with other pulmonary hygiene interventions if possible, for example, administration of bronchodilators or chest physical therapy. Ensure adequate pain management for surgical patients, because the vigorous coughing induced by suctioning can be extremely painful.
Suction oropharynx before suctioning tracheostomy.
Prepare sterile equipment needed, using strict sterile technique.
    Use sterile gloves and catheter.
    Use sterile container and water.
    Put on protective face shield or goggles before suctioning.
Hyperoxygenate the patient before suctioning. Ventilator hyperoxygenation is preferable to the use of an Ambu bag for mechanically ventilated patients.
Hyperinflate the airway before suctioning if possible. Ventilator hyperinflation via the sigh mechanism is preferable to the use of an Ambu bag for mechanically ventilated patients.
Lubricate catheter with sterile water or water-soluble lubricant before insertion.

Do *not* instill saline before suctioning. It is *not* effective in liquefying secretions.
Insert catheter *without suction* about 8 inches, or deep enough to produce an effective cough.
Apply intermittent suction and withdraw catheter slowly, rotating while withdrawing. Suction for no longer than 10-15 seconds at one time.
Rinse catheter in sterile water between insertions.
Hyperoxygenate again between insertions. Allow patient to rest for 1-3 minutes between suctionings.
Repeat procedure if needed.
Monitor blood pressure, pulse, pulse oximetry, heart rhythm, and intracranial pressure if appropriate during suctioning. Bradycardia is common.
Auscultate lungs at conclusion to ensure effectiveness.
Clean inner cannula (if present) every 4 hours or as necessary.

TRACHEOSTOMY CARE

After suctioning, unlock and remove inner cannula if present.
Immerse in H_2O_2 and cleanse with brush.
Rinse in sterile water or saline, shake dry, reinsert, and lock in place.
Cleanse around stoma with H_2O_2 and saline on applicators or 4 × 4 inch gauze pads.
Apply povidone-iodine (Betadine) solution or ointment around tracheostomy if part of hospital protocol.
Change tracheostomy dressing as needed.
Change ties as needed. (Figure 8-10).
    Insert ties through slits to secure to outer cannula.
    Tie tapes with double knot at side of neck.
    NOTE: Tracheostomy tube should be manually secured in place whenever tapes are not in place.
    Tapes should be snug but allow passage of fingertips beneath them when tied.

A   B   C

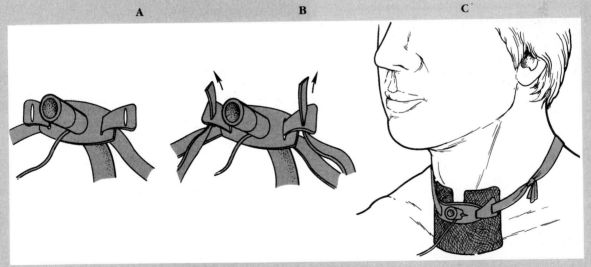

FIGURE 8-10 Changing tracheostomy ties.

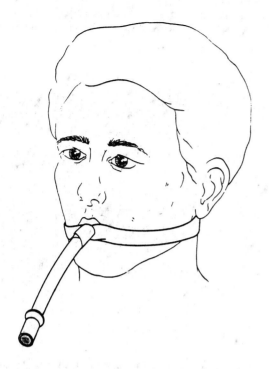
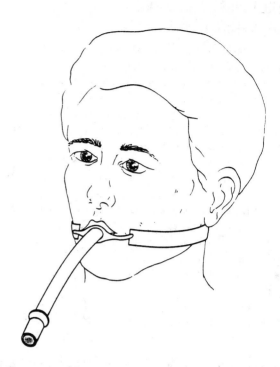

A

B

FIGURE 8-11 Options for securing an endotracheal tube. **A,** Comfit tube holder. **B,** Dale tube holder. (From Kaplow R, Bookbinder M: *Heart Lung* 23 [1]: 59-66, 1994.)

BOX 8-17	Indications for Mechanical Ventilation

RESPIRATORY RATE
<10 breaths/min or >40 breaths/min
Extreme work of breathing, use of accessory muscles

VITAL CAPACITY
<10-20 ml/kg

BLOOD GASES
pH <7.25
pCO_2 >50 mm Hg
pO_2 <50 mm Hg on supplemental oxygen

HEART RATE
>120, presence of dysrhythmia

MENTAL STATUS
Confusion, somnolence, delirium

Encourage involvement with CF support groups.
Refer for genetic or career counseling as indicated.
Ensure patient understanding and skill in managing daily pulmonary treatments, use of aerosol medications.

Reinforce teaching concerning adequate nutrition, use of pancreatic enzyme supplement, and importance of daily weight records.

Reinforce the nature of symptoms that indicate the need for medical evaluation: increased shortness of breath, change in amount or character of the sputum, fever, increased fatigue.

Refer patient to Cystic Fibrosis Foundation and other social services for cost assistance, disability assistance, and support.

Reinforce the importance of respite care for primary caretakers.

◆ EVALUATION

Successful achievement of expected outcomes for the patient with CF admitted with a respiratory infection is indicated by the following:

Clear breath sounds to auscultation; thin, clear sputum

Independence in self-care; resumption of normal daily activities

Stable body weight within 10% to 20% of ideal

Correct description and demonstration of all required aspects of management regimen; open communication between patient and family supports

RESPIRATORY FAILURE

Etiology/Epidemiology

Respiratory *insufficiency* occurs when the exchange of oxygen and carbon dioxide is inadequate to meet body needs during normal activities. It is usually accompanied by dyspnea. *Failure* occurs when the exchange of oxygen and carbon dioxide is inadequate to meet body needs at rest and hypoxemia, hypercapnia, and acidosis exceed predetermined levels.

These conditions may occur as a result of any of the disorders discussed in this chapter as well as a variety of other acute or chronic, surgical, neurologic, and neuromuscular disorders. Diagnosis is made from blood gas results, pulmonary function testing, and the patient's clinical status. The following criteria are used:

pO_2 <50 to 60 mm Hg on room air
pCO_2 >45 to 50 mm Hg
pH ≤7.35
Vital capacity <15 ml/kg
Respiratory rate >30/min or <8/min

In acute failure there is often a marked decrease in vital capacity. The signs and symptoms of failure often depend more on the rate of change than on absolute values, since in patients with COPD the basic imbalances are present chronically.

BOX 8-18 — **Oxygen Therapy in Respiratory Failure**

Severe hypoxemia is incompatible with life. Supplemental oxygen is given to maintain a pO_2 of at least 60 mm Hg as established via blood gases.

OXYGEN TOXICITY

Prolonged exposure to high oxygen concentrations damages lung tissues. Atelectasis, alveolar collapse, and the development of ARDS are significant risks. General parameters include the following:

Use the lowest concentration of oxygen that will sustain an acceptable pO_2 level.

Utilize 60% or greater oxygen concentration for no more than 36 hours and 100% oxygen for no more than 6 hours if possible.

BOX 8-19 — **Oxygen Therapy**

Oxygen therapy prevents or reverses hypoxemia and reduces the work of breathing. Options for oxygen delivery (Figure 8-12) follow.

LOW-FLOW SYSTEMS

Nasal Prongs or Cannula (Fig. 8-12, *A*)

Can deliver 0.5-6 L/min
Inexpensive, disposable, and easy to use
Permits talking, eating, and easy movement
Easily dislodged; can cause nasal drying
Concentration delivered to patient depends on patient's respiratory rate and breathing pattern

Simple Face Mask (Fig. 8-12, *B*)

Delivers oxygen through entry port
Efficient for rapid, short-term delivery
Poorly tolerated by patients because it requires a tight seal around the mouth for accurate delivery, which interferes with talking and eating and frequently causes claustrophobic feelings
Concentration delivered to patient depends on breathing pattern

Partial Rebreather Mask (Fig. 8-12, *C*)

Allows patient to rebreathe the first one third of exhaled air, which contains primarily oxygen, increasing concentration delivered
Uses reservoir bag to mix incoming oxygen with exhaled air
Poorly tolerated because of need for tight seal around mouth (see information on simple face mask)

Transtracheal Catheter (Fig. 8-12, *D*)

Small catheter inserted directly into trachea between tracheal cartilage
Permits highly efficient oxygen delivery on continuous basis throughout respiratory cycle, which allows delivered concentration to be lower

Does not interfere with talking, eating, or mobility
Risk of infection low but realistic

HIGH-FLOW SYSTEMS

Control concentration of patient's inspired air and are not affected by changes in respiratory pattern or rate

Nonrebreather Mask (Fig. 8-12, *E*)

Mask and reservoir separated by one-way valve
Can deliver up to 100% oxygen
Extensive humidification of inspired air not possible
Poorly tolerated because of need for tight seal (see information on simple face mask)

Venturi Mask (Fig. 8-12, *F*)

Mask connected to Venturi device that mixes specific volume of air and oxygen; delivers most precise oxygen concentrations
Oxygen passes through restricted port that increases velocity of gas flow
Poorly tolerated because of need for tight seal (see discussion of simple face mask)

GENERAL CARE CONSIDERATIONS

Flow rates and pulse oximetry results should be checked at specified intervals throughout the therapy, especially for patients with COPD.
Oxygen therapy is drying and irritating to the mucous membranes.
Humidification of oxygen is recommended, especially with higher concentrations.
Delivery equipment must be changed regularly to prevent or contain bacterial growth.
Warning signs concerning oxygen use should be clearly posted.

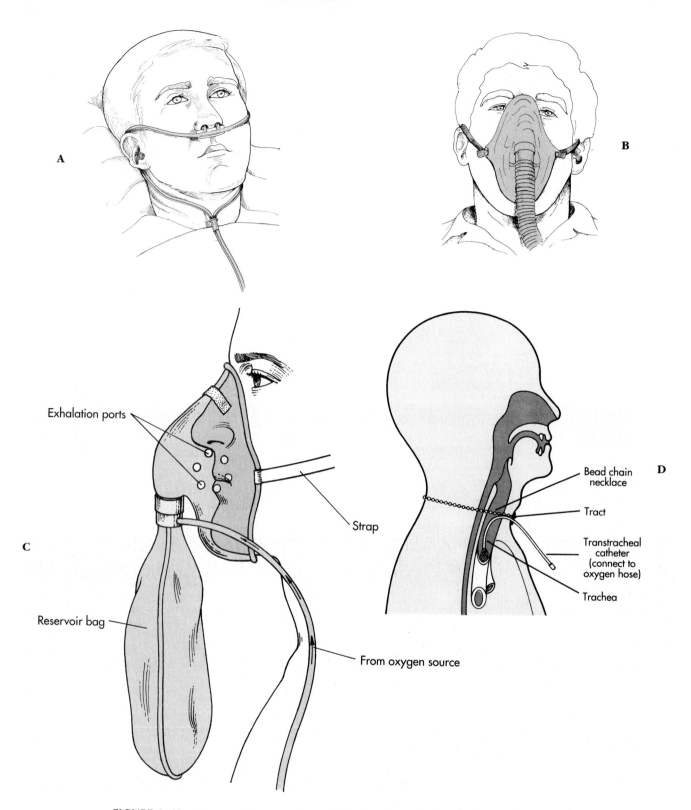

FIGURE 8-12 Oxygen delivery systems. **A,** Nasal cannula. **B,** Simple face mask. **C,** Partial rebreather mask, **D,** Transtracheal catheter. **E,** Nonrebreather mask. **F,** Venturi mask.

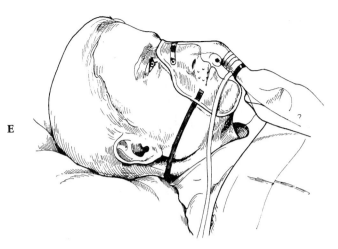

E

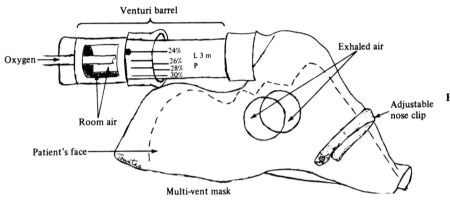

Venturi barrel

Oxygen

24%
26%
28%
30%

L 3 m
P

Exhaled air

Room air

Patient's face

Adjustable
nose clip

F

Multi-vent mask

FIGURE 8-12 Continued.

BOX 8-20 | **Pulse Oximetry**

Pulse oximetry is a noninvasive way of measuring arterial oxygen saturation. Saturation represents the percentage of hemoglobin-binding sites that are occupied by oxygen. If all the binding sites are occupied, the hemoglobin is considered to be 100% saturated. The oximeter uses fiberoptics to measure the amount of oxygenated hemoglobin in the arterial blood. The probe can be applied to the ear, finger, or bridge of the nose.

O_2 saturation is *not* synonymous with blood oxygen pressure (pO_2). Arterial blood gases measure the amount of oxygen in the plasma, which is only 3% of the total. The rest is carried on the hemoglobin and replenished as needed. Hemoglobin saturation needs to be maintained between 90% and 100% to adequately replenish the plasma. Levels below 70% are life threatening. The following rough relationships apply:

>96% O_2 saturation yields a pO_2 >90 mm Hg
96% O_2 saturation yields a pO_2 >80 mm Hg
90% O_2 saturation yields a pO_2 >60 mm Hg
50% O_2 saturation yields a pO_2 >30 mm Hg

Guidelines for Inflating an Endotracheal Tube Cuff

The cuff is inflated to a volume that adequately occludes the trachea for ventilation yet prevents pressure-related complications. Pressures less than 18 mm Hg are recommended. The exact pressure can be measured with a hand-held meter attached to the pilot balloon.

Slowly inject air into the cuff using a 10 to 20 ml syringe.

When the airway is sealed (no air passage from the nose or mouth), 0.5 ml of air is *removed* to create a "minimal leak seal."

Auscultate the tracheal area while ventilating the patient. A small amount of air should be heard gurgling past the cuff.

Notify the physician if a seal cannot be obtained with 25 ml of air.

BOX 8-21	Mechanical Ventilation

Ventilators are classified according to the mechanism that cycles the machine cycle. The four main types follow.

NEGATIVE PRESSURE

Negative pressure ventilators work by alternately removing and replacing air from a container. Removing air creates a negative pressure that forces the chest to expand, pulling air into the lungs. Restoring air to the container allows the chest wall to fall, causing exhalation. The device can contain the patient's chest and upper abdomen or the entire body (iron lung).

PRESSURE CYCLED

Pressure-cycled ventilators stop inspiration when a preset pressure is reached, regardless of the volume of air that has been delivered. Exhalation then occurs passively. Examples include the Bird and Bennett models, which are primarily used today for IPPB treatments.

VOLUME CYCLED

Volume-cycled ventilators stop inspiration when a preset volume of air has been delivered, regardless of the amount of pressure required to deliver it. Expiration is passive. These are the ventilators in most common use. Examples include Bennett MA series, Air-Shields, Ohio, BEAR 2, and Siemens-Servo.

HIGH FREQUENCY

High-frequency ventilators use high respiratory rates and small tidal volumes to keep the alveoli ventilated. They utilize low pressures.

BOX 8-22	Modes and Adjuncts to Mechanical Ventilation

Mechanical ventilators are adjusted to the unique needs of each individual patient. A wide variety of options exists.

MECHANICAL VENTILATION MODES

Continuous Mandatory Ventilation (CMV)

A preset tidal volume is delivered at a preset rate regardless of the patient's inspiratory effort. Spontaneous breathing is not possible. CMV is typically used only with unconscious patients, because the respiratory muscles atrophy, making weaning extremely difficult.

Assist Control Ventilation (ACV)

The patient initiates the breath. Any decrease in pressure triggers the machine to deliver a breath at a preset volume. Breaths will also be delivered at a preset rate if the patient does not initiate any breaths spontaneously.

Intermittent Mandatory Ventilation (IMV)

The ventilator delivers a set number of breaths per minute of a preset volume. The patient may initiate spontaneous breaths between the preset ones. IMV is frequently used as a weaning tool.

Synchronized Intermittent Mandatory Ventilation (SIMV)

SIMV is similar to IMV, but the machine synchronizes the ventilator breaths with the patient's spontaneous efforts. A mandatory breath will be delivered if the patient does not spontaneously initiate a breath within a preset time interval. SIMV is used frequently in weaning.

Pressure Support Ventilation (PSV)

The machine supports a spontaneous breath with positive pressure. The patient controls the length and volume of inspiration. PSV is used primarily during weaning. Pressure support can also be combine with PEEP or CPAP. This use is termed *biphasic airway pressure*.

Pressure-Controlled Inverse Ratio Ventilation (PCIRV)

PCIRV increases the inspiratory time by reversing the normal inspiratory/expiratory ratio. It is useful in ARDS when patients have marked O_2 desaturation and do not respond to conventional approaches.

High-Frequency Adjuncts

High-frequency, positive pressure ventilation, jet ventilation, and oscillation ventilation all remain under research investigation. They deliver small tidal volumes at low pressure and extremely high rates. The lower airway pressures support tissue healing after fistula formation or reconstructive surgery.

MECHANICAL VENTILATION ADJUNCTS

Positive End-Expiratory Pressure (PEEP)

The addition of PEEP maintains a positive pressure in the airway rather than allowing pressure to return to atmospheric at the end of expiration. Alveoli are held open, increasing the chance for ongoing gas exchange across the capillary membrane. PEEP plays a major role in the treatment of ARDS.

Continuous Positive Airway Pressure (CPAP)

CPAP is based on the same principle as PEEP but allows the maintenance of positive airway pressure in patients who are able to breathe spontaneously. It is used most often with neonates. The work of breathing is increased because of the resistance present against airflow.

BOX 8-23   Common Ventilatory Terms

Fio$_2$ Fraction of oxygen the patient receives during inhalation.

functional residual capacity (FRC) Amount of air remaining in lungs at the end of a normal expiration.

Inspiratory time (length of inspiration) Time elapsed from the beginning to the end of inspiration.

mode of ventilation Mechanism that initiates inspiration by the mechanical ventilator.

peak inspiratory pressure (PIP) Amount of pressure required to deliver a preset tidal volume; may be digitally displayed on the ventilator or may be determined by checking the needle on an airway pressure gauge.

tidal volume (Vt) Volume of air inhaled or exhaled with each breath; normal: 10-15 ml/kg.

BOX 8-24   Troubleshooting the Ventilator

VOLUME OR PRESSURE ALARM ON

The alarm will sound if the patient becomes disconnected from the ventilator, the patient experiences a decrease in patient-initiated breaths, or there is a leak in the ventilator delivery system.

  Check all tubing for loss of connection, beginning with the patient.

  Recheck all ventilator settings.

  Check or tighten humidifier connections.

  Occlude the endotracheal tube adaptor. If the alarm sounds, the problem is with the patient; if not there is a ventilator problem.

  Auscultate for leaks around the endotracheal tube.

  Evaluate the patient methodically; respiratory rate, sedation, ABGs.

  If ventilatory problem cannot be corrected promptly, the patient should be hand ventilated until the ventilator is fixed.

HIGH OR PEAK PRESSURE ALARM ON

The peak pressure alarm will sound if the tubing becomes kinked or water filled or if there is an increase in dynamic or static patient lung pressures. It also commonly sounds when the patient and ventilator are not in synchrony.

  Suction patient if indicated.

  Try a position change.

  Evaluate the ABGs.

  Sedate the patient if synchrony cannot be established.

  Check all tubing, and drain standing water into a receptacle.

  Recheck all settings.

Pathophysiology

The two major components of respiration include the effective movement of air in and out of the lungs and the effective exchange of gases inside the lungs. Any pulmonary pathologic condition can result in respiratory insufficiency or failure if either or both of the components of respiration fail to a significant degree. Regardless of the underlying mechanism, the results are very similar. Arterial oxygen levels fall, the tissue cells become increasingly hypoxic, carbon dioxide accumulates, arterial blood pH falls, and respiratory acidosis occurs. The process can occur abruptly or very slowly over a period of many years. The underlying blood gas abnormalities are the basis of the primary symptoms of respiratory failure. Classic signs and symptoms associated with respiratory failure include the following:

  Headache
  Irritability
  Confusion
  Tachycardia
  Somnolence, stupor advancing to coma
    Asterixis (flapping tremor)
  Hypotension
    Cardiac dysrhythmia
  Cyanosis

If the respiratory failure develops acutely, the patient will initially exhibit tachypnea and dyspnea. As the condition worsens, however, the breathing rate slows and muscles become exhausted. Patients with chronic long-standing COPD, on the other hand, typically exhibit few actual symptoms until the failure is well advanced. The key in all cases is prevention of the failure state by early recognition and prompt treatment of high-risk patients who exhibit a declining respiratory status.

Medical Management

Medical therapy is based on the severity of the failure and involves ongoing bedside assessment of arterial blood gases, reversing or treating the underlying cause if possible, and interventions with oxygen therapy and intubation for mechanical ventilation if needed.

NURSING MANAGEMENT

The nursing role is highly collaborative and involves implementing the ongoing bedside monitoring, instituting oxygen therapy, and keeping the airway open and clear through positioning, suctioning, and chest physiotherapy. Support for the patient and family is an essential intervention, especially if intubation and mechanical ventilation are required. Specific elements of airway management are presented in Boxes 8-15 to 8-21.

Guidelines for Nursing Care of the Mechanically Ventilated Patient

GENERAL MEASURES

Explain the treatment to the extent possible, including sensations that will be experienced. Include family members.

Establish an acceptable communication system with patient. The presence of the endotracheal tube in the larynx makes speech impossible.

Monitor vital signs, ABGs, and pulse oximetry as ordered.

Position the patient in a semi-Fowler's position if permitted. Change positions every 2 hours. Perform chest physiotherapy if ordered.

Secure a bite block to prevent the patient from chewing on the tube and obstructing the flow of gas. Do not use an oral airway for this purpose.

Suction the patient as indicated by the breath sounds.

Monitor for signs of pneumothorax and oxygen toxicity.

Provide emotional support and assist the patient not to fight the ventilator if possible.

Use soft restraints if absolutely necessary to prevent extubation.

Administer a sedative and/or neuromuscular blocking agent if ineffective ventilation results from ventilator fighting. Mivacurium chloride (Mivacron), pancuronium bromide (Pavulon), and vecuronium bromide (Norcuron) are used for neuromuscular relaxation; and midazolam hydrochloride (Versed) is frequently used as the sedative.

VENTILATOR MANAGEMENT

Check all connections between ventilator and patient.

Make sure that all alarms are turned on and set properly: low and high pressure alarms, volume alarms.

Verify all ventilator settings with orders. Visually confirm that all rates and volumes are being delivered to the patient.

Check the humidifier and refill as necessary.

Check all tubing for condensation, and drain into receptacle.

Change all tubing with aseptic technique every 24-48 hours.

Check all temperature gauges.

SELECTED REFERENCES

Arbour R: Weaning a patient from a ventilator, *Nurs 93* 23(2):52-56, 1993.

Avalos-Bock S: Getting a rise out of tuberculosis with the PPD skin test, *Nurs 94* 24(8):51-53, 1994.

Avey MA: TB skin testing: how to do it right, *Am J Nurs* 93(9):42-45, 1993.

Barnes P et al: Tuberculosis in patients with human immunodeficiency virus infection, *N Engl J Med* 324:1644-1649, 1991.

Barry MA et al: Tuberculosis infection in urban adolescents: results of a school based testing program, *Am J Public Health* 80:439-441, 1990.

Benner KL: Terminal weaning: a loved one's vigil, *Am J Nurs* 93(5):22-25, 1993.

Bloch AB et al: Nationwide survey of drug-resistant tuberculosis in the United States, *JAMA* 271(9):665-671, 1994.

Bolton PJ, Kline KA: Understanding modes of mechanical ventilation, *Am J Nurs* 94(6):36-43, 1994.

Boutotte J: TB the second time around . . . , *Nurs 93* 23(5):42-49, 1993.

Bradley RB: Adult respiratory distress syndrome, *Focus Crit Care* 14:48-59, 1989.

Carroll P: Safe suctioning prn, *RN* 57(5):32-38, 1994.

Caruthers DD: Infectious pneumonia in the elderly, *Am J Nurs* 90:56-60, 1990.

Casey KM: Fighting MDR-TB, *RN* 56(9):26-30, 1993.

Colditz GA et al: Efficacy of BCG vaccine in the prevention of tuberculosis, *JAMA* 271:698-702, 1994.

Davis PB: Pathophysiology of pulmonary disease in cystic fibrosis, *Semin Respir Med* 6(4):261-269, 1985.

DeVito-Dabbs A, Olslund L: New alternatives to intubation, *Am J Nurs* 94(8):42-45, 1994.

Dowling PT: Return of tuberculosis: screening and preventive therapy, *Am Fam Physician* 43(2):457-467, 1991.

Ehrhardt BS, Graham M: Pulse oximetry: an easy way to check oxygen saturation, *Nurs 90* 20(3):50-54, 1990.

Falco R: Taking the fight to the street, *RN* 56(9):34-39, 1993.

Ferguson GT, Cherniack RM: Management of chronic obstructive pulmonary disease, *N Engl J Med* 328:1017-1022, 1993.

Freichels T: Orchestrating the care of mechanically ventilated patients, *Am J Nurs* 93(10):26-35, 1993.

Gift AG, Bolgiano CS, Cunningham J: Sensations during chest tube removal, *Heart Lung* 20(2):131-137, 1991.

Harvey JC, Beattie EJ: Lung cancer, *Clin Symp* 45(3):1-32, 1993.

Hayden RA: What keeps oxygenation on track? *Am J Nurs* 92(12):32-43, 1992.

Howard BA: Guiding allergy sufferers through the medication maze, *RN* 57(4):26-33, 1994.

Hunter FC, Mitchell S: Managing ARDS, *RN* 56(7):52-57, 1993.

Kaplow R, Bookbinder M: A comparison of four endotracheal tube, *Heart Lung* 23(1):59-66, 1994.

Lavin J, Haidorfer C: Anergy testing: a vital weapon, *RN* 56(9):31-32, 1993.

McKinney B: COPD & depression, treat them both, *RN* 57(4):48-50, 1994.

Miller WE: The role of the outpatient nurse in endoscopic sinus surgery, *ORL Head Neck Nurs* 10(3):20-24, 1992.

O'Brien LM, Bartlett KA: TB plus HIV spells trouble, *Am J Nurs* 92(5):28-34, 1992.

Reinke LF, Hoffman LA: Breathing space: teaching asthma comanagement, *Am J Nurs* 92(10):40-49, 1992.

Repasky TM: Emergency: tension pneumothorax, *Am J Nurs* 94(9):47-48, 1994.

Rodman MJ: Asthma medication, *RN* 56(4):40-47, 1993.

Spyr J, Preach MA: Pulse oximetry: understanding the concept, knowing the limits, *RN* 53(5):38-43, 1990.

Stiesmeyer JK: What triggers a ventilator alarm? *Am J Nurs* 91(10):60-65, 1991.

Steismeyer JK: A four step approach to pulmonary assessment, *Am J Nurs* 93(8):22-31, 1993.

Tobin MJ: Mechanical ventilation, *N Engl J Med* 330:1056-1061, 1994.

U.S. Department of Health and Human Services, Public Health Service, National Heart, Lung, and Blood Institute: *Teach your patients about asthma: a clinician's guide,* Bethesda, Md, 1992, The Institute.

Weilitz PB, Dettenmeier PA: Back to basics: test your knowledge of tracheostomy tubes, *Am J Nurs* 94(2):46-50, 1994.

Weixler D: Correcting metered-dose inhaler misuse, *Nurs 94* 24(7):62-65, 1994.

Wetta M: When gauging respiratory status is critical, *RN* 56(11):40-48, 1993.

Yeaw EMJ: Positioning and oxygenation, *Am J Nurs* 92(3):26-43, 1992.

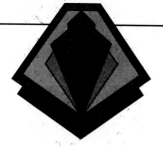

CHAPTER 9

Disorders of the Endocrine System

◆ ASSESSMENT

SUBJECTIVE DATA

Health history
  Prior history of endocrine disorder
    Treatment, surgery
  Family history of:
    Obesity
    Abnormal patterns of growth and development
    Diabetes, thyroid disorders, infertility
  Medication use
    Prescription and over the counter (OTC)
  Current symptoms
    Degree of impairment of activities of daily living
      (ADL) or usual life-style
Energy level
  Fatigue
    Impact on self-care or usual life-style
  Generalized weakness
    Severity and duration
  Sleep pattern changes
  Tolerance to and response to physical and emotional
    stress
  Increased frequency of infection
Nutrition
  Changes in food or fluid intake
    Anorexia, chronic hunger or thirst, nausea
    Food cravings
  Weight changes: loss or gain
  Usual daily food intake
Elimination patterns
  Urinary elimination
    Frequency, volume, nocturia, dysuria
    Use of diuretics
  Bowel elimination
    Constipation or diarrhea
    Abdominal cramping or discomfort
    Use of stool softeners or laxatives
Sexual and reproductive function
  Reproductive history
    Menstruation
      Onset, cycle length
      Amount and duration of flow, menorrhagia
      Changes in normal pattern

GERONTOLOGIC PATIENT CONSIDERATIONS: PHYSIOLOGIC CHANGES IN ENDOCRINE SYSTEM FUNCTIONING

A variety of changes in endocrine functioning are associated with the aging process. The changes are frequently subtle, may be overlooked as part of the diagnostic workup, and may lead to incorrect diagnoses regarding other organs and systems. Basic changes include the following:

- Decreased ovarian function with menopause causing widespread tissue changes in the body
- Increased secretion of antidiuretic hormone (ADH) in response to serum osmolality
- Thyroid gland atrophy and fibrosis
  Decreased T_4 secretion and metabolism
  Decreased serum T_3 levels
- Altered calcium metabolism by the parathyroid gland
- Decreased cortisol and androgen secretion
- Impaired glucose tolerance: delayed insulin secretion and altered hepatic metabolism
- Impaired hypothalamic secretion
- Anterior pituitary fibrosis

    Perceived problems with fertility
      Pregnancy history
      Birth control methods, duration of use
  Sexual history
    Changes in libido
    Impotence
Perceptions of changes in physical self or personality
  Body proportions, size of hands or feet
  Facial appearance
  Hair distribution and texture
  Skin pigmentation, texture, and quality
  Voice quality
  Secondary sex characteristics
  Emotional stability: mood swings, depression, anger

OBJECTIVE DATA

Inspection
  NOTE: Careful inspection is the key to physical assessment, since only the thyroid gland is accessible for palpation.
  General
    Overall appearance, body proportions

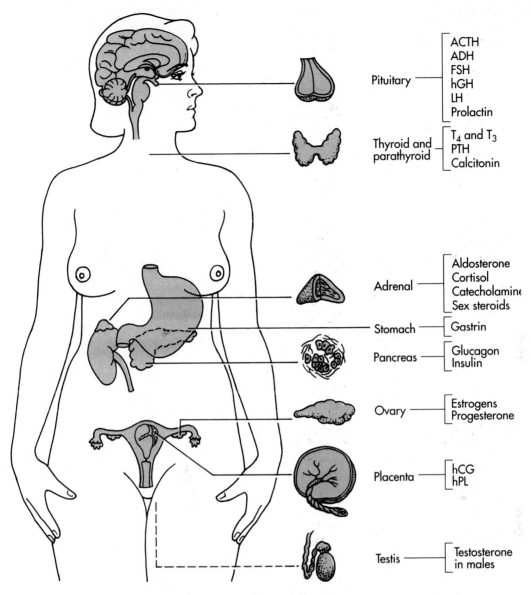

FIGURE 9-1   Sites of hormonal secretion.

Truncal obesity
Moon face, supraclavicular or cervicodorsal fat
    pad (buffalo hump)
Presence of goiter
Height and weight
Presence of exophthalmos
Skin
    Turgor, texture
    Pigmentation
    Presence of edema, striae, ecchymoses
Hair and nails
    Distribution, texture
    Nail brittleness, configuration
Cardiovascular
    Vital signs, orthostatic changes
        Tachycardia, palpitations, angina
Musculoskeletal

    Muscle mass, strength
Nervous system
    Alertness and responsiveness
    Tremors
Palpation of thyroid gland
    Size, symmetry, presence of nodules

✍ DIAGNOSTIC TESTS

LABORATORY TESTS
Blood Tests

Most diagnostic tests involving the endocrine system are blood tests. Tests are performed to evaluate the level of hormone in the blood, the response of glands to the effects of stimulation, and the relationships among the hypothalamus, anterior pituitary gland, and other endo-

TABLE 9-1 Tests of Pituitary Function

NORMAL VALUES	INTERPRETATION
SERUM GROWTH HORMONE	
Men: 0-5 ng/ml Women: 0-10 ng/ml	↑ levels result from pituitary or hypothalamic tumor ↓ levels result from pituitary dysfunction
PROLACTIN	
0-23 ng/dl in nonlactating females	↑ levels result from pituitary adenoma causing autonomous secretion ↓ levels in lactating mothers represent postpartum pituitary dysfunction
ADH	
1-5 pg/ml in normal serum osmolality	↑ levels indicate syndrome of inappropriate antidiuretic hormone (SIADH) ↓ levels indicate diabetes insipidus

TABLE 9-2 Tests of Thyroid Gland Function

NORMAL VALUES	INTERPRETATION
SERUM T_4	
5-13.5 µg/dl	↑ levels found in primary and secondary hyperthyroidism ↓ levels found in primary or secondary hypothyroidism
SERUM T_3	
90-230 ng/dl	↑ levels found in primary hyperthyroidism ↓ levels found in hypothyroidism and in euthyroid persons with severe systemic illness or malnutrition
T_3 RESIN UPTAKE	
25%-35%	High resin uptake with elevated T_4 levels indicates hyperthyroidism Low resin uptake with low T_4 levels indicates hypothyroidism
FREE T_3/T_4	
FT_3: 0.2-0.6 ng/dl FT_4: 0.8-3.3 ng/dl	Elevated levels of free T_3/T_4 indicate hyperthyroidism Low levels of free T_3/T_4 usually indicate hypothyroidism
SERUM TSH	
0-15 µIU/ml	TSH levels >20 suggest primary hypothyroidism Low levels may be normal but can indicate secondary hypothyroidism or Graves' disease/thyroiditis

crine glands. Several tests are usually required to obtain the desired profile of gland function.

Tests of pituitary function

The pituitary gland as the master gland secretes multiple stimulating and suppressing hormones. Tests that measure these substances are presented with the target glands. Table 9-1 presents the major blood tests of primary pituitary function.

Tests of thyroid function

Tests of thyroid function can be made at the hypothalamic, pituitary, or thyroid level. Basic tests of thyroid function are summarized in Table 9-2. The major tests of the processes of thyroid stimulation and suppression are summarized in Table 9-3.

Tests of parathyroid function

The maintenance of normal calcium and phosphorus levels in the body involves the parathyroid gland and multiple other systems, particularly the renal. Serum calcium, phosphorus, and alkaline phosphatase are all

TABLE 9-3 Stimulation and Suppression Tests of Thyroid Function

PROCEDURE AND PREPARATION	INTERPRETATION
TRH STIMULATION TEST TRH is given intravenously (IV) and then serum thyroid-stimulating hormone (TSH) levels are repeatedly measured. Patient may feel facial flushing, the urge to urinate, or nausea for 5 min after injection. These are self-limiting and not complications.	Normal serum TSH begins to rise at 10 min and peaks at 45 min; subnormal tests reflect diminished TSH reserve; supranormal response occurs in patients with hypothyroidism of thyroid origin; no response occurs in most patients with thyrotoxicosis except when it is caused by excess TSH.
TSH STIMULATION TEST Baseline levels of radioactive iodine uptake (RAIU) and protein-bound iodine (PBI) are taken, TSH injection is given, and repeat RAIU and PBI levels are taken.	Test assists in differentiating between primary and secondary hypothyroidism; in primary hypothyroidism repeat level of RAIU and PBI stays the same; if they become normal, this indicates hypothyroidism caused by too little TSH (secondary).
THYROID SUPPRESSION TEST RAIU test and serum T_4 levels are done. Patient is given thyroid hormone for 7-10 days, and RAIU and serum T_4 tests are repeated.	If euthyroid (normal), repeat RAIU and serum T_4 levels will be low; failure of hormone therapy to suppress RAIU and serum T_4 indicates hyperthyroidism.

TABLE 9-4 Stimulation and Suppression Tests of Adrenal Gland Function

PROCEDURE AND PREPARATION	INTERPRETATION
ACTH STIMULATION TEST (VARIOUS TESTS AVAILABLE)	
Synthetic adrenocorticotropic hormone (ACTH) given in 500-1000 ml of normal saline at 2 U/24 hr; then 17-OHCS and plasma cortisol levels are measured; alternative method: infuse 25 units of ACTH over 8-hr period on 2-3 days and measure 17-OHCS and plasma cortisol levels on these days	Normally 17-OHCS excretion increases to 25 mg/24 hr, and plasma cortisol increases to 40 µg/dl or greater; in patients with secondary adrenal insufficiency, 17-OHCS rate is 3-20 mg/24 hr, and cortisol level is 10-40 µg/dl
SCREENING ACTH STIMULATION TEST; COSYNTROPIN TEST	
Cosyntropin, 250 ng, given IV and plasma cortisol level measured before and 30-60 min after this dose	Normally plasma cortisol increases >18 µg/dl; increase confirms functional hypothalamic-pituitary-adrenal (HPA) axis and rules out adrenal insufficiency
CORTISONE SUPPRESSION TEST	
24-hour urine specimen for 17-OHCS collected for baseline; dexamethasone, 0.5 mg, given every 6 hr for 2 days; 24-hr urine collected for these 2 days	Dexamethasone suppresses pituitary secretion of ACTH and thus steroid levels; normally by second day of dexamethasone, 24-hr urinary level of OHCS should drop more than 50% below baseline; patients with adrenocortical excess (primary) will not show decrease in 24-hr urine levels; patients with secondary adrenocortical excess will have drop but less than 50%
SCREENING SUPPRESSION TEST	
Dexamethasone, 1 mg, given at 12 PM; at 8 AM cortisol level is drawn	Normally cortisol should be less than 5 µg/dl
MINERALOCORTICOID SUPPRESSION TEST (VARIOUS TESTS AVAILABLE)	
Saline, 500 ml/hr, for 4 hr is infused intravenously; alternative: patient is placed on normal sodium diet (100 mEq) or high sodium diet (200 mEq); after patient is in sodium balance, deoxycorticosterone acetate (DOCA) (10 mg q 12 hr) is administered intramuscularly (IM) for 3-5 days	Normally saline infusion depresses plasma aldosterone to <8 µg/dl if patient has been on sodium-restricted diet and to <5 µg/dl if patient has been on normal sodium diet; normal persons on sodium diet of 100 mEq/day will have 70% decrease in aldosterone
CLONIDINE SUPPRESSION TEST	
Clonidine, 0.3 mg, is administered orally after baseline sample drawn; another catecholamine sample collected after 3 hr	Clonidine normally suppresses secretion of catecholamines; in presence of tumor pheochromocytoma, levels are not suppressed by administration of clonidine

measured along with urine calcium. The primary hormone value measured is parathyroid hormone (210 to 310 pg/ml). This measurement must be interpreted in conjunction with serum calcium. Elevated levels indicate hyperparathyroidism, whereas low levels result from hypoparathyroidism and malignant disease.

Tests of adrenal function

Adrenal function tests are designed to test both cortical function and medullary function. A variety of stimulation and suppression tests are summarized in Table 9-4. The major hormones measured include the following:

1. Cortisol (7 to 28 µg/dl): elevated levels may indicate hypersecretion associated with Cushing's disease/syndrome; low levels may indicate adrenal hypofunction.
2. Catecholamines (resting: epinephrine, 0 to 110 pg/ml; norepinephrine, 70 to 750 pg/ml; and dopamine, 0 to 3 pg/ml): high levels are associated with pheochromocytoma and other tumors; low levels suggest autonomic system dysfunction.
3. Aldosterone (1 to 16 ng/dl): elevated levels are associated with tumor or hyperplasia or occur

secondary to a systemic disease such as cirrhosis or heart failure. Low levels indicate primary deficiency or adrenal hypofunction.

Tests of pancreatic endocrine function

Tests involving the endocrine function of the pancreas primarily involve the various tests for blood glucose and the body's ability to effectively metabolize it. The major tests are outlined in Table 9-5.

Urine Tests

Twenty-four–hour urine collections are frequently used to measure the amount of a hormone or its breakdown product excreted from the body during an entire day's cycle. These tests are used most commonly for evaluating levels of catecholamines and other adrenal hormones and metabolites. Several of these urine tests are summarized in Table 9-6.

RADIOLOGIC TESTS

Computed tomography (CT) and magnetic resonance imaging (MRI) tests are frequently employed in the evaluation of pituitary and adrenal structure. They assist

TABLE 9-5 Tests of Pancreatic Endocrine Function

NORMAL VALUES	INTERPRETATION

FASTING GLUCOSE

70-100 mg/dl	Normal level should be at 60-120 mg/dl; elevated level indicates need for further study to rule out diabetes mellitus

TWO-HOUR POSTPRANDIAL GLUCOSE

<145 mg/dl	Blood glucose should be within normal limits; levels above 120 mg/dl should be investigated further

GLUCOSE TOLERANCE TEST (GTT)

Differs according to source of blood, method of analysis, and critical levels established by various authorities; levels established by National Diabetes Data Group (as diagnostic for diabetes mellitus in nonpregnant adults are as follows:

Source	Fasting (mg/dl)	2 hr after glucose load (mg/dl)
Venous plasma	>140	>200
Venous whole blood	>120	>180
Capillary whole blood	>120	>200

CORTISONE GLUCOSE TEST

140 mg/dl considered a positive test	Used when GTT results are inconclusive; cortisone increases blood glucose levels and decreases peripheral glucose utilization

C-PEPTIDE TEST

0.9-4.2 ng/ml	C-peptide levels normally parallel those of insulin; levels help to determine beta cell functioning and indirectly measure insulin secretion

GLYCOSYLATED HEMOGLOBIN (HbA$_{1c}$)

Values reported as percentage of total hemoglobin; HbA$_{1c}$ values normally about 5%	Measures glucose levels over 120-day period and provides stable values that average daily glucose levels over time; useful for ongoing diabetic monitoring

TABLE 9-6 Urine Tests of Adrenal Function

NORMAL VALUES	INTERPRETATION

URINE ALDOSTERONE

2-16 µg/24 hr	Elevated levels suggest aldosteronism; low levels found with adrenal hypofunction

URINE CATECHOLAMINES

0-135 µg/24 hr	Elevated levels following hypertensive episode suggest pheochromo-cytoma; in absence of hypertension, tumor is likely; low levels indicate autonomic dysfunction

URINE 17-HYDROXYSTEROIDS

Men: 4.5-12 mg/24 hr Women: 2.5-10 mg/ 24 hr	Elevated levels may indicate Cushing's disease or tumor; low levels indicate adrenal hypofunction

URINE 17-KETOSTEROIDS

Men: 6-21 mg/24 hr Women: 4-17 mg/ 24 hr	Elevated levels indicate adrenal hyperplasia, cancer, or ovarian disease; low levels result from adrenal or pituitary hypofunction

URINE VANILLYLMANDELIC ACID

0.7-6.8 mg/24 hr	Elevated levels associated with cate-cholamine-secreting tumor (pheo-chromocytoma); no pathologic condition associated with low levels

with detection and evaluation of microadenomas and tumors of all varieties. In addition, ultrasonography can be useful in the evaluation of the thyroid gland. The thyroid gland is also evaluated using radioactive trace elements that can be measured as they bind to the gland.

Radioactive Iodine Uptake Test

Purpose—RAIU is used to evaluate thyroid function and distinguish between primary and secondary disorders.

Procedure—A tracer dose of radioactive iodine is administered orally and followed at 2-, 6-, and 24-hour intervals with scintillation scanning. The amount of accumulated iodine is measured. Urine is also collected for 24 hours to measure the amount of iodine excreted.

Patient preparation and aftercare—The patient is instructed to fast the night before the test and is reassured about the safety of the brief half-life iodine. The patient is able to resume a normal diet about 2 hours after the administration of the isotope. No special follow-up care is needed. The test is painless.

Radionuclide Thyroid Imaging

Purpose—Radionuclide thyroid imaging utilizes a radionuclide to assess the size, structure, and position of the thyroid gland.

Procedure—An oral dose of radioactive iodine is administered 24 hours before the test, or an IV injection of labeled pertechnetate is administered 30 minutes before the test. Scintillation scanning is performed, and the image of the thyroid is captured on x-ray film.

Patient preparation and aftercare—The patient is instructed to fast before the administration of the oral isotope. Thyroid hormones, antagonists, and iodine solutions are discontinued several weeks before the test. Salicylates and antihistamines are discontinued 1 week before the test. The patient should also strictly limit or eliminate the ingestion of iodized salt or seafood. The patient is reassured about the safety of the use of the very brief half-life isotopes. The patient may resume all medications and normal diet and activity after the test. No special aftercare is required.

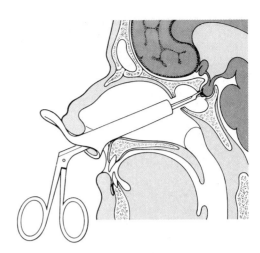

FIGURE 9-2 Transsphenoidal surgical approach. (From Beare PG, Myers JL: *Principles and practice of adult health nursing,* ed 2, St Louis, 1994, Mosby.)

DISORDERS OF THE ENDOCRINE SYSTEM

DISORDERS OF THE PITUITARY GLAND

Pituitary gland disorders can involve hyperfunction or hypofunction of either the anterior or posterior gland. An overview of the various disorders is presented in Table 9-7, and the regulating hormones of the pituitary are summarized in Table 9-8.

Anterior Gland Disorders: Hyperpituitarism
Etiology/epidemiology

Hyperpituitarism may result from a primary problem in the pituitary gland or occur secondary to a dysfunction of the hypothalamus. Pituitary adenomas are the most common cause, and the tumors are almost always secreting or functioning tumors. They are usually benign but may grow aggressively. They are typically classified based on the type of hormone secreted, and prolactin-secreting tumors account for 60% to 80% of the total. Hyperfunction can also result from glandular hyperplasia, usually as a result of failure of normal feedback mechanisms.

Pathophysiology

Adenomas produce symptoms related to the hypersecretion of hormones or from pressure on the surrounding brain tissue as the tumor grows. Patients often delay seeking help until symptoms of increasing intracranial pressure occur. The growing tumor may put pressure on the surrounding brain tissue or the cranial nerves. The optic chiasm lies above the sella turcica and is often compressed when the tumor enlarges. The dysfunction may also be identified during a workup for adrenal, menstrual, or thyroid dysfunction. Depending on which hormone or hormones are being oversecreted, a wide variety of effects may be seen (see Table 9-7).

Medical management

Serum and urine tests reveal elevated hormone levels, and CT or MRI scans may be used to confirm the presence and size of the adenoma. Treatment is aimed at decreasing the abnormal levels and/or removing the adenoma. Bromocriptine (Parlodel) may be used with prolactin-secreting tumors to restore normal hormone levels, restore fertility, and reduce tumor size. No further treatment may be necessary. GH- and ACTH-secreting tumors are treated surgically via transsphenoidal hypophysectomy in which the tumor is removed from the sella turcica from below through the sphenoid sinus (Figure 9-2). Patients treated surgically require either temporary or long-term replacement of the anterior pituitary hormones after surgery.

Radiation therapy may be used as an adjunct treatment or as an alternative. It is commonly used for tumors that have extended beyond the sella turcica and cannot be completely resected. The response to radiation is slow, and hypopituitarism develops in many patients. Careful monitoring of hormone levels is essential, because the deficits may not show up for years after the treatment.

NURSING MANAGEMENT

The nurse assists with patient education about the disease process and treatment options. The prospect of intracranial surgery of any type is extremely frightening to patients and families. Prolactin-associated sexual changes are usually reversible with effective treatment, and the patient needs to be reassured about this and the return of fertility. The specific care delivered to patients undergoing pituitary surgery is presented in the Guidelines box on p. 177. The risk of postoperative infection and the potential for fluid imbalance related to disruption of ADH secretion are of particular concern.

Anterior Gland Disorders: Hypopituitarism

Panhypopituitarism results most commonly from surgical removal of the gland. Selected deficiencies can also

TABLE 9-7   Pituitary Gland Dysfunction

ALTERATION IN SECRETION	ETIOLOGY	SIGNS AND SYMPTOMS
ANTERIOR PITUITARY		
Growth hormone (GH) excess	Pituitary tumors Pituitary hyperplasia	Gigantism in children Acromegaly in adults: growth of soft tissues, cartilages, bones Enlargement and coarsening of facial features Enlarged tongue Visceral enlargement (liver, spleen, heart, kidneys) Warm, moist, coarse skin; increased sweating Husky voice Hypertension
GH deficit	Infection Granuloma Trauma Congenital tumor	Dwarfism in children Immature voice and facial features Sensitivity to insulin Hypoglycemia No symptoms in adults
ACTH excess	Pituitary tumors or hyperplasia Nonpituitary secreting tumor Iatrogenic from chronic steroid use	Similar to Cushing's syndrome (adrenocortical excess)
ACTH deficit	Same as GH deficit Iatrogenic suppression of hypothalamic-pituitary axis by exogenous corticosteroids	Similar to Addison's disease (adrenocortical deficiency) Asthenia (weakness) Nausea, vomiting Hypotension, hypoglycemia Hyponatremia, hyperkalemia
TSH excess	Pituitary tumor or hyperplasia	Same as hyperthyroidism (thyroid hormone excess)
TSH deficit	Same as GH deficit	Same as hypothyroidism (thyroid hormone deficit) Cretinism in newborn Myxedema in adult
Prolactin excess	Pituitary tumor Idiopathic Side effect of certain drugs that interfere with secretion	Amenorrhea, galactorrhea, depressed libido, infertility, impotency, change in secondary sex characteristics
Prolactin deficit	Same as GH deficit	Usually no clinical symptoms in adults
Gonadotropic hormone excess	Same as GH deficit	Hirsutism in female

Gonadotropic hormone deficit	Same as GH deficit	Delayed sexual development in children
		In adults
		   Amenorrhea, infertility in female
		   Impotence in male
		   Changes in secondary sex characteristics in both males and females

POSTERIOR PITUITARY		
ADH excess	Pituitary disease Central nervous system (CNS) trauma or surgery Cancer, particularly oat cell cancer of lung, which secretes ADH	Water retention without edema Weight gain Oliguria Sodium deficit: weakness, lethargy, seizures, coma Serum hypoosmolality
ADH deficit	Pituitary surgery CNS trauma or surgery Trauma or other extreme stressor	Polyuria: >10 L daily; specific gravity <1.005 Thirst Weight loss Signs of dehydration if intake inadequate

occur idiopathically or as a result of vascular lesions, infection, or trauma. The clinical picture varies dramatically based on the nature and severity of the hormone deficiency and the age of the patient. Failure of synthesis and secretion of gonadatropins are the most commonly encountered problem, followed by deficiency of growth hormone. Medical management is directed toward identifying the underlying deficiency and providing appropriate hormone replacement or supplementation. Biosynthetic human GH (somatrem [Protropin],

somatropin [Humatrope]) is now available for clinical use in deficiency states. The nurse assists the patient to achieve knowledgeable self-care and to accept the hormone-related changes in body image associated with the disease and its treatment.

Posterior Gland Disorders: Hyperpituitarism
Etiology/epidemiology

Excess secretion of the posterior pituitary gland hormone ADH creates the syndrome of inappropriate ADH

TABLE 9-8 Hormones of the Pituitary Gland

HORMONE	FUNCTIONS
ANTERIOR PITUITARY	
Thyroid-stimulating hormone (TSH)	Stimulates thyroid to secrete thyroxin
Adrenocorticotropic hormone (ACTH)	Stimulates adrenal cortex to secrete cortisol
Gonadotropic hormones Luteinizing hormone (LH)	Induces ovulation and stimulates formation of corpus luteum and progesterone secretion in female
Follicle-stimulating hormone (FSH)	Stimulates follicle growth in ovary and secretion of estrogen in female
Interstitial cell-stimulating hormone (ICSH)	Stimulates secretion of testosterone in male
Growth hormone (GH) (somatotropin)	Stimulates body growth; influences protein, carbohydrate, and fat metabolism
Prolactin	Stimulates mammary gland development
POSTERIOR PITUITARY	
Antidiuretic hormone (ADH, vasopressin)	Major regulator of osmolality and body water volume
	Increases permeability of collecting ducts in kidney to water, resulting in increased H_2O reabsorption
	May stimulate H_2O intake by stimulating perception of thirst
Oxytocin	Results in milk "letdown" in lactating breast
	Causes increased uterine contraction after labor has begun; role in initiating labor unclear

Guidelines for Nursing Care Following Pituitary Surgery

GENERAL MEASURES

Encourage frequent deep breathing.
  Remind patient *not* to cough.
Encourage patient to be active to tolerance.
Provide analgesics and other comfort measures for headache.

FLUID BALANCE

NOTE: Diabetes insipidus usually occurs within the first 24 hours after surgery.
Maintain accurate intake and output records; weigh daily.
Assess for signs of fluid imbalance:
  Polyuria (output >200 ml/hr)
  Decreased skin turgor, dry mucous membranes
  Low urine specific gravity (1.000-1.005)
  Postural hypotension, tachycardia
Encourage daily fluid intake of 2500-3000 ml.
Administer vasopressin or desmopressin as ordered.

PREVENTING INFECTION

Instruct patient to rinse the mouth with saline or mouthwash several times each day.
Clean teeth using a toothette. Do *not* use a toothbrush until incisional healing occurs.
Avoid rough foods that could irritate the incision.
Avoid activities that increase intracranial pressure.
NOTE: The defect in the sella turcica is repaired with a muscle plug, bone, or cartilage. This patching is strong but can be easily disrupted in the early days by increased intracranial pressure.
  No bending over, straining, coughing, sneezing, or nose blowing is permitted.
  Head of bed is maintained at 30 degrees.
Monitor for signs of cerebrospinal fluid (CSF) leakage:
  Complaints of postnasal drip despite nasal packing
  Appearance of halo ring on nasal drip pad
Test any drainage for presence of CSF; will test positive for glucose. If leakage is discovered:
  Send specimen to laboratory.
  Place patient on bed rest.
  Notify physician immediately for initiation of antibiotics.
  Monitor for signs of infection or meningitis.

PATIENT EDUCATION

Teach patient about any needed hormone replacement:
  Lifelong cortisol replacement may be needed.
  Glucocorticoid supplement may be indicated.
Teach patient about monitoring for complications and the importance of ongoing medical follow-up:
  Hormone imbalances
  Recurrent tumor

(SIADH). The syndrome is associated with a variety of diseases, trauma, and surgery of the nervous system. It also occurs with the use of certain drugs, in situations of extreme physiologic stress, and with certain malignancies, particularly oat cell carcinoma of the lung where the cells develop the capacity to secrete ADH. The continual hormone release is unrelated to the normal feedback mechanism of serum osmolality. Water is retained, extracellular fluid volume expands, and dilutional hyponatremia occurs.

Pathophysiology

In SIADH a hypoosmolar state results from extreme water retention in response to ADH. The intravascular volume increases dramatically, but edema does not occur because of ongoing sodium excretion. The hypoosmolarity of the fluid creates an osmotic gradient across cell membranes and the blood-brain barrier. Water follows the osmotic gradient into the cells and brain, creating swelling and overhydration. Most individuals become symptomatic when serum sodium falls below 125 mEq/L and may experience seizures or coma at levels below 115 mEq/L. Classic symptoms of SIADH include the following:

Falling urine output
Weight gain without apparent edema
Anorexia progressing to nausea and vomiting
Lethargy and headache progressing to disorientation, seizures, and coma
Decreased serum sodium and osmolality

Medical management

Treatment focuses on controlling the underlying primary pathologic condition and restoring the serum sodium level. Water intake is restricted to no more than 800 to 1000 ml/day depending on the severity of the sodium deficit, and oral salt intake is increased if the patient is able to take oral nutrients. Patients with severe hyponatremia may be treated with hypertonic saline (3%) in combination with diuretic therapy. The solution is administered with great care to prevent too rapid fluid shifts. The syndrome is usually self-limiting and responds well to treatment with fluid restriction.

NURSING MANAGEMENT

Nursing care focuses on meticulous assessment and support of the patient. All fluid intake and output parameters are carefully monitored and recorded, particularly if treatment with hypertonic saline is required. The nurse assists the patient to adhere to the fluid restriction and balances the available fluid throughout the day and in consideration of meals. Ice chips can be used effectively to deal with the discomfort of thirst. Daily weights, intake and output, and serum and urine osmolalities are all assessed frequently. Clinical signs of sodium imbalance are monitored with great care and documented frequently. Patients with chronic disease will be taught to enrich sodium in their diet, maintain a restricted fluid intake, and monitor their fluid status through ongoing assessment of body weight.

Posterior Gland Disorders: Hypopituitarism
Etiology/epidemiology

Hypofunction of the posterior pituitary creates the condition of diabetes insipidus from the lack of sufficient ADH to control fluid balance. True primary disease is rare, but diabetes insipidus is a common secondary problem following surgery or trauma or with pituitary tumor. The problem may be temporary or permanent.

Pathophysiology

Without sufficient ADH to stimulate water reabsorption from the renal tubules, as much as 15 L of fluid can be excreted daily, creating the potential for serious fluid and electrolyte disturbance and vascular collapse. The polyuria triggers intense thirst and if the patient is able to take oral liquids, severe changes in serum osmolality do not usually occur. Classic symptoms include the following:

Polyuria: specific gravity of 1.005 or less
Polydipsia
Slightly elevated serum osmolality
Symptoms of fluid and electrolyte disturbance if unable to consume adequate quantities of replacement fluids

Medical management

Treatment is aimed at correcting the underlying condition if possible and providing adequate hormone re-placement if needed. Temporary diabetes insipidus is treated with subcutaneous aqueous vasopressin followed by nasal administration of lysine or DDVP when appropriate. Chronic disease states are managed with desmopressin (DDAVP), which is more potent and has a longer duration of effect. Replacement of fluid is planned if the patient is unable to meet fluid needs orally.

NURSING MANAGEMENT

Nursing interventions focus on assisting the patient to maintain a balance of fluid and electrolytes. Careful intake and output records are maintained, and daily weights are recorded. Fluid parameters such as vital signs, mental status, and skin and mucous membrane condition are assessed frequently. The nurse works with the patient to plan an appropriate response to the thirst, and the nurse ensures that adequate quantities of acceptable fluids are always available at the bedside. Chronic conditions require careful teaching for safe self-care, especially the adjustments needed to respond to changes in temperature, humidity, and activity.

DISORDERS OF THE THYROID GLAND
Hyperthyroidism
Etiology/epidemiology

Hyperthyroidism is a condition that results from the excessive secretion of thyroxine (T_4) and/or triiodothyronine (T_3). Thyroid problems are relatively common and can be caused by a variety of pathologic processes. Graves' disease and toxic nodular goiter are the most common. The following discussion uses Graves' disease as a model. Toxic nodular goiter is summarized in Box 9-2, and other causes of hyperthyroidism are summarized in Box 9-1.

Graves' disease occurs primarily in women and typically affects individuals under the age of 40 years. Although the etiology is unknown, the disease frequently appears after a period of extreme physiologic and psychologic stress. It also appears to have a hereditary component. Graves' disease is often associated with a familial incidence of autoimmune disease. The disease is characterized by the presence of one or more of the following: diffuse goiter, hyperthyroidism, and infiltrative ophthalmopathy.

Pathophysiology

Research supports the theory that Graves' disease is caused by autostimulation of the thyroid gland by a group of immunoglobulins of the IgG class called thyroid-stimulating immunoglobulins. The normal regulatory control of thyroid function is lost, and there is an increased concentration of thyroid hormone. The multiple functions of the thyroid hormones are listed in Box 9-3. The effects of hyperthyroidism on body systems are well known and occur in large part because of the interaction of the hypermetabolic state, increased circu-

BOX 9-1 Causes and Definitions of Types of Hyperthyroidism

GRAVES' DISEASE
See text

TOXIC MULTINODULAR GOITER
See Box 9-2

TOXIC ADENOMA
Single or occasionally multiple adenomas of follicular cells that secrete and function independent of TSH

THYROIDITIS
Increased amount of thyroxine (T_4) and triiodothyronine (T_3) released during acute inflammatory process; transient hyperthyroid state followed by return to euthyroid state, and eventually to hypothyroid state as gland is destroyed by recurring inflammatory exacerbations; hyperthyroid state usually requires no treatment

T_3 THYROTOXICOSIS
T_3 level elevated but cause unknown; T_4 normal or low; should be suspected in patients who have normal T_4 but have signs and symptoms of thyrotoxicosis

HYPERTHYROIDISM CAUSED BY METASTATIC THYROID CANCER
Rare because thyroid cancer cells do not usually concentrate iodine efficiently; may occur with large follicular carcinomas

PITUITARY HYPERTHYROIDISM
Rare; pituitary adenomas may secrete excess TSH; treatment involves removal of pituitary tumor

CHORIONIC HYPERTHYROIDISM
Chorionic gonadotropin has weak thyrotropin activity; tumors such as choriocarcinoma, embryonal cell carcinoma, and hydatidiform mole have high concentrations of chorionic gonadotropins that can stimulate T_4 and T_3 secretion; hyperthyroidism disappears with treatment of tumor

STRUMA OVARII
Ovarian dermoid tumor made up of thyroid tissue that secretes thyroid hormone

FACTITIOUS HYPERTHYROIDISM
Results from ingestion of exogenous thyroid extracts

IODINE-INDUCED HYPERTHYROIDISM (JOD-BASEDOW)
Overproduction of thyroid hormone resulting from administration of supplemental iodine to person with endemic goiter

BOX 9-2 Toxic Nodular Goiter

Toxic nodular goiter is characterized by the presence of multiple nodules within the thyroid gland that secrete thyroxine and trigger hyperthyroidism that is usually fairly mild. Goiters result from increased stimulation of the thyroid gland by TSH. The disease primarily affects persons over the age of 50 years, particularly persons who have had a nodular goiter for a period of years. The disorder is probably triggered by a mild iodide deficiency. There is no evidence of autoimmune involvement. The disorder may be treated medically or with surgery.

BOX 9-3 Functions of Thyroid Gland Hormones

THYROXINE (T_4) AND TRIIODOTHYRONINE (T_3)
Regulates protein, fat, and carbohydrate catabolism in all cells
Regulates metabolic rate of all cells
Regulates body heat production
Insulin antagonist
Necessary for muscle tone and vigor
Maintains cardiac rate, force, and output
Affects CNS development
Maintains secretion of gastrointestinal tract
Affects respiratory rate and oxygen utilization
Maintains calcium mobilization
Affects red blood cell production
Stimulates lipid turnover, free fatty acid release, and cholesterol synthesis

THYROCALCITONIN
Lowers serum calcium and phosphorus levels by inhibiting osteoclastic activity
Decreases calcium and phosphorus absorption in gastrointestinal tract

lation, and excess adrenergic stimulation. Classic symptoms are presented in Box 9-4.

The ophthalmopathy of Graves' disease can occur at any time. The classic visible outcome is exophthalmos. The protrusion of the eyes results from expansion of muscle and tissue volume caused at least in part by fluid accumulation. The eye is forced forward, which stretches the extraocular muscles and impairs their functioning. The condition is considered to be a parallel autoimmune process to Graves' disease and usually is controlled with treatment of the hyperthyroidism. It does not occur with other forms of hyperthyroidism.

Medical management

A variety of laboratory tests are used to diagnose Graves' disease, including serum hormone levels, sensitive TSH assays, and stimulation and suppression tests. Ultrasound or CT will be employed to rule out structural problems and cancer.

Treatment is designed to decrease the synthesis and release of thyroid hormones and block the effects of the hormones on body tissues. Options include drug therapy, surgery, and radioactive iodine treatment. Drug therapy is usually employed first to return the patient to a euthyroid condition before definitive treatment is undertaken. The choice of treatment is based on the patient's age and sex, the size of the goiter, duration and severity of the disease, and the patient's reproductive status. Radioactive iodine is the treatment of choice for most older patients for whom childbearing is not a consideration. Precautions for patients receiving radio-

BOX 9-4	Classic Symptoms of Graves' Disease

GASTROINTESTINAL

Increased appetite	Weight loss
Abdominal cramping/discomfort	Increased number of stools

CARDIOVASCULAR

Tachycardia	Increased blood pressure
Palpitations	Angina
Atrial fibrillation	Heart failure

MUSCULOSKELETAL

Muscle weakness	Muscle wasting
Fine, rhythmic tremors	Mild osteoporosis

INTEGUMENT

Warm, moist skin	Heat intolerance
Fine, fragile hair	Increased body temperature

EMOTIONAL/BEHAVIORAL

Nervousness/restlessness	Fatigue
Decreased attention span	Insomnia
Emotional lability	

SEXUAL/REPRODUCTIVE

Altered menstrual pattern	Change in libido
Infertility	

LABORATORY RESULTS

Elevated blood glucose	Hypercalcemia
Decreased cholesterol/ triglycerides	Elevated liver enzymes

TABLE 9-9	Drugs Used in Treatment of Hyperthyroidism

DRUG	ACTIONS
ANTITHYROID DRUGS	
Propylthiouracil (PTU) Methimazole (Tapazole)	Block thyroid hormone synthesis; slow-acting drugs that may take 2-4 wk to produce noticeable improvement; approximately 50% achieve remission
IODINE PREPARATIONS	
Lugol's solution Saturated solution of potassium iodide (SSKI)	Block synthesis and release of thyroid hormone, producing rapid reduction in metabolic rate; do not have a sustained effect but reduce gland vascularity and are frequently given preoperatively
BETA-ADRENERGIC BLOCKERS	
Propranolol (Inderal)	Used to treat tachycardia, arrhythmia, and angina symptoms that may accompany hyperthyroidism; used for all patients in thyroid storm
CALCIUM CHANNEL BLOCKERS	
Verapamil Diltiazem	Similar to beta-adrenergic blockers; fewer adverse side effects

active treatment are presented in the Guidelines box. The drugs used to treat Graves' disease are summarized in Table 9-9.

Surgery is the treatment of choice for patients with large goiters and is the primary therapy in children and during pregnancy. Subtotal thyroidectomy with removal of 75% to 80% of the gland is the preferred procedure. The risks of hypothyroidism are eliminated, but some patients experience a return of hyperthyroidism from hypertrophy of the remaining tissue over time.

NURSING MANAGEMENT

♦ ASSESSMENT

Subjective Data

History of symptoms and severity
Family history of thyroid disease
Patient's complaints of the following:
    Nervousness and irritability
    Exaggerated emotions and mood swings
    Heat intolerance
    Palpitations, anginal pain
    Fatigue and muscle weakness
    Increased hunger plus weight loss
    Menstrual irregularities, decreased libido and fertility
    Abdominal discomfort, frequent soft stools

 Guidelines for Nursing Care Following Radioactive Iodine Therapy

The dose is administered orally on an outpatient basis. The patient is held in the nuclear medicine area until it is certain that vomiting will not occur. Symptoms decrease gradually over about 3 weeks, but a euthyroid state is not achieved for about 6 months. Repeat treatment is often necessary. Radiation precautions are dose dependent. The isotope is excreted in the urine, saliva, sweat, and feces.

TEACHING

Isotope is eliminated within about 2 days.
Flush the toilet two or three times after each use.
Increase the intake of fluids to aid in excretion of the isotope.
Void every 2 hours to minimize the stagnant time in the bladder.
Avoid prolonged physical contact, particularly with infants. Sleeping alone may be advised with high doses.
Wash sinks and tubs after use, and wash hands well after urination or defecation.
Expect some neck soreness or dysphagia after treatment. Discomfort should be controllable with mild analgesics.
Maintain adequate follow-up care to evaluate effectiveness of treatment. Major adverse side effect is hypothyroidism, which occurs in most persons within 5 to 7 years after treatment.

Objective Data

Body weight and proportions
Skin appearance and texture
    Dermopathy
    Presence of sweating or reddening
    Fine, thin hair
Tachycardia; signs of congestive heart failure
Elevated systolic blood pressure
Fine tremors
Exophthalmos
Goiter
Elevated serum T_3, T_4; decreased TSH assay

■   ■   ■

The remainder of the nursing management of the patient with Graves' disease undergoing surgery is presented in the nursing care plan. A critical pathway for a patient with Graves' disease and atrial fibrillation is also included.

Hypothyroidism
Etiology/epidemiology

Hypothyroidism is a metabolic state resulting from deficiency of thyroid hormone. It can occur at any age. The disease can be idiopathic or result from a congenital deficiency, iodine deficiency, or the effects of drugs. Congenital hypothyroidism can produce a condition known as cretinism. Myxedema is the severe adult form of the disease. Iodine deficiency is the most common worldwide cause of hypothyroidism, whereas autoimmune thyroiditis and treatment effects from surgery and radioactive iodine administration are the most common causes in the United States.

Hashimoto's thyroiditis is the most common form in which autoimmune changes occur in the thyroid, which leads first to goiter and then to hormone deficiency. The problem tends to occur in older persons.

GERONTOLOGIC PATIENT CONSIDERATIONS FOR HYPERTHYROIDISM

Older patients rarely present with the full-blown syndrome of Graves' disease, and the problem may be overlooked in the management of other ongoing health problems. The term *apathetic hyperthyroidism* is often applied to the disease in elders, since patients rarely exhibit the classic cardiovascular effects. Fatigue, irritability, and muscle weakness are common, and weight loss may occur. GI complaints are typical but may not be prominent or severe. Goiter and exophthalmos are also rare. New-onset atrial fibrillation or angina may be the first symptom.

Serum hormone levels may remain within normal limits, making the diagnosis complex. Sophisticated assays may be necessary to establish the diagnosis. Radioactive iodine treatment is the approach of choice in older patients.

Pathophysiology

Goiter, or enlargement of the thyroid gland, occurs as the pituitary gland secretes more TSH in response to perceived lower levels of thyroid hormone in the blood. When the enlarging gland is unable to maintain a sufficient hormone output the symptoms of hypothyroidism begin. In Hashimoto's thyroiditis the initial autoimmune response may trigger episodes of hyperthyroidism with inappropriate release of hormone from the gland. Over time, however, atrophy occurs along with hormone deficiency.

Lack of adequate thyroid hormone causes a general depression of metabolic rate and activity. Alterations occur in every major body system. Early signs may go unrecognized, particularly in elderly persons. Weakness, tiredness, and lethargy are common and may be attributed to many other causes, particularly psychologic ones such as depression. The full range of clinical symptoms is presented in Box 9-6.

Medical management

The diagnosis of hypothyroidism can be established through examination of serum values of thyroid hormones, free T_4, and "sensitive" TSH. Antithyroid antibodies will be examined in the diagnosis of Hashimoto's thyroiditis. Drug therapy is the foundation of care and involves the administration of replacement thyroid hormone. The treatment is lifelong. Synthroid is the drug of choice in most situations, but Cytomel, Trionine, and Euthroid are other options that may be selected in different circumstances. Symptom relief will begin within 2 to 3 days of treatment, but it may take a period of trial and error to establish the optimal dosage. Surgical treatment may be needed for large goiters.

NURSING MANAGEMENT

Nursing care primarily involves patient teaching for self-care and monitoring the patient's response to therapy. Adjustments must be made slowly in elderly

BOX 9-5   Thyroid Crisis/Storm

Thyroid crisis is a rare medical emergency in which patients develop severe manifestations of hyperthyroidism. The crisis is usually precipitated by a major stressor such as severe infection, trauma, or surgery. Thyroid crisis typically affects patients who are poorly controlled or who stop taking their prescribed therapy. The associated mortality is high, and patients are managed in a critical care area. Symptoms of thyroid crisis include the following:
    Elevated temperature
    Tachycardia, dysrhythmia, elevated blood pressure
    Tremors and restlessness
    Declining mental status, delirium, coma
The crisis is treated with meticulous monitoring of all vital functions and administration of oral propylthiouracil and IV iodides and beta blockers. Supportive measures include control of body temperature with cooling devices, oxygen, cardiac glycosides, and general comfort measures.

NURSING CARE PLAN

THE PATIENT WITH GRAVES' DISEASE UNDERGOING THYROIDECTOMY

■ **NURSING DIAGNOSIS**

Injury, high risk for (related to postoperative edema and hypocalcemia)

Expected Patient Outcome	Nursing Interventions

Patient will maintain a patent airway and be free of overt symptoms of hypocalcemia.	1. Maintain a semi-Fowler's position to reduce stress on the incision line.
	2. Teach patient the importance of supporting the head with the hands when moving and changing position to prevent suture line stress.
	3. Assess frequently for:
	  a. Bleeding on dressings behind neck and on pillow
	  b. Difficulty in speaking or persistent hoarseness
	  c. Dysphagia or choking sensation
	  d. Sensation of constriction or tightness of dressings
	  e. Persistent or worsening respiratory distress, dyspnea, crowing sound
	4. Assess for signs of calcium imbalance:
	  a. Numbness and tingling around the mouth and fingertips
	  b. Positive Chvostek's and Trousseau's signs
	  c. Muscle twitching, spasm, tetany
	5. Report any positive findings from assessment to surgeon immediately.
	6. Administer calcium chloride or gluconate as ordered.
	7. Ensure ready access to emergency equipment: oxygen, suction, tracheostomy set.

■ **NURSING DIAGNOSIS**

Nutrition, altered: less than body requirements (related to persistent excess in metabolic rate; early postoperative dysphagia)

Expected Patient Outcome	Nursing Interventions

Patient will ingest sufficient nutrients to meet body needs and maintain desired weight.	1. Introduce fluids and soft diet with caution; supervise first efforts at swallowing. Advance diet as tolerated.
	2. Provide high-calorie, high-protein diet.
	  a. Keep snacks at bedside.
	  b. Maintain adequate fluid intake.
	  c. Encourage patient to avoid caffeine.
	3. Use a humidifier if indicated to prevent drying of secretions.
	4. Remind patient to monitor weight twice weekly as metabolism stabilizes.

NURSING CARE PLAN—CONT'D

THE PATIENT WITH GRAVES' DISEASE UNDERGOING THYROIDECTOMY

■ NURSING DIAGNOSIS

Sensory/perceptual alterations, risk of (visual) (related to eye changes of exophthalmos)

Expected Patient Outcome	Nursing Interventions

Patient will employ measures to prevent eye damage.	1. Assess visual acuity, ability to close eyes, degree of photophobia.
	2. Restrict dietary sodium.
	3. Keep head of bed elevated 30 degrees for sleep.
	4. Protect cornea from irritation and infection:
	  a. Patch eyes for sleep if lid closure is inadequate.
	  b. Use artificial tears to keep eyes moist.
	  c. Teach patient to use wraparound sunglasses to protect the eyes from wind, sun, and particles when outdoors.
	5. Teach patient to report any episode of double vision or other visual problem.

■ NURSING DIAGNOSIS

Activity intolerance (related to easy fatigability of muscles)

Expected Patient Outcome	Nursing Interventions

Patient will regain muscle strength and endurance and resume preillness activity pattern.	1. Establish a calm, quiet environment.
	  a. Keep temperature cool.
	  b. Assign patient to room away from major activities.
	2. Help patient plan activities to foster rest.
	3. Patient should avoid activities needing fine coordination.
	4. Encourage activity. After 5 to 7 days, initiate range of motion exercises for the neck.

■ NURSING DIAGNOSIS

Anxiety and nervousness (related to excess nervous system activity)

Expected Patient Outcomes	Nursing Interventions
Patient will understand reason for changes in behavior. Emotional lability will be minimized. Patient will successfully control emotions.	1. Help patient understand physiologic basis for nervousness and moods. 2. Maintain calm, relaxed environment. Teach and reinforce relaxation strategies. 3. Encourage visitors who promote relaxation. 4. Provide privacy (such as single room). 5. Explain all interventions. 6. Avoid stimulants such as coffee, tea, cola, alcohol. 7. Decrease known stressors, explain planned interventions, and listen to patient's concerns.

CRITICAL PATHWAY   **Hyperthyroidism with Atrial Fibrillation**

DRG #: 300; expected LOS: 7

	Day of Admission **Day 1**	**Day 2**	**Day 3**
Diagnostic Tests	CBC; UA; SMA/18*, serum TSH and free T_4 index or free T_4 concentration; total T_4 or T_3 concentrations as necessary; ECG; C & S blood/UA/sputum if necessary; O_2 saturation on room air, ABGs if necessary	CBC; O_2 saturation on room air, ABGs if necessary	SMA/18*, ECG
Medications	IV @ TKO; propylthiouracil; antiatrial fibrillation medication (possibly including digitalis, coumadin, propranolol, or calcium channel blockers); medication for congestive heart failure (CHF) as necessary; eye drops OU q 2 hr PRN for dryness; multivitamins; medication for rest/sleep if necessary; stool softener	IV @ TKO; propylthiouracil; antiatrial fibrillation medication; medication for CHF as necessary; eye drops OU q 2 hr PRN for dryness; multivitamins; medication for rest/sleep if necessary; stool softener	IV @ TKO; propylthiouracil; antiatrial fibrillation medication; medication for CHF as necessary; eye drops OU q 2 hr PRN for dryness; multivitamins; medication for rest/sleep if necessary; stool softener
Treatments	I & O q 4 hr; VS q hr 4 times, then q 2 hrs; O_2 PRN; cardiac monitor; weight; record food intake; assess moisture to eyes q 2 hr; assess neuro-cardio-pul-circ systems q 2 hr 4 times then q 4 hr	I & O q 8 hr; VS q 4 hr; O_2 PRN; cardiac monitor; weight; record food intake; assess moisture to eyes q 2 hr; assess neuro-cardio-pul-circ systems q 4 hr	I & O q 8 hr; VS q 4 hr; O_2 PRN; cardiac monitor; weight; record food intake; assess moisture to eyes q 2 hr; assess neuro-cardio-pul-circ systems q 4 hr
Diet	Soft diet with high calories, protein, and CHO; serve 6 meals; *no stimulants*	Soft diet with high calories, protein, and CHO; serves 6 meals; *no stimulants*	Soft diet with high calories, protein, and CHO; serve 6 meals; *no stimulants*
Activity	Bed rest with BRP; minimize environmental stressors (keep room cool, calm, quiet; provide rest periods)	Bed rest with BRP; minimize environmental stressors	Up in room 4 times; minimize environmental stressors
Referral/Consultation	Social services	Dietary, home health if necessary	

NOTE: Acknowledge that patients recover at varying rates; therefore specified daily actions should be based solely on patient need.
*Serum calcium, phosphorus, triglycerides, uric acid, creatinine, blood urea nitrogen (BUN), total bilirubin, alkaline phosphate, aspartate aminotransferase (AST) (formerly serum glutamic oxaloacetic transaminase [SGOT]), alanine aminotransferase (ALT) (formerly serum glutamic pyruvate transaminase [SGPT]), lactic dehydrogenase (LDH), total protein, albumin, sodium, potassium, chloride, total CO_2, glucose.

persons, who can have strong cardiac responses to the increased level of thyroid hormone. The patient is instructed about the lifelong need for replacement hormone, the importance of taking the medication every day, and the symptoms of both overmedication and undermedication. Ongoing medical follow-up is stressed.

Thyroid Cancer

Thyroid nodules develop in about 4% of the population, but only 1 in 1000 of these nodules is cancerous. Malignant nodules tend to occur in children and elderly persons, with a 4:1 ratio of female to male. A history of irradiation to the head and neck is the primary identified risk factor. The diagnosis is typically confirmed through radionuclide imaging and fine needle biopsy. Most patients are euthyroid and do not develop symptoms of either gland hyperactivity or hypoactivity. Treat-

GERONTOLOGIC PATIENT CONSIDERATIONS FOR HYPOTHYROIDISM

Hypothyroidism is a common problem in elderly persons that is frequently overlooked until the disease is very advanced. Depression and lethargy are common early symptoms that are frequently attributed to the aging process, declining abilities, or loss of a partner. The disease can dramatically worsen existing coronary artery and vascular disease, which makes treatment difficult, because the replacement hormones can precipitate cardiac problems. Myxedema coma (Box 9-7) is also more common in this age-group.

ment of the cancer employs partial and total thyroidectomy, radiation, hormonal gland suppression, and occasionally chemotherapy depending on the cell type, size of the tumor, and age and health status of the patient.

CRITICAL PATHWAY   Hyperthyroidism with Atrial Fibrillation

DRG #: 300; expected LOS: 7

Day 4	Day 5	Day 6	Day of Discharge Day 7
	CBC, SMA/18*		
IV saline lock; adjust propylthiouracil, antiatrial fibrillation medication, and other medications for home use; eye drops OU q 2 hr PRN for dryness; multivitamins; medication for rest/sleep PRN; stool softener	IV saline lock; adjust propylthiouracil, antiatrial fibrillation medication, and other medications for home use; eye drops OU q 4 hr PRN for dryness; multivitamins; medication for rest/sleep PRN; stool softener	IV saline lock; adjust propylthiouracil, antiatrial fibrillation medication, and other medications for home use; eye drops OU q 2 hr PRN for dryness; multivitamins; medication for rest/sleep PRN; stool softener	Discontinue saline lock; continue propylthiouracil, antiatrial fibrillation medication, and other medications for home use; eye drops OU q 2 hr PRN for dryness; multivitamins; medication for rest/sleep PRN; stool softener; provide info for ^{131}I radioactive isotope as outpatient in 6 wk
I & O q 8 hr; VS q 6 hr; discontinue O$_2$; cardiac monitor; weight; record food intake; assess moisture to eyes q 4 hr; assess neuro-cardio-pul-circ systems q 6 hr	Discontinue I & O; VS q 8 hr; weight; discontinue cardiac monitor; assess moisture to eyes q 8 hr; assess neuro-cardio-pul-circ systems q 8 hr	VS q 8 hr; weight; assess moisture to eyes q 8 hr; assess neuro-cardio-pul-circ systems q 8 hr	VS q 8 hr; weight; assess moisture to eyes q 8 hr; assess neuro-cardio-pul-circ systems 8 q hr
Regular diet with high calories, protein, and CHO; serve 6 meals; *no stimulants*	Regular diet with high calories, protein, and CHO; serve 6 meals; *no stimulants*	Regular diet with high calories, protein, and CHO; serve 6 meals; *no stimulants*	Regular diet with high calories, protein, and CHO; serve 6 meals; *no stimulants*
Up in room ad lib; minimize environmental stressors	Up in room ad lib	Up ad lib	Up ad lib

DISORDERS OF THE PARATHYROID GLAND

The parathyroid glands secrete parathyroid hormone (PTH), which maintains serum calcium and phosphorus levels by controlling bone resorption, GI absorption, and urinary excretion of these minerals. Disorders of the parathyroid glands are extremely rare but are being diagnosed more often as a result of the increased frequency of routine calcium measurement.

Hyperparathyroidism
Etiology/epidemiology

The most common cause of primary hyperparathyroidism is benign adenoma, but the problem also occurs secondary to chronic hypocalcemia associated with renal disease and malabsorption. Hyperplasia and malignant disease can also occur. The primary disease is seen most commonly in women over 40 years of age, although no link with postmenopausal estrogen deficiency has been proven. It is found with increasing frequency in older individuals. Most people are asymptomatic and are identified secondary to routine screening for another purpose. A history of radiation to the neck is one of the few identified risk factors.

Pathophysiology

Hypersecretion of parathyroid hormone produces an elevation of the serum calcium level and a decreased phosphorus level. The increased calcium can increase bone resorption and accelerate osteoporosis. The reabsorption of calcium by the kidney can also predispose the patient to kidney stones. Mild symptoms of malaise, muscle weakness, and mental depression are reported most commonly, although most individuals are unaware of any symptoms at all. Relatively small changes *can* trigger GI symptoms and mental status changes, particularly in elderly persons.

Medical management

The diagnosis of primary hyperparathyroidism is established through an elevated level of serum PTH plus persistent hypercalcemia. The physician will attempt to rule out other common causes for hypercalcemia such

BOX 9-6	Symptoms of Hypothyroidism

GASTROINTESTINAL

| Decreased appetite | Weight gain |
| Constipation | |

CARDIOVASCULAR

| Bradycardia | Heart enlargement |
| Pericardial/pleural effusion | Possible hypertension |

MUSCULOSKELETAL

| Muscle weakness | Activity intolerance |

INTEGUMENT

Cool, pale, dry scaly skin	Thin, dry hair
Myxedema skin changes	Cold intolerance
Puffy face	Yellow cast to skin/nails
Enlarged tongue	Thickened vocal cords/deep voice
Peripheral edema	
Slow wound healing	

EMOTION/BEHAVIOR

Apathy	Slow, slurred speech
Somnolence	Slowed mental processes
Paresthesias	Decreased tendon reflexes

SEXUALITY/REPRODUCTIVE

Decreased libido	Infertility
Anovulation	Menstrual changes
Oligospermia	Impotence

LABORATORY

Hypoalbuminemia	Low blood glucose
Increased cholesterol/	Anemia
triglycerides	

BOX 9-7	Myxedema Coma

Myxedema coma is the most severe and life-threatening form of hypothyroidism. It can occur in any inadequately treated patient but is usually precipitated by surgery, use of narcotics or sedatives, trauma, or infection. In addition to the standard symptoms of hypothyroidism the patient lapses into coma and is severely hypothermic. The associated mortality runs as high as 25%, usually from respiratory failure. The diagnosis is established clinically, and treatment begins before conclusive laboratory results are available.

Treatment is grounded in meticulous supportive care and monitoring, particularly of respiratory and cardiac functioning. Thyroid hormone is administered IV but in cautious doses while the patient's response, particularly of the cardiovascular system, can be assessed. Mechanical ventilation may be necessary. Improvement is generally seen after about 24 hours.

as malignancy. X-rays will be taken of the skeletal system to evaluate bone density.

Control of hypercalcemia is the treatment priority, but therapy is not typically initiated until the serum calcium rises above 13 mg/dl or higher. Immediate treatment involves normal saline infusion to support calcium excretion by the kidney. This may be supplemented by diuretic administration. Anticalcemic drugs may be used for actively symptomatic patients, but they are highly toxic and their use is limited. Choices include mithramycin, edidrate, and calcitonin.

Once the patient is stabilized, surgical intervention may be planned if the problem is an adenoma. Surgery typically involves the removal of at least three glands and a portion of the fourth. Severe hypocalcemia is common in the immediate postoperative period while calcium is taken up again by the bones.

NURSING MANAGEMENT

Postoperative care for the patient treated surgically is very similar to that outlined for the thyroidectomy patient (see above). The patient's airway is monitored carefully for signs of obstruction, and the vital signs are monitored for adverse effects of calcium shifts. A liberal fluid intake should be maintained. Cardiac monitoring may be ordered, particularly if the patient is receiving digitalis therapy. Sharp drops in calcium level will occur within the first 24 hours, and the patient is carefully monitored for signs of hypocalcemia, such as paresthesias. Calcium is replaced orally if hypocalcemia occurs. Parathyroid function usually stabilizes within 5 to 7 days. Patient teaching is provided concerning any ongoing diet or medication requirements.

Hypoparathyroidism
Etiology/epidemiology

Hypoparathyroidism is a metabolic disorder that results in hypocalcemia. It typically occurs following surgery to the neck or thyroid gland, but it can also occur as an idiopathic primary disease process. It shows up at an early age and may be genetic or autoimmune. The outcomes of the disease may be serious, because chronically decreased calcium levels can leave the patient vulnerable to tetany.

Pathophysiology

The deficiency of PTH leads to decreased bone resorption, decreased calcium absorption from the intestine, and increased renal calcium excretion. The end result is hypocalcemia and hyperphosphatemia. Low calcium levels increase neuromuscular excitability. Patients are often asymptomatic with mild disease, and the degree of symptoms often directly reflects the severity of the calcium deficiency. Symptoms include the following:

Numbness and tingling around the mouth and fingertips

Spasms of the fingers, wrists, forearms, and feet leading to full tetany

Convulsions (tonic or tonic/clonic spasms)

Irritability, anxiety, confusion

Dysrhythmia and decreased cardiac output

GI malabsorption and steatorrhea

Medical management

Treatment begins with correction of the calcium levels with IV calcium gluconate or chloride. The diagnostic workup attempts to determine a cause if possible and treat or reverse it. Calcium balance is maintained through diet, mineral supplement, and restriction of phosphate in the diet. Vitamin D therapy may be used to increase GI absorption.

NURSING MANAGEMENT

Patients with hypoparathyroidism will only be hospitalized during episodes of acute hypocalcemia. Monitoring is the key nursing intervention. Factors include subjective symptoms, mental status, vital signs, airway patency, and physical assessment signs of hypocalcemia, such as Chvostek's and Trousseau's signs. The physiologic imbalance resolves slowly, and ongoing assessment is critical. The nurse also assists the patient to deal with anxiety, since the physical symptoms are frightening and the close monitoring can also increase the patient's anxiety. Seizure precautions may be ordered.

DISORDERS OF THE ADRENAL GLANDS

Disorders of the adrenal glands can involve hyperfunction or hypofunction of either the adrenal cortex or adrenal medulla. The hormones of the cortex are essential to life through the stress response. The hormones of the medulla are duplicated, although less efficiently, through the actions of the sympathetic nervous system. The hormones of the adrenal gland are summarized in Box 9-8.

Hypersecretion of the Adrenal Cortex: Cortisol Excess

Etiology/epidemiology

Excessive levels of glucocorticoids produce a classic group of symptoms called Cushing's syndrome. Primary Cushing's syndrome typically results from adenoma or carcinoma of the adrenal glands and primarily affects females from 20 to 40 years of age. Secondary causes of cortisol excess include the following:

Increased release of ACTH from the pituitary

Increased release of ACTH from an ectopic source such as bronchogenic or pancreatic cancer

Iatrogenic Cushing's syndrome as a complication of chronic corticosteroid therapy, which is the most frequent cause seen in clinical practice; the end result is cortisol excess with a loss of normal diurnal secretory patterns

Iatrogenic Cushing's syndrome is by far the most common cause with up to 10 million Americans receiving glucocorticoid treatment each year. The ectopic variety is primarily related to oat cell carcinoma of the lung.

Pathophysiology

The basic pathology of Cushing's syndrome involves overproduction of cortisol. The noniatrogenic forms are characterized by a loss of the normal diurnal secretory pat-

---

BOX 9-8 — **Hormones of the Adrenal Gland and Their Functions**

ADRENAL CORTEX

Glucocorticoids (Cortisol)

Overall effect is to maintain blood glucose level by increasing gluconeogenesis and decreasing rate of glucose utilization by cells

Increase protein catabolism

Promote lipolysis

Promote sodium and water retention

Antiinflammatory, decrease new antibody release

Decrease T-lymphocyte participation in cell-mediated immunity by decreasing circulating level of T-lymphocytes

Increase neutrophils by increasing release and decreasing destruction

Decrease scar tissue formation, degrade collagen

Increase gastric acid and pepsin production, stimulate appetite

Maintain emotional stability

Mineralocorticoids (Aldosterone)

Major stimulus in renin-angiotensin system

Primarily responsible for maintenance of normovolemic state by increasing sodium and water retention in distal tubules

Cause potassium excretion

Androgens

Same functions as gonadal sex hormones

ADRENAL MEDULLA

Epinephrine and Norepinephrine

Necessary for maintenance of neuroendocrine integrating functions of body

Elevate blood pressure, increase heart rate, and cause vasoconstriction

Stimulate conversion of glycogen to glucose for emergency fuel

Stimulate gluconeogenesis

Increase lipolysis

---

terns. The hormone is not so much oversecreted as continually secreted. Excess cortisol exaggerates the multiple known effects of the hormone and produces widespread changes in body appearance and function. Metabolism, immune response, water balance, and emotional stability are all affected. In addition, the patient is placed at greater risk for a variety of chronic illnesses including peptic ulcer disease, osteoporosis, hypertension, and diabetes mellitus.

Adrenal tumors may also cause oversecretion of the other adrenal hormones. Aldosterone excess will produce hypokalemia, hypernatremia, and hypertension from fluid volume excess. Excess androgen will result in masculinizing effects in the female.

The major effects of glucocorticoid excess are summarized in Box 9-9.

Medical management

The diagnosis of cortisol excess is determined through serum cortisol levels and elevated levels of urinary

<table>
<tr><td colspan="2">

BOX 9-9   **Major Effects of Glucocorticoid Excess**

</td></tr>
</table>

CORTISOL

Gastrointestinal/Metabolic

Increased secretion of
  pepsin and HCl
Hunger
Postprandial hyperglycemia
Altered fat metabolism

Weight gain	Moon face
Truncal obesity	Deposits of adipose tissue on back of neck and shoulders (buffalo hump)

Integument

Loss of collagen support	Thinning of skin
Pale, purplish striae	Bruises and petechiae
Flushed face	

Musculoskeletal

Muscle wasting	Thin extremities
Easy fatigability	Osteoporosis

Cardiovascular

Fluid retention	Hypertension
Congestive heart failure	

Immune/Inflammatory Response

Suppression of immune
  response
Suppression of local
  inflammatory response
Decreased lymphocytes
Impaired wound healing

Emotional/Behavioral

Euphoria	Irritability
Excitability	Depression

ALDOSTERONE

Extreme sodium and water
  retention
Potassium excretion

ANDROGENS

Hirsutism in females
Menstrual irregularities
Changes in libido
Acne

17-hydroxysteroids and ketosteroids. Suppression tests may also be performed to test the gland response. Electrolyte and hematology abnormalities may also be found. Effective treatment of Cushing's syndrome depends on identifying and removing the cause of hypersecretion. Surgical treatment may involve transsphenoidal hypophysectomy of a pituitary tumor or unilateral or bilateral adrenalectomy. Drug treatment, which may be used as an adjunct to surgery or radiation, uses mitotane, aminoglutethimide, or metyrapone, which block cortisol synthesis. Adrenalectomy will necessitate life-long hormone replacement. Skilled supportive care is essential while hormonal balance is being reestablished. Care in iatrogenic Cushing's syndrome is aimed at reducing the steroid dose or controlling symptoms.

NURSING MANAGEMENT

◆ ASSESSMENT

Subjective Data

History and severity of symptoms
Patient's perception of the problem
Perceived changes in body appearance and proportions: skin, hair, body weight
Patient's complaints of the following:
  Fatigue—onset, severity, interference with activities of daily living
  Edema or weight gain
  Changes in appetite and thirst; indigestion
  Mood swings or instability
  Menstrual irregularities
Recent infections, slowed wound healing
Change in normal dietary pattern
Medications in use
History of other chronic health problems

Objective Data

Daily weights
Vital sign patterns, hypertension
Intake and output balance, daily food intake
Urine and blood glucose levels
Body appearance (see Box 9-9)
Muscle mass and strength
Energy level, self-care abilities
Skin integrity
Laboratory values showing increased cortisol; hypokalemia
Secondary sex characteristics
Elevated serum cortisol and urinary steroids
Hypokalemia, hyperglycemia

◆ NURSING DIAGNOSES

Nursing diagnoses for the person with Cushing's syndrome may include, but are not limited to, the following:
  Fluid volume excess (related to sodium and water retention)
  Nutrition, altered: more than body requirements (related to increased appetite and altered metabolism)
  Infection/bleeding, risk of (related to decreased immune response and excess acid secretion)
  Activity intolerance (related to muscle fatigability)
  Body image disturbance (related to changes in appearance)
  Home maintenance management, risk of impaired (related to inadequate knowledge concerning disease, treatment, and prevention of complications)

◆ EXPECTED PATIENT OUTCOMES

Patient will maintain a stable weight and show no signs of peripheral edema.

Patient will adjust diet pattern to compensate for hyperglycemia and fluid excess characteristic of the disease.

Patient will take measures to prevent infection and bleeding.

Patient will balance rest and activity while muscle strength and endurance improve.

Patient will maintain a positive body image while waiting for physical changes to reverse or lessen.

Patient will be knowledgeable about disorder and treatment and comply with treatment regimen.

◆ NURSING INTERVENTIONS

Promoting Fluid Balance

Maintain accurate intake and output records.

Record daily weights.

Monitor patient for edema or early symptoms of congestive heart failure and hypertension.

Restrict fluids if ordered; balance fluid intake throughout the day. Provide ice chips to reduce thirst.

Follow serum potassium levels and monitor for signs of hypokalemia.

Modifying the Diet

Teach patient principles of, and purpose of, diet modification. Diet should be low in calories, high in protein, low in sodium, and high in potassium.

Measure blood glucose as ordered every 4 to 8 hours. Administer sliding scale insulin as ordered.

Preventing Infection and Bleeding

Monitor vital signs frequently.

Administer antacids as prescribed. Guaiac test stools for blood.

Teach patient importance of good hygiene. Assess for early signs of infection.

Protect patient from staff, other patients, and visitors with infections.

Promoting Activity

Balance rest and activity.

Encourage patient to take short walks to combat osteoporosis.

Assist patient with ADL as needed.

Keep environmental stimuli at low levels.

Decrease physical and emotional stressors where possible.

Supporting a Positive Body Image

Teach patient about widespread disease effects and proposed treatment.

Encourage patient to verbalize feelings about body changes.

Provide ongoing support. Teach and reassure about reversibility of most symptoms.

Assist patient to control and understand mood swings.

Teaching for Effective Home Management

Teach patient signs and symptoms of complications.

Teach patient with iatrogenic Cushing's syndrome measures that will minimize effects of steroid therapy:

Always take steroids with food or antacid, because the risk of peptic ulcer is high.

Weigh daily and report any abrupt weight gain or edema.

Exercise and walk regularly to reduce bony demineralization.

Have regular follow-up and eye examinations (drugs stimulate cataract formation).

Obtain and wear a Medic Alert bracelet.

Teach patient that steroid drugs must be withdrawn slowly; it takes time for the adrenal glands to recover from suppression (Box 9-10).

NOTE: Interventions for patients being treated with adrenalectomy are outlined in the Guidelines box.

◆ EVALUATION

Successful achievement of expected outcomes for the patient with Cushing's syndrome is indicated by the following:

Absence of signs of fluid excess, stable blood pressure and weight

Adherence to a low-calorie, low-sodium diet; absence of weight gain

Meticulous personal hygiene, freedom from infection

Ability to engage in normal activities without undue fatigue

BOX 9-10 Adrenal Crisis

Adrenal crisis (addisonian crisis) occurs when there is a severe exacerbation of the insufficiency. It is a sudden, life-threatening condition that may be precipitated by the sudden cessation of steroid therapy or situations that create a sudden need for more cortisol than is available, usually in a previously undiagnosed individual who experiences a major stressor. Hypovolemia, which can represent a loss of up to 20% of the circulating fluid volume, can lead quickly to hypovolemic shock and acidosis.

The syndrome is characterized by severe hypotension, cardiovascular collapse (shock), hyperpyrexia (extremely high fever), hypoglycemia, hyponatremia, and coma. Treatment of the crisis involves the IV administration of glucocorticoids and mineralocorticoids (hydrocortisone, fludrocortisone), volume replacement with normal saline, and provision of glucose IV if nausea or vomiting prevents oral replacement. Vasopressors may be needed if the patient does not respond to the outlined initial measures.

> **BOX 9-11** **Iatrogenic Cushing's Syndrome and Adrenal Insufficiency**
>
> High blood levels of glucocorticoids cause negative feedback to the hypothalamus and anterior pituitary gland, suppressing the production of ACTH. The lack of ACTH causes a gradual adrenal atrophy. If glucocorticoids are given for a prolonged period they must be withdrawn slowly to prevent adrenal insufficiency because the adrenal gland is unable to suddenly assume responsibility for renewed production. It may take as long as 9 months to restore full natural hypothalamic-pituitary-adrenal balance.
>
> Iatrogenic steroids must be slowly tapered to allow the body to begin natural production again. This same process also makes it imperative that patients never abruptly discontinue their steroid medication, regardless of the side effects. Use must be tapered. Some patients successfully produce sufficient hormone to meet the body's need for everyday activities but are unable initially to meet the needs of stress, infection, or trauma. A Medic Alert ID is essential during steroid therapy. Symptoms are discussed under the presentation of adrenal insufficiency.

> **Guidelines for Nursing Care of the Patient Experiencing Adrenalectomy**
>
> **PREOPERATIVE**
> Teach patient about proposed surgery and care routines to be followed postoperatively.
> Teach usual coughing and deep breathing exercises.
>
> **POSTOPERATIVE**
> Monitor vital signs frequently, because adrenal function tends to be very labile. Vasopressors may be needed.
> Maintain infusions of cortisol as prescribed.
> Maintain accurate records for intake and output and blood glucose.
> Observe patient for signs of hypoglycemia.
> Monitor for signs of adrenal crisis, which include severe weakness, nausea and vomiting, and hypotension.
> Monitor adequacy of urine output regularly.
> Monitor wound healing (a major surgical complication).
> Maintain strict asepsis.
> Introduce activity gradually and assess patient's response.
> Maintain adequate pain relief and effective splinting to facilitate coughing.
> Initiate teaching concerning medication regimen prescribed:
> Medication may be needed for lifelong replacement.
> Close supervision is needed during initial months to adjust dose.
> Patient should be alert for signs of hormone excess or deficit.
> Patient should be cognizant of situations that will increase need for hormone, such as physical or emotional stress or illness.

Positive references to self

Correct description of disease process, management regimen, and signs indicating need for medical evaluation

Hyperfunction of the Adrenal Cortex: Aldosterone Excess

Primary aldosteronism and secondary aldosteronism are rare disorders that primarily affect the hypertensive population from disruption of the renin-angiotensin-aldosterone system. Primary disease can occur from hyperplasia or adenoma. Excessive aldosterone secretion results in profound sodium reabsorption, fluid volume expansion, and hypertension. Potassium is excreted and may cause cardiac problems. Surgical resection is performed for adenomas. Other problems are treated medically with sodium restriction, potassium replacement, and spironolactone (Aldactone) for diuresis.

Hyposecretion of the Adrenal Cortex

Etiology/epidemiology

A deficiency in adrenocortical hormones can result from a primary disease process of the adrenal cortex (Addison's disease), insufficient ACTH secretion by the pituitary, or glandular atrophy from long-term suppression of the glands with glucocorticoid therapy. All forms of adrenal insufficiency are rare, but iatrogenic disease is the most common cause. Addison's disease has a genetic component and tends to occur in families. Deficiencies in glucocorticoids lead to impairments in metabolism and an inability to maintain a normal blood glucose. Deficiencies in mineralocorticoids produce fluid and electrolyte imbalances. The deficiency can be life threatening and may appear slowly or abruptly. In Addison's disease the patient remains clinically asymptomatic until up to 90% of both glands is destroyed.

Pathophysiology

Addison's disease involves autoimmune destruction of the gland. It deprives the body of both glucocorticoids and mineralocorticoids. The losses decrease the body's ability to conserve sodium and excrete potassium, which leads to fluid volume depletion and decreased cardiac output. The loss of glucocorticoids impairs hepatic gluconeogenesis with the subsequent loss of muscle strength. Secondary insufficiency creates the same types of problems, but the fluid and electrolyte problems are typically not as severe. The signs of adrenal insufficiency are summarized in Box 9-12.

Medical management

Adrenal insufficiency is treated by hormone replacement. Dosages are modified and adjusted to help the patient achieve a symptom-free state. Oral cortisone and fludrocortisone are typically used and administered twice daily. Only glucocorticoid replacement is typically needed for secondary insufficiency states. Dosages may need to be doubled or tripled to deal with situations of extreme physiologic or mental stress or infection. Knowledgeable self-care is critical to prevent extreme imbalances.

BOX 9-12	Signs of Adrenal Insufficiency

APPEARANCE

Patient has lost weight; appears fatigued

SKIN

Bronze coloration of skin and mucous membranes from increased levels of melanocyte-stimulating hormone

MUSCULOSKELETAL

Severely weak and fatigued muscles

CARDIOVASCULAR

Hypotension
Risk of complete vascular collapse

GASTROINTESTINAL

Anorexia
Cramping abdominal pain
Diarrhea
Nausea and vomiting, weight loss

METABOLISM

Hypoglycemia

FLUID AND ELECTROLYTES

Hyponatremia
Hyperkalemia
Fluid deficit

MENTAL-EMOTIONAL

Lethargy, depression
Loss of vigor

NURSING MANAGEMENT

Nursing management focuses on meticulous patient monitoring during any acute disease exacerbations and careful teaching to support the patient in efforts to maintain successful self-care. Patients must be helped to understand the serious nature of the disorder and the importance of taking their medications regularly and avoiding situations of undue stress. Patients are instructed to take their medication with food or antacid and to be certain that they always have a sufficient supply of medication on hand, particularly when traveling. Medic Alert identification is critical.

Hypersecretion of the Adrenal Medulla

Pheochromocytoma is a rare catecholamine-producing tumor of the adrenal medulla that can occur in individuals in middle age. It is usually unilateral and benign. The tumor releases excessive quantities of both epinephrine and norepinephrine. The hormones stimulate both the alpha and beta receptors, triggering massive vasoconstriction. The hormone release may be constant or occur in episodic fashion, creating malignant hypertension. A hypertensive crisis can be precipitated by any activity that increases intraabdominal pressure. The diagnosis is usually made during a workup for labile severe hypertension that is unresponsive to therapy.

Initial treatment is aimed at controlling blood pressure through alpha- and beta-adrenergic blocking agents. Surgical resection of the tumor is the treatment of choice for a stabilized patient. Blood pressure instability is a common problem in the postoperative period, and the patient requires careful monitoring. The remainder of the care is similar to that for any adrenalectomy patient. Most individuals have a complete recovery.

PANCREATIC HORMONE DYSFUNCTION
Diabetes Mellitus
Etiology/epidemiology

Diabetes mellitus is a complex chronic disease involving disorders in carbohydrate, fat, and protein metabolism. Its symptoms are caused by either a decrease in the secretion of insulin or a decrease in the effectiveness and utilization of insulin by the tissues. There are several forms of the disease (Box 9-13), but the vast majority of cases are either insulin-dependent diabetes mellitus (IDDM) or non-insulin-dependent diabetes mellitus (NIDDM).

Over 14 million persons are affected by diabetes today, and it is estimated that millions more have the disease but are unaware of it. It is the fourth leading cause of disease-related death. The prevalence increases with age, and over 750,000 new cases are diagnosed each year, the majority being NIDDM. Diabetes is associated with a greatly increased risk of macrovascular, microvascular, and neuropathic problems and complicates the management of most other chronic illnesses. Treatment costs exceed 20 million dollars annually.

The etiology of each type of diabetes is still under investigation, with factors such as genetics, heredity, environment, and immunity believed to play a different role in each. Genetics appears to play a permissive role in IDDM that allows environmental factors to trigger the onset of the disease by stimulating an autoimmune process that attacks the islet cells. In NIDDM, being chronically overweight appears to increase insulin resistance, especially in adults with a family history of diabetes, and provides a stimulus for disease onset. The pancreas initially compensates for this resistance by secreting more insulin, but over time it can become exhausted. Aging also results in an increase in insulin resistance, and most persons with NIDDM are in late middle age. Table 9-10 compares the major characteristics of IDDM and NIDDM.

Pathophysiology

The primary function of insulin is to promote the transport of serum glucose and amino acids across the cell membrane where they can be used for energy, stored as glycogen, or converted into fat. In diabetes there is an absolute or relative deficiency of insulin and its action that results in significant abnormalities in the

BOX 9-13 Classification System for Diabetes Mellitus

INSULIN-DEPENDENT DIABETES MELLITUS (IDDM): TYPE 1

Persons are deficient in insulin and depend on exogenous insulin to prevent ketoacidosis and sustain life.

Onset of symptoms is abrupt, usually occurring while a youth and almost always before 30 years.

With certain HLA types, an autoimmune mechanism and precipitation by an environmental factor, such as a viral infection, have been associated with susceptibility and onset.

NON-INSULIN-DEPENDENT DIABETES MELLITUS (NIDDM): TYPE 2

Persons do not depend on insulin to sustain life but may be treated with insulin in special circumstances; they are resistant to ketoacidosis except during periods of excessive stress.

Onset is usually after 40 years, without classic symptoms.

Associated with endogenous insulin levels that may be mildly depressed, normal, or high and with tissue resistance to insulin.

Obesity and heredity have been associated with susceptibility and onset.

GESTATIONAL DIABETES MELLITUS (GDM)

Persons have onset of glucose abnormality during pregnancy.

Women with known diabetes mellitus who become pregnant are not classified in this group.

After delivery, the woman is reclassified on the basis of blood or plasma glucose testing.

MALNUTRITION-RELATED DIABETES MELLITUS

Persons require insulin.

Diabetes mellitus found in tropical areas.

It occurs in young adults with histories of nutritional deficiencies.

Ketosis is not usually present.

OTHER TYPES OF DIABETES MELLITUS

Diabetes mellitus may be associated with other disorders such as pancreatic disease, other endocrine diseases, drugs, and genetic syndromes.

IMPAIRED GLUCOSE TOLERANCE (IGT): OBESE, NONOBESE, OR OTHER CONDITIONS

Persons have glucose levels higher than normal but lower than those considered diagnostic for diabetes mellitus.

TABLE 9-10 Characteristics of IDDM and NIDDM

IDDM	NIDDM
INCIDENCE	
10% of total	90% of total
INSULIN SECRETION	
Decreased insulin secretion	Insulin secretion increased, decreased, or normal
AGE	
Usually in young but can occur at any age	Usually over 35 yr but can occur at any age
RACE	
More common in Whites	More common in African-Americans and Hispanics; highest in Native Americans
FAMILY HISTORY	
Questionable	Strong link
Body Build	
Lean	80%-90% overweight
SYMPTOMS	
Polyuria, polydipsia, polyphagia, weight loss	None, or the same as IDDM, especially under stress
TREATMENT	
Insulin, diet, exercise	Diet, exercise, oral hypoglycemics, insulin
KETOSIS	
Prone	Resistant except with infection or stress
COMPLICATIONS (VASCULAR/NEUROLOGIC)	
After 5 or more yr	Frequent, may be present at diagnosis

metabolism of body fuels. Insulin is the only metabolic hormone that lowers blood glucose. All the others are counterregulatory in action and elevate blood glucose. Insulin binds with receptors on the cell surface and triggers reactions that allow for entry of glucose and amino acids. Without insulin, glucose and other metabolic products accumulate in the blood. During fasting states the counterregulatory hormones allow glycogen in the liver and lipids released from the fat cells to be metabolized for energy.

A relative or absolute deficiency of insulin results in hyperglycemia and impaired fat metabolism. Glycogenesis (Box 9-14) is inhibited and cellular starvation triggers the liver to continue to produce glucose through glycogenolysis, worsening hyperglycemia. Peripheral tissues cannot extract glucose and must metabolize their own glycogen and then break down protein for energy. Since amino acid transport also requires insulin, tissue proteins are broken down to be used for gluconeogenesis. Fat metabolism is also impaired. The liver continues to produce ketone bodies from fatty acids, but lipolysis occurs instead of lipogenesis.

When the glucose level exceeds the renal threshold (usually about 180 mg/dl), glucose is excreted in the urine, producing glycosuria. Since glucose is hyperosmolar, it creates an osmotic diuresis and carries large amounts of water and electrolytes with it, producing polyuria, which can lead to dehydration and electrolyte imbalance. This fluid loss triggers thirst in the patient and polydipsia. Cellular starvation leads to hunger and increased food intake (polyphagia). Weight loss can occur rapidly in IDDM. The relative deficiency of NIDDM leads to fatigue and listlessness. Ketone bodies,

---

BOX 9-14 · Metabolic Pathways

GLUCONEOGENESIS

The building of glucose from new sources such as amino acids, lactate, and glycerol. The process occurs in the liver when intake of carbohydrate is inadequate to meet the body's metabolic needs. Process is stimulated by the counterregulatory hormones, for example, epinephrine, glucagon, cortisol.

GLYCOGENESIS

The conversion of glucose to glycogen. This process is promoted by insulin.

GLYCOLYSIS

The breakdown of glucose to CO_2 and water. Insulin is needed for cells to take up glucose and the liver to initiate the metabolic pathways.

GLYCOGENOLYSIS

The breakdown of glycogen to glucose by the action of glucagon and epinephrine. Insulin opposes this process.

LIPOGENESIS

The conversion of excess fuel to fat. Insulin supports this process.

LIPOLYSIS

The breakdown of triglycerides; encouraged by cortisol and the absence of insulin.

KETOGENESIS

The metabolism of fatty acids to ketones by the liver; encouraged by an absence of insulin.

---

the acid metabolites of fats, can accumulate in the blood and cause ketosis and ketonuria.

The severity of the altered metabolism depends on the degree of insulin deficiency, but altered lipid metabolism resulting in elevated serum triglycerides occurs in even mildly deficient states. High production of ketones is usually seen only in the severe insulin-deficient states associated with IDDM but can exist in NIDDM during the stress response.

Complications—Chronic insulin deficiency leads to a number of pathologic changes in the blood vessels and nerves that can result in hypertension, coronary artery and cerebrovascular disease, renal failure, blindness, and both autonomic and peripheral vascular problems. The pathologic changes occur at variable rates and are rare in the first 5 to 10 years for IDDM but are often present at the time of diagnosis in NIDDM.

Macrovascular changes are primarily related to earlier and more severe onset and progression of atherosclerosis. Diabetes is associated with several atherogenic factors, particularly disordered lipid metabolism, which is found in 25% to 75% of all diabetics. Changes cause a decrease in lumen size, compromised blood flow, and decreased delivery of oxygen to the tissues. Coronary artery disease (CAD), peripheral vascular disease (PVD),

and cerebral vascular disease (CVD) are the usual outcomes. These problems are much more prevalent in NIDDM.

The classic microvascular changes associated with diabetes do not occur in disease-free persons. The cause is not understood, but the result is thickening of the capillaries and damage to the basement membrane. Nephropathy is extremely common, and diabetics account for 30% of persons receiving chronic renal dialysis. Hypertension accelerates the nephropathy and must be controlled. Diabetic retinopathy is a leading cause of blindness and affects 50% to 80% of diabetics within 10 to 15 years of diagnosis. Microaneurysms form and bleed, or the vessels can become proliferative with repetitive episodes of bleeding. Cataracts are also more common in persons with diabetes.

Neuropathies are extremely common in diabetics. It is theorized that metabolic imbalances cause sorbitol to be deposited in the nerve cells, resulting in fluid shifts, swelling, nerve dysfunction, and altered nerve conduction. Peripheral polyneuropathy is the most common problem. Sensory changes and loss in the lower extremities are typical. Autonomic neuropathies are also common (Box 9-15). They are slow developing but progressive, and a patient may experience some or all of them.

Medical management

Although controversy exists over the exact diagnostic criteria for diabetes it is generally agreed that a random glucose above 200 mg, a fasting glucose above 140 mg, or a positive glucose tolerance test plus the presence of polyuria, polydipsia, polyphagia, and weight loss can be considered presumptive of IDDM in adults. Asymptomatic cases of NIDDM are occasionally more controversial, particularly if the laboratory values are borderline.

Research data seem to indicate that long-term complications can be prevented or delayed by consistent

---

BOX 9-15 · Autonomic Neuropathies of Diabetes Mellitus

BLADDER

Hypotonic or atonic; neurogenic bladder

SEXUAL FUNCTION

Male impotence; female loss of lubrication

GI TRACT

Delayed gastric emptying; constipation or diarrhea

CARDIOVASCULAR

Orthostatic hypotension; fixed heart rate (unresponsive to activity demands)

SWEATING

Poor response to environmental changes; excessive or diminished

BOX 9-16 The Diabetic Foot

Macrovascular, microvascular, and neuropathic changes all contribute to the classic problems inherent in the "diabetic foot." *Sensory neuropathy* may lead to painless trauma, ulceration, or infection. *Motor neuropathies* contribute to bone changes that change gait and pressure distribution on the foot. *Autonomic neuropathies* contribute to anhidrosis with resultant drying and cracking of the skin. *Vascular changes* lead to tissue ischemia and skin changes that can precipitate ulceration and infection. The interrelationship of these factors can lead to gangrene and eventually amputation. Prevention is the key to management. It is theorized that the need for amputation can be reduced by 50%-75% with proper preventive care.

TABLE 9-11 Commonly Used Insulins

INSULIN	ONSET (HR)	PEAK (HR)	DURATION (HR)
SHORT ACTING			
(clear)			
Regular Iletin/Humulin/ Novolin	½-1	2-4	6-8
INTERMEDIATE			
(cloudy)			
NPH Iletin/Humulin/ Novolin	1-2	4-12	12-14
Lente Iletin/Humulin/ Novolin	2	8-12	12-16
LONG ACTING			
(cloudy)			
Ultralente Humulin/ Standard	8	18	24-36
MIXTURES			
(cloudy)			
70/30 Humulin/ Novolin	Effects are a combination of short and intermediate		
50/60 Humulin			
70/30 Mixtard			

normalizing of the metabolic environment. This is not always a realistic goal for all patients, however, and does increase the risk of hypoglycemia in the IDDM patient. Decisions about the degree of control desired are made collaboratively with the patient and consider the patient's life circumstances and resources as well as the burden of the regimen. The major aspects of the regimen include medication, diet, exercise, and the promotion of optimal general health.

Medications—Insulin is necessary for every patient with IDDM. Insulin or a hypoglycemic agent *may* be necessary for patients with NIDDM. Insulin is available from beef, pork, and human sources. Human insulin (a biosynthetic recombinant product derived from bacteria or yeast) is least antigenic and is recommended for all newly diagnosed diabetics. It is available in a variety of short- and long-acting preparations. Insulin of all types is standardly available in U-100 strength (100 units of insulin per milliliter). Common types of insulin and their onset, peak, and duration of effect are summarized in Table 9-11. The administration of insulin is coordinated to ensure that insulin is available when food is consumed and that food is available while insulin is acting. Most insulin regimens for IDDM are planned to mimic the normal endogenous secretion of insulin (Box 9-17). This means basal secretion between meals with a meal-related increase. Attempts to replicate this pattern have meant that the single once-daily insulin injection that was standard in the past is no longer the regimen of choice in IDDM. The use of an insulin pump allows for continuous insulin delivery. The pump is programmed for a basal delivery and can be manually triggered to deliver an insulin bolus in the preprandial period.

Oral hypoglycemic agents are used in the treatment of NIDDM patients who cannot be controlled through diet and exercise alone (Table 9-12). They are believed to work by increasing islet cell secretion of insulin, increasing tissue insulin sensitivity, and decreasing glucose production by the liver. Their use has been controversial because of a series of studies that appeared to show a significantly increased death rate from cardiovas-

BOX 9-17 Examples of Possible Insulin Regimens

1. One daily injection of an intermediate-acting insulin

   - Convenient
   - Does not mimic normal secretion

2. Two injections of intermediate-acting insulin daily

   - Used primarily in NIDDM
   - Does not mimic normal secretion

3. Two injections daily of mixed regular and intermediate-acting insulin

   - Widely used in IDDM
   - Theoretically covers both basal and mealtime needs

4. Multidosage regimen including regular insulin before each meal and intermediate-acting insulin at bedtime

   - Regular insulin covers mealtime increases
   - Covers basal needs of night and prebreakfast rise

cular disease associated with tolbutamide use. Most patients today are prescribed a second-generation sulfonylurea drug. Hypoglycemia is the major complication of both insulin and oral hypoglycemic therapy (Box 9-18).

Diet—Nutritional therapy is the cornerstone of diabetes management. The overall goal is the development of a flexible meal plan that fits the patient's life-style, maintains reasonable weight, and controls blood glucose and lipid levels. The recommended diet is similar to "heart healthy" approaches suggested for all Ameri-

BOX 9-18 Hypoglycemia

DEFINITION

A plasma glucose level <50 mg/dl

NOTE: Any hypoglycemic episode is serious, because it interferes with the oxygen consumption of nerve tissue. Prolonged hypoglycemia can cause irreversible brain damage.

CAUSES

Excessive dose or prolonged action of insulin or oral hypoglycemic agent

Too little food, vomiting, or diarrhea

Excessive exercise in relation to food intake and medication doses

Ingestion of other hypoglycemic agent, such as alcohol

SYMPTOMS

NOTE: Symptoms are highly individualized and vary among diabetics. The most commonly experienced symptoms are marked with an asterisk.

Pallor	Palpitation	Weakness*
Perspiration*	Nervousness*	Trembling
Tachycardia	Irritability	Hunger
Headache	Fatigue	Blurred vision
Numbness (lips, tongue)	Mental confusion (convulsion*)	Emotional changes

NOTE: The symptoms are related to both sympathetic nervous system activity and loss of a steady glucose supply for the CNS. Hypoglycemia can occur during sleep, creating nightmares, sweating, and headache on awakening.

TREATMENT

10-15 g of rapid-acting carbohydrate. If questions about the diagnosis exist, draw a blood glucose and treat immediately. Examples include:

½ C fruit juice
½ C sugared soda
½ C gelatin dessert
4 cubes or 2 packets of sugar
2 squares of graham crackers
2 or 3 pieces of hard candy
1 tsp. corn syrup or honey can be placed between gum and cheek if patient is too groggy to swallow safely
50% glucose IV if patient is unconscious

NOTE: When symptoms have cleared, patient is given a snack consisting of complex carbohydrates and proteins, such as cheese or peanut butter and crackers.

TABLE 9-12 Oral Hypoglycemic Agents

DRUG	ONSET	PEAK (HR)	DURATION (HR)
FIRST GENERATION			
Tolbutamide (Orinase)	1 hr	4-6	6-12
Tolazamide (Tolinase)	1 hr	4-8	~24
Acetohexamide (Dymelor)	1-2 hr	8-12	~18
Chlorpropamide (Diabinese)	1 hr	3-6	Up to 60
SECOND GENERATION			
Glyburide			
Nonmicronized: Micronase, Diabeta	1 hr	4-8	12-24
Micronized: Glynase	1 hr	2-6	12-24
Glipizide (Glucotrol)	10-30 min	1-3	12-24

BOX 9-19 Somogyi Phenomenon

The Somogyi phenomenon is a condition of alternating hypoglycemic reactions and hyperglycemia that is seen most frequently during initial attempts at blood glucose regulation. Both the peak effect of the longer-acting insulin and the counterregulatory hormone effects to hypoglycemia are exaggerated. The hypoglycemia frequently occurs at night followed by an early-morning hyperglycemia that can be mistaken for a need for more insulin.

The signs and symptoms are the same as for hypoglycemia from any cause, and if they occur at night the patient may report only night sweats, nightmares, and early-morning headache. Blood glucose levels may fluctuate widely.

Treatment consists of decreasing the insulin dose until the patient stabilizes. It is critical to accurately monitor and record all objective and subjective symptoms of hypoglycemia along with laboratory results and timing and consistency of meals to create an accurate metabolic picture.

cans, such as 55% to 60% carbohydrates with an emphasis on complex carbohydrates, 12% to 20% protein, and less than 30% fat, primarily polyunsaturated. Fiber is increased to a recommended level of 25 to 40 g daily from plant sources. Fiber has been found to delay gastric emptying, increase satiety, and decrease both fasting and postprandial glucose levels and cholesterol. Nutrients are distributed on a consistent basis to match the blood level of insulin or oral hypoglycemic agent, and consistency in the timing of meals is also important. The calories are distributed over 24 hours to prevent large increases in postprandial blood glucose.

Although a variety of dietary teaching plans are now available the American Dietetic Association and American Diabetes Association (ADA) Exchange System approach is still used most commonly. Foods are divided into six groupings called exchange lists based on their protein, fat, and carbohydrate content. Serving sizes are indicated to provide approximately equal proportions of the nutrients. The physician prescribes the overall calorie count and number of each exchange to be used each day. The patient then is able to make a wide number of food choices from this overall plan to meet individual preferences (Table 9-13). Other meal planning systems in current use include point systems, tracking only total available carbohydrates, and food guide pyramids.

Exercise—Exercise is an important component of the diabetic treatment plan, because exercise increases the uptake of glucose by active muscle cells and can increase tissue sensitivity to insulin. Overall, exercise has a hypoglycemic effect. Controversy exists as to whether exercise should be recommended for all IDDM

TABLE 9-13 Examples of Food Exchanges

EXCHANGES	FOOD SERVING SAMPLE

STARCH/BREAD EXCHANGE

(includes starchy vegetables)
Calories—80
CHO (g)—15
Protein (g)—3
Fat (g)—trace

1 slice bread
½ hamburger bun
⅓ C corn, ½ C peas
½ C cooked pasta
6 saltines

½ bagel, 1 tortilla
½ small baked potato
½ C oatmeal
⅓ C rice

MEAT EXCHANGE

Lean

Calories—55
CHO (g)—0
Protein (g)—7
Fat (g)—3

Lean

1 oz lean beef, pork, veal, or poultry without skin
2 oz fish
¼ C dry cottage cheese
¼ C tuna, mackerel
1 oz diet cheese (<55 calories/oz)

Medium

Calories—75
CHO (g)—0
Protein (g)—7
Fat (g)—5

Medium-Fat

1 oz 15%-fat beef, boiled ham, or liver
1 egg

High

Calories—100
CHO (g)—0
Protein (g)—7
Fat (g)—8

High-Fat

1 oz 20%-fat beef, ground pork, duck, or regular cheeses
1 frankfurter
1 oz lunch meat
1 T peanut butter (contains unsaturated fats)

VEGETABLE

Calories—25
CHO (g)—5
Protein (g)—2
Fat (g)—0

½ C cooked or 1 C raw of beets, carrots, brussels sprouts,
   onions, sauerkraut, eggplant, asparagus, cabbage, green or
   wax beans, or mustard greens
1 medium tomato

FRUIT EXCHANGE

Calories—60
CHO (g)—15
Protein (g)—0
Fat (g)—0

1 small apple, orange, peach, tangerine, or pear
½ C applesauce
½ banana or grapefruit
⅓ cantaloupe
⅛ honeydew melon

MILK EXCHANGE

Calories—80
CHO (g)—12
Protein (g)—8
Fat (g)—trace if skim

1 C skim or nonfat milk
1 C plain nonfat yogurt
1 C skim buttermilk

Calories— 120, Fat (g)—5:
1 C low-fat (2%) milk
1 C low-fat (2%) yogurt

FAT EXCHANGE

Calories—45
CHO (g)—0
Protein (g)—0
Fat (g)—5

1 t margarine
1 t oil
1 t regular mayonnaise
1 T cream cheese

⅛ avocado
1 strip crisp bacon
1 T reduced-calorie mayonnaise

FREE EXCHANGE

Calories—0
CHO (g)—0
Protein (g)—0
Fat (g)—0

Unsweetened gelatin
Calorie-free beverages
Coffee, tea, spices, bouillon

C, Cup; *CHO,* carbohydrate; *T,* tablespoon; *t,* teaspoon.
From American Diabetes Association and American Dietetic Association: *Exchange lists for meal planning,* Alexandria, Va, 1986, The Association.

Guidelines for Teaching Patients About Exercise in Diabetes*

Begin with light-level aerobic exercise.
   NIDDM patients should use low-impact varieties.
Exercise 3-5 times per week.
Exercise for approximately 1 hour.
   Include warm-up, 30 minutes at target intensity, and cool down.
Be sure to take daily insulin dose or oral hypoglycemic agent.
   Avoid exercise during peak insulin times.
   Avoid injection into muscle groups stressed during exercise.
Eat a meal 1-3 hours before exercise.
   Take additional carbohydrates if exercise is strenuous or over 30 minutes in duration.
Carry a rapid-acting source of glucose during exercise.
Check blood glucose before, during, and after exercise to establish baselines.
   Check urine ketones; do not exercise if positive.
   Avoid extreme heat and cold.
   Inspect feet carefully after exercise; ensure proper-fitting footwear.

---

*NOTE: Disease should be stabilized before exercise is initiated, and all patients should undergo thorough cardiac evaluation before the start of an exercise program, usually including a stress test.

---

patients, because it is associated with risks such as hypoglycemia, cardiovascular problems, and worsening of long-term complications. The benefits are clear in NIDDM, however. Exercise assists in weight loss and decreases insulin resistance. General guidelines for exercise are summarized in the Guidelines box above.

NURSING MANAGEMENT

◆ ASSESSMENT
Subjective Data

Knowledge of, attitude toward, and meaning of diagnosis of diabetes
Presence of other chronic diseases, such as vascular, metabolic, renal
Presence of classic "poly" symptoms: polyuria, polydipsia, polyphagia
Life-style patterns: food buying and preparation, smoking history, activity and exercise
Changes or problems with sexuality: libido, impotence
Coping strategies and support systems, financial security, insurance
Presence of paresthesias or pruritus, blurred vision
Fatigue, weakness, lethargy
Nausea, abdominal discomfort, weight loss, indigestion, constipation, diarrhea
Formerly diagnosed: current diabetic regimen and degree of adherence

Hypoglycemic agents in use
Insulin preparation/administration
ADA exchange system diet management
Exercise
Blood and urine testing
Foot care
Management of illness episodes and complications
Hypoglycemia
Ketoacidosis

NOTE: Many NIDDM patients experience only very subtle overt symptoms despite significant metabolic imbalance, for example, extreme fatigue, blurred vision, or falling asleep inappropriately.

Objective Data

Body weight: history of obesity
Vital signs: blood pressure, peripheral pulses
Changes in touch, pain, and temperature sensation
Skin: appearance, intactness, hair distribution, presence of lesions
Visual acuity or changes
Fluid intake, urine output, and specific gravity
Laboratory results: hyperglycemia, increased postprandial glucose
   Elevated serum lipids
   Glycosylated hemoglobin twice normal value
   Positive urine glucose or ketones

◆ NURSING DIAGNOSES

Nursing diagnoses for the person with diabetes may include, but are not limited to, the following:
Nutrition, altered: high risk for more than or less than body requirements (related to impaired glucose utilization and/or the presence of obesity)
Injury or infection, risk of (related to impaired circulation and peripheral neuropathies)
Knowledge deficit: disease, self-care skills, management of illness, and prevention or treatment of complications (related to lack of exposure to new information and skills)
Coping, risk of ineffective individual (related to the life-style changes mandated by diabetic regimen)

◆ EXPECTED PATIENT OUTCOMES

Patient will achieve and maintain desired body weight and meet nutritional needs through appropriate use of ADA diet and medication.
Patient will practice scrupulous hygiene and foot care, will take measures to compensate for sensory losses, and will not develop skin infections or ulceration.
Patient will demonstrate an adequate knowledge of disease, correct insulin preparation and administration, glucose and urine monitoring, ADA exchange system, exercise plan and precautions, management of sick days, and prevention of complications.

Patient will demonstrate positive coping behaviors, express commitment to effective disease management, and maintain full involvement in preferred life-style.

♦ NURSING INTERVENTIONS

Promoting Adequate Nutrition

Prepare teaching plan in collaboration with teaching dietitian and diabetes nurse specialist if available.

Obtain baseline diet history, including meal patterns, food likes and dislikes.

Negotiate nutrition goal with patient:
Target body weight and weight loss plan
Distribution of food throughout the day
Cultural or social food factors, such as fast food, vegetarianism
Role of alcohol and sweets

Reinforce the principles of the ADA exchange system or other individualized diet pattern.
Encourage consistency of meal spacing and meal times to avoid hypoglycemia.
Reinforce that special or dietetic foods are not required to use the diet plan.

Teach patient how to adapt food choices to shift work, eating in restaurants, vacation and business travel, and social events.

Teach patient how to incorporate small amounts of alcohol into the diet if desired. High-calorie alcoholic beverages such as beer and cordials should be avoided.

Teach patient how to adapt diet during GI upset or illness.

Provide multiple opportunities for patient to choose foods from sample menus.

Encourage patient to honestly verbalize the perceived impact of diet plan on normal life-style.

Preventing Injury and Infection

Teach patient the effect of diabetes on skin defenses and importance of scrupulous hygiene:
Loss of subcutaneous fat deposits and catabolism of body proteins
Impaired inflammatory response and wound healing from decreased peripheral circulation and impaired leukocyte function, that is, migration, phagocytosis, and cell kill

Reinforce the importance of patient not smoking.

Keep skin supple and dry, particularly in warm moist areas (between toes, under breasts, axilla, groin).

Treat all minor skin trauma thoroughly with cleansing and cover. Seek medical attention promptly if injury does not heal.

Assess feet daily, and teach patient to do the same:
Color, temperature, pulses
Sensory function: pinprick and vibratory function
Presence of lesions: calluses, corns, cuts, cracks, redness, blisters

Guidelines for Teaching Patients Diabetic Foot Care

Inspect feet daily. Use a mirror if needed to see soles of feet.
Wear proper-fitting shoes:
Shoes should allow for free toe movement.
Add soft insoles if protective sensation is impaired.
Break in new shoes gradually.
Wear clean socks when ambulating.
Never walk barefoot.
Bathe feet daily and dry well, paying particular attention to areas between toes.
Cut nails immediately after bathing when soft. Cut straight across and smooth with an emery board.
If skin is dry, apply bland cream or petroleum jelly to heels and feet. Do *not* apply to toes.
Do not self-treat calluses, corns, or ingrown toenails; consult a podiatrist if these are present.
Bath water should be 30° to 32° C (84° to 90° F) and should be tested with a bath thermometer or elbow before immersing the feet.
Heating pads and hot-water bottles should not be used; wear socks if feet are cold.
Measures that increase circulation to the lower extremities should be instituted, including the following:
Avoid smoking.
Avoid crossing legs when sitting.
Protect extremities when exposed to cold.
Avoid immersing feet in cold water.
Use socks or stockings that do not apply pressure to the legs at specific sites.
Institute an exercise regimen.
Do not walk or jog in the dark; have a light source.
Obtain proper shoes before jogging.

Teach patient to seek podiatric consultation if neuropathy develops and for treatment of minor problems such as calluses and corns.
Teach the principles of preventive foot care (see Guidelines Box above).

Encourage patient to obtain regular monitoring from dentist and ophthalmologist to prevent complications if possible.

Supporting Effective Coping

Encourage patient to verbalize feelings, fears, or frustrations about the diagnosis and regimen (loss of job, health insurance, driving and flying licenses; injections; relationships).

Convey permission to grieve for actual and potential losses.

Avoid overwhelming the patient with regimen teaching. Focus initially on survival skills and plan for future community-based education to increase knowledge base.

Provide sufficient opportunity for patient to master needed skills through repetition.

Include family members as appropriate and acceptable to patient.

Refer to local community support services for information and financial and emotional support.

Guidelines for Teaching Patients Self-care Management

MEDICATIONS

Teach patient and family about prescribed insulin.
  Explain onset, peak, and duration of action.
  Explain that food must be taken within the time of onset for insulin prescribed.
  Explain importance of planning a snack for time of peak action of insulin.
  Explain importance of bedtime snack for patients on long-acting insulin to provide glucose coverage for the night.
Teach patient the proper preparation and administration of insulin (see Guidelines box).
Encourage patient to utilize all available sites to avoid the development of lipodystrophies (see Figure 9-3 for acceptable insulin sites).
  Insulin absorption varies with different body areas: abdomen is greater than arm, which is greater than thigh. Some researchers encourage patients to avoid use of extremities if active exercise is planned.
  Increased purity of insulin has decreased the severity of lipodystrophy problems, but hypertrophy from frequent injections is still a concern, and site rotation is recommended.
Teach patient to safely dispose of used syringes in a resealable container such as a coffee can.
Include appropriate family members or friends in teaching sessions as acceptable to patient.
  At least one close support person should know how to safely inject insulin in an emergency situation.
Teach patient receiving oral hypoglycemic drug the onset, dose, peak effect, and duration of action of drug. Patients are usually encouraged to eat about 30 minutes after taking their medication.
  Reinforce the hypoglycemic effects of alcohol with medications, particularly chlorpropamide (Diabinese).

MONITORING

Teach patient technique of blood and urine testing.
Test strips provide a glucose range; glucose meters provide a more precise numeric value.
Regimens for blood testing vary with the stage of treatment and stability of the patient's condition.
  Initially: before and after meals and at bedtime
  If stable: after meals and at bedtime for one day each week and whenever patient is ill
  If manipulating insulin doses daily: four times per day
Reinforce importance of accurate record keeping for results.
Teach patient to follow product or glucose meter instructions carefully.
Establish parameters with physician for notification of abnormal results.
Urine glucose testing is no longer recommended. However, all patients should be taught to monitor for urine ketones whenever they are ill or blood glucose is above 240 mg/dl.

MANAGING SICK DAYS

Teach patient relationship of insulin need and illness.
  Insulin needs are greater during illness; patient should never skip a dose.
  Patient should adjust diet to liquids if necessary but maintain intake.
  Patient should increase frequency of blood and urine testing and contact physician if hyperglycemia worsens.
Patient should contact physician if he or she is ill for more than 1 or 2 days, is unable to eat food for more than 1 day, experiences vomiting or diarrhea for more than 6 hours, or develops urine ketones. The development of ketoacidosis is a medical emergency and cannot be self treated. Ketoacidosis is presented in Box 9-20.

BOX 9-20 Ketoacidosis

Diabetic ketoacidosis occurs with severe insulin deficiency and is primarily associated with IDDM. Ketoacidosis may occur in the undiagnosed person or in situations in which the patient's insulin needs are greatly increased because of infection, trauma, or severe stress. The pathophysiology mimics the pattern of basic diabetic insulin deficiency, but it is worsened by secretion of the counter-regulatory hormones. This creates a constant state of hyperglycemia with profound osmotic diuresis, protein breakdown with the liberation of potassium, and massive ketone formation, which leads to severe metabolic acidosis, dehydration, and electrolyte imbalance. The patient will lapse into coma if the process is not interrupted, and this usually requires hospitalization. The onset is relatively slow.

SYMPTOMS

Increased thirst
Nausea, vomiting, anorexia*
Abdominal cramping
Lethargy and weakness*
Polyuria leading to oliguria as dehydration progresses

SIGNS

Kussmaul respirations (deep and rapid)
Fruity, acetone odor to the breath*

Hot, dry, flushed skin*
Loss of skin turgor
Decreasing level of consciousness to coma
Signs of shock: tachycardia, hypotension
Serum glucose: 300-800 mg/dl
Arterial pH: <7.2
Serum K: normal to high
Urine ketones: large

TREATMENT

Medical management involves fluid and electrolyte replacement, initially with isotonic saline, and insulin therapy with low-dose, continuous infusion of regular insulin to reduce blood glucose by about 75-100 mg/dl each hour. Potassium replacement is governed by blood values and the adequacy of the urine output.

Nursing management consists of monitoring vital signs, intake and output, level of consciousness, and all blood parameters including arterial blood gases. A Foley catheter, nasogastric tube, and invasive monitoring lines may be inserted based on the severity of the imbalance. Nursing also focuses on comfort measures and reassurance of the patient and family.

---

*Classic signs and symptoms.

Guidelines for Teaching Patients Insulin Administration

Always use an insulin syringe calibrated in the same unit/ml scale that matches the scale of the insulin.

Select insulin according to type, strength, species, and brand name as specified by the prescription.

Rotate or gently roll the bottle if it is other than regular or globin insulin.

Examine *intermediate* and *long-acting* insulin vials for appearance and expiration dates; do not use unless solution is cloudy.

Check for and remove any air bubbles after insulin is drawn into the syringe (do not use an air bubble to clear the needle after injection).

When mixing insulins, do not vary the sequence in which two insulins are drawn into the same syringe; usually air is injected into both bottles (regular and intermediate); the insulin is with- drawn first from the regular vial and then from the longer-acting insulin vial.

Rotate injection sites using all sites in one geographic area before moving to another. Document sites on rotation grid (see Figure 9-3).

Do not use one geographic area more than once every 4 to 6 weeks. Injection sites should be 1 to 1½ inches apart.

Insert the needle into the area beneath the fatty tissue using a 45- to 90-degree angle. Use a 45-degree angle when fatty tissue is less than 1 inch.

Store currently used insulin at room temperature; refrigerate extra supplies.

Keep extra supplies on hand and immediately available when traveling.

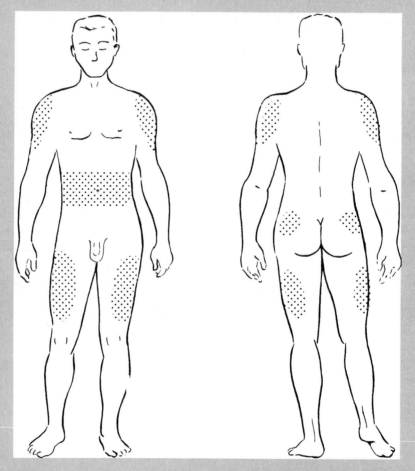

FIGURE 9-3   Arms, legs, buttocks, or abdomen can be used for insulin injections. A different site (indicated by each dot) should be used for each injection. No individual site should be used more than once every 4 to 6 weeks. All sites in one geographic region are used before one moves on to another. Injection sites should be 1 to 1½ inches apart.

Assist patient to identify and problem solve for anticipated difficulties in incorporating regimen into life-style.

Support and reinforce all positive coping behaviors.

Provide patient and family with access to printed resource materials from drug companies and American Diabetes Association.

Assist patient to obtain a Medic Alert tag or bracelet and explain importance of wearing it at all times.

◆ EVALUATION

Successful achievement of expected outcomes for the patient with diabetes is indicated by the following:

Maintenance of desired body weight; correct description of food types, amounts, and distribution; glycosylated hemoglobin, blood glucose, and lipids within established parameters

Demonstration of good foot care and absence of signs of skin breakdown or irritation

Correct verbalization of nature of diabetes, use of oral agents, signs of hypoglycemia and its management, principles of safe exercise, management of minor illness; and demonstration of insulin administration and blood/ketone monitoring

Demonstration of effective coping behaviors and commitment to ongoing disease management

---

BOX 9-21	Hyperglycemic, Hyperosmolar, Nonketotic Coma (HHNC)

HHNC is seen primarily in elderly patients with NIDDM when the action of insulin is severely inhibited. The initial process is similar to any situation of hyperglycemia, but it is worsened by a failure of the normal osmotic diuretic effect of hyperglycemia. The patient may not receive enough fluid, may not respond to thirst, or may experience vomiting or diarrhea. Glomerular filtration and excretion of glucose are impaired. The increasing osmolarity also osmotically depletes the intracellular spaces and causes profound CNS dysfunction. It is not associated, however, with either ketosis or acidosis. Acute infection is a common precipitating factor, and the onset is gradual.

SIGNS AND SYMPTOMS

Initial polyuria leading to oliguria
Poor fluid intake
Dehydration: hypotension, circulatory collapse
Lethargy, confusion leading to coma
Focal neurologic deficits, seizures
Laboratory values
    Blood glucose: >600-2000 mg/dl
    Osmolarity: >350 mOsm/L

Arterial pH: >7.3
Serum Na: normal to high
Serum potassium: normal

TREATMENT

Fluid replacement, usually with 0.5% normal saline, is the cornerstone of therapy. Replacement is initially aggressive and then adjusted based on laboratory values and the patient's response. Insulin therapy is similar to that used in ketoacidosis with low-dose, continuous infusion of regular insulin. Five to ten units per hour will be given. Electrolytes will be continuously monitored and adjusted once the patient is rehydrated.

The mortality associated with HHNC is extremely high, and patients require critical care monitoring of all parameters, particularly cardiovascular ones, during fluid replacement. The patient will be on a cardiac monitor, have a Foley catheter inserted, and be monitored with a Swan-Ganz or arterial line. The nurse will also attempt to ensure patient comfort and reorient the patient as metabolic indicators stabilize. A critical pathway for a patient with HHNC is included.

CRITICAL PATHWAY	Hyperglycemic, Hyperosmolar, Nonketotic Coma (HHNC)

DRG #: 294; expected LOS: 5

	Admission to ICU Day of Admission Day 1	Day 2	Transfer out of ICU Day 3	Day 4	Day of Discharge Day 5
Diagnostic Tests	CBC; SMA/18*; UA; ECG; ABGs; urine, blood, and sputum C & S; Chest x-ray film; ? CT scan	FBS and 2-hour post-prandial SMA/6†	FBS and 2-hour post-prandial	FBS and 2-hour post-prandial with SMA/6†	FBS
Medications	IVs (0.5% NS at rate of 1.5 L first hour, 1 L over next hour, then 500 ml for 1 hr; when serum osmolarity is <320 mOsm/L, switch to NS); IV insulin bolus and gtt; add dextrose (5% saline) when glucose is 250-300 mg/dl; K^+ replacement to maintain serum levels of 4-5 mEq/L; IV antibiotics; evaluate home medications	Continue with appropriate IV solutions and medications; IV antibiotics; continue with appropriate home medications	IV to saline lock; return to prehospital treatment for diabetes mellitus and insulin on sliding scale; IV antibiotics	IV saline lock; return to prehospital treatment for diabetes mellitus; antibiotics; evaluate medications for home use	Discontinue saline lock; adjust medications for home use
Treatments	VS q hr until neurologic status stable, then q 2 hr for 12 hr; I & O including Foley q hr for 4 hr then q 2 hr for 12 hr; weight; capillary blood glucose (CBG) q hr while range <60 and/or >200, then q 4 hr; monitor hemodynamic parameters q hr; assess cardiovascular, pulmonary, and neurologic systems q hr; assess skin and feet and give special care q 2 hr	VS q 2 hr; I & O q 4 hr; weight; CBG q 4 hr and PRN; assess cardiovascular, pulmonary, and neurologic systems q 2 hr; assess skin and feet and give special care q 2 hr	VS q 6 hr; I & O q 8 hr; discontinue Foley and central lines; wt; CBG AC and HS and PRN; assess cardiovascular, pulmonary, and neurologic systems q 4 hr; assess skin and feet and give special care q 4 hr	VS q 8 hr; discontinue I & O; weight; CBG AC and HS and PRN; assess cardiovascular, pulmonary, and neurologic systems q 8 hr; assess skin and feet and give special care q 6 hr	VS q 8 hr; weight: CBG AC and HS and PRN; assess cardiovascular, pulmonary, and neurologic systems q 8 hr; assess skin and feet and give special care q 8 hr
Diet	NPO, clear liquids when fully awake	Full liquid American Diabetes Association (ADA) with appropriate calorie restriction	ADA diet with appropriate calorie restriction; add between meal snacks as appropriate	ADA diet with appropriate calorie restriction; add between-meal snacks as appropriate	ADA diet with appropriate calorie restriction; add between-meal snacks as appropriate
Activities	Bedrest, T & DB q 2 hr, patient safety considerations (bed in lowest position, suction ready, etc.) until neurologic status stable	Up in chair with help, T & DB q 2 hr; continue with patient safety considerations	Up in room and walk in hallway with help	Up in room ad lib and walk in hallway with help	Up ad lib
Referral/ Consultation	Endocrinologist		Dietary, social service, home health, diabetes education		

NOTE: Acknowledge that patients recover at varying rates; therefore specified daily actions should be based solely on patient need.

*Serum calcium, phosphorus, triglycerides, uric acid, creatinine, BUN, total bilirubin, alkaline phosphate, aspartate aminotransferase (AST) (formerly serum glutamic oxaloacetic transaminase [SGOT]), alanine aminotransferase (ALT) (formerly serum glutamic pyruvate transaminase [SGPT]), lactic dehydrogenase (LDH), total protein, albumin, sodium, potassium, chloride, total CO_2, glucose.

†Serum sodium, potassium, chloride, total CO_2, glucose, BUN.

GERONTOLOGIC PATIENT CONSIDERATIONS FOR DIABETES

NIDDM is primarily associated with older adults, and its complications are major concerns for elderly persons. Target blood glucose ranges are generally more liberal for elderly persons, and attention is paid to preventing hypoglycemia. Elderly patients are more likely to already experience cardiovascular problems such as CAD, hypertension, or PVD, and the presence of these problems will complicate diabetes management. They are also at greater risk for developing HHNC during periods of acute illness.

Working with elderly patients requires some adaptation of patient teaching approaches. Instruction should be self-paced and low key and utilize short sessions with multiple opportunities to review and reemphasize learning. Any visual or auditory deficits should be acknowledged and planned for with appropriate materials. Learning new psychomotor skills can be troublesome, and the patient may require more practice opportunities. Teaching about foot care will be particularly important with this population. With today's short stays, it will be unlikely for the patient to have learned sufficient self-care strategies while hospitalized. The nurse will initiate referrals for home care or community education programs and support groups based on availabilities in the local area. If visual impairment exists it may be necessary to enlist home health assistance for the preparation and administration of needed insulin. The elder's natural support network should be included in as much of the education as feasible, and appropriate written materials should be supplied to the patient at discharge to serve as references for all concerned participants.

BOX 9-22   The Surgical Patient with Diabetes

Many surgical patients have their surgery complicated by the presence of diabetes. The disease affects both perioperative management and wound healing. The enormous stress of surgery also affects the control and management of the diabetic process during this period. The patient faces the risk of both hypoglycemia and hyperglycemia. NPO status decreases the need for insulin, but the stressors of surgery cause catecholamine release, which increases blood glucose.

The diabetic patient should be in good control before surgery and should be scheduled for an early-morning procedure if possible. There are several approaches in use for managing glucose, fluid, and insulin needs. A common technique is the administration of an IV with glucose the morning of surgery plus half the standard insulin dose. The IV is continued until the patient can resume an oral diet. Insulin needs are met by dividing the normal daily dose equally over the 24-hour period and substituting regular insulin in the IV. Boluses of regular insulin can be administered based on blood glucose checks performed every 4-6 hours. Patients normally regulated by diet or oral hypoglycemic agents often need supplemental insulin while hospitalized and should also receive frequent blood glucose checks and sliding scale boluses as indicated.

SELECTED REFERENCES

Batcheller J: Disorders of antidiuretic hormone secretion, *Crit Care Nurs* 3(2):370-378, 1992.

Cagno J: Diabetes insipidus, *Crit Care Nurs* 9(6):86-93, 1989.

Chin R: Adrenal crisis, *Crit Care Clin* 7:23-41, 1991.

Christensen MH et al: How to care for the diabetic foot, *Am J Nurs* 91(3):50-56, 1991.

Deakins DA: Teaching elderly patients about diabetes, *Am J Nurs* 94(4):38-42, 1994.

Fox MA et al: Blood glucose self-monitoring usage and its influence on patients' perceptions of diabetes, *Diabetes Educator* 10:27-31, 1984.

Guthrie DW, Guthrie RA: *Nursing management of diabetes mellitus,* ed 3, New York, 1991, Springer.

Isley WL: Thyroid disorders, *Crit Care Nurs Q* 13(3):39-49, 1990.

Juliano J: *When diabetes complicates your life,* Minneapolis, 1993, Chronimed Publishing, Inc.

Kestel F: Using blood glucose meters, *Nurs 93* 26(3):34-41, 1993.

Kestel F: Are you up to date on diabetes medications? *Am J Nurs* 94(7):48-52, 1994.

Lee L, Gumowski J: Adrenocortical insufficiency: a medical emergency, *AACN Clin Issues Crit Care Nurs* 3(2):319-330, 1992.

Lumey W: Controlling hypoglycemia and hyperglycemia, *Nursing* 18:34-41, 1988.

Macheca MKK: Diabetic hypoglycemia: how to keep the threat at bay, *Am J Nurs* 93(4):26-30, 1993.

Murray R: Home before dark, *Am J Nurs* 93(11):36-42, 1993.

Nath C et al: Lessons in living with Type II diabetes mellitus, *Nurs 88* 18:44-49, 1988.

Peterson A, Drass J: How to keep adrenal insufficiency in check, *Am J Nurs* 93(10):36-39, 1993.

Reasner II CA, Isley WL: Thyrotoxicosis in the critically ill, *Crit Care Clin* 7:57-73, 1991.

Robertson C, Cerrato PL: Managing diabetes, *RN* 56(10):26-29, 1993.

Sarsany S: Thyroid storm, *RN* 51(7):46-48, 1988.

Sawin CT: Thyroid dysfunction in older persons, *Adv Intern Med* 37:223-247, 1991.

Shapiro B, Gross MD: Pheochromocytoma, *Crit Care Clin* 7(1):1-2, 1991.

Smith-Rooker JL, Garrett A, Hodges LC: Case management of the patient with pituitary tumor, *Med Surg Nurs* 2:265-274, 1993.

Spittle L: Diagnoses in opposition: thyroid storm and myxedema coma, *AACN Clin Issues Crit Care Nurs* 3(2):300-308, 1992.

Steil CF, Deakins DA: Oral hypoglycemics, *Nurs 92* 25(11):34-39, 1992.

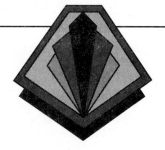

Disorders of the Gastrointestinal System

◆ ASSESSMENT

Health history
  Past/family history
    Previous gastrointestinal (GI) problems, hospitalization, surgery
    Past and current medication use: prescription and over the counter (OTC)
    GI problems in nuclear or extended family: peptic ulcer, bowel problems, inflammatory bowel disease (IBD), cancer
  Diet and nutrition
    Usual eating pattern
    24-hour diet recall
    Food preferences and intolerances, allergies
    Ingestion of alcohol, sugar and salt substitutes, caffeine
    Use of vitamins or other dietary supplements
    Planned and unplanned weight changes
    Social/cultural factors
      Financial resources
      Access to food preparation and storage
      Personal or religious beliefs about diet
  Gastrointestinal symptoms (presence, severity, self-treatment)
    Abdominal pain (onset, duration, character; relationship to eating, activity, and stress)
      Heartburn or indigestion
      Cramping
    Dysphagia
    Anorexia, bloating, nausea, or vomiting
    Fatigue or weakness
  Elimination
    Normal bowel elimination pattern
      Changes in pattern
      Use of laxatives, suppositories, bran, or other aids
    Presence and severity of constipation or diarrhea
    Color and consistency of stool
      Steatorrhea
      Clay color
      Tarry/melena
      Overt bleeding

Physical Assessment
  Mouth (gloves should be worn for direct examination)
    Lips
      Symmetry
      Moisture
      Color
      Cracking/fissures
      Herpes simplex (cold/fever sore)
      Erythroplakia or leukoplakia
    Teeth and gums
      Color of enamel
      Presence/degree of stains
      Existence of loose, broken, or absent teeth or dentures
      Condition of gingivae: color, irritation, ulceration, recession
    Tongue, cheeks, and palate
      Mucosal moisture
      Presence of debris, lesions, inflammation, or ulceration
      Tongue mobility and function (cranial nerve XII)
      Symmetry and movement of palate (cranial nerve X): swallowing
      Mouth odor
      Palpation for tenderness, ulcers, lumps
  Abdomen (patient in supine position, knees slightly bent, pillow under head, and good light)
    Inspection
      Color, texture, turgor, and integrity of skin
      Contour: flat, rounded, scaphoid, distended
      Presence and location of scars, rashes, lesions, visible masses, engorged veins, spider angioma
      Visible pulsations or peristalsis
      Abdominal girth
    Auscultation
      Presence, location, frequency, and intensity of bowel sounds
        Normally occur 5 to 35 times per minute
          Hypoactive: 1 to 5 per minute
          Hyperactive: >35 per minute
          High pitched and gurgling: borborygmi (excessively loud)

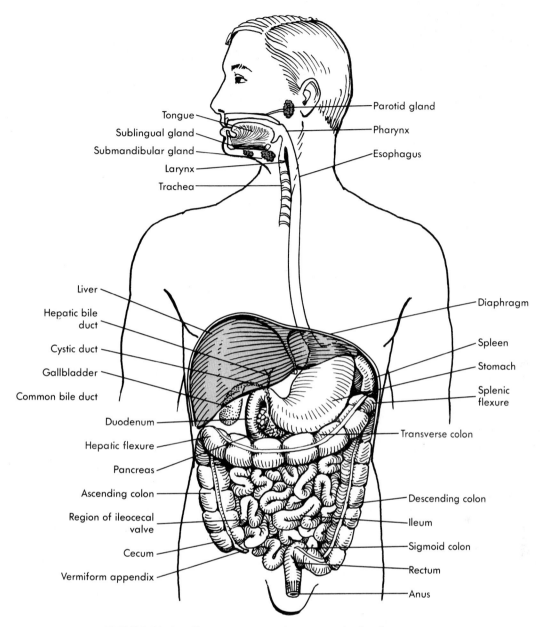

FIGURE 10-1   The gastrointestinal system and related structures.

Best heard below umbilicus to the right; use stethoscope diaphragm

Vascular sounds: bruit over aorta, renal or iliac arteries

Not normally present

Use stethoscope bell

Percussion (limited value in abdomen)

Confirm size of various organs

Determine presence of excess fluid or air

Sounds are normally tympanic with dullness over solid organs

Palpation (deep palpation requires special training)

Determines outlines of organs, presence of masses; presence and degree of tenderness, guarding, and pain

Abnormal findings

Murphy's sign: liver palpation elicits sharp pain and brief inspiratory arrest; associated with gallbladder disease

Blumberg's sign: palpation over a tender region induces acute pain on withdrawal (rebound tenderness); reflects peritoneal inflammation

Rectum: presence of inflammation, fissure, fistula, hemorrhoids, or prolapse

✍ DIAGNOSTIC TESTING
BLOOD TESTS

Major blood tests for the gastrointestinal system are summarized in Table 10-1.

TABLE 10-1 Major Gastrointestinal Blood Tests	
RANGE OF NORMAL VALUES	**DESCRIPTION AND PURPOSE**
GASTRIN	
<200 pg/ml (200 ng/L)	Gastric hormone that is a powerful stimulus for gastric acid secretion; elevated levels found in pernicious anemia and Zollinger-Ellison syndrome
TOTAL PROTEIN (ALBUMIN/GLOBULIN)	

Total protein:6-8 g/dl
  Albumin:3.2-4.5 g/dl
  Globulin:2.3-3.4 g/dl
	Primarily a reflection of liver function but serum protein is also a measure of nutrition; malnourished patients have greatly decreased levels of blood protein

D-XYLOSE ABSORPTION TEST	
Blood levels of 25-40 mg/dl 2 hr after ingestion	Monosaccharide that is easily absorbed by normal intestine but not metabolized by body and does not require biliary or pancreatic function; administered orally and assists in diagnosis of malabsorption
LACTOSE TOLERANCE TEST	
Rise in blood glucose >20 mg/dl	Oral dose of lactose administered; in absence of intestinal lactase, lactose is neither broken down nor absorbed and plasma glucose levels do not rise; assists in diagnosis of lactose intolerance
CARCINOEMBRYONIC ANTIGEN (CEA)	
<5 ng/ml	Protein normally present in fetal gut tissue; typically elevated in persons with colorectal tumors; although not useful as a screening tool it is useful in determining prognosis and response to therapy

---

GERONTOLOGIC PATIENT CONSIDERA-TIONS FOR GI ASSESSMENT

Careful exploration of:
  Adequacy of diet
  Food intolerances and digestive complaints
  Presence and fit of dentures
  Financial resources and access to shopping and facilities for
    cooking
  Elimination patterns and problems
  Use of antacids, laxatives, suppositories, and other aids to
    digestion or elimination

STOOL TESTS

Stool specimens are collected to examine for ova, parasites, blood, fat, and bacterial culture.

Stool Color

Fecal color changes may provide insight into the nature of GI problems. Color may also vary in response to diet and artificial colors in foods. Common variations include the following:

White	Residual barium
Gray/tan	Lack of bile, biliary obstruction
Red	Lower GI bleeding
Black	Upper GI bleeding
Green	Rapid peristalsis and bile content

Occult Blood

Tests for occult blood vary in sensitivity and stringency of patient preparation.

The guaiac (Hemoccult) test is least sensitive. No special preparation is required. Multiple false-positive results occur.

The benzidine and orthotoluidine (Occultest) test involves 3-day restrictions of meat, poultry, and fish and high intake of vitamin C. Results are more sensitive and accurate.

RADIOLOGIC TESTS

Upper GI Series

Description—An upper GI series is a fluoroscopic/x-ray test that allows visualization of the esophagus, stomach, duodenum, and upper jejunum through the use of a contrast medium (usually barium).

Procedure—The patient ingests the barium orally in a milkshake form. X-rays are taken at intervals throughout the test, which takes about 45 minutes.

Patient preparation and aftercare—No special preparation is necessary. The patient is NPO for at least 6 hours before the test. A laxative is administered after the test to eliminate the residual barium.

Barium Enema

Description—Barium enema is a fluoroscopic/x-ray test that visualizes most of the large intestine through administration of a contrast medium.

Procedure—Barium is instilled through a rectal tube with an inflatable balloon to help retain the barium in the colon. Fluoroscopic observation is maintained while the patient's position is shifted to move the barium. The test takes about 30 minutes.

Patient preparation and aftercare—The bowel is thoroughly cleansed with laxatives and/or enemas before the test, and the patient is NPO for at least 8 hours. The patient is informed that the instillation and retention of the barium may cause considerable discomfort. Laxatives are again administered *after* the test to facilitate removal of the barium.

Radionuclide Imaging (GI bleeding scan, scintigraphy)

Description—GI scintigraphy may be used to help localize the site of GI bleeding that is not found in the esophagus or stomach.

Procedure—An intravenous injection of ^{99m}Tc sulfur colloid is administered in the nuclear medicine department. The radionuclide pools at the bleeding site and is detected on scan, which takes about 30 minutes.

Patient preparation and aftercare—No pretest preparation or aftercare is required, and no discomfort is experienced. Patients should be reassured concerning the brief half-life of the isotope and test safety.

SPECIAL TESTS
Esophageal Function Tests

Description—Several diagnostic tests may be performed in a series to evaluate the functioning of the esophagus:

- Manometry: measures the pressure in the lower esophageal sphincter (LES) and records the duration and sequence of peristaltic movements in the esophagus
- pH: measures the acidity or alkalinity of the lower esophagus to evaluate the function of the LES
- Clearance: the rate and efficiency of acid clearance from the esophagus are measured

Procedure—The patient swallows two or three tiny tubes attached to an external transducer. Sedation is not required unless gagging is severe. The test is complete in 30 to 40 minutes unless 24-hour pH monitoring is planned.

Patient preparation and aftercare—No special preparation is required, but the patient is kept NPO for 8 hours. Medications that may affect acidity and LES pressure are held if possible. No posttest care is needed.

Gastric Analysis

Description—The test involves the aspiration of gastric contents in the fasting and stimulated state to quantify gastric output and acidity.

Procedure—A nasogastric tube is inserted to aspirate gastric contents. Repeated aspirates are taken over 1½ hours as the response to various stimulating agents is assessed.

Patient preparation and aftercare—The patient is NPO and instructed not to smoke for 8 to 12 hours before the test. The patient is prepared for the possibility of reactions such as warmth, flushing, itching, and headache in response to stimulating agents such as histamine. No aftercare is required.

Schilling Test

Description—The test evaluates the body's ability to absorb vitamin B_{12} from the intestine. In the absence of gastric intrinsic factor, ingested B_{12} cannot be absorbed.

Procedure—Parenteral B_{12} is administered first to saturate tissue-binding sites. This is followed by oral ingestion of B_{12} with a radioactive tracer. With normal absorption processes, the B_{12} is excreted in the urine. In pernicious anemia, little or no B_{12} will be detectable in the urine.

Patient preparation and aftercare—The patient is kept NPO for 8 to 12 hours and reassured concerning the brief half-life and safety of the isotope. No aftercare is required.

ENDOSCOPY
Esophagogastroduodenoscopy

Description—A flexible fiberoptic endoscope is inserted into the esophagus, stomach, and/or duodenum to evaluate ulcers, biopsy tissue, remove polyps, or control bleeding.

Procedure—The endoscope is inserted after the patient is sedated (with diazepam or midazolam) and administered a topical anesthetic. Air may be instilled to improve visualization and may create a feeling of fullness or pressure. The test lasts 15 to 30 minutes.

Patient preparation and aftercare—The patient is instructed about the test and planned sedation and is asked to remain NPO for 8 hours before the test. Aftercare involves frequent vital sign monitoring and assessment for dyspnea, bleeding, and acute dysphagia. Oral food and fluid are held until the gag reflex returns. A temporary sore throat is a common complaint.

Proctoscopy, Sigmoidoscopy, and Colonoscopy

Description—A rigid proctoscope/sigmoidoscope or flexible fiberoptic endoscope may be inserted through the anus to visualize variously the rectum, sigmoid colon, or colon. The test may be used to evaluate the mucosa, localize bleeding, remove polyps, and take biopsy specimens.

Procedure—The endoscope is inserted after the patient is premedicated with diazepam or midazolam. Air is introduced as the colonoscope is inserted to improve visualization. The procedure takes from 20 to 60 minutes. Proctoscopy and sigmoidoscopy are shorter procedures, and sedation is not generally used.

Patient preparation and aftercare—Thorough bowel cleansing is performed before the test. This may involve laxative and enema administration but increasingly entails the ingestion of an oral osmotic solution (polyethylene glycol [Colyte]), which induces a profuse watery diarrhea within 1 hour. The patient is NPO for 8 hours. After the test the patient is carefully monitored for vital signs changes and the development of abdominal pain, fever, or rectal bleeding.

DISORDERS OF THE UPPER GASTROINTESTINAL TRACT

Problems involving the GI system include a wide variety of common and uncommon, acute and chronic disorders. Ingestion and digestion are essential to health and survival and are closely linked to enjoyment of life. Because they are also closely linked with cultural habits and values, disorders involving the GI tract present challenging situations for medical and nursing management.

Disorders presented in this chapter include problems of both the upper and lower GI tract and encompass infections, obstructions, and tumors, as well as structural alterations.

MOUTH INFECTIONS

Infection may affect virtually any structure of the mouth. Mouth infections may be primary or occur as a secondary effect of vitamin deficiencies or other systemic diseases and treatments. Although they are usually fairly mild, mouth infections can seriously affect the patient's ability to ingest oral food and fluids. Table 10-2 summarizes the common mouth infections and their treatment.

ORAL CANCER
Etiology/Epidemiology

Cancers involving the lips, oral cavity, and the tongue represent 4% of all cancers in men and 2% of all cancers in women. Over 90% of oral cancers occur in people over 45 years of age, and the incidence increases with age. The incidence of oral cancer is clearly linked to a history of smoking and alcohol consumption. Although it is difficult to separate the effects of these agents, current research seems to point to chronic alcohol intake as the critical factor. The mortality for cancer of the tongue and floor of the mouth is high because of the vascularity and extensive lymph drainage of the area.

Pathophysiology

Most oral cancers develop from the squamous cells that line the oral epithelium. Most lesions are asymptomatic in their early stages and may go unnoticed at the base of the tongue or floor of the mouth. Metastasis is present in 60% of patients by the time the diagnosis is made. The exception is cancer of the lip with its high visibility.

Premalignant mouth lesions include leukoplakia (white patches), erythroplakia (red patches), and erythroplasia (white patches within red patches). They usually develop in response to a chronic irritant such as cigarette or pipe smoke or chewing tobacco. Premalignant lesions may progress toward malignancy. Many heal completely with removal of the irritant.

Parotid tumors often present as painless lumps that can be easily palpated. They cause minimal interference, if any, with function in early stages.

TABLE 10-2 Mouth Infections		
ETIOLOGY	**CLINICAL MANIFESTATIONS**	**MANAGEMENT**
APHTHOUS STOMATITIS (CANKER SORE)		
Autoimmune disorder	Painful small ulceration on oral mucosa; heals in 1-3 wk; is recurrent	Palliative: mouthwashes, hydrocortisone-antibiotic ointment, fluocinonide (Lidex) ointment in Orabase
HERPETIC STOMATITIS (COLD SORE, FEVER BLISTER)		
Herpes virus type I	Painful vesicles and ulcerations of mouth, lips, or edge of nose; fever, malaise, lymphadenopathy may occur	Palliative: mouthwashes, fluids, soft diet, topical or systemic acyclovir (Zovirax) in severe cases
VINCENT'S GINGIVITIS (TRENCH MOUTH)		
May be caused by overgrowth of normal oral spirochetes or fusiform bacilli	Painful hemorrhagic gums with ulceration, fever, lymphadenopathy	Oral antibiotics, analgesics, topical hydrogen peroxide, good oral hygiene, referral to dentist for removal of plaque or tartar
CANDIDIASIS (THRUSH)		
Candida albicans	Creamy white, curdlike patches closely adherent to mucosa; bleeds and ulcerates when scraped off	Oral nystatin, ketoconazole, clotrimazole; amphotericin B for immunocompromised person
PAROTITIS		
Viral and nonviral forms (surgical mumps)	Fever, swelling, and pain in glands with abrupt onset	Local heat and cold, frequent oral hygiene, adequate hydration; broad-spectrum antibiotics occasionally needed

Medical Management

Treatment depends on the location and staging of the tumor, and tissue biopsy is the primary diagnostic test. Most oral cancers are treated initially with surgery, external radiation, or the implant of radioactive seeds or needles. The treatment for advanced disease is basically palliative. Surgery usually includes wide excision that significantly interferes with major oral functions such as eating and speaking. Prosthetic reconstruction to gradually restore appearance and function is a common adjunct to this type of surgery.

NURSING MANAGEMENT

◆ ASSESSMENT
Subjective Data

History of smoking and alcohol use: amount and duration

History of mouth soreness, pain, or irritation

Oral and dental hygiene practices

Patient's understanding of proposed surgery or treatment plan and its expected outcomes, including the following:

Extent of tissue destruction

Degree of interference with communication

Loss of or interference with eating function

Planned method for postoperative nutrition maintenance

Objective Data

Condition of mouth and teeth

Presence of leukoplakia, ulcerated lesion, or palpable lump

General health and nutritional status

◆ NURSING DIAGNOSES

Possible nursing diagnoses for the person with oral cancer may include, but are not limited to, the following:

Communication, impaired verbal (related to destruction of structures essential for speech)

Nutrition, altered: less than body requirements (related to chewing and swallowing difficulties or pain)

Oral mucus membranes, altered (related to surgical wounds or effects of radiation and chemotherapy)

Body image disturbance (related to visible structural changes in mouth and throat)

◆ EXPECTED PATIENT OUTCOMES

Patient will successfully communicate with staff and family and begin vocal therapy as healing progresses.

Patient will ingest all needed fluid and nutrients and maintain a stable weight.

Patient's mouth and neck will heal without complications or infection.

Patient will incorporate body changes into an altered but positive body image.

◆ NURSING INTERVENTIONS
Preoperative Care

Teach patient about proposed surgery and its outcomes.

Be specific and honest about the resulting changes in appearance and function, particularly communication and feeding.

Clarify misconceptions.

Ensure that patient's perceptions are accurate.

Encourage patient and family to verbalize their feelings and concerns about body changes. Support appropriate grieving.

Explain expected postoperative measures such as suctioning, nasogastric (NG) tube, drains, tube feedings.

Begin prescribed preoperative mouth preparation.

Facilitating Verbal Communication

Establish effective communication with patient.

Use magic slate or pad and pencil.

Use yes or no questions initially.

Initiate speech retraining when healing occurs.

Encourage patient to speak slowly and use the throat rather than the lips to achieve clarity.

Reassure patient that speech is possible as long as vocal cords are intact.

Listen carefully and validate messages.

Refer to speech therapy for retraining.

Promoting Adequate Nutrition

Provide nutrition through a liquid diet administered with a catheter, tube, or syringe.

Teach patient technique for feeding. Place syringe or spoon on back of tongue to facilitate swallowing. Avoid use of fork, which may injure healing tissue.

Advance patient to soft foods as healing progresses.

Provide privacy during feeding if patient prefers.

Teach patient to rinse mouth carefully after meals.

Encourage self-care for feedings and mouth care as soon as physically possible.

Promoting Oral Hygiene

Provide frequent oral hygiene care with mouth irrigations. Avoid use of toothbrush.

Use saline, water, or dilute hydrogen peroxide and sterile equipment to avoid introducing infection.

Teach patient technique for oral hygiene. Encourage patient participation as able. A cotton-tipped applicator may be used to reach difficult or painful areas.

NOTE: Oral irradiation causes inflammation and tissue sloughing of mucous membranes, bad odor, and dry mouth. Meticulous oral hygiene and diet modifications are mandatory. Care of the patient with radioactive needle implants is summarized in the Guidelines box below.

Position patient to maintain airway and promote drainage of secretions from the mouth—usually in side-lying and then semi-Fowler's position when reactive. Maintain oral suction at the bedside.

Assist patient to remove saliva from mouth with suction, gauze wick, or emesis basin. Provide constant monitoring if patient cannot swallow.

Maintain patency of drainage tubes.

Facilitating Adaptation to Body Image Changes

Encourage patient to express feelings about surgery in order to reach grief resolution.

Encourage family to include patient in family gatherings and social events to foster acceptance of changed appearance.

Put patient and family in contact with community agencies that can provide assistance.

◆ EVALUATION

Successful achievement of expected outcomes for the patient undergoing surgery for oral cancer is indicated by the following:

Ability to communicate needs effectively and maintain social interaction

Ability to feed self effectively and maintenance of a stable body weight

Healing of all surgical incisions without complications

Guidelines for Nursing Care of the Patient with Radioactive Needle Implants in Oral Tissue

IMPLANT CARE

Do not pull on the strings. Any movement could alter the placement or direction of the radiation or cause the needles to loosen.

Check needle patency several times each day.

Monitor linens, bed areas, and emesis basin for needles that may dislodge.

Ensure that a protective container is present in the room to contain any needles that might dislodge.

Patient Care

Assist with gentle oral hygiene every 2 hours while awake.

Encourage patient to avoid hot and cold foods and beverages and smoking.

If patient has dentures encourage their removal at night for comfort.

Assess gums for irritation and bleeding whenever dentures are removed.

Provide viscous lidocaine (Xylocaine) solutions or lozenges as needed when oral discomfort interferes with nutrition.

Provide patient with an alternate means of communication, because talking around implanted needles is frequently difficult or impossible.

Assist patient to implement mouth care regimen prescribed by physician.

Ability to perform mouth care and control oral secretions and odor

Expressed acceptance of body changes

Resumption of family, social, and occupational roles

TRAUMA OF THE MOUTH AND JAW

Traumatic injury of the mouth and jaw may be limited to the soft tissues or extend to the bony structures. Most soft tissue injuries, although temporarily disfiguring, resolve with rest and supportive care. Fractures create greater challenges, because ensuring mandibular continuity is essential for normal chewing.

Jaw fractures are treated by closed or open reduction with intermaxillary fixation. The teeth are connected with rubber bands or tie wires. Care must be taken to prevent aspiration, and scissors or wire cutters should be kept readily available at the bedside. The patient is usually restricted to a liquid diet and may experience considerable pain from muscle spasms in the immobilized jaw.

ESOPHAGEAL DISORDERS

Most esophageal disorders are fairly uncommon. The primary exception is gastroesophageal reflux disease, which is usually referred to by the patient as simple heartburn. Other structural and functional disorders of the esophagus are summarized in Table 10-3.

Gastroesophageal Reflux Disease
Etiology/epidemiology

Gastroesophageal reflux disease (GERD) can occur in any age-group and is estimated to cause daily symptoms in as much as 10% of the general population. Most cases are attributable to the inappropriate relaxation of the lower esophageal sphincter (LES), which allows reflux of gastric and duodenal contents into the distal esophagus. LES pressure may be influenced by dietary factors, pharmacologic agents, and elevated intraabdominal pressure.

Pathophysiology

Periodic reflux occurs normally in most people and is usually asymptomatic. Persistent reflux, however, breaks down the mucosal barrier of the esophagus and causes an inflammatory response to occur. Over time, repeated episodes of inflammation and healing can result in fibrotic tissue changes that can result in stricture or increase the risk of cancer.

The clinical manifestations of GERD are directly related to the irritation of reflux. They include heartburn, regurgitation of sour- or bitter-tasting fluid up the throat, water brash (reflex salivary hypersecretion), and dysphagia in severe cases.

Medical management

GERD can frequently be diagnosed from its classic symptoms. The gold standard for diagnosis includes

TABLE 10-3   Esophageal Disorders

DESCRIPTION	MEDICAL MANAGEMENT
ACHALASIA (CARDIOSPASM)	
Absence of peristalsis in esophagus Failure of esophageal sphincter to relax after swallowing, creating acute muscle spasm Esophagus dilates above constriction Dysphagia is major symptom	Forceful dilation of constricted sphincter Esophagomyotomy Peristalsis not restored
ESOPHAGEAL DIVERTICULA	
Bulging of esophageal mucosa through weakened portion of muscular layer Portions of ingested food may enter diverticula Causes regurgitation of food from diverticula	Surgical excision if symptoms are severe
ESOPHAGEAL TUMORS	
Incidence highest in elderly males, particularly African-Americans, and is associated with heavy alcohol and tobacco use Tumors rare but usually fatal, because early diagnosis is seldom possible	Radiation therapy for palliation Esophageal dilation Surgical excision (esophagogastrostomy) is preferred procedure
DIAPHRAGMATIC (HIATAL) HERNIA	
Causes progressive dysphagia to solid food and weight loss Protrusion of part of stomach through diaphragm and into thoracic cavity Precipitated by any condition increasing intraabdominal pressure, usually congenital Causes heartburn and reflux of gastric contents, especially when patient is recumbent	Minor problems treated with antacids, small frequent feedings, bland diet, and avoiding lifting Surgery to repair hernia via thoracic or abdominal route (fundoplication: wrapping stomach fundus around distal esophagus)

24-hour pH monitoring that records the number, duration, and severity of reflux episodes (see p. 207).

Drug therapy is the cornerstone of management. It usually begins with PRN antacid use. Histamine receptor antagonists may be added for more severe cases. They do not directly influence reflux but support tissue healing by reducing gastric acid secretion. The new proton pump inhibitors, which reduce acid secretion by 90%, are being used experimentally. They support rapid healing but are not approved for long-term use, and their use is accompanied by frequent relapses. Bethanechol (Urecholine) or metoclopramide (Reglan) may be tried in severe cases. Bethanechol directly increases LES pressure, and metoclopramide facilitates gastric emptying. Both drugs are associated with frequent side effects and need careful monitoring.

Drug therapy is accompanied by prescribed changes in diet, eating patterns, and life-style that are discussed under nursing management. Fundoplication surgery may be recommended if conservative measures fail, particularly if a hiatal hernia can be documented.

NURSING MANAGEMENT

◆ ASSESSMENT
Subjective Data

Heartburn: severity and duration
Presence of regurgitation or water brash
Diet and meal pattern

Relationship of symptoms to meal pattern, position, and activity
Self-treatment strategies: use of OTC medications

Objective Data

Body weight
Results of 24-hour pH monitoring or endoscopy

◆ NURSING DIAGNOSES

Possible nursing diagnoses for the person with GERD may include, but are not limited to, the following:
Pain (related to the effects of acid reflux in the esophagus).
Knowledge deficit (related to diet and life-style modifications to control reflux).

◆ EXPECTED PATIENT OUTCOMES

Patient will report minimal or no episodes of heartburn.
Patient can accurately list diet and life-style changes to control reflux.

◆ NURSING INTERVENTIONS
Promoting Comfort

Teach patient about safe use of antacids and expected side effects.
Take antacids 1 hour before and 2 to 3 hours after meals, at bedtime, and PRN.
Suggest use of combination mixtures (Maalox, Mylanta) to minimize bowel problems.

Modifying the Diet

Teach patient to reduce intake of foods that lower
  LES pressure:
  Fatty foods
  Chocolate
  Beverages with caffeine
Encourage patient to eat four to six small meals daily.
Encourage patient to avoid lying down after eating.
Encourage patient to avoid nighttime snacking and
  any food consumption for 2 to 3 hours before
  bedtime.
Encourage patient to eat slowly and chew food
  thoroughly.

Promoting Life-Style Changes

Teach patient to do the following:
  Elevate the head of bed 8 to 12 inches for sleep. A
    foam wedge may be used instead of blocks.
  Avoid increases in intraabdominal pressure caused
    by constrictive clothing, heavy lifting, or work-
    ing in a stooped or bent over position.
  Reduce body weight if obese.
  Reduce or eliminate smoking (drops LES pressure).

◆ EVALUATION

Successful achievement of expected outcomes for the
patient with GERD is indicated by the following:
  Absence of episodes of heartburn
  Successful diet modification and appropriate body
    weight
  Incorporation of recommended changes into life-
    style

Hiatal Hernia
Etiology/epidemiology

Hiatal (diaphragmatic) hernias develop when the distal
esophagus and possibly a portion of the stomach move
into the thorax through the esophageal hiatus. Sliding
hernias, which move freely between the thorax and
abdomen, account for over 90% of all cases. They are
believed to develop from muscle weakness that may be
congenital or associated with aging, trauma, obesity, or
chronic elevations in intraabdominal pressure. Hiatal
hernias are common in adults and may affect 30% of the
general population and up to 60% of elderly persons.

**GERONTOLOGIC PATIENT
CONSIDERATIONS FOR GERD**

Elderly patients tend to underreport heartburn and need to be
specifically assessed. They are particularly vulnerable to alkaline reflux from the duodenum, which typically occurs at night
and causes the patient to awaken with paroxysmal coughing,
choking, or wheezing. The risk of aspiration is high.

Pathophysiology

Hiatal hernias are asymptomatic until the development of
gastroesophageal reflux. The low-pressure environment of
the thorax significantly impairs the function of the LES.
Hiatal hernias are usually diagnosed as part of a workup for
severe reflux, and the clinical manifestations are quite
similar. Acute hernia-related complications are rare.

Medical and nursing management

Hiatal hernias are treated initially with the medication,
diet, and life-style interventions outlined for treatment
of GERD. Surgical repair is considered when conservative therapy is ineffective. Procedures are designed to
repair the defect in the diaphragm and restore LES
pressure. The Nissen repair, which involves wrapping
the fundus 360 degrees around the distal esophagus, is
the most common (Figure 10-2).

Postoperative care initially focuses on pulmonary
interventions to prevent complications. Many patients
experience some initial problems with eating and swallowing following the repair. The food storage area is
reduced, and temporary dysphagia is fairly universal.
Small soft meals and an upright position for eating are
helpful for most patients. The patient may have persistent difficulties with belching and is taught to avoid
carbonated beverages, gas-producing foods, and drinking through a straw.

Cancer of the Esophagus
Etiology/epidemiology

Cancer of the esophagus is rare but almost always fatal
within 5 years. The tumors are rarely diagnosed early
enough to allow for effective treatment. The disease
typically affects men between 50 and 80 years of age. It
occurs four times more commonly in African-Americans.
The long-term heavy ingestion of alcohol in combination with cigarette smoking appears to be the primary
etiologic factor.

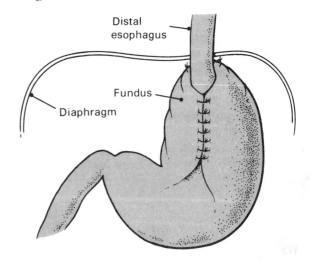

FIGURE 10-2 Nissen fundoplication for repair of hiatal hernia. (From Lewis SM, Collier IC: *Medical-surgical nursing*, ed
3, St Louis, 1992, Mosby.)

Pathophysiology

The majority of esophageal tumors are squamous cell and develop in the middle and lower two thirds. The process is believed to begin with initially slow tissue changes that gradually accelerate in growth and infiltrate the rich local lymphatic supply. Tumors tend to both encircle the esophagus and extend up and down its length.

Early diagnosis is rare, and tumors of less than 10 cm are considered small. Most patients experience gradually progressive dysphagia that is continuous and worsens steadily from solids to liquids. Dysphagia does not usually appear until the diameter of the esophagus is at least 60% obstructed.

Medical and nursing management

Radical surgery is the only definitive treatment for esophageal cancer and is the treatment of choice for otherwise healthy people. The surgeries are extensive and involve subtotal or total esophagectomy. The esophagogastrostomy is the current preferred choice (Figure 10-3). Significant risks are associated with the operative procedure, leakage from the anastomosis site, and aspiration caused by loss of the protective barrier of the LES. Chemotherapy may be used as part of the total treatment plan or with radiation therapy for disease palliation. Esophageal dilation may be needed at intervals to control obstructive dysphagia.

Patients with esophageal cancer present multiple nursing care challenges. Initial postoperative care focuses on protecting the airway and supporting healing

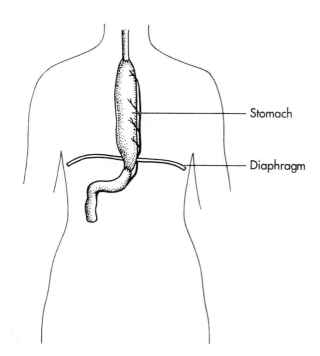

FIGURE 10-3 Esophagogastrostomy for esophageal cancer.

of the multiple incisions. Oral nutrition is gradually resumed with sips of water and progresses according to the patient's tolerance. Small meals and an upright position at all times are emphasized. The nurse also helps the patient accept the terminal diagnosis, begin the process of grieving, and make realistic plans for future care needs.

PEPTIC ULCER DISEASE
Etiology/Epidemiology

Peptic ulcers are one of the most common GI disorders, affecting 1% of the total adult population. There are several types and multiple causes. They are frequently chronic in nature and follow a pattern of remission and exacerbation. Genetic predisposition, environmental factors, and infection are currently believed to be the major factors involved in ulcer development.

Peptic ulcers occur two to three times more often in families with a history of ulcers. Analysis of racial and cultural factors has not, however, revealed any clear trends. Smoking impairs ulcer healing, but its role in initial etiology is not clear. Alcohol causes direct mucosal injury, but its place in long-term management is again unclear. Caffeine is an acid secretagogue, but its role in ulcer etiology is uncertain. No other dietary factor is linked with ulcer development. The role of life stress in ulcer disease has been studied for over a century with few supportable conclusions. Persons with ulcers do not experience more stress, but they seem to react to it more negatively.

The chronic use of aspirin, nonsteroidal antiinflammatory drugs (NSAIDs), and corticosteroids is felt to be a direct cause of peptic ulcers. They impair mucosal defenses, damage the surface mucosa, and stimulate increased acid secretion. Infection with *Helicobacter pylori* bacteria is also believed to play a causative role. The bacteria appear to render the mucosa more vulnerable to damage from other factors.

Duodenal ulcers are more common than gastric ulcers, and they affect men much more frequently than women. These classic patterns have been steadily shifting, however. Ulcer patients who are older and women are comprising an ever increasing percentage. A bimodal pattern still exists, however, with duodenal ulcers primarily affecting younger persons and gastric ulcers affecting older adults.

Pathophysiology

The basic pathology of peptic ulcer disease is an imbalance between acid secretion and the protective mechanisms of the mucosa, which include both the thick mucous layer and the secretion of bicarbonate to maintain a protective pH gradient.

Acid oversecretion is almost exclusively related to duodenal ulcers and is associated with an increase in parietal cell mass and an elevated level of gastrin secretion postprandially. The defenses of the mucosa can be affected in several ways. NSAIDs are prostaglandin inhibitors, and their chronic use blocks the mucosal production of mucus. They also impair bicarbonate secretion. Infection with *H. pylori* also interferes with mucus production and bicarbonate secretion. The net effect is a back diffusion of acid into the mucosa, triggering an inflammatory response.

The clinical manifestations of peptic ulcer disease are very variable and range from asymptomatic to "classic" symptom patterns. Classic symptoms include the following:

1. Duodenal
   a. Epigastric pain that may radiate around costal border
   b. Pain described as burning, gnawing, aching
   c. Pain occurs 2 to 4 hours after meals and at night
   d. Pain typically relieved by food or antacid
2. Gastric
   a. Epigastric pain that may radiate around costal border
   b. Pain described as burning, gnawing, aching
   c. Pain occurs 1 to 2 hours after meals
   d. Pain may be worsened by food or antacids
   e. Vague nausea, bloating, distention

Medical Management

Peptic ulcers can frequently be diagnosed from the pattern of symptoms. An ulcer is clearly visible by GI series, but endoscopy is typically employed to biopsy the ulcer and rule out malignancy.

Drug therapy is the foundation of treatment for peptic ulcer disease and is typically employed for 6 to 8 weeks. Antacids, H$_2$ receptor antagonists, and sucralfate are the primary agents. They are summarized in Table 10-4. With 8 weeks of drug therapy 85% to 90% of ulcers will heal.

Diet therapy plays no significant role in ulcer healing. Individuals are encouraged to restrict or eliminate foods that cause discomfort and experiment with the effectiveness of six small meals per day.

Rest appears to facilitate ulcer healing, but no significant change in daily activities is necessary. Surgery no longer plays a major role in peptic ulcer disease management. It is primarily used to treat ulcer complications or deal with ulcers that are resistant to standard therapy or continue to relapse. Common surgical procedures are illustrated in Figure 10-4 and include the following:

Truncal vagotomy and drainage: severs the vagus where it enters the stomach and reduces acid secretion

TABLE 10-4 Drug Therapy in Peptic Ulcer Disease		
DRUG	**ACTION**	**COMMENTS**
ANTACIDS Amphogel Basalgel Maalox Gelusil Mylanta	Neutralize free hydrochloric acid Aluminum hydroxide products preferred because they also decrease pepsin activity and may stimulate prostaglandin synthesis	Administered 1-3 hr after meals, at bedtime, and PRN Tablet form administration prolongs effect Can *heal* ulcers when used alone but takes longer Bowel problems (constipation) common

HISTAMINE (H$_2$) RECEPTOR ANTAGONISTS
Cimetidine (Tagamet)
Ranitidine (Zantac)
Famotidine (Pepcid)
Nizatadine (Axid)
	Inhibit HCl secretion by binding to histamine H$_2$ receptor sites on stomach cells, blocking histamine-mediated secretion of acid	Variable dosage schedules including:
		   Throughout the day with meals
		   Single massive bedtime dose
		Low drug side effects and excellent safety record

SUCRALFATE (CARAFATE)	Coats ulcer to provide sealant against effects of acid; increases prostaglandin synthesis	Administered 30-60 min before meals and at bedtime May be dissolved in water if difficult to swallow Constipation only common side effect
MISOPROSTOL (CYTOTEC)	Synthetic prostaglandin analogue that replaces gastric prostaglandins and has some antisecretory activity; used preventively at present with NSAID use; has no current role in ulcer healing	Administered orally QID Crampy abdominal pain and diarrhea: reported side effects
H. PYLORI therapy Bismuth compounds (Pepto-Bismol) Amoxicillin or tetracycline Metronidazole (Flagyl)	Triple therapy recommended to ensure eradication of bacteria and to prevent development of resistant strains	Therapy still controversial Used primarily when peptic ulcers relapse GI side effects common and may be severe Therapy continued for minimum of 3 wk

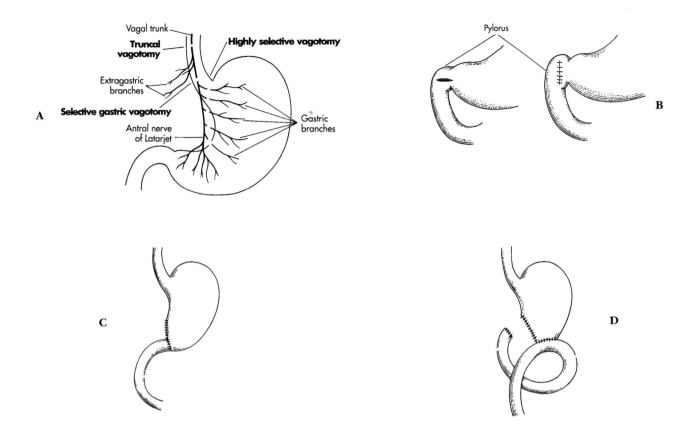

FIGURE 10-4 Surgery for peptic ulcer disease. **A,** Vagotomy. *A,* Truncal vagotomy; *B,* selective vagotomy; *C,* highly selective vagotomy. **B,** Pyloroplasty. Longitudinal incision across pylorus is pulled apart and closed in transverse position to widen pyloric outlet. **C,** Billroth I: gastroduodenostomy. Anastomosis of gastric segment to duodenum. **D,** Billroth II: gastrojejunostomy. Anastomosis of gastric segment to proximal jejunum.

by 70%. A pyloroplasty is performed for drainage, because the procedure creates gastric stasis. The vagotomy may also be performed more selectively, which preserves gastric function but increases the incidence of relapse.

Subtotal gastrectomy: procedures will remove varying amounts of the distal stomach. Reconstruction is performed with anastomosis to the duodenum (Billroth I) or the side of the proximal jejunum (Billroth II). Patients experience varying degrees of difficulty with relapse and dumping syndrome.

NURSING MANAGEMENT

◆ ASSESSMENT
Subjective Data

Pain: presence, location, severity, nature, and relationship to meals and activity
Nausea or bloating

Smoking and alcohol history
Use of potentially ulcerogenic drugs: aspirin, steroids, antiinflammatory drugs (NSAIDs)
OTC drugs used to manage ulcer symptoms
Diet and meal pattern
Life-style: work, leisure, perceived stress level
Knowledge of peptic ulcer disease and treatment

Objective Data

Guaiac-positive stools
Iron deficiency anemia
Hematemesis—frank GI bleeding
Weight loss or gain
Positive results from upper GI series or endoscopy

■ ■ ■

Nursing management of peptic ulcer disease is summarized in the nursing care plan.

NURSING CARE PLAN

PERSON WITH PEPTIC ULCER DISEASE

■ NURSING DIAGNOSIS
Pain (related to the action of gastric secretions on the inflamed mucosa)

Expected Patient Outcome	Nursing Interventions

Patient's pain decreases or resolves.	1. Give prescribed medications:
	  a. Antacids: 1 and 3 hr after meals and at bedtime for best effect; may be given as often as every 30 min for severe pain
	  b. Histamine H_2 blockers with meals and at bedtime or single large bedtime dose
	  c. Sucralfate: 1 hr before meals and at bedtime
	  d. Do not give antacids concurrently with cimetidine or sucralfate
	2. Avoid substances high in caffeine.
	3. Eliminate foods that trigger gastric pain. Beer is a strong acid secretagogue.
	4. Use a five- to six-meal pattern if it reduces incidence of ulcer pain. Avoid bedtime snacking.
	5. Assist patient to rest. Explore use of relaxation strategies.

■ NURSING DIAGNOSIS
Injury, high risk for (related to ulcer perforation or hemorrhage)

Expected Patient Outcome	Nursing Interventions

Patient does not experience bleeding.	1. Monitor patient for signs of complications:
	  a. Signs of overt bleeding: hematemesis, tarry stools
	  b. Signs of shock
	  c. Signs of perforation: severe sharp abdominal pain
	2. If signs of complications occur, give patient nothing by mouth and prepare to insert NG tube for lavage.
	3. Eliminate ulcerogenic medications if possible, particularly aspirin, anti-inflammatories, steroids.

GERONTOLOGIC PATIENT CONSIDERATIONS FOR PEPTIC ULCER DISEASE

The incidence of peptic ulcer disease is steadily increasing in the elderly population. Elders are most likely to be hospitalized and experience the majority of complications and mortality. The disease is frequently related to chronic NSAID use and often presents in an atypical fashion. Standard pain symptoms are rarely present, and the problem is often not diagnosed until it presents with complications.

Complications of Peptic Ulcer Disease

The major complications of peptic ulcer disease are hemorrhage, perforation, or obstruction of the pyloric outlet.

Hemorrhage

Peptic ulcers account for 80% of all GI bleeds. Hemorrhage is by far the most common disease complication. It affects 15% to 20% of all ulcer patients, primarily elderly persons. It is more common in gastric ulcers and ranges in severity from slight oozing to frank hemorrhage. The management of GI bleeding is discussed in

NURSING CARE PLAN

PERSON WITH PEPTIC ULCER DISEASE

■ NURSING DIAGNOSIS
Coping, ineffective individual (related to life stresses)

Expected Patient Outcome	Nursing Interventions

Patient is able to understand and identify stressors and effectively problem solve to reduce them.	1. Help patient identify:
	  a. Any present stressors in daily life
	  b. Feelings and responses to identified stressors
	  c. Usual coping mechanisms
	  d. Individuals who can serve as support persons when new stressors occur
	2. Assist patient to explore alternative ways of coping.
	3. Teach patient stress management techniques, such as relaxation response, as appropriate.
	4. Encourage activities that promote relaxation (recreation, hobbies).
	5. Assist patient to do the following:
	  a. Identify specific health-risking behaviors that may aggravate the ulcer (e.g., smoking, caffeine, alcohol, stressful situations)
	  b. Explore ways of modifying the behaviors, such as ways to stop smoking or drinking or to avoid certain stressful situations

■ NURSING DIAGNOSIS
Knowledge deficit (related to peptic ulcer treatment regimen)

Expected Patient Outcome	Nursing Interventions

Patient is knowledgeable concerning prescribed medications and life-style modifications necessary to promote healing.	1. Teach patient the following:
	  a. Nature of peptic ulcers
	  b. Factors that contribute to healing and decreased occurrence of ulcers
	  c. Medication regimens
	  d. Methods to reduce stress and promote relaxation
	  e. Need to report symptoms of bleeding, perforation, and pyloric obstruction to physician immediately

the Guidelines box. It is estimated that ulcer bleeding will stop spontaneously in up to 85% of patients. Endoscopy is used to isolate and evaluate the bleeding site. Thermal coagulation by heater probe, cautery, or laser may be used to treat the bleeding site. Injection therapy with epinephrine, absolute alcohol, or another sclerosing agent may also be utilized. Surgery is employed if the bleeding cannot be controlled by other means.

Perforation

Perforation involves erosion of the ulcer through the muscular wall with spillage of gastric secretions into the peritoneal cavity. It is more common with duodenal ulcers. A chemical peritonitis develops almost immediately followed by bacterial peritonitis. The classic clinical picture includes the following:

- Severe, sharp abdominal pain
- Rigid, boardlike abdomen with rebound tenderness
- Tachycardia, tachypnea, diaphoresis

The symptoms are often much less dramatic in elderly persons. Emergency surgery is indicated. It may involve patching the defect or definitive ulcer correction.

Guidelines for Nursing Care of Ulcer Hemorrhage (GI Bleeding)

SYMPTOMS

Vomiting of bright red or coffee ground blood (usually occurs with gastric ulcers)

Tarry stools (more common with duodenal ulcers)

Signs of early and progressive hypovolemic shock

Faint feeling, dizziness, thirst

Feelings of apprehension, restlessness

Dyspnea, pallor, rising pulse, falling blood pressure

INTERVENTIONS

Place patient on bed rest.

Patient should receive nothing by mouth.

Monitor vital signs frequently (every 15 minutes).

Administer IV fluids and blood transfusions as prescribed.

Record accurate intake and output; assess response to treatment.

Provide supplemental O_2 by nasal cannula, particularly for elderly persons.

Administer histamine H_2 receptor antagonist IV as ordered.

Position patient to the side and keep head of bed elevated at least 45 degrees.

Keep suction available.

If bleeding is acute, insert NG tube and irrigate with room temperature tap water or saline until clear.

Provide mouth care after patient vomits—a weak solution of hydrogen peroxide helps remove blood from oral mucous membranes.

Monitor stools for increasing blood content after episode.

Prepare patient for endoscopy procedure if indicated.

Explain all procedures, keep calm, and reassure patient as much as possible.

Obstruction

Effective drug therapy for peptic ulcer disease has dramatically decreased the incidence of obstruction. Repeated episodes of ulceration and scarring may gradually obstruct the pylorus. The patient develops dyspepsia symptoms as the stomach fails to empty completely and gradually progresses to vomiting as the obstruction becomes complete. Surgery is performed after the patient is adequately stabilized.

STRESS ULCERS

Mucosal inflammation, erosion, and bleeding can develop within hours of major stressors such as trauma, burns, sepsis, and shock. The classic pattern is the development of painless upper GI bleeding, usually within 3 days. Acute hemorrhage is the most common complication, but perforation may also result. Overproduction of acid is rarely a causative factor except in central nervous system (CNS) trauma and sepsis. Instead, the stress state decreases blood flow to the mucosa, inducing cellular hypoxia and necrosis. Mucosal resistance to acid injury is therefore felt to be the key.

Aggressive prevention is the key to stress ulcer management. Gastric acidity is reduced through continuous IV infusion of histamine H_2 receptor antagonists, possibly supplemented by antacids to keep the gastric pH

above 3.5. Therapeutic endoscopy, vasopressin administration, and laser photocoagulation may be used to attempt to control bleeding if it occurs. The mortality associated with bleeding is quite high. The nursing role focuses on continuous bedside monitoring of at risk patients and gastric pH monitoring through manual aspiration, continuous pH probe, or the use of a tonometer that measures the pH of the mucosa rather than just the secretions.

CANCER OF THE STOMACH
Etiology/Epidemiology

The incidence of cancer of the stomach has shown a steady decline in the United States over the last 50 years, but the disease presents a highly erratic worldwide incidence pattern. Environmental and dietary factors appear to be crucial, because the incidence rate of immigrants from high-risk areas such as Japan drops sharply by the second generation. It is typically a disease of later middle age and affects more men than women. Cigarette smoking is clearly implicated in the cancer's etiology as are diets high in nitrates and nitrites and deficient in fresh fruits and vegetables.

Pathophysiology

Gastric cancers are typically primary adenocarcinomas that develop in the pyloric and antral regions. The cancer spreads directly to adjacent tissue and through the rich lymphatic networks of the region. The tumor is usually asymptomatic in early stages and is typically incurable by the time of diagnosis. Gastric distress and heartburn, weight loss, fatigue, and weakness are common symptoms.

Medical Management

Gastric cancer is diagnosed through endoscopy with multiple biopsies. The only potentially curative treatment is surgical resection, and the procedure depends on the location and extent of the tumor. Total gastrectomy is no longer recommended because of the serious digestive problems that may develop. Radiotherapy has no proven effectiveness, and chemotherapy is utilized primarily for palliation.

NURSING MANAGEMENT

The care outlined is tailored for the patient undergoing gastric surgery.

PREOPERATIVE INTERVENTIONS
Teaching about the Proposed Surgery and Postoperative Care Routines

High abdominal incision increases risk of respiratory complications.

Demonstrate deep breathing, effective coughing, use of incentive spirometer, incisional splinting, and position changes.

Discuss need for and use of NPO status and NG tube.

Promote optimal nutritional status before surgery.

POSTOPERATIVE INTERVENTIONS
Maintaining a Patent Airway

Initiate frequent position changes: use mid-Fowler's to high Fowler's position to facilitate chest excursion.

Encourage patient to cough and deep breathe. Ensure adequate analgesia. Splint the incision.

Supporting Adequate Nutrition

Maintain NPO status until peristalsis is well established and initial healing is ensured.

NOTE: NG tubes are not routinely irrigated after stomach surgery. Clarify order before irrigating. Drainage should contain no fresh blood after first 12 hours. Do not reposition NG tube.

Administer IV fluids and monitor for signs of electrolyte imbalance.

Record intake and output accurately.

Introduce liquid and small amounts of bland food after NG tube is removed—about 7 days after surgery—usually as three to six small meals daily.

Monitor for signs of early satiety and dumping syndrome (Box 10-1). Avoid stress after meals; rest after eating.

Avoid lying flat in bed to prevent reflux.

Managing Complications

Monitor NG tube drainage for blood.

Monitor for signs of anastomosis leakage (peritonitis): severe abdominal pain and rigidity.

Teach patients to report incidence of steatorrhea and weight loss.

Supplement intake of fat-soluble vitamins.

Teach patient about risk of pernicious anemia (loss of intrinsic factor necessary for B_{12} absorption).

SURGERY FOR OBESITY

Obesity surgery is performed for individuals with massive or morbid obesity who have tried and failed at all standard methods of weight control. Obesity has multiple effects on the body and is implicated as a risk factor in hypertension, coronary artery disease (CAD), arthritis, stress incontinence, non–insulin dependent diabetes mellitus (NIDDM), and sleep apnea.

BOX 10-1	Dumping Syndrome

DEFINITION

A group of unpleasant vasomotor and GI symptoms that occur after gastric surgery in up to 50% of patients. It is a complex process involving the following:

Rapid entry of hypertonic food boluses into the duodenum/jejunum causing abrupt fluid shifts and hypotension

Rapid gastric emptying initiating an intense gastrocolic reflex

Excessively rapid absorption of glucose triggering excess insulin release and hypoglycemia

SYMPTOMS

Weakness, faintness, diaphoresis, gastric fullness, nausea, and possibly diarrhea

Appear 5-30 minutes after meals and again 2-4 hours after meals and may last 20-60 minutes

SYMPTOM MANAGEMENT

Focus is on prevention rather than treatment.

Teach patient to eat meals low in simple carbohydrates, high in protein, and moderate in fat.

Teach patient to avoid simple sugars.

Teach patient to take fluids only between meals.

Teach patient to eat small, frequent meals.

Teach patient to lie down on left side after eating for 20-30 minutes.

Teach patient to avoid very hot and very cold foods and beverages.

Anticholinergic or antispasmodic drugs may be used.

Surgical correction may be necessary.

BOX 10-2	Nausea and Vomiting

DEFINITIONS

Vomiting is a complex physical phenomenon. Nausea is a subjective experience. They frequently occur together but may be present independently.

VOMITING

Vomiting center is located in the medulla. It is stimulated by the vagus nerve and sympathetic nervous system.

Vomiting can be produced *directly* by:

Spasms or inflammation in the GI tract that triggers visceral receptors

Increased intracranial pressure

Vomiting can be produced *indirectly* by:

Stimulation from chemoreceptive trigger zone (CTZ) at the base of the fourth ventricle

Cerebral cortex responses to pain or stress by poorly understood mechanisms; includes conditioned responses to specific sensations or situations

MANAGEMENT OF VOMITING

Discontinue stimulating medications if possible.

Experiment with diet and meal pattern and utilize relaxation strategies.

Administer antiemetic medications as indicated: use drugs preventively and use oral route if possible.

DRUG CATEGORIES

Antihistamines (e.g., Dimenhydrinate, hydroxyzine, meclizine): primarily useful for motion sickness and vertigo

Phenothiazine (e.g., prochlorperazine, trimethobenzamide): depresses the CTZ and used primarily for postoperative problems; produces significant sedation

Metoclopramide (Reglan): increases GI mobility; effective with some chemotherapy protocols

Ondansetron (Zofran): prevents serotonin binding, aborting the emetic impulse; excellent results for chemotherapy and being researched for postoperative use

BOX 10-3 — Constipation

DEFINITION

The term *constipation* refers to an abnormal infrequency of defecation, or the passage of abnormally hard stools, or both. Lack of dietary fiber, lack of fluids, and lack of physical activity are all common causes. Normal patterns vary widely from more than once daily to once every 2-4 days. Chronic constipation leads to decreased intestinal muscle tone, increased use of Valsalva's maneuver, and an increased incidence of hemorrhoids.

PREVENTION

1. Diet
   a. Eat a high-fiber diet: whole grains, fresh fruits and vegetables.
   b. Avoid highly refined cereals, breads, pastries.
   c. Drink 2500-3000 ml of fluid daily.
   d. Use supplemental bran only in moderation and begin with a low dose (6-10 tsp/day).
2. Activity
   a. Participate in daily active exercise.
   b. Do not suppress the natural defecation reflex.
   c. Set aside a regular daily time for defecation.

TREATMENT

Suppositories, laxatives, or enemas are for occasional use only. Stool softeners and bulk formers are recommended for routine problems.

1. Stool softeners (emollients) act as detergents in the colon, reducing surface tension of the stool.
   a. Dioctyl sodium sulfosuccinate (Colace)
   b. Docusate calcium (Surfak)
2. Bulk formers (polysaccharide and cellulose derivatives) mix with intestinal fluids, swell, and stimulate peristalsis.
   a. Psyllium (Metamucil)
   b. Methylcellulose (Citrucil)
   c. Bran
3. Lubricants lubricate the intestinal mucosa for easy stool passage (for example, mineral oil).
4. Stimulants/irritants directly stimulate and irritate the intestine to promote peristalsis.
   a. Cascara (Cas-Evac)
   b. Bisacodyl (Dulcolax)
   c. Senna (Senokot)
   d. Castor oil
5. Saline/osmotics draw water into the intestine osmotically to alter stool consistency and promote peristalsis.
   a. Milk of magnesia
   b. Magnesium citrate
   c. Lactulose (Cephulac)

BOX 10-4 — Diarrhea

DEFINITION

The term *diarrhea* refers to watery stool. It is not a reflection of the number of stools per day. It primarily results from infection and disease of the GI tract, food allergy, hypermetabolism, and malabsorption. Acute diarrhea may cause severe fluid and electrolyte imbalances (hypokalemia and hyponatremia) and metabolic acidosis from bicarbonate loss.

GENERAL TREATMENT

1. Correct underlying cause if possible.
2. Diet:
   a. Withhold food for 24 hours if severe.
   b. Continue oral fluids (Gatorade or other electrolyte-rich solution) if tolerated.
   c. Initiate oral diet with low-fiber, low-fat, bland foods and avoid milk products (transient lactase deficiency is common).
   d. Avoid very hot and cold foods and beverages.
3. Activity: rest after meals to avoid stimulating peristalsis.
4. Comfort: keep perianal tissue clean and dry. Use protective ointments (zinc oxide) and sitz baths for excoriation.
5. Drug therapy:
   a. Local acting: soothe intestinal mucosa to increase water and nutrient absorption
      (1) Kaolin and pectate (Kaopectate)
      (2) Bismuth subsalicylate (Pepto-Bismol)
   b. Systemic acting: reduce peristalsis and motility
      (1) Loperamide (Imodium)
      (2) Tincture of opium (Paregoric)
      (3) Diphenoxylate hydrochloride with atropine (Lomotil)

A number of surgical approaches have been used in the past, but only two are currently approved. Jaw wiring has been demonstrated to achieve no lasting effects, and the placement of intragastric balloons has been discontinued because of the high incidence of side effects. Roux-en-Y gastric bypass is still in use but is often associated with prolonged dumping syndrome and malabsorption. Gastric stapling/partitioning (gastroplasty) is the preferred option. It significantly reduces the food storage area of the stomach and creates minimal adverse effects. Nursing care focuses on the prevention of the complications of abdominal surgery in obese persons. Wound healing and atelectasis are primary concerns. Patients typically need extensive psychosocial support and may be referred to peer support groups for continued weight loss.

DISORDERS OF THE LOWER GASTROINTESTINAL TRACT

ACUTE INFECTION/INFLAMMATION

Appendicitis

Acute inflammation of the appendix occurs most commonly in people between 10 and 30 years, more often in males than females. No specific causes of the disease have been identified, but the lumen of the appendix is small and vulnerable to incomplete emptying or obstruction by hardened feces. An inflammatory reaction is initiated that may progress to abscess formation or perforation. Classic symptoms include the following:

Pain in right lower quadrant of the abdomen, which
  may localize at McBurney's point

Rebound tenderness

Pain initially intermittent but rapidly becomes steady
  and severe

Anorexia, nausea and vomiting

Fever of 38° to 38.5° C

White blood cell count >10,000

Some patients may have less defined symptoms and require a more careful diagnostic workup. This is often true in elderly persons.

Prompt surgical intervention is required, because delay could lead to perforation. The appendix is removed through a small incision, and healing is usually prompt. Drains may be inserted if an abscess is found. Bowel function returns promptly after surgery, and the convalescence is short.

Nursing management involves monitoring and supportive care while the diagnosis is being established and general postoperative surgical care. The hospitalization is usually brief.

Diverticular Disease/Diverticulitis

Diverticula are small outpouchings of the mucosal lining of the bowel that develop through weakenings or defects in the muscular wall. Diverticulitis occurs when trapped fecal material and bacteria produce acute inflammation and infection. Abscess formation or microperforation is possible.

Diverticular disease is rare before middle age. The incidence then increases steadily with aging. It primarily affects the descending and sigmoid colon and is attributed to chronic ingestion of a low-fiber diet. Classic symptoms include the following:

Crampy pain in the left lower quadrant

Low-grade fever

Nausea and vomiting

The diagnosis is made from the history and symptoms. Computed tomography (CT) scans can be used to rule out abscess. Treatment is conservative. The patient is made NPO during an acute exacerbation and monitored carefully for signs of perforation that would necessitate emergency surgery. Teaching is provided concerning the prevention of constipation through a high-fiber, high-fluid diet and the use of hydrophilic bulk-forming laxatives to increase the mass and water content of stool.

Peritonitis

Peritonitis involves a local or general inflammation of the peritoneum. Primary peritonitis typically results from bacterial infection that follows ulcer perforation, pelvic inflammatory disease (PID), ruptured appendix, or bowel obstruction. Secondary peritonitis is triggered by trauma, surgical injury, or chemical irritation. Bacterial invasion occurs within hours of the initiating event.

The body may successfully wall off the acute inflammation with adhesions and abscess formation or progress rapidly to massive fluid and electrolyte shifts and hypovolemia. Local symptoms include the following:

Acute local or diffuse pain and rebound tenderness

Intense abdominal rigidity and guarding

Paralytic ileus and abdominal distention

Hypovolemic shock: tachycardia, tachypnea, oliguria,
  and restlessness

Symptoms are often suppressed or masked in elderly persons, delaying diagnosis and treatment.

The diagnosis is made from symptoms and x-rays showing abnormal abdominal gas and air patterns. Treatment is primarily surgical to remove infected material and correct the underlying problem. Surgical healing is delayed, and the mortality is about 40%. The nursing role involves careful monitoring and standard postoperative interventions for critically ill patients. Preventing respiratory complications and wound care will be priorities for care.

INFLAMMATORY BOWEL DISEASE
Etiology/Epidemiology

Crohn's disease and ulcerative colitis are the two classic forms of inflammatory bowel disease (IBD). Although distinctly different disease processes, they have many overlapping features and are both characterized by inflammation. A clear familial link is present, but no genetic markers have been identified. Erratic worldwide incidence patterns also point to environmental factors, but their exact nature remains elusive. No clear patterns have emerged from research into infectious or dietary causes as well.

Ulcerative colitis is more prevalent, but the incidence of Crohn's disease has shown a steady increase in recent years. IBD is much more prevalent in Caucasians, particularly females. It can occur at any age, but the peak period of onset is in young adulthood.

Pathophysiology

Although inflammation is the hallmark of both diseases, they vary substantially in nature and location of the inflammation, distribution pattern, and degree of mucosal penetration. Table 10-5 compares the major features of the two disorders. Both diseases follow a pattern of exacerbation and remission.

Crohn's disease is characterized by cobblestone granulomas along the mucosa, thickening of the intestinal wall, and scar tissue formation. Lesions commonly perforate and form fissures with the intestinal wall or other hollow organ. Scar tissue interferes with normal bowel absorption. Lesions may occur in an ascending pattern throughout the bowel, often separated by patches of normal tissue.

Ulcerative colitis consists primarily of mucosal ulcerations that begin in the rectosigmoid colon and spread

TABLE 10-5   Comparison of Crohn's Disease and Ulcerative Colitis

CROHN'S DISEASE	ULCERATIVE COLITIS
AGE OCCURRING	
20-30 yrs 40-50 yrs	Young adults
AREA AFFECTED	
Mainly terminal ileum, cecum, and ascending colon; can occur anywhere in GI tract	Colon and rectum only, primarily the descending portion
EXTENT OF INVOLVEMENT	
Segmental areas of involvement	Continuous, diffuse areas of involvement
CHARACTER OF STOOLS	
No blood; may contain fat; three to five semisoft stools per day	Blood present; frequent liquid stools; no fat content
ABDOMINAL PAIN	
Colicky cramping pain in right lower quadrant, which may be severe	May occur, usually before defecation
COMPLICATIONS	
Fistulas; perianal disease; strictures; vitamin and iron deficiencies	Pseudopolyps; hemorrhage; cachexia; infrequently perforation
REASONS FOR SURGERY	
Fistulas; obstruction	Poor response to medical therapy; hemorrhage; perforation
TYPE OF SURGERY	
Colon resection with anastomosis	Total proctocolectomy with permanent ileostomy; continent ileostomy

---

BOX 10-5   Irritable Bowel Syndrome

DEFINITION

Irritable bowel syndrome/spastic colon/mucous colitis is a syndrome of abdominal pain and altered bowel habits, usually diarrhea, that occurs in the absence of any demonstrable organic disease. It is the most common GI condition.

In United States most treated patients are women, but opposite is true worldwide. No changes can be seen in bowel mucosa and inflammation is not present.

SYMPTOMS

Symptoms often begin in middle and late adolescence.
Symptoms vary, but two major patterns predominate:
    Colicky abdominal pain relieved by passing gas or stool, periodic constipation and diarrhea
    Urgent, painless diarrhea during or after meals

MANAGEMENT

Avoid excess intake of rich fatty foods.
Limit intake of gas-producing foods and carbonated beverages.
Reduce or eliminate alcohol, smoking, and other gastric irritants.
Assess response to high-fiber diet or use of bulk-forming hydrophilic laxatives.
Use stress reduction and relaxation strategies.

---

upward through the colon. The ulcers may bleed or perforate. The bowel mucosa becomes edematous and thickened. The formation of scar tissue thickens the colon and causes loss of elasticity.

Extraintestinal symptoms also occur in patients with IBD. Their etiology is unknown. Arthritis is extremely common, but cholelithiasis, renal stones, cirrhosis, uveitis, and skin problems appear with a frequency that is not present in the general population.

Medical Management

The diagnosis of IBD is established from the pattern of symptoms, barium enema to evaluate physical changes in the bowel, and endoscopy to establish the spread of the disease or evaluate premalignant lesions. There is no definitive treatment for IBD. Medications are the cornerstone of treatment and are used in an attempt to induce remission, increase comfort, relieve symptoms, and improve the quality of life. Commonly prescribed medications include the following:

1. *Sulfasalazine (Azulfidine)* combines bacterial suppression with the antiinflammatory effects of aspirin. It is the cornerstone of treatment for mild to moderate ulcerative colitis and may be used in Crohn's disease as well. It may also be administered topically as an enema or suppository when disease is confined to the rectosigmoid area.

2. *Corticosteroids* are primarily used to induce remission in acute Crohn's disease. Their potent antiinflammatory action is restricted by severe systemic side effects, which limit their use. Research is proceeding to develop less absorbable drug forms that can be administered rectally (budesonide and beclomethasone).

3. *Antibiotics* play a supportive role in disease management. They are used during acute exacerbations to

procedures for ulcerative colitis involve total colectomy and are therefore curative. Options are summarized in Box 10-6.

BOX 10-6 **Surgical Options for Ulcerative Colitis**

The removal of the entire colon and rectum cures ulcerative colitis, and the effectiveness of these procedures is well supported (Figure 10-5).

PROCTOCOLECTOMY AND ILEOSTOMY

This is the oldest procedure. It involves removal of the colon, rectum, and anus with permanent closure of the anus. The end of the terminal ileum is brought out though the abdominal wall to form a continuously draining stoma.

CONTINENT ILEOSTOMY (KOCK POUCH)

This procedure modifies the traditional ileostomy by creating an abdominal reservoir to store feces using the terminal ileum. A portion of the ileum is intussuscepted to create a nipple valve that is catheterized to empty the pouch. No drainage bag is required. Chronic problems with the nipple valve have decreased the use of this procedure.

COLECTOMY AND ILEOANAL ANASTOMOSIS

During the colectomy a 12-15 cm rectal stump is preserved, and the small bowel is inserted into this sleeve for anastomosis. It preserves continence but retains the risk of disease recurrence in the stump and an increased risk of cancer.

COLECTOMY WITH ILEOANAL RESERVOIR

This is the current procedure of choice. The anal sphincter and a 1-inch section of rectum are preserved but stripped of mucosa. A reservoir is constructed from the ileum. Continence is preserved, and the risks of disease recurrence or cancer are negligible.

---

control bacterial overgrowth and infection. Some studies using metronidazole (Flagyl) indicate that it may be an alternative to sufasalazine in certain situations.

Patients also frequently require vitamin supplementation when absorption is impaired by inflammation and oral nutrition is difficult to maintain.

Diet does not cause IBD and cannot alter the course of the disease, but it plays a role in patient comfort. Patients are encouraged to restrict intake of raw fruits and vegetables, fatty or spicy foods, and dairy products since lactose intolerance is common. Constipation may develop from strictures, scarring, and loss of motility. Bulk hydrophilic laxatives may be used. Bowel rest is considered important during exacerbations of Crohn's disease but appears to have little effectiveness in ulcerative colitis. Total parenteral nutrition (TPN) may be needed to maintain nutrition during acute exacerbations of IBD.

Surgery is indicated when the patient does not respond to medical management. Surgery is performed in Crohn's disease for obstruction, fistula, or abscess drainage. It usually consists of bowel resection and anastomosis but may involve a newer procedure, strictureplasty, which allows for release of strictures without loss of bowel tissue. Since disease recurrence must be anticipated, surgical management of Crohn's disease focuses on preserving as much bowel as possible. Most surgical

NURSING MANAGEMENT

◆ ASSESSMENT
Subjective Data

Patient's knowledge base and understanding of the disorder

Pain: location, nature, severity, frequency; relationship to eating; measures used to self-treat

Bowel elimination pattern: constipation or diarrhea, frequency and character of stools; presence of blood, fat, mucus, or pus

Nutritional status: usual meal pattern and intake; recent weight changes, food intolerance and allergies, appetite, fatigue or weakness, nausea

Social relationships: support network; impact of illness on family, employment, life-style, and sexuality

Perceived life stress and usual coping patterns

Medications in current use (prescribed and OTC): dosage and side effects; perceived effectiveness in managing disease and symptoms

Objective Data

Body weight
Skin turgor and condition of mucous membranes
Presence of fever
Bowel sounds: presence, character
Condition of perianal skin

▪ ▪ ▪

The nursing management of the patient with IBD is summarized in the Nursing Care Plan. Care for the patient undergoing ileostomy is summarized in the Guidelines box.

MALABSORPTION AND MALNUTRITION

Malnutrition is a multifaceted problem that may result when the body experiences increased need or increased losses of nutrients through open wounds or suctioning, in situations of deficient intake for physical or psychosocial reasons, and from malabsorption of nutrients in the GI tract.

GERONTOLOGIC PATIENT CONSIDERATIONS: INFLAMMATORY BOWEL DISEASE

Although IBD usually appears in young adulthood, it can occur after 60 years of age. The presentation and clinical course are quite similar. Ulcerative colitis usually appears as proctitis and is responsive to treatment after a typically severe first attack. Crohn's disease also tends to be localized to the distal colon and rectum. Complications are frequently related to comorbid conditions rather than the primary IBD.

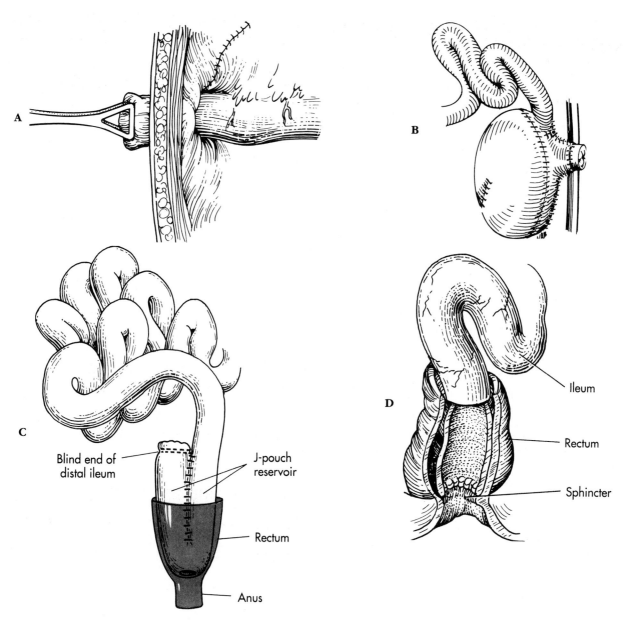

FIGURE 10-5 Surgeries for ulcerative colitis. **A,** Ileostomy. **B,** Kock pouch. **C,** Ileoanal reservoir. **D,** Ileoanal anastomosis.

Protein-calorie malnutrition is a common problem in acute and chronic care situations. Some research indicates an incidence of 25% to 50% among hospitalized adults, particularly elderly patients. Intake of nutrients may be deficient in all areas or just protein, which is critical since the process of protein synthesis in the body is constant and depends on ingested sources. Ongoing deficits lead to losses in both muscle and visceral mass and failure of cell-mediated immunity. Serum albumin levels below 3.5 g/dl indicate malnutrition. Management is based on identifying patients at risk and diet supplementation through PO, enteral, or parenteral feedings.

Malabsorption results when nutrients cannot be broken down adequately for absorption; nutrients cannot be effectively transported across cell membranes; or nutrients cannot be transported into the lymphatic or circulatory system. A wide variety of diseases and conditions can result in malabsorption, including gastrectomy, pancreatic insufficiency, IBD, intestinal resection, celiac disease, tropical sprue, and lactase deficiency. Medical treatment depends on the cause and may involve diet restrictions or modifications, diet supplements, and enteral or parenteral nutrition.

Enteral Nutrition

Enteral nutrition involves delivery of nutrients directly to the GI tract. It is used only when both GI motility and absorption are intact. Feedings may be delivered to the stomach (nasogastric) or the distal duodenum/jejunum (nasointestinal). The nasointestinal route is used primarily for patients at risk for aspiration. A wide variety of tubes exist ranging from 8 to 10 Fr (small

NURSING CARE PLAN

PERSON WITH INFLAMMATORY BOWEL DISEASE

■ NURSING DIAGNOSIS

Pain, chronic, and abdominal cramping (related to bowel inflammation and perianal irritation)

Expected Patient Outcomes	Nursing Interventions
Patient reports improvement in frequency and severity of abdominal discomfort. Patient utilizes dietary and noninvasive pain relief strategies to manage pain.	1. Facilitate easy access to toilet, commode, or bedpan (abdominal cramping is relieved by bowel movements). Empty promptly. 2. Provide soft toilet tissue or medicated wipes (Tucks). 3. Keep anal area clean with mild soap and water and dry well. Apply zinc oxide or other protective ointments after cleaning. 4. Provide sitz baths for rectal comfort, as necessary. 5. Use analgesic ointments (Nupercaine) as needed. 6. Protect and massage pressure areas developing from prolonged toilet/bedpan sitting. Keep sheepskin or eggcrate mattress on bed. 7. Use room deodorizers, as needed. 8. Examine anus at intervals for signs of perianal fissures.

■ NURSING DIAGNOSIS

Diarrhea (related to inflammation and ulceration of the bowel)

Expected Patient Outcomes	Nursing Interventions
Patient experiences fewer episodes of diarrhea. Patient identifies dietary and activity factors that worsen or improve diarrhea.	1. Monitor stools for characteristics and frequency. 2. Give prescribed antiinflammatory medications (sulfasalazine, corticosteroids) and monitor for side effects. 3. Give prescribed antidiarrheals or antibiotics as ordered. 4. Encourage patient to lie quietly after meals to reduce peristalsis. 5. Encourage fluid intake of at least 2500 to 3000 ml daily. Use Gatorade or other electrolyte-rich liquid if tolerated. 6. Monitor intake and output and daily weigh.

Continued.

bore) to 16 to 18 Fr (large bore). They are usually made of silicone or polyurethane. Small-bore tubes tend to collapse with the application of suction and make aspiration for residuals difficult or impossible.

Parenteral Nutrition

Parenteral nutrition allows for the administration of highly concentrated solutions (1800 to 2200 mOsm/L) intravenously to meet all of a patient's nutritional needs for growth, maintenance, and repair. It is used as a supplement or when oral/enteral nutrition is not feasible. It is typically administered via a central venous route but can in short-term situations be administered via peripheral vein if lower osmolality solutions are used. A variety of central venous access devices and peripheral lines are in use. (See Chapter 4 for a discussion of these devices and their management.)

Infection is a major concern related to TPN administration and is believed to develop primarily from catheter contamination at the skin entry site, with migration of bacteria along the catheter. Rigorous dressing protocols are followed, but research has not established clear guidelines for intervals for dressing changes or the effectiveness of various dressing materials.

NURSING CARE PLAN—CONT'D

PERSON WITH INFLAMMATORY BOWEL DISEASE

■ NURSING DIAGNOSIS

Nutrition altered: less than body requirements (related to anorexia, nausea, and malabsorption of nutrients)

Expected Patient Outcomes	Nursing Interventions
Patient follows a high-calorie, low-fat diet with limited intake of raw fruits, vegetables, and dairy products. Patient maintains stable body weight and positive nitrogen balance.	1. Give nothing by mouth or only prescribed feedings during acute episode. 2. If elemental feedings are required, chill the fluids and offer a variety of flavors, because taste is poor. 3. Provide a high-protein, low-residue, high-carbohydrate diet after acute episode subsides. 4. Identify foods, such as those high in fats or fiber, spicy foods, or milk products, that are poorly tolerated by patient and eliminate these foods from the diet. Limit use of intestinal stimulants: alcohol and caffeine. 5. Use measures to encourage increased food intake (pleasant environment, reduction of stress at mealtime, between-meal snacks). 6. Give supplemental vitamins and minerals. 7. Monitor weight two to three times per week. 8. Record accurate intake and output. 9. Encourage fluids to 2500 ml/day if patient is on oral diet. 10. Assess skin turgor and status of mucous membranes daily.

■ NURSING DIAGNOSIS

Coping, high risk of ineffective individual (related to frequent exacerbations and lack of cure)

Expected Patient Outcomes	Nursing Interventions

Patient identifies factors that increase disease-related anxiety and stress.
 	
Patient verbalizes coping strategies and support mechanisms to handle stressors.
	1. Give patient opportunities to express feelings about condition (frustration, depression, anger) and identify content related to these feelings.
	2. Discuss effects of stress on disease exacerbations.
	3. Help patient identify the following:
	  a. Life stressors and usual response to the stressors
	  b. Usual coping mechanisms and alternative methods of coping
	4. Refer to IBD support group after discharge.
	5. Encourage rest during exacerbations. Space activities to conserve energy.
	6. Assist with activities of daily living as needed.
	7. Encourage patient to gradually resume responsibility for self-care as condition improves.
	8. Discuss need for independence with family.

NURSING CARE PLAN—CONT'D

PERSON WITH INFLAMMATORY BOWEL DISEASE

■ NURSING DIAGNOSIS
Health maintenance, high risk of altered (related to lack of knowledge of condition and treatment)

Expected Patient Outcomes	Nursing Interventions

Patient describes:
  Nature of illness and planned treatment
  Side effects of all prescribed medications
  Symptoms requiring medical supervision
	1. Assess patient's knowledge of disorder and provide information as needed.
	2. Encourage patient to participate in planning activities and assuming self-care.
	3. Provide patient with written material about all drugs and associated side effects.
	4. Utilize prepared teaching materials from the National Foundation for Ileitis and Colitis.
	5. Ensure that plans are made for medical follow-up.
	6. Teach symptoms requiring medical attention: fever, rectal discharge, abrupt change in pattern or severity of abdominal pain, or diarrhea.

Guidelines for Administering an Enteral Tube Feeding

Feeding schedules may be intermittent, bolus, or continuous.
Check placement of feeding tube.
  Aspirate gastric secretions if possible.
  Measure gastric residual and return to stomach.
  Inject 10-30 ml of air into feeding tube and auscultate over left upper quadrant of abdomen.
Place patient in high Fowler's position if permitted.
Attach syringe to feeding tube (for intermittent feedings).
  Elevate syringe 18 inches above patient's head.
  Fill syringe with formula.
  Allow solution to instill by gravity.
  Avoid infusion of air.
Hang feeding bag 18 inches above patient's head (for continuous feedings). Set prescribed flow rate.
Flush tube with 30-50 ml of water at the end of the feeding or every 4 hours if continuous. Always flush tube thoroughly before and after medication administration.
Record all volumes and residuals accurately.

BOX 10-7 Percutaneous Endoscopic Gastrostomy: PEG Tubes or "G" Buttons

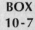
Gastrostomies create an opening into the stomach through the abdominal cavity for long-term feeding administration.

PEG TUBE
This gastrostomy is created endoscopically rather than surgically and does not require extensive incision into the abdominal cavity (Figure 10-6). It is fast and safe to create with the patient under only local anesthesia and sedation.

BUTTON GASTROSTOMY OR "G" TUBE (FIGURE 10-7)
This gastrostomy is created by making a small tube from the wall of the stomach and creating an intussusception valve that is brought to the skin surface to form a flat stoma. No dressings are needed. A tube is inserted for administration of feedings. The small mushroom dome button lies almost flush with the skin.

Home parenteral nutrition
The administration of TPN in the home is now a routine intervention for patients who will need long-term or lifelong nutritional support. Most patients requiring home TPN have severe IBD or advanced cancer. Over time, most families can successfully master the complex protocol demanded by home TPN. (See care plan on p. 232.)

INTESTINAL OBSTRUCTION
Etiology/Epidemiology

Any factor or condition that either narrows the intestinal passageway or interferes significantly with peristalsis can result in bowel obstruction. Obstructions are typically classified as mechanical (affecting the lumen) or nonmechanical (related to peristalsis) and can be partial or complete. Common causes of mechanical obstruction include (see Figure 10-8) the following:

Hernias: wall defect strangulates bowel segment
Tumor: bowel cancer accounts for 80% of obstructions in large bowel
Adhesions: most common cause of obstruction in the small bowel; fibrous bands of scar tissue loop around the bowel, kinking it or compressing it
Volvulus: twisting of bowel on itself, creating acute obstruction

Guidelines for Nursing Care of the Patient with an Ileostomy

PREOPERATIVE CARE

Teach patient in detail about the proposed surgery:
 Size and appearance of stoma
 Amount and consistency of drainage
 Appliances used and their basic care, if any
Encourage patient to ask questions and express feelings about major alteration in body appearance and function.
Provide emotional support for stage of grief or acceptance patient exhibits.
Provide for initiation of teaching and visits by enterostomal therapist. Therapist usually does stoma site selection.
Assist with complete bowel preparation as ordered: laxatives, enemas, antibiotics (Neomycin).
Assist with nutritional preparation; TPN may be used to improve postoperative healing.
Explain need for and function of all tubes and drains: IV lines, NG tubes, wound drains.

POSTOPERATIVE CARE

Provide routine care for major abdominal surgery.
Monitor fluid and electrolyte balance carefully:
 Measure all output accurately.
 Maintain patency of IV lines and NG drainage system.
 Weigh patient daily.
 Teach patient symptoms of dehydration.
Monitor stoma and suture line carefully:
 Stoma should be pink–bright red; dark blue–red indicates impaired circulation and should be reported immediately.
 Note amount and type of drainage
  Mucous and serosanguineous discharge occurs for first 24-48 hours.
 Liquid drainage occurs with returning peristalsis—may initially be as much as 1500 ml per day. Terminal ileum will begin absorption in about 2 weeks, and drainage will then thicken.
 Maintain liberal fluid intake (2500-3000 ml daily).

Teach patient stoma management:
 Teach technique for pouch application and skin care.
 Teach emptying and disposal or cleansing of pouch; empty pouch when one third to one half full.
Protect skin around stoma from fecal drainage:
 Cleanse skin carefully and dry.
 Apply skin barrier. Ileostomy drainage is erosive.
 Change pouch as needed if leaking occurs—never simply add tape. Do routine changes every 5-7 days. Encourage and reinforce all self-care efforts.
Advance diet and fluids as prescribed:
 Begin with bland, low-residue diet.
 Avoid foods that cause increased gas or odor, such as corn, celery, cabbage, onions, and spiced foods.
Teach patient that some foods and substances (seeds, kernels, enteric or slow-release medications) will pass through stoma unchanged. Use liquid or chewable medications when available.
Discuss with patient the following modifications in lifestyle necessitated by ileostomy:
 Modify clothing.
 Adjust recreational pursuits—contact sports should be avoided, but most other activities may be resumed.
 Make adaptations for traveling.
  Hand carry all necessary ostomy supplies.
  Use disposable equipment and take extra supplies.
  Eat moderately—use restraint with new foods and water.
Put patient in touch with local ostomy associations.
Encourage patient to discuss concerns regarding resumption of sexual activity.
Teach patient importance of reporting any early signs of complications. Patient should be alert to the following:
 Changes in color, consistency, or odor of stool
 Bleeding from stoma
 Persistent diarrhea or lack of stool
 Changes in stoma contour (prolapse or inversion) or signs of infection
 Skin irritation that does not respond to basic treatment

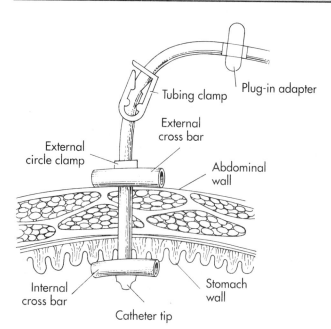

FIGURE 10-6 PEG tube in place in stomach.

Intussusception: telescoping of a segment of bowel within itself

Nonmechanical obstruction is usually caused by adynamic or paralytic ileus in response to surgery, trauma, or sepsis.

Pathophysiology

When the forward movement of chyme is obstructed, intestinal secretion continues, at least initially, and fluid and air accumulate significantly proximal to the site of obstruction. An increase in peristalsis occurs near the obstruction in an effort to move intestinal contents. As intraluminal pressure increases, the proximal intestine dilates, smooth muscle becomes atonic, and peristalsis ceases. Large amounts of isotonic fluid then move from the plasma into the distended bowel, and normal reabsorption of intestinal gas and fluid is impeded. The tissue becomes edematous, and mucosal blood flow is decreased. The stagnant distended bowel becomes in-

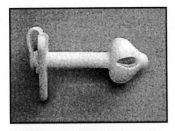
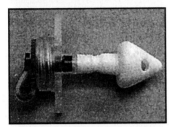
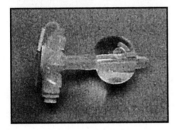

FIGURE 10-7 Button gastrostomies. (From Faller N, Lawrence KG: Comparing low-profile gastrostomy tubes, *Nurs 93,* pp 46-48, Dec 1993.)

creasingly permeable to bacteria, which enter the peritoneal cavity.

The end result may be severe dehydration and electrolyte imbalance with possible perforation or strangulation of the bowel. The severity of the symptoms will depend on the site and degree of obstruction and the amount of time that elapses before the patient seeks help.

Although symptoms vary with location and acuity, abdominal pain is a consistent feature. The pain, however, decreases as the obstruction worsens. Small bowel obstructions cause vomiting, which may be profuse. As the patient becomes increasingly dehydrated from fluid shifts the signs of hypovolemic shock can appear.

Medical Management

Bowel obstruction is diagnosed primarily from the pattern of symptoms and x-rays that show air and fluid entrapment in the obstructed segment. Treatment of intestinal obstruction may include NG or intestinal intubation and decompression, fluid and electrolyte replacement, and surgical relief of the source of obstruction if necessary. The operative procedure will vary with the cause and location but may include release of adhesions, bowel resection, and temporary or permanent colostomy.

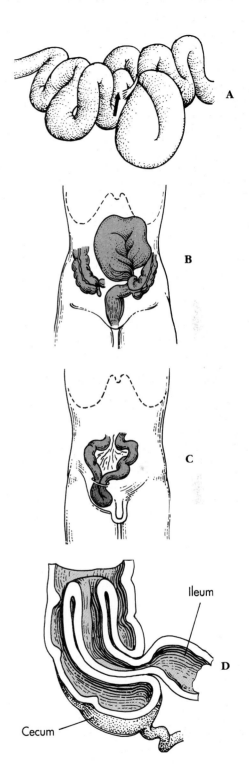

FIGURE 10-8 Common causes of intestinal obstruction. **A,** Constriction by adhesions. **B,** Volvulus of sigmoid colon. **C,** Strangulated inguinal hernia. **D,** Ileocecal intussusception.

BOX 10-8 · Tube Feeding Solutions

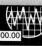 All formulas contain some balance of the essential nutrients. They vary in both nutrient balance and the amount of digestion required before absorption. Most commercial formulas contain 1 Kcal/ml in the standard formula.

PROTEIN CONTENT

Intact nutrients in pureed form
Hydrolyzed proteins from meat or soy predigested to dipeptides and amino acids
Crystalline amino acid solutions that require no digestion

CARBOHYDRATE CONTENT

Typical components: starch, polysaccharides, disaccharides, and monosaccharides
Most solutions lactose free

FAT CONTENT

Primary source of concentrated calories and essential fatty acids
Usually derived from vegetable oils

Dependent on intact bile salt and pancreatic enzyme production for digestion

CALORIC DENSITY

One of major considerations in solution osmolality
High-density formulas must frequently be diluted to ensure patient tolerance

OSMOLALITY

Primarily a reflection of carbohydrate and protein concentration
Additional free water needed with all types
  Isotonic (280-300 mOsm/kg): can usually be administered at full strength
  Hypertonic (400-1100 mOsm/kg): typically need significant dilution and slow administration to prevent serious hyperosmolar diarrhea

Guidelines for Troubleshooting Tube Feeding Problems

TUBE OBSTRUCTION

Flush tube with 30-50 ml of water before and after feedings, medication administration, and checking residuals and at least every 4 hours.
Administer medications in elixir form if possible. Crush pills thoroughly and dissolve before administration.
Attempt to irrigate obstructed tube with carbonated cola. Do not use meat tenderizer.

REGURGITATION/ASPIRATION

Confirm tube placement by x-ray after insertion and as needed if position is questioned.
Keep head of bed elevated 30-40 degrees if permitted.
Aspirate for residuals if possible. Sounds heard by injection of air reverberate throughout abdomen and can be inaccurate.
Use weighted tip or nasointestinal tubes for patients who cannot protect their airway.
Add food coloring to formula for high-risk patients.

DIARRHEA

Begin with diluted formula strength and advance slowly.
Administer at slow rate and advance slowly.

Ensure adequate supplemental free water.
Consider *Lactobacillus acidophilus* preparation if patient is receiving antibiotics.
Avoid use of lactose-based solutions.
Consider adding fiber or bulking agents.

BACTERIAL CONTAMINATION

Use prefilled, ready-to-use sets if possible.
Follow strict aseptic technique in handling.
Rinse delivery set before adding new solution.
Limit hang time for commercial formulas to 8-12 hours (no more than 6 hours for hospital-prepared formulas if possible).

HYPERGLYCEMIA (ELDERLY PATIENTS ARE AT GREATER RISK)

Monitor blood and urine glucose at intervals.
Utilize sliding-scale insulin if ordered.
Monitor respiratory rate. High carbohydrate content yields high carbon dioxide production, which may stress the respiratory system in ventilated or critically ill patients.

NURSING MANAGEMENT

◆ ASSESSMENT

Subjective Data

History and course of the symptoms
Location and severity of pain, cramping, tenderness
Patient's complaints of bloating or distention, nausea
Timing and consistency of latest bowel movement
Passage of flatus

Objective Data

Auscultation of the abdomen for the following:
  Loud, high-pitched sounds early in obstruction (borborygmi)
  Diminished or absent sounds late in obstruction
Vomiting
  Profuse, nonfecal if proximal small bowel
  Infrequent fecal type if distal bowel
Abdominal distention and increasing girth; taut, shiny skin

BOX 10-9 TPN Solutions

 Solutions are individually tailored and prepared to balance the protein, carbohydrate, fat, vitamin, and mineral components to meet the patient's unique needs for wound healing, anabolism, weight maintenance or gain, and growth in children.

PROTEIN CONTENT

Typically provides 42 g of protein per liter (3%-5% of total) as amino acids for tissue anabolism

CARBOHYDRATE CONTENT

Typically provides 25%-35% dextrose (5%-15% for peripheral solutions) content, providing about 250 g of glucose with 25% concentration

FAT CONTENT

Lipid emulsions provide major source of nonprotein calories Concentrations of 10%-20% (1.1-2.2 Kcal/ml) usually administered separately to limit incompatibility problems but may be added to TPN solution; provide twice the caloric density of dextrose and exert minimal osmotic pressure

OTHER

Balanced electrolytes
Vitamins and minerals, trace elements
Insulin may be added to the solution

 Guidelines for Administering TPN

Avoid using the TPN catheter for any other purpose if possible.
Administer TPN with volume-controlled infusion pump.
Provide frequent oral hygiene.
Preventing infection
Maintain strict aseptic technique.
Keep solutions refrigerated; use within 24-36 hours. Remove solution from refrigerator 1 hour before use.
Observe solution for cloudiness. All additions to TPN solutions should be performed under sterile laminar flow conditions.
Administer through tubing with an in-line 0.22 µm filter (1.2 µm filter if solution contains lipids or albumin). Lipids are attached below the filter.
Follow institutional protocol for handling tubing, catheter, and dressing changes.
Change tubing per institutional protocol (usually with each new bag or every 24 hours).
Attach tubing directly to central line catheter; do not attach with a needle.
Monitor insertion site for redness, swelling, or drainage.
Preventing air embolism
Tape all system connections securely.
Position patient as flat as possible for all dressing and tubing changes.
Clamp central line catheter before opening the catheter hub.
Instruct patient to perform Valsalva maneuver whenever catheter hub is open to the air.
Cover catheter insertion site with an air-occlusive dressing or transparent polyurethane (OpSite) dressing.
Managing/preventing complications
Fluid and electrolyte balance
Maintain a uniform infusion rate. Do not attempt to "catch up" if infusion falls behind schedule for any reason.
Maintain accurate intake and output.
Weigh patient daily. Suspect fluid imbalance if weight gain exceeds 1.1 lb/day.
Hyperglycemia
Monitor for nausea, weakness, thirst, headache, rapid respirations.
Check blood glucose by fingerstick every 6 hours.
Administer sliding-scale insulin as ordered.
Hypoglycemia
Monitor for pallor, diaphoresis, tachycardia, trembling, and anxiety when TPN not infusing.
Always administer glucose solution if administration of TPN is interrupted.

Signs of dehydration
Abdominal x-ray studies showing air and fluid in the bowel and a gradually worsening electrolyte profile

◆ NURSING DIAGNOSES

Possible nursing diagnoses for the person with an intestinal obstruction may include, but are not limited to, the following:
Fluid volume deficit (related to accumulation of excess fluid in the bowel)
Pain (related to pressure and accumulation of fluid and gas in the bowel)

◆ EXPECTED PATIENT OUTCOMES

Patient will exhibit physical signs of fluid balance:
Vital signs in normal range
Good skin turgor and moist mucous membranes
Serum hematocrit and electrolytes within normal limits
Urine specific gravity of 1.010 to 1.025
Stable body weight
Patient will experience relief of pain and distention.

◆ NURSING INTERVENTIONS
Promoting Fluid and Electrolyte Balance

Maintain accurate intake and output records.
Assess for fluid and electrolyte imbalance.
Monitor IV fluids carefully.

Monitor vital signs for indications of shock, fluid overload, or peritonitis.
Assess for edema and measure abdominal girth every 4 hours.
Assess for passage of flatus; auscultate for bowel sounds.
Maintain patency of intestinal tubes (Box 10-10).

Relieving Discomfort

Provide good supportive care.
Position patient comfortably and change positions frequently. Side lying is often most comfortable.

Home Care Consideration for TPN

KNOWLEDGE BASE

Review purpose and procedures for home TPN.
Review physician's instructions:
  Solution
  Dressing changes
  Tubing changes
  Monitoring
Validate understanding and skill with aseptic technique.
Review understanding of all equipment and functioning. Supplies available for home health are often different from those used in acute care.
Develop acceptable record-keeping system for body weights, temperature, and blood glucose monitoring.

SUPPLIES AND EQUIPMENT

Evaluate adequacy of home refrigeration and storage.
Establish system for regular supply monitoring and reordering.
Provide social service referral for completion of reimbursement paperwork.
Ensure safe disposal of equipment.

MANAGING COMPLICATIONS

Post list of pertinent emergency telephone numbers.
Encourage patient to acquire and use a Medic Alert ID.
Internal catheter leak: swelling, pain, heat near or over insertion site
  Stop using catheter and tape securely.
  Contact physician or home health nurse.
Leaking external catheter: leakage of blood or fluid from catheter or cap
  Clamp catheter.
  Change heparin lock and cap.
  Contact physician or emergency room for repair.
Air embolism: shortness of breath, chest pain, cough
  Stop flow of solution.
  Lie on left side.
  Contact physician immediately.
Infection: redness or swelling at insertion site or general chills, fever, hyperglycemia
  Avoid general bathing until implanted catheter is completely healed.
  Change dressings promptly if soiled or wet.
  Contact physician.

BOX 10-10 — Intestinal Tubes

Intestinal tubes are used to drain fluids and gas that accumulate above a mechanical obstruction and thereby decompress the bowel (Figure 10-9).

TYPES

Cantor tube: a single-lumen, 300 cm tube with a single opening for drainage. Its balloon is injected with 4-5 ml of mercury before insertion.
Harris tube: a single-lumen, 180 cm tube with a metal tip. Its single lumen is used for drainage or irrigation and is weighted with a prefilled mercury balloon.
Miller-Abbott tube: a double-lumen, 300 cm tube with distance markings. One lumen leads to the mercury balloon, which is filled after insertion. The second has openings along its length for drainage and irrigation.
Dennis tube: a three-lumen, 300 cm tube with one lumen for suction, one for irrigation and venting, and one for inflation of the balloon with mercury after insertion.
NOTE: The balloons act like a bolus of food, stimulating peristalsis and advancing the tube. The weight of the mercury propels the tube in the complete absence of peristalsis.

PATIENT CARE

Special care is taken during insertion, because the presence of the balloon makes passage through the nose quite difficult.
After tube passes into the stomach, its progression is aided by positioning the patient.
  Encourage patient to lie on right side for 2 hours.
  Patient switches to lying on back for 2 hours with head elevated.
  Patient lies on left side for 2 hours.
  Walking about stimulates further movement by increasing peristalsis.
Advance tube 2 to 10 cm (1 to 4 inches) at specified intervals to provide slack for peristaltic action.
Never tape tube in place until it reaches desired position.
Use intermittent suction with single-lumen tubes to prevent mucosal injury. Constant suction may be used with sump tubes.
Irrigate tube for patency if ordered—return aspiration is often not feasible.
If tube is well advanced in bowel, light food and fluid may be permitted.
Monitor patient for return of bowel sounds, passage of flatus, or spontaneous bowel movement.
Pin excess tubing to clothing.
Provide comfort measures for nose and throat: throat lozenges, ice chips.

Use Fowler's position to support ventilation.
Assist patient as needed with activities of daily living.
Provide regular skin care.
Offer frequent, scrupulous mouth care, especially if patient is vomiting.
Ensure adequate pulmonary ventilation; encourage deep breathing.
Patient should avoid mouth breathing and air swallowing.
Provide nasal care and prevent crusting of nares.
Assess degree of abdominal pain and record. Explore nonpharmacologic pain relief.

◆ EVALUATION

Successful achievement of expected outcomes for the patient with a bowel obstruction is indicated by the following:
  Fluid balance is normalized.
    Body weight is stable.
    Skin turgor is good, and mucous membranes are moist.
    Vital signs are stable.

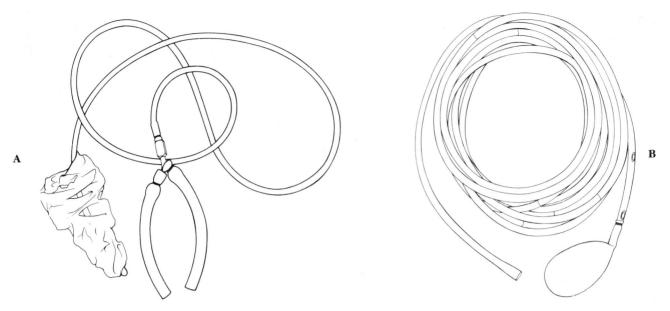

FIGURE 10-9   Intestinal tubes. **A,** Miller-Abbott tube. **B,** Cantor tube.

Blood values are all within normal limits.
Urine specific gravity is 1.010 to 1.025.
Abdominal pain and nausea are absent.

ABDOMINAL HERNIAS
Etiology/Epidemiology

A hernia occurs when an organ or other structure protrudes through a congenital or acquired defect in the muscle of the abdominal wall. Hernias can occur at any age and are more common in men and elderly persons. Hernias of the groin account for 80% of the total.

Indirect inguinal hernias develop from weaknesses in the abdominal wall acquired congenitally during fetal development of the spermatic cord in the male and round ligament in the female.

Direct inguinal hernias are located at the posterior inguinal wall and are typically caused by increased intraabdominal pressure. They are most common in elderly males.

Femoral hernias develop in women, usually in response to pregnancy-related muscle and abdominal pressure changes.

Pathophysiology

The major pathologic condition related to hernias is the risk of strangulation of the herniated segment and bowel obstruction. *Sliding hernias* move freely in and out of the hernia sac. A *reducible hernia* can be manually returned to its proper position. An *irreducible hernia* cannot be restored to its natural position and is termed *incarcerated* if bowel obstruction occurs. If the blood flow to the trapped segment is compromised, the hernia is *strangulated* and creates an acute surgical emergency.

Hernias rarely cause major symptoms beyond the

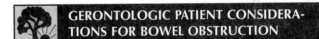

GERONTOLOGIC PATIENT CONSIDERATIONS FOR BOWEL OBSTRUCTION

Elderly persons are at particular risk for large bowel obstruction by tumor, since bowel cancer primarily affects older adults. The obstruction is rarely severe or complete, however, and the primary concern is with the cancer diagnosis. The care does not vary in any major way from that offered younger persons.

palpable protrusion that worsens with coughing or lifting. Vague discomfort and a feeling of heaviness or a "dragging" sensation are common. Incarcerated and strangulated hernias produce the acute symptoms of bowel obstruction.

Medical Management

Hernias are repaired surgically on an elective basis if possible. The procedure is straightforward, and most patients are discharged directly home. The surgeon either simply corrects the defect in the fascia or muscle or reinforces the weakened segment with fascia or synthetic material.

NURSING MANAGEMENT

Recovery from hernia surgery is usually rapid and without incident. The nurse teaches the patient to avoid all lifting for about 6 weeks. Driving and stair climbing may also be restricted.

Ice bags are applied after surgery to minimize edema, and "jockey" style underwear may be recommended to provide gentle scrotal support. The patient is taught to monitor wound healing, walk upright with good posture, and use a stool softener to prevent straining until healing occurs.

COLORECTAL CANCER

Etiology/Epidemiology

Cancer of the colon and rectum is the third most common cancer in men and the second most common in women. Its mortality is second only to lung cancer, and the 5-year survival rate remains about 52%. The incidence of the disease varies significantly worldwide, and the rates are much higher in industrialized countries, which supports a strong diet and environmental link. The mean age at onset is 65 years.

The etiology of colorectal cancer remains elusive. Research is focusing on the effect of diets high in fat and low in fiber-rich foods, but the results remain inconclusive. The presence of a mutant gene that promotes mutation in other genes and may lead to cancer is receiving considerable attention. Some researchers estimate that 95% of persons carrying the gene defect will develop some form of cancer, 60% of these cancers being colorectal. The development of colorectal cancer is also associated with long-term ulcerative colitis and the presence of adenomatous colon polyps. About 70% of all colorectal cancers develop in the distal portions of the colon, and 50% occur in the sigmoid colon and rectum. Cancer involving the small bowel is extremely rare.

Pathophysiology

Colorectal cancer may develop as a polyplike lesion or as an annular lesion that encircles the lumen of the colon. Polyps may ulcerate but rarely obstruct. In the descending and rectosigmoid portion of the colon, the constricting tumor may present with symptoms of bowel obstruction. Specific symptoms vary with position and type of tumor growth pattern. The tumor may alter bowel elimination patterns, trigger nausea or vomiting, or produce blood in the stool. Weakness, anorexia, and weight loss are nonspecific symptoms that occur frequently with colorectal cancer. There are frequently *no* early symptoms.

Early diagnosis of colorectal cancer is critical. It is estimated that 75% of cases would be curable if detected early, but little agreement exists over screening guidelines. The American Cancer Society currently recommends the following:

Annual digital rectal examination after 40 years
Annual occult blood screening after 50 years
Proctoscopy/sigmoidoscopy every 5 years after 50 years
Accuracy and cost of testing are major factors. Sigmoidoscopy is very accurate with distal tumors but expensive and very unacceptable to patients. The effectiveness of occult blood screening is less clear. Extremely contradictory study results exist. The standard tests are fairly insensitive in identifying disease in asymptomatic persons. The carcinoembryonic antigen (CEA) tumor marker is also not sensitive for diagnosis but is useful in monitoring for recurrences.

BOX 10-11	Types of Colostomies

END STOMA
The proximal bowel is brought out through the incision and sutured to the skin.

LOOP STOMA
The bowel segment is brought intact through the incision with a support under it. The upper wall is opened, creating one stoma with two openings. It is usually temporary.

LOOP END STOMA
The loop procedure is used, and the distal loop is oversewn with an end stoma created from the proximal portion.

MUCOUS FISTULA
The distal bowel is preserved and a second stoma created that secretes mucus.

Medical Management

Surgery remains the primary treatment approach. Chemotherapy plays no role in primary treatment but is used for metastatic disease. Radiation is extensively used for rectal cancer but is ineffective as a primary treatment for colon tumors.

The surgical approach has typically involved removal of the tumor, surrounding colon, and lymph nodes. Resection with anastomosis is possible in the ascending, transverse, or descending colon but was not generally considered possible for rectal tumors. Abdominoperineal resection has been standard with removal of the entire rectum and anus and creation of a permanent colostomy. Options for colostomy formation are summarized in Box 10-11. Newer sphincter-sparing approaches are now being used with patients who have early localized rectal disease. They involve regional rectal resection, reanastomosis, and supplemental radiotherapy and chemotherapy to prevent recurrence. Early studies show promising results.

NURSING MANAGEMENT

♦ ASSESSMENT
Subjective Data

Emotional response to need for surgery, usual coping strategies
Knowledge of planned surgical procedure
Previous exposure to ostomies or ostomy care
Available support mechanisms

Objective Data

Nutritional status
Cognitive ability, vision, memory
Manual dexterity
Ostomy site planning and marking (if indicated)

A wide variety of materials are available commercially to care for ostomies. Patients need to explore factors such as convenience, cost, and local availability as they develop a self-care plan.

POUCH OPTIONS

An effective system protects the skin, contains odor and stool, permits movement, and is inconspicuous. Options include the following:

One-piece and two-piece systems, with or without attached skin barriers

Drainable (reusable) and nondrainable (disposable) (Figure 10-10) systems

Drainable pouches are changed about every 3-7 days and must be rinsed carefully, especially around the drainage spout, to prevent odor.

SKIN CARE PRODUCTS

Peristomal skin is vulnerable to irritation from stool, tape, and pouch adhesives. Prevention of skin problems is essential.

SKIN BARRIERS

Skin barriers exist in several forms and are an important means for protecting the skin:

Powder (karaya or stoma-adhesive powder): must be sealed for pouch to adhere

Paste: used around stoma and to fill in skin creases

Wafers: used with a variety of pouches to protect the skin from stool (Figure 10-11)

Sealants: sprays, liquids, gels that coat the skin and are useful under pouch adhesives

BOX 10-13	Pouch Change Procedure

Measure stoma carefully. Size varies slightly during early months.

Appliance is cut ⅛ to ¼ inch larger than stoma.

Prepare skin barrier the same way.

Remove old pouch. Gently peel away wafer top to bottom.

Cleanse peristomal skin with warm water and pat dry.

Center pouch opening over stoma and gently press in place.

Change nondrainable pouches when half full.

Change drainable pouches every 4-7 days.

Never "prick" a pouch to release gas, because this destroys odor-proof quality.

Consult with enterostomal therapist if problems occur.

◆ NURSING INTERVENTIONS

Preoperative Care

Reinforce all teaching about surgery and ostomy procedure.

Provide written materials from American Cancer Society.

Include family in teaching sessions if possible.

Refer patient to enterostomal therapist if available.

Assist with site selection and marking.

Clarify understanding of surgery's impact on sexuality.

Implement bowel-cleansing protocol.

Reduce diet from low residue to clear fluids.

Administer laxatives and enemas as ordered.

Administer oral antibiotic to reduce bowel flora.

Postoperative Care

Managing the perineal wound

Maintain patency of perineal drains.

Assess nature and quantity of drainage (copious serosanguineous drainage is common).

Perform wound irrigations as ordered by catheter or Water Pik and assess for healing.

Change absorbent dressings as needed.

Assist patient to find comfortable position—use foam pads or pillows for sitting. Side lying limits stress on incision and discomfort.

Monitoring the stoma

Assess color and degree of edema.

Report color changes or presence of dark or dusky brown color.

Adjust opening as needed for changes from edema (resolves in 5 to 7 days).

Report any frank bleeding.

Assess anchoring sutures for intactness. Initially secretions are mucus. Fecal drainage resumes in 4 to 7 days.

◆ NURSING DIAGNOSES

Possible nursing diagnoses for the person undergoing colostomy surgery for colorectal cancer may include, but are not limited to, the following:

Health maintenance, high risk of altered (related to lack of knowledge concerning stoma and skin care)

Self-concept disturbance, high risk of (related to impact of ostomy on life-style and body image)

Grieving (related to diagnosis of cancer, uncertain prognosis, and altered body function)

◆ EXPECTED PATIENT OUTCOMES

Patient will demonstrate understanding of components of ostomy care including the following:

Pouch changes, skin care, irrigation

Diet modifications to control odor and flatus

Symptoms requiring medical attention

Patient will verbalize feelings about the need for the ostomy and actively participate in stoma care.

Patient will express grief and discuss the personal meaning of the diagnosis and surgery.

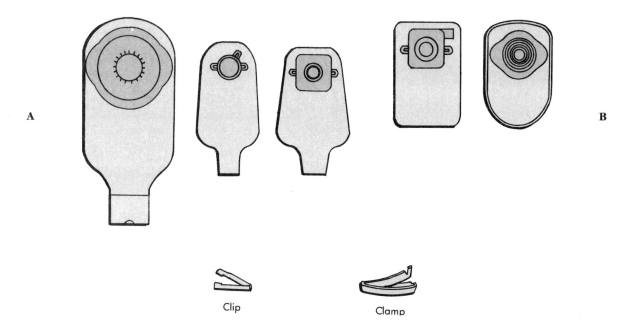

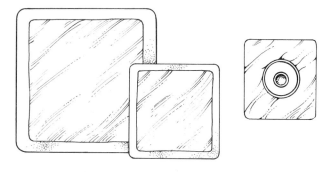

FIGURE 10-10 Common ostomy products. **A,** Drainable pouches. **B,** Nondrainable pouches.

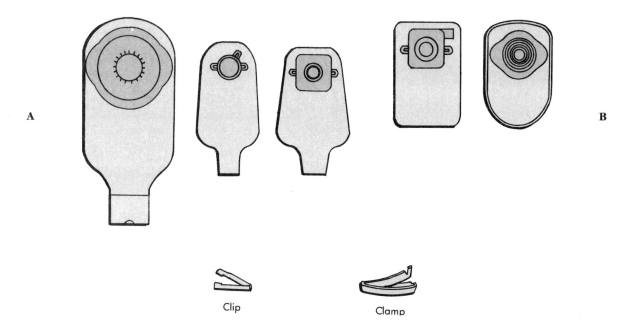

FIGURE 10-11 Skin barrier products.

NOTE: Loop colostomies may be opened on the unit. Procedure is frightening, but the bowel has no sensory nerve endings and causes no pain.

Teaching for self-care

Teach the basic principles of ostomy management: stoma care, skin care, pouch changes, irrigations.

Provide opportunity to handle, assemble, and use all equipment. Allow time for practice.

Coordinate teaching plan with enterostomal therapist and make referrals for community ostomy services.

Encourage patient to look at and touch the stoma. Reinforce all efforts at self-care involvement. Provide written resources for home use. See Boxes 10-12 and 10-13 and Guidelines box on p. 237 for specifics about teaching.

Promoting a positive self-concept

Encourage patient to view stoma and become involved with self-care.

Use a matter-of-fact approach, but offer emotional support.

Encourage patient to meet with a peer visitor from the Ostomy Association.

Discuss issues openly with patient, for example, clothing, hygiene, exercise and recreation, impact of stoma on body image and sexuality.

Discuss diet modifications to control gas and odor.

Resolving grief

Encourage patient to express sense of loss.

Explore coping resources.

Refer to community support groups.

Encourage open discussion between patient and spouse or partner, particularly over sexual concerns.

Guidelines for Teaching Patient Colostomy Irrigation

The procedure involves administering an enema through the stoma to stimulate bowel emptying at a predictable time. The procedure is no longer routinely recommended but may be taught if the patient chooses.

PROCEDURE

Position patient on toilet or on padded chair next to toilet if perineal wound has not healed.
Remove old pouch.
Clean skin and stoma with water.
Apply irrigating sleeve and belt.
Fill bag with desired amount of tepid water (250-1000 ml).
Hang bag so bottom of bag is at shoulder height.
Remove air from tubing.
Gently insert irrigating cone snugly into stoma, holding it parallel to floor. Insert catheter no more than 2-4 inches.
Let water run in slowly until patient identifies need to expel stool. Halt irrigation if cramping occurs.
Remove cone and allow solution to drain into container.
When most of stool is expelled (about 15 minutes), rinse sleeve with water and close up bottom end.
Encourage activity to complete bowel emptying (about 30-45 minutes).
Remove sleeve and apply clean pouch.

◆ EVALUATION

Successful achievement of expected outcomes for the patient undergoing colostomy surgery or colorectal surgery is indicated by the following:

Accurate performance of ostomy care
Description of symptoms indicating stoma problems
Successful liaison with community resources
Expressed acceptance of ostomy
Verbalization of concerns between sexual partners
Return to presurgical life-style pattern

■ ■ ■

A critical pathway for a patient undergoing colon resection without colostomy is presented.

ANORECTAL LESIONS
Etiology/Epidemiology

A variety of common disorders can affect the perianal region, including the following:

GERONTOLOGIC PATIENT CONSIDERATIONS FOR COLOSTOMY SURGERY

The incidence of bowel cancer is highest in the elderly population. The issues of general health and comorbidity are extremely important to the outcome. The challenges of learning an ostomy self-care regimen are significant in older individuals who may have difficulty processing new information or acquiring psychomotor skills. The hospitalization will be brief, and referral to community support and ostomy services will be essential for success.

Hemorrhoids are masses of dilated blood vessels that lie beneath the skin in the anal canal. They affect up to 50% of the population by 50 years of age. There are two main types. Internal hemorrhoids lie above the anal sphincter, and external ones lie below. Pregnancy, obesity, chronic constipation, and portal hypertension are all causative factors.

Anal fissure is an elongated laceration between the anal canal and perianal skin. It may be idiopathic or occur in response to chronic constipation or ulceration.

Anal abscesses result typically from obstruction of gland ducts in the anal region by feces. Stasis leads to infection in adjacent tissue.

Anal fistula involves the development of an abnormal communication between the anal canal and outside skin. It may form from the rupture of an abscess.

Pathophysiology

Hemorrhoids have been compared to varicose veins but are actually composed of spongy vascular tissue with direct arteriovenous connections. External hemorrhoids are readily apparent with an exterior skinfold. They rarely bleed and seldom cause pain unless they become thrombosed or inflamed. Internal hemorrhoids are the most common cause of painless rectal bleeding. They remain basically asymptomatic unless they prolapse or thrombose. Pain and itching are not present except when complications occur.

Most anal fissures heal spontaneously and are superficial. The severity of the infection typically determines the course of abscesses and fistulas. Pain is the primary symptom, because there is a rich network of somatic nerves in the perianal area. Constipation develops in an effort to avoid defecation, and local swelling, tenderness, and pruritus are common. Purulent drainage may signify an abscess or fistula.

Medical Management

A variety of treatment options exist for hemorrhoids:

Sclerotherapy involves injection of a sclerosing agent into small internal hemorrhoids. It produces fibrous induration of the distended veins. The treatment is palliative.

Cryosurgery or *photocoagulation* is use of intense heat or cold to destroy the hemorrhoidal tissue and produce tissue necrosis. A prolonged discharge as the tissue sloughs makes this an unpopular approach.

Ligation with latex bands is a very effective approach to internal hemorrhoids. The tissue necroses and sloughs off within 1 week (Figure 10-12).

Hemorrhoidectomy is surgical excision of external hemorrhoids and those that do not respond to conservative treatment.

Anal fissures are usually treated supportively, with analgesics, stool softeners, and sitz baths, until the tissue heals. Abscesses are usually opened and drained, and fistulas may require extensive surgical repair.

CRITICAL PATHWAY   **Colon Resection Without Colostomy**

DRG #: 152; expected LOS: 8

	Day of Admission Day 1	Day of Surgery Day 2	Day 3	Day 4
Diagnostic Tests	CBC, UA, SMA/18,* chest x-ray films, ECG, T & X	CBC, electrolytes		CBC, electrolytes
Medications	IV saline lock; IV antibiotics; colon cleansing, e.g., oral laxatives, enemas	IVs, IV antibiotics, IV analgesic	IVs, IV antibiotics, IV analgesic	IVs, IV antibiotics, IV analgesic
Treatments	Wt, VS q 8 hr	I & O q 8 hr, including NG and Foley; check drainage on dressing q 2 hr; elastic leg stockings; mouth and nares care q 2 hr	I & O q 8 hr, including NG and Foley; check dressing for drainage q 4 hr, VS q 4 hr; wt; elastic leg stockings; mouth and nares care q 2 hr; assess bowel sounds q 4 hr	I & O q 8 hr, including NG and Foley; check dressing for drainage q 4 hr, VS q 6 hr; elastic leg stockings; mouth and nares care q 2 hr; assess bowel sounds q 4 hr
Diet	Clear liquids; NPO p MN	NPO	NPO	NPO
Activity	Up ad lib	Bed rest; up in chair with assistance x 1; T, C & DB q 2 hr	Bed rest; up in room with assistance x 4; T, C & DB q 2 hr	Bed rest; up in chair with assistance x 6; T, C & DB q 2 hr
Consultations	Anesthesiologist; other specialists as needed for other medical problems			SNU care/or home health

NOTE: Acknowledge that patients recover at varying rates; therefore specified daily actions should be based solely on patient need.
CBC, Complete blood cell count; *Disc*, discontinue; *I & O*, intake and output; LOS, length of stay; *p MN*, after midnight; *SMA*, sequential multiple analysis; *SNU*, skilled nursing unit; *T, C & DB*, turn, cough, and deep breathe; *T & X*, type and crossmatch; *UA*, urinalysis; *VS*, vital signs; *Wt*, weight.

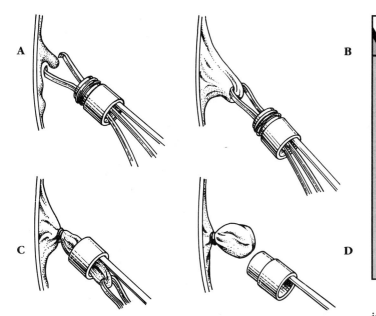

FIGURE 10-12   Rubber band ligation of internal hemorrhoid.

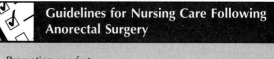

Guidelines for Nursing Care Following Anorectal Surgery

Promoting comfort
    Administer analgesics as prescribed.
    Position patient prone or side lying.
    Provide sitz baths every 4 hours.
Restoring normal elimination
    Administer laxatives and stool softeners as ordered.
    Administer analgesics before defecation.
    Monitor for hypotension or dizziness.
    Cleanse rectal area carefully after defecation.
Discharge teaching
    Avoid constipation with high-fiber diet and liberal fluid intake.
    Use stool softeners until healing is complete.
    Do not strain at defecation.
    Contact surgeon if bleeding or foul drainage develops.

NURSING MANAGEMENT

Conservative approaches to hemorrhoids may prevent the need for any definitive interventions. The nurse encourages the patient to follow a fiber-rich diet, increase fluid intake, exercise regularly, and utilize bulk laxatives and stool softeners as needed to prevent straining at stool. During periods of flare-up, local applications of ice, heat, and analgesic ointments may increase comfort. Careful hygiene is important, and sitz baths may increase the success of cleansing.

Similar interventions are used to increase comfort with fissures and abscesses. Diet and life-style changes will help to prevent recurrences. Care of the patient undergoing anorectal surgery is summarized in the Guidelines box.

CRITICAL PATHWAY	Colon Resection Without Colostomy

DRG #: 152; expected LOS: 8

Day 5	Day 6	Day 7	Day of Discharge Day 8
	CBC, electrolytes		
IV rate decreased as PO fluid increased; IV antibiotics; IM to PO analgesic	IV to saline lock; IV antibiotics; PO analgesic, stool softener	Discontinue antibiotic; PO analgesic, stool softener	Discontinue saline lock
I & O q 8 hr (?discontinue NG and Foley); check dressing for drainage q 6 hr, VS q 6 hr; elastic leg stockings; mouth and nares care q 2 hr; assess bowel sounds q 4 hr	I & O q 8 hr, VS q 8 hr; wt; assess bowel sounds q 8 hr; elastic leg stockings	Discontinue I & O; VS q 8 hr; assess bowel sounds q 8 hr; elastic leg stockings	VS q 8 hr; elastic leg stockings
Begin clear liquids	Clear liquids; advance to soft diet	Soft	Soft
Up walking in hallway with assistance x 3; up in chair x 6	Up walking in hallway with assistance x 4; up in chair ad lib	Up ad lib; walking in hallway	Up ad lib; walking in hallway

*Serum calcium, phosphorus, triglycerides, uric acid, creatinine, BUN, total bilirubin, alkaline phosphate, asparate aminotransferase (AST) (formerly serum glutamic-oxaloacetic transaminase [SGOT]), alanine aminotransferase (ALT) (formerly serum glutamate pyruvate transaminase [SGPT]), lactic dehydrogenase (LDH), total protein, albumin, sodium, potassium, chloride, total CO_2, glucose.

SELECTED REFERENCES

Ahern H, Rice K: How do you measure gastric pH, *Am J Nurs* 91:70-73, 1991.

Ahlquist DA et al: Accuracy of fecal occult blood screening for colorectal neoplasia, *JAMA* 269(10):1262-1267, 1993.

Beck ML: Percutaneous endoscopic gastrostomy, *Am J Nurs* 89(6):76-78, 1989.

Benedict P, Haddad A: Postop teaching for the colostomy patient, *RN* 52(3):85-90, 1989.

Black J, Mangan M: Body contouring and weight loss surgery for obesity, *Nurs Clin North Am* 26(3):777-789, 1991.

Black M: Crohn's disease, pathophysiology, diagnosis and management, *Gastroenterol Nurs* 2(4):259-262, 1989.

Blaylock B: Enhancing self care of the elderly client: practical teaching tips for ostomy care, *J ET Nurs* 18(4):118-121, 1991.

Bockus S: Troubleshooting your tube feedings, *Am J Nurs* 91(5):24-30, 1991.

Bockus S: When your patient needs tube feedings, *Nurs 93* 23(7):34-42, 1993.

Bruckstein DC: Percutaneous endoscopic gastrostomy, *Geriatr Nurs* 9(2):32-33, 1988.

Bryant GA: When the bowel is blocked, *RN* 55(1):58-66, 1992.

Bufalino J, Kolisetty L, McCaskey GW, Stratton KL: Surgery for morbid obesity: the patient's experience, *Appl Nurs Res* 2(1):16-22, 1989.

Burris J, McGovern P: Mass colorectal cancer screening, *AAOHN J* 41(4):186-191, 1993.

DiIorio C, Price ME: Swallowing: an assessment guide, *Am J Nurs* 90(7):38-46, 1990.

Eisenberg P: Enteral nutrition: indications, formulas and delivery techniques, *Nurs Clin North Am* 24(2):315-337, 1989.

Eisenberg P: Monitoring gastric pH to prevent stress ulcer syndrome, *Focus Crit Care* 17:316-322, 1990.

Faller N, Lawrence KG: Comparing low profile gastrostomy tubes, *Nurs 93* 23(12):46-49, 1993.

Feikert DM, Jillson E, Palazzo T: Gastrectomy for stomach carcinoma, *AORN J* 47:1396-1406, 1988.

Gardner SS, Messner RL: Gastrointestinal bleeding, *RN* 12:43-46, 1992.

Hennessy KA: Now TPN therapy begins at home, *RN* 51(6):81-84, 1988.

Hennessy KA: Nutritional support and gastrointestinal disease, *Nurs Clin North Am* 24(2):373-381, 1989.

Holmgren C: Abdominal assessment, *RN* 55(3):28-33, 1992.

Irwin M: Managing leaking gastrostomy sites, *Am J Nurs* 88:359-360, 1988.

Jess LW: Acute abdominal pain: revealing the source, *Nurs 93* 23(9):34-41, 1993.

Johndrow PD: Making your patient and family feel at home with TPN, *Nurs 88* 18(10):65-69, 1988.

Johns JL: When the patient has an ulcer, *RN* 11:44-50, 1991.

Kinash RG: IBD: implications for the patient, challenges for the nurse, *Rehab Nurs* 34(12):82-89, 1989.

Kohn CL, Keithley JK: Enteral nutrition: potential complications and patient monitoring, *Nurs Clin North Am* 24(2):339-350, 1989.

Konopad E, Noseworthy T: Stress ulceration: a serious complication in critically ill patients, *Heart Lung* 17:339-348, 1988.

Krasner D: Six steps to successful stoma care, *RN* 56(7):32-38, 1993.

Lindsey M: Abdominal assessment, *Orthop Nurs* 8(4):34-38, 1989.

Long LV: Ileostomy care: overcoming the obstacles, *Nurs 91* 21(10):73-75, 1991.

Massoni M: GI handbook, *Nurs 90* 20(11):65-80, 1990.

McConnell E: Auscultating bowel sounds, *Nurs 90* 20(6):76-79, 1990.

McMillan SC: Validity and reliability of the constipation assessment scale, *Ca Nurs* 12(3):183-188, 1989.

McShane RE: Constipation: impact of etiological factors, *J Gerontol Nurs* 14(4):31-34, 46-47, 1988.

McVey L: A direct assault on abdominal cancers, *RN* 55(2):46-52, 1992.

Meehan M: Nursing Dx: potential for aspiration, *RN* 55(1):30-34, 1992.

Meize-Grochowski AR: When the Dx is Crohn's disease, *RN* 54(2):52-55, 1991.

Mertes JE: Action stat! GI bleeding, *Nurs 89* 19(8):37, 1989.

Morton PG: Improving your palpation techniques, *Nurs 89* 19(12):32C-32F, 1989.

Neill KM, Rice KT, Ahern HL: Comparison of two methods of measuring gastric pH, *Heart Lung* 22(4):349-355, 1993.

Novak LT: Accelerated recovery technique: a new approach to abdominal surgery, *Nurs 92* 22(7):48-55, 1992.

O'Toole MT: Advanced assessment of the abdomen and gastrointestinal problems, *Nurs Clin North Am* 25(4):771-775, 1990.

Patras A: Managing GI bleeding: it takes a two tract mind, *Nurs 88* 18(4):68-74, 1988.

Paulford-Lecher N: Teaching your patient stoma care, *Nurs 93* 23(9):47-49, 1993.

Perkins SB, Kennally KM: The hidden danger of internal hemorrhage, *Nurs 89* 19(7):34-41, 1989.

Prevost SS, Oberle A: Stress ulceration in the critically ill patient, *Crit Care Nurs Clin North Am* 5(1):163-169, 1992.

Renkes J: GI endoscopy: managing the full scope of care, *Nurs 93* 23(6):50-55, 1993.

Roberts MK: Assessing and treating volvulus, *Nurs 92* 22(2):56-58, 1992.

Smith CE: Assessing bowel sounds, *Nurs 88* 18(2):42-44, 1988.

Starkey JF, Jefferson PA, Kirby DF: Taking care of a percutaneous endoscopic gastrostomy, *Am J Nurs* 88:42-45, 1988.

Wadle KR: Diarrhea, *Nurs Clin North Am* 25(4):901-910, 1990.

Wang JF: Stomach cancer, *Semin Oncol Nurs* 4:257-264, 1988.

Wardell TL: Assessing and managing a gastric ulcer, *Nurs 91* 21(3):34-41, 1991.

Webber-Jones J: How to declog a feeding tube, *Nurs 92* 22(4):62-64, 1992.

Wilkinson M: Nursing implications after endoscopic cholangiopancreatography, *Gastroenterol Nurs* 13(2):105-109, 1990.

Worthington PH, Wagner BA: Total parenteral nutrition, *Nurs Clin North Am* 24(2):355-369, 1989.

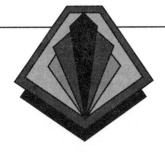

Disorders of the Liver, Biliary System, and Pancreas

◆ ASSESSMENT

SUBJECTIVE DATA

Health history
  Previous biliary, hepatic, or pancreatic disorders or surgery
  Medication use, both prescribed and over the counter (OTC)
  Concurrent illnesses, health risks
    Alcohol use, drugs of abuse
    Smoking history
    Occupational risks and exposure to potential toxins
    Recent foreign travel
Diet and nutrition
  Usual dietary patterns, nutritional adequacy
    24-hour diet recall assessment
  Use of special diet (e.g., low sodium) and adherence
  Cultural and religious influences on diet
  Changes in appetite
  Food tolerances and intolerances (e.g., fatty foods)
Current health problem
  Abdominal pain
    Location, nature, severity, and duration
    Relationship to food and alcohol intake

Factors that alleviate or exacerbate discomfort
    Self-treatment measures attempted and effectiveness
  Nausea and vomiting
    Presence, frequency, and severity
    Precipitating factors, association with food intake
    Self-treatment measures attempted and effectiveness
  Pruritus
    Presence, duration, and severity
    Factors that alleviate or exacerbate the itching
  Energy level
    Presence and severity of fatigue or weakness
    Impact on occupation, social, and activities of daily living (ADL) abilities
  Fluid and electrolytes
    Presence, location, and severity of edema
      Hands, feet, legs, abdominal girth
      Weight changes
  Elimination patterns
    Changes in color of urine or stool
    Presence of blood
    Change in urine volume

OBJECTIVE DATA

Inspection
  General appearance
    Chronic illness
    Nutritional status
    Presence and severity of tremor
  Skin and mucous membranes
    Presence and severity of jaundice
    Presence of bruising or palmar erythema
  Abdomen
    Contour, degree of enlargement
    Presence of distended or dilated periumbilical veins (caput medusae)
    Ascites: glistening skin, protruding umbilicus
Fluid status
  Vital signs, orthostatic blood pressure, temperature
  Skin turgor
  Condition of mucous membranes
  Intake and output balance
  Weight

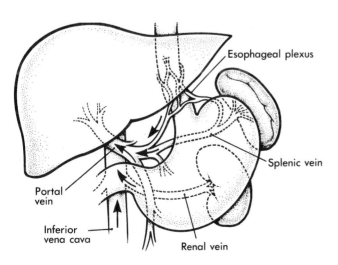

FIGURE 11-1 Portal circulation.

GERONTOLOGIC CONSIDERATIONS: PHYSIOLOGIC CHANGES IN HEPATIC, BILIARY, AND PANCREATIC FUNCTION

LIVER

Decrease in number and size of hepatic cells, which decreases organ size and weight

Increase in fibrous tissue in liver

    Decreased protein synthesis

    Possible decrease in enzyme production for drug metabolism

Liver function studies normal unless pathologic condition present

BILIARY SYSTEM

Increased cholesterol content of bile

Increased incidence of gallstones

PANCREAS

Hyperplasia of ducts and increase in fibrous tissue

Decreased production of pancreatic enzymes

Documented changes occur in all three organs with aging, but the changes are relatively minor and cause little or no disruption of normal function in an otherwise healthy elder. Drug metabolism must be considered with the use of all drugs cleared by the liver, and the increased incidence of gallstones is noteworthy in this population.

Mental status

    Level of consciousness, alertness

    Affect and responsiveness

    Confusion or disorientation

    Handwriting or drawing sample

Palpation

    Hepatic size, consistency, and tenderness

    Presence of fluid

    Abdominal girth

✍ DIAGNOSTIC TESTS

LABORATORY TESTS

Multiple tests may be used to evaluate the functioning of the liver, biliary system, and pancreas. Tests are often performed repetitively to obtain data concerning functioning over time. Major blood and urine tests are summarized in Table 11-1.

Peritoneal Fluid Analysis

Purpose—Peritoneal fluid analysis is performed to help determine the cause of ascites and to detect the presence of abdominal trauma. The fluid sample is obtained by paracentesis.

Procedure—The patient is positioned seated or in a high Fowler's position. The puncture site or sites are prepared, and a local anesthetic is injected. The site is usually 1 to 2 inches below the umbilicus. The needle is inserted, the fluid sample is removed, and a pressure dressing is applied to the site. The procedure takes about 30 minutes. The paracentesis may be combined with peritoneal lavage in instances of abdominal trauma to evaluate for bleeding.

Patient preparation and aftercare—No special pretest preparation is required except careful teaching to ensure informed consent. Baseline vital signs and abdominal girth are recorded, and the patient is encouraged to void before the test. Vital signs are monitored after the test until they are stable, and the puncture site is monitored for bleeding or drainage. Abdominal girth recordings may be ordered, and the urine is assessed for signs of bleeding. If a large amount of fluid has been removed, the patient is carefully monitored for signs of hypovolemic shock or peritonitis and may receive IV fluids.

RADIOLOGIC TESTS

Many of the tests used to evaluate functioning of the liver, biliary system, and pancreas overlap those used in a general gastrointestinal (GI) workup (see Chapter 10).

Ultrasonography

Purpose—Ultrasonography involves the use of high-frequency sound waves that are transmitted into the abdomen and create echoes that vary with tissue density. It reveals organ size, position, and shape and is extremely useful in diagnosing cysts, tumors, and stones. It has become the procedure of choice for evaluating jaundice and gallbladder disease, because it readily distinguishes obstructive and nonobstructive forms. It is also useful in visualizing the pancreas and does not expose the patient to radiation.

Procedure—The patient is placed in a supine position. A water-soluble lubricant is applied to the transducer, and multiple scans are taken of the targeted organ. The patient may be asked to exhale deeply and hold his or her breath during each scanning pass. The test is both safe and painless and takes about 15 to 30 minutes to complete.

Patient preparation and aftercare—The patient is usually instructed to fast for 8 to 12 hours before the test. A low-fat evening meal is prescribed if the gallbladder is the focus of the test to allow bile to accumulate in the gallbladder and enhance visualization. No after-test care is required.

Computed Tomography (CT Scan)

Purpose—CT scanning may also be used for all three organs and is useful in identifying problems similar to ultrasonography. It provides more accurate images in obese individuals, however, when increased tissue density limits the effectiveness of ultrasound transmission. Contrast medium may be used to enhance visualization of vascular structures and liver parenchyma.

Procedure—The patient is placed in a supine position, and the table is positioned within the scanner. A series of films are taken and reconstructed into images by a computer. The total test takes about ½ hour.

TABLE 11-1 Blood and Urine Tests of the Liver, Biliary System, and Exocrine Pancreas

TEST	NORMAL RANGE OF VALUES	DESCRIPTION
BLOOD TESTS		
Biliary System		
Total bilirubin	0.1-1.0 mg/dl	Bilirubin is excreted in the bile. Obstruction in the biliary tract contributes primarily to a rise in conjugated (direct) values.
Conjugated (direct)	0.1-0.3 mg/dl	
Unconjugated (indirect)	0.1-0.8 mg/dl	
Alkaline phosphatase	30-85 ImU/ml	Alkaline phosphatase is found in many tissues with high concentrations in bone, liver, and biliary tract epithelium. Obstructive biliary tract disease and carcinoma may cause significant elevations.
Pancreas		
Amylase	80-150 Somogyi units	Amylase is secreted normally by the acinar cells of the pancreas. Damage to these cells or obstruction of the pancreatic duct causes the enzyme to be absorbed into the blood in significant quantities. It is a sensitive yet nonspecific test for pancreatic disease.
Lipase	0-110 units/L	Lipase is a pancreatic enzyme normally secreted into the duodenum. It appears in the blood when damage occurs to the acinar cells. It is a specific test for pancreatic disease.
Calcium	9.0-11.5 mg/dl	Calcium levels may be low in cases of severe pancreatitis or steatorrhea, because calcium soaps are formed from the sequestration of calcium by fat necrosis.
Liver		
Serum enzymes	8-20 units/L	An enzyme found in large quantities in the liver. Elevated levels occur with necrosis of liver cells and enzyme release into the blood. Also present in high levels in skeletal and cardiac muscle.
Aspartate aminotransferase (AST), formerly called serum glutamic-oxaloacetic transaminase (SGOT)	5-40 IU/L 8-20 units/L (SI units)	
Alanine aminotransferase (ALT), formerly called serum glutamic-pyruvic transaminase (SGPT)	5-35 IU/L	Same as AST. Primarily found in the liver.
Lactic dehydrogenase (LDH)	45-90 units/L 115-225 IU/L 0.4-1.7 μmol/L (SI units)	Same as AST. Found in cardiac, kidney, and skeletal muscle as well as liver. Tissue source can be determined by isoenzymes.
Gamma-glutamyl transpeptidase (GGT) (γ-glutamyltransferase)	8-38 units/L	Same as AST. Also found in high levels in kidney cells. Elevates early in liver disease and stays elevated as long as damage persists.
Alkaline phosphatase	30-85 ImU/ml	Enzyme originates in liver, bone, and intestine. Elevated in liver disease but much greater elevation in biliary disease.
Albumin	3.4-5.0 g/dl	Made only in liver; in hepatocellular disease there may be a decrease in serum albumin level.
Blood urea nitrogen (BUN)	10-20 mg/dl	In severe hepatocellular disease if portal venous flow is obstructed, level may decrease; varies with dietary protein intake and fluid volume.
Immunoglobulins	IgG: 565-1765 mg/dl IgA: 85-385 mg/dl IgM: 55-375 mg/dl IgD and IgE: minimal	Five classes of antibodies (IgA, IgG, IgM, IgE, and IgD): IgA and IgG are often increased in the presence of cirrhosis; IgG is elevated in the presence of chronic active hepatitis; biliary cirrhosis and hepatitis A cause an increase in the IgM component.
Ammonia	15-110 μg/dl 47-65 μmol/L (SI units)	Ammonia, a by-product of protein metabolism, is converted into urea by the liver. Ammonia levels rise when the liver is unable to catabolize it.
Antigens and antibodies of viral hepatitis	—	Hepatitis antigens are not normally present. Antibodies appear in the acute and early convalescent period and are used to confirm diagnosis of hepatitis A. Type B has many associated serum particles.
URINE TESTS		
Urine bilirubin	None	Bilirubin is not normally excreted in the urine. Biliary stricture, inflammation, or stones may cause its presence.
Urobilinogen	24-hr collection: 0.2-1.2 units 24-hr collection: 0.05-2.5 mg	A sensitive test for hepatic or biliary disease. Decreased levels are seen in biliary obstruction and pancreatic cancer.
Urine amylase	10-80 amylase units/hr	A rise in level usually mimics the rise in serum amylase. The level remains elevated for 7-10 days, however, which allows for retrospective diagnosis.

Patient preparation and aftercare—The patient is kept NPO for 8 to 12 hours before the test and receives instructions about the test. The patient is carefully assessed for any history of allergy to contrast media, iodine, or shellfish. The patient is instructed to keep very still during the test and hold his or her breath when requested. The injection of the contrast medium may cause a transient feeling of warmth or flushing. The development of nausea or headache should be reported. No special aftercare is needed.

Radionuclide Imaging

Purpose—Liver scanning may be employed to detect focal disease or tumors, screen for hepatic metastases, or detect hepatomegaly. Its use is being largely replaced by CT scanning or ultrasonography.

Procedure—The patient receives an injection of a radioactive colloid and then is placed in a supine position. The liver is scanned, and determination is made of the amount of radiation coming from the organ. Nonfunctioning areas show decreased activity, whereas tumors usually show increased activity. The test takes about 1 hour.

Patient preparation and aftercare—The patient receives instructions about the test and reassurance about the brief half-life and safety of the radioactive isotope. No specific pretest preparation is required. The patient is monitored for any adverse reaction to the injection. No posttest care is required.

Oral Cholecystography

Purpose—Oral cholecystography involves the radiographic examination of the gallbladder after administration of a contrast medium. It is used to detect gallstones and aid in diagnosis of inflammatory disorders or tumors. Once considered the standard test it has now been largely replaced by ultrasonography.

Procedure—A healthy liver removes radiopaque drugs and stores them in the gallbladder. The abdomen is scanned fluoroscopically from several directions during the test. A high-fat food or drink may be administered during the test to stimulate the emptying of the gallbladder. The procedure takes about 45 minutes.

Patient preparation and aftercare—The patient is carefully assessed for allergies to contrast media, iodine, or shellfish. The patient is instructed to eat a low-fat evening meal and then is restricted to only water orally. Radiopaque tablets are administered 2 to 3 hours after the evening meal, and the dose is based on the patient's body weight. The pills are taken one at a time at 5- to 10-minute intervals with liberal amounts of water. The tablets can produce abdominal discomfort, vomiting, or diarrhea. No specific aftercare is required.

Cholangiography

Purpose—Cholangiography involves examination of the bile ducts to demonstrate the presence of stones,

strictures, or tumors. The dye may be administered intravenously (IV), percutaneously, or through a T-tube after surgery.

Procedure—The patient is positioned supine for the scanning portion of the test. The dye is injected by one of the methods outlined, and the movement of the dye is tracked fluoroscopically. The procedure takes about 30 minutes.

Patient preparation and aftercare—The patient is kept NPO for 8 hours before the test. The patient is instructed about the test and evaluated for risk of hypersensitivity. The injection of the dye may cause temporary pain and a sense of epigastric fullness. Vital signs are monitored, and the patient rests in bed for about 6 hours after the test, usually on the right side. The insertion site is monitored for signs of bleeding or infection.

LIVER BIOPSY

Purpose—Liver biopsy involves needle aspiration of a core of tissue for histologic analysis. It is used to diagnose liver infection, disease, or malignancy.

Procedure—The patient is positioned supine and instructed to remain absolutely still during the procedure. A local anesthetic is injected, and the biopsy site is selected. The patient is instructed to hold his or her breath during the insertion and removal of the needle from the liver. The entire procedure takes about 10 to 15 minutes.

Patient preparation and aftercare—Patient teaching is critical because a formal consent is usually required. The patient fasts for 4 to 8 hours. Prothrombin times and platelet counts are obtained before the biopsy, and the patient may receive a bolus of vitamin K to support clotting. The patient is informed that a painful "punching" sensation may be perceived in the shoulder as the needle penetrates the liver. Posttest care focuses on careful assessment for signs of bleeding or complications. The patient is positioned on the right side for about 2 hours over pillows or sandbags to put pressure on the biopsy site. Vital signs are monitored frequently, and the patient is assessed for persistent shoulder pain, respiratory difficulty, and a rise in temperature. Bed rest is maintained for about 24 hours.

ENDOSCOPIC RETROGRADE CHOLANGIOPANCREATOGRAPHY

Purpose—Endoscopic retrograde cholangiopancreatography (ERCP) involves the examination of the pancreatic ducts and hepatobiliary tree after injection of a contrast medium. It is used to evaluate pancreatic disease, locate calculi and stenosis of the pancreatic ducts, or diagnose cancer.

Procedure—A small, side-viewing endoscope is inserted through the mouth and esophagus and advanced through the pylorus and into the duodenum with the patient under local anesthesia and sedation. The viewing port is positioned by the ampulla of Vater, and a contrast medium is injected. The pancreas is visualized fluoroscopically, and tissue or fluid specimens may be obtained. The hepatobiliary tree may be visualized as part of the same test, which takes from 30 to 60 minutes.

Patient preparation and aftercare—Patient teaching is an essential aspect of preparation and includes reassurance about the use of local anesthesia and sedation, although the patient is conscious during the test. The patient is kept NPO after midnight. The patient is carefully assessed for a history of allergy to contrast media, iodine, or shellfish and is informed that the administration of anticholinergics during the test may cause dry mouth and thirst. Vital signs are carefully monitored after the test, and the patient is assessed for signs of respiratory difficulty. Fluids are withheld until the gag reflex is intact. A sore throat is a common complaint following the test. Patients are instructed to report the incidence of fever, chills, or left upper quadrant pain after the test, which could indicate the development of complications.

DISORDERS OF THE LIVER
HEPATITIS
Etiology/Epidemiology

Hepatitis is defined as any acute inflammatory disease of the liver. Although viral forms of hepatitis are by far the most common, the disease can also be triggered by toxic substances such as drugs and alcohol, industrial toxins, and plant poisons. Although the causes can be quite different and the pathologic findings may vary, there is great similarity in the presentation and clinical management. Hepatitis usually resolves without incident, but any form of hepatitis can result in postnecrotic cirrhosis if it does not respond to treatment.

Viral hepatitis is a major worldwide health problem. Five major categories of viruses have currently been identified. Forty percent of all cases of hepatitis are caused by type A virus. Hepatitis B is of primary concern to health care workers, and hepatitis C is clearly related to the development of chronic disease states. The major forms of the disease are summarized in Table 11-2.

TABLE 11-2   Characteristics of Different Types of Hepatitis

CHARACTERISTIC	HEPATITIS A	HEPATITIS B	HEPATITIS C	HEPATITIS D	HEPATITIS E
Onset	Abrupt, febrile	Insidious, seldom febrile	Insidious, often nonicteric	Insidious	Abrupt, resembles hepatitis A
Incubation period	15-50 days	45-180 days	14-150 days	Unknown	15-60 days
Transmission	Primarily person to person through oral-fecal contamination; rare by blood; *not* transmitted by kissing or sharing utensils	Infected blood or body fluids; introduced by contaminated needles and sexual contact; spread by direct household contact is possible; *not* transmitted by oral-fecal route or contaminated water	Infected blood transfusion or parenteral drug abuse	Same routes as hepatitis B	Oral-fecal contamination; water
Mortality	Less than 0.5%	1%-5%	Unknown	Increased	Unknown
Age-groups	Older children, young adults, particularly custodial or day-care situations	Young adults, particularly immigrants and refugees from endemic areas, drug abusers, and hemodialysis patients and personnel About 10%	All ages, particularly those receiving frequent blood transfusions	Same as hepatitis B	All ages; immigrants and travelers from endemic regions
Incidence of chronic disease	Virtually absent		20%-70%	Frequent with superinfections	No
Carrier state	Does not occur	6%-10%	8%	80% with superinfections	Unknown
Protective immunity	IgG class and anti-HAV antibodies confer immunity	Anti-HB antibodies confer immunity	No test available; people experience repeated infections	No test available; can only occur if hepatitis B is present	No test available

Pathophysiology

Viral hepatitis causes diffuse inflammatory infiltration of hepatic tissue with local necrosis. Inflammation, degeneration, and regeneration occur simultaneously, distorting the normal lobular pattern, creating pressure within the portal vein areas, and obstructing the bile channels. The liver cells become extremely swollen, creating hepatomegaly. Bile flow is interrupted, bile salts accumulate under the skin, and bilirubin diffuses into the tissues and is excreted by the kidney. The disease occurs in three stages, termed *preicteric, icteric,* and *posticteric,* and may take months to completely resolve. Classic clinical manifestations include jaundice, dark amber urine, grayish white stools, profound weakness, malaise, anorexia, plus fever, chills, nausea, and vomiting in the preicteric phase.

Medical Management

The disease is diagnosed based on characteristic results of liver transaminases, bilirubin, alkaline phosphatase, and the presence of viral antigens, antibodies, or actual viral particles. There is no specific medical therapy for hepatitis. Rest is the foundation of care to allow the liver to heal itself. Other supportive measures include a well-balanced diet with limited fats and sodium plus elimination of alcohol, vitamin K to support clotting factor synthesis, and possibly the use of antihistamines for severe pruritus. Corticosteroids may be administered in severe fulminant cases, but their use is controversial.

NURSING MANAGEMENT

◆ ASSESSMENT

Subjective Data

Knowledge of the disease and its treatment
History of exposure to hepatotoxic agents, infected persons, injections, or blood transfusions
Complaints of:
Severe anorexia, nausea, possibly vomiting
Fever and chills (preicteric phase)
Severe fatigue and malaise, weakness
Tenderness or aching in the right upper quadrant (RUQ) of abdomen
Generalized pruritus

Objective Data

Jaundice, yellowed sclera
Dark amber urine, clay-colored stools
Hepatomegaly
Abnormal laboratory tests
Elevated direct and indirect bilirubin
Elevated ALT and AST
Elevated alkaline phosphatase
Bilirubinuria

◆ NURSING DIAGNOSES

Nursing diagnoses for the person with hepatitis may include, but are not limited to, the following:

| BOX 11-1 | Hepatitis Prevention and Prophylaxis |

PREVENTION

Universal precautions for all body fluids for all patients constitute the primary prevention strategy for all forms of hepatitis for hospitalized patients.

Treat *all* feces, urine, blood, and other body fluids as potentially infectious.

Handle all contaminated needles and syringes as potentially infectious, and follow institutional policy for the disposal of contaminated material. *Do not attempt to recap needles.*

Employ enteric precautions during period of infectivity.

Practice frequent careful hand washing.

Use separate bagging for all linens (type A).

Disposable dishes and utensils are recommended (type A).

Abstain from sexual contact during period of infectivity.

Instruct patient not to donate blood.

PROPHYLAXIS

Type A

Preexposure: recommended for travelers to developing countries. Immune globulin (0.02 ml/kg) is the recommended therapy.

Postexposure: immune globulin is recommended for selected persons exposed to type A through close household or sexual contact, and staff and attenders of day-care centers or residential facilities if given within 2 weeks of exposure.

Type B

Preexposure: hepatitis B vaccine is recommended for health care workers, hemodialysis patients, persons with multiple sex partners (particularly homosexual men), IV drug abusers, and recipients of frequent blood products. The vaccine is administered as a series of three intramuscular (IM) injections over a period of about 8 months.

Postexposure: hepatitis B vaccine plus anti-HB immune globulin may be administered to close household or sexual contacts or to persons exposed to contaminated blood or equipment. Previously vaccinated persons may be given a booster dose.

Type C

Preventive measures are the best policy. Immunoglobulin may be given, but its effectiveness is unknown.

Type D

Since this disease requires the presence of type B the best prevention lies in vaccination for type B.

Type E

Prevention is emphasized for travelers, because the value of immune globulin is unknown.

Activity intolerance (related to extreme fatigue)
Nutrition, risk of altered: less than body requirements (related to pronounced anorexia and nausea)
Skin integrity, high risk for impaired (related to severe pruritus)
Knowledge deficit: prevention of spread, reinfection (related to lack of exposure to information about the disease process)

◆ EXPECTED PATIENT OUTCOMES

Patient will gradually resume a normal activity level as energy increases.

Patient will resume a normal nutritional intake that meets all basic body needs.

Patient will maintain an intact skin.

Patient will correctly describe precautions to be followed at home to prevent spread of the disease or reinfection.

◆ NURSING INTERVENTIONS

Reducing Fatigue

Maintain patient on bed rest during acute phase.

Caution patient to resume activity very gradually.

Relapses are believed to be frequently related to too rapid increases in activity.

Promote patient comfort while on bed rest.

Provide frequent position changes.

Keep environment cool and quiet with low levels of stimuli.

Encourage the restriction of visitors during acute phase.

Group care activities and assist patient with ADL as needed. Provide for periods of uninterrupted rest.

Provide diversionary activities to prevent boredom.

Maintaining Adequate Nutrition

Encourage oral fluid intake (to 3000 ml/day). Use IV route if nausea or vomiting is severe.

Administer antiemetics if nausea and vomiting are severe.

Maintain accurate intake and output records.

Discuss food preferences with patient.

Fruit juices, carbonated beverages, and hard candy are usually well tolerated.

Diet high in protein and carbohydrates but low in fats is optimal.

Provide frequent mouth care—keep environment pleasant and odor free.

Reducing Pruritus

Provide or encourage good skin care.

Implement measures to treat pruritus.

Give tepid water baths; avoid use of heat and rubbing, because they increase vasodilation and itching sensation.

Use lotions and creams for dry skin.

Avoid use of wool or any constricting clothing.

Encourage patient to keep nails trimmed short.

Administer medications if prescribed—antiemetics, antihistamines, vitamins.

Teaching about Disease Management

Maintain precautions appropriate to the source of the virus.

Provide separate toilet facilities if feasible.

Use disposable dishes and utensils.

Take special precautions with excreta, blood, and blood-drawing equipment.

Avoid direct contact.

Teach patient importance of continuing to restrict activity during home convalescence, and provide follow-up care to monitor blood values.

Teach family measures for continuing care at home.

Describe symptoms indicative of relapse—increasing fatigue, return of nausea and vomiting, incidence of bleeding or easy bruising.

Encourage patient to avoid alcohol during the recovery period.

Teach patient the importance of using safe sex practices until the laboratory studies return to normal.

Several months are often needed for resolution of the disease process.

Address need for vaccination among family and friends.

◆ EVALUATION

Successful achievement of expected outcomes for the patient with hepatitis is indicated by the following:

Return of energy level to preillness levels

Consumption of a balanced diet and maintenance of a stable body weight

Presence of an intact skin and an absence of pruritus

Correct description of all precautions to be followed at home to prevent disease spread or reinfection

LIVER CANCER

Etiology/Epidemiology

Malignant tumors of the liver can be primary or metastatic. The liver is a common site of metastasis because of its highly vascular structure. Primary liver cancer is relatively rare in the United States (1% to 2% of total), but it is much more common in regions of the world where chronic liver diseases such as hepatitis A and B are endemic.

Pathophysiology

Primary tumors arise from the liver cells, bile ducts, or both and may be single or multiple. They compress the surrounding tissue and grow by direct infiltration or invasion of the portal veins. Many tumors are rapid growing and display few if any early symptoms. Initial symptoms frequently mimic hepatitis, but the accompanying weight loss is often profound.

Medical Management

Although ultrasonography and CT scanning may outline lesions in the liver, a biopsy is necessary to make the definitive diagnosis. Depending on the stage of the disease, treatment may consist primarily of supportive care similar to that used for advanced cirrhosis. Chemotherapy is often administered to induce tumor regression and may be administered by arterial infusion into the hepatic artery. Radiotherapy has not been shown to prolong survival. Solitary primary tumors may be treated surgically because of the liver's remarkable regenerative capacity.

NURSING MANAGEMENT

Nursing management of the patient with liver cancer varies with the stage of the disease and the treatment measures employed. Psychosocial support for the patient and family is needed throughout care, because the prognosis is grave. General measures are aimed at supporting comfort, maintaining nutrition, reducing pruritus, and preventing bleeding-related injury or infection. Managing pain can be a particular challenge, since there are no safe analgesics to use in the presence of liver dysfunction. The patient undergoing surgery will receive standard but meticulous care and may be monitored initially in an intensive care unit.

Chemotherapy is being used in treatment with increasing frequency. Nursing management of the patient receiving chemotherapy is discussed in Chapter 1. The use of a hepatic artery catheter is presented in Box 11-2.

CIRRHOSIS OF THE LIVER
Etiology/Epidemiology

Cirrhosis is a general term applied to a group of chronic diseases of the liver that are characterized by diffuse liver inflammation and fibrosis that leads to severe structural changes and loss of liver function. Table 11-3 summarizes the major forms of cirrhosis. Although alcoholism and malnutrition are the two most common causes of cirrhosis, the disease can result from any chronic liver disorder, including hepatitis, and is frequently of unknown etiology.

Laennec's cirrhosis is by far the most common type in the United States and accounts for over 75% of the cases. Cirrhosis can occur at any age but is most common in white males between 45 and 65 years of age and in nonwhites of both sexes. Although the role of

BOX 11-2	Implanted Pump Chemotherapy

The Infusaid pump allows the patient to be treated at home. A catheter is surgically inserted into the hepatic artery and connected to an implanted infusion pump. The pump can be programmed to deliver chemotherapy at a desired dose over a desired time interval. The pump is filled with a heparin solution between rounds of chemotherapy to keep the catheter patent. The pump usually needs to be refilled about every 2 weeks. The patient is instructed to monitor for any signs of redness or inflammation around the insertion site (Figure 11-2).

alcohol is incompletely understood, the volume consumed appears to be the key factor. Most alcoholics who develop Laennec's cirrhosis report a history of consumption equal to 1 pint of whiskey daily for 15 years.

Pathophysiology

The basic changes in cirrhosis are liver cell death and replacement of the normal tissue with regenerated cell masses and scar tissue that produce nodules of normal liver tissue surrounded by fibrous tissue. Fatty infiltration is the first step. Acute inflammation follows and leads to cell death. The structural changes eventually obstruct portal blood flow. The body attempts to compensate for the changes through establishing collateral circulation, but pressure gradually builds in the portal system and creates increased venous pressure, splanchnic congestion, splenomegaly, fluid retention, and esophageal varicosities.

As much as three fourths of the liver is effectively destroyed before the person with cirrhosis develops active symptoms. A wide variety of symptoms occur. Early in the disease process the person may experience general signs of failing health such as anorexia, nausea and vomiting, and indigestion. Later problems include jaundice, ascites, clotting problems, and frequent infections.

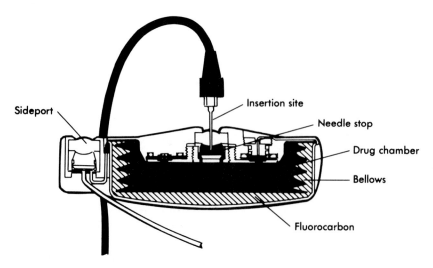

FIGURE 11-2 Infusaid (implantable infusion) pump.

TABLE 11-3 Types of Cirrhosis	
ETIOLOGY	**DESCRIPTION**
LAENNEC'S CIRRHOSIS (nutritional, portal, or alcoholic cirrhosis)	
Alcoholism, malnutrition	Massive collagen formation; liver in early fatty stage is large and firm; in late stage is small and nodular
POSTNECROTIC CIRRHOSIS	
Massive necrosis from hepatotoxins, usually viral hepatitis	Liver is decreased in size, with nodules and fibrous tissue
BILIARY CIRRHOSIS	
Biliary obstruction in liver and common bile duct	Chronic impairment of bile drainage; liver is first large and then becomes firm and nodular; jaundice is a major symptom
CARDIAC CIRRHOSIS	
Right-sided congestive heart failure (CHF)	Liver is swollen and changes are reversible if CHF is treated effectively; some fibrosis with long-standing CHF
NONSPECIFIC, METABOLIC CIRRHOSIS	
Metabolic problems, infectious diseases, infiltrative diseases, GI diseases	Portal and liver fibrosis may develop; liver is enlarged and firm

Medical Management

Cirrhosis is typically quite advanced before diagnosis. The symptoms are not definitive, and the diagnosis is supported by the findings of abnormal liver function studies; impaired clotting factors; decreased red blood cells (RBCs), white blood cells (WBCs), and platelets; and classic electrolyte imbalances. CT scanning and liver biopsy may also be performed for confirmation of the diagnosis.

There is no specific treatment for cirrhosis. Care is primarily supportive and focuses on treating causative factors such as alcohol and preventing further liver damage. Treatment elements include diet modification, drug therapy with vitamin supplementation and possibly diuretics, balancing rest and exercise, preventing bleeding and infection, and treating complications.

NURSING MANAGEMENT

◆ ASSESSMENT
Subjective Data

Knowledge of disease process and relationship to alcohol or other toxins
　　Alcohol history
History and severity of symptoms
　　Anorexia, nausea, indigestion
　　Weight loss
　　Elimination problems: constipation, flatus
　　RUQ abdominal pain or heaviness
　　Pruritus: presence and severity
　　Weakness and fatigue
Other concurrent health problems
Normal dietary pattern and adequacy
Menstrual irregularities
Changes in libido or sexual functioning

Objective Data

Presence and severity of edema or ascites:
　　abdominal girth
Jaundice: color of urine or stool
Muscle wasting: decreased muscle strength
Orientation, alertness, memory:
　　presence of tremor (asterixis)
Presence of:
　　Dilated visible abdominal veins (caput medusae)
　　Gynecomastia and/or testicular atrophy
　　Palmar erythema
　　Spider angiomas (small, red, pulsing arterioles)
　　Hemorrhoids
　　Skin bruising
　　Abnormal liver function studies
　　Anemia, leukopenia, thrombocytopenia
　　Hepatomegaly and splenomegaly
The remainder of the nursing management of cirrhosis is summarized in the "Nursing Care Plan."

Complications of Cirrhosis

Disease complications tend to occur in patients with long-standing cirrhosis. Portal hypertension is typically the primary stimulus, which then may progress to ascites, esophageal varices, and hepatic encephalopathy.

Ascites

Ascites is one of the most common complications of cirrhosis and is associated with portal hypertension. The mechanisms of ascites are poorly understood but seem to be related to the following:
　　Decreased hepatic synthesis of albumin necessary for adequate colloid osmotic pressure
　　Increased portal vein pressure, which moves fluid into the peritoneal space

NURSING CARE PLAN

THE PATIENT WITH CIRRHOSIS

■ NURSING DIAGNOSIS

Activity intolerance (related to chronic fatigue, anemia, weight of ascites, and peripheral edema)

Expected Patient Outcomes	Nursing Interventions
Patient will have sufficient energy to maintain independence in self-care activities.	1. Encourage bed rest during acute phase. 2. Encourage increasing activity, but space activity to allow for uninterrupted rest. 3. Encourage moderate planned exercise within patient's tolerance. 4. Intervene if patient shows fatigue after prolonged visits by family and/or friends. 5. Encourage patient to remain independent in activities of daily living.

■ NURSING DIAGNOSIS

Nutrition, altered: less than body requirements (related to fatigue and anorexia)

Expected Patient Outcomes	Nursing Interventions

Patient will eat sufficient balanced nutrients to meet the body's basic needs.	1. Assess nutrient intake.
	2. Teach patient how to plan and implement a well-balanced, high-carbohydrate diet that limits fat and total protein. Diet should include the following:
	  a. Sufficient protein to meet body repair needs (approximately 40 g of high biologic value)
	  b. Carbohydrates for energy
	  c. Low fat
	3. Restrict sodium intake and explore use of alternate seasonings or salt substitutes.
	4. Make environment pleasant to encourage patient to eat.
	  a. Try frequent small feedings.
	  b. Incorporate food preferences where possible.
	5. Give antiemetics and mouth care if nausea is present.
	6. Administer vitamins as prescribed.

■ NURSING DIAGNOSIS

Fluid volume excess (related to increased intraabdominal pressure, hypoalbuminemia, and impaired aldosterone metabolism)

Expected Patient Outcomes	Nursing Interventions
Patient will reestablish a normal fluid and electrolyte balance. Patient will maintain a stable body weight, and edema and ascites will decrease.	1. Keep accurate intake and output records. Check weight and abdominal girth daily. Monitor for signs of peripheral edema. 2. Restrict fluids if prescribed; provide fluids that are best tolerated, and space these fluids throughout the day. 3. Administer diuretics if ordered (spironolactone or furosemide). 4. Administer potassium replacement as ordered.

NURSING CARE PLAN—CONT'D

THE PATIENT WITH CIRRHOSIS

5. Teach patient rationale for sodium restriction (usually 1 g). Encourage bed rest when ascites is severe.
6. Administer salt-poor albumin if ordered.
7. Assist with paracentesis if ordered (see page 242).

■ **NURSING DIAGNOSIS**

Skin integrity, high risk for impaired (related to decreased activity, ascites, and peripheral edema)

Expected Patient Outcomes	Nursing Interventions
Patient will maintain an intact skin.	1. Use antipressure foam mattresses if on bed rest.
	2. Assess skin daily for signs of pressure or breakdown.
	3. Provide or encourage good skin care. Keep skin clean and moisturized.
	4. Implement measures to control pruritus.
	a. Provide a cool environment.
	b. Apply antipruritic lotion to skin after bathing.
	c. Keep fingernails cut short.
	d. If patient must scratch, provide a soft cloth to prevent excoriations.
	5. Support abdomen when positioned on side.

■ **NURSING DIAGNOSIS**

Injury and infection, high risk for (related to thrombocytopenia and leukopenia)

Expected Patient Outcomes	Nursing Interventions
Patient will not experience bleeding or infection related to depressed blood values of white cells and platelets.	1. Patient should maintain good hygiene and avoid exposure to infections and toxins.
	2. Monitor for signs of infection. Auscultate lungs every 4 hours.
	3. Encourage pulmonary hygiene.
	4. Use high Fowler's position to support gas exchange. Encourage frequent position changes and regular deep breathing.
	5. Use sterile technique for all intrusive procedures.
	6. Monitor for bleeding:
	a. Check urine and stool for blood.
	b. Check skin and mucous membranes for signs of bleeding.
	c. Assess regularly for petechiae and easy bruising.
	7. Avoid injections, if possible; apply pressure at all puncture sites for several minutes.
	8. Give prescribed vitamin K.
	9. Teach patient the following bleeding precautions to be observed if patient is thrombocytopenic:

Continued.

NURSING CARE PLAN—CONT'D

THE PATIENT WITH CIRRHOSIS

> a. Use gentle mouth care and soft toothbrush.
> b. Avoid use of straight razor.
> c. Check for bruises and petechiae daily.
> 10. Encourage patient to prevent constipation and avoid foods that may traumatize esophageal varices (spicy, hot, raw).

■ NURSING DIAGNOSIS

Home maintenance management, high risk for impaired (related to insufficient knowledge and nonadherence to disease regimen)

Expected Patient Outcomes	Nursing Interventions
Patient will be knowledgeable about diet and life-style changes required by treatment regimen and will make a positive adjustment to disease.	1. Teach patient: a. Basis of symptoms and therapeutic regimen b. Dietary and fluid restrictions c. Medication therapy d. Avoidance of infection and substances toxic to liver; clarify use of all OTC medications e. Importance of avoiding alcohol use f. Signs requiring immediate medical follow-up g. Importance of regimen adherence, because disease requires lifelong management 2. Discuss measures to increase compliance with treatment regimen. Remind patient that controlling disease will be a lifelong process. 3. Encourage patient to verbalize concerns over changes in body image and function. 4. Help patient identify personal strengths and give positive feedback. 5. Encourage patient to participate in goal setting and decision making.

Obstructed hepatic lymph flow
Increased serum aldosterone level

A vicious cycle is established as escaped albumin further aggravates the osmotic balance. Fluid is retained in the abdomen and throughout the body. The abdominal fluid accumulation may be profound.

The general management of ascites is discussed in the care plan under fluid volume excess. If conservative measures fail, diuretics may be administered. Albumin may be administered in an attempt to maintain or restore an adequate vascular volume. If other measures fail to control the severity of the ascites, a peritoneal venous shunt may be surgically placed to allow for continuous reinfusion of the fluid back into the venous circulation (Box 11-3).

BOX 11-3 Peritoneal Venous Shunting for Ascites

A *LeVeen* or *Denver* peritoneal venous shunt may be surgically placed to support the continuous reinfusion of ascitic fluid back into the venous system (Figure 11-3). One end of the tube is implanted into the peritoneal cavity, and the other is channeled through the subcutaneous tissue and inserted into the superior vena cava. A one-way pressure valve opens whenever the pressure gradient is greater than 3 mm of water, allowing for flow of the fluid. The Denver pump also contains a pump that can be manually compressed to irrigate the tubing and help keep it patent. Deep breathing is encouraged every 1 to 2 hours when shunts are in place to facilitate the opening of the valve when pressure gradients have stabilized.

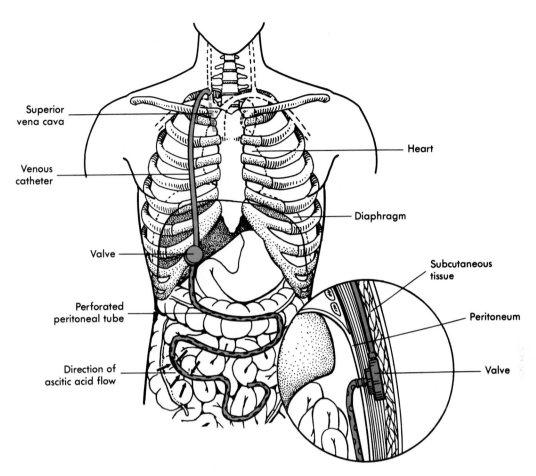

FIGURE 11-3   LeVeen shunt, showing placement of catheter.

Esophageal varices

Bleeding esophageal varices are the most dangerous complication of portal hypertension. Obstruction within the portal system causes the blood to be forced into smaller collateral vessels that drain the stomach, spleen, and esophagus, which were not designed to carry this volume or pressure. The vessels become dilated, tortuous, and fragile and are prone to injury from minor trauma such as that associated with coarse foods, coughing, or vomiting. Abrupt, copious, and painless bleeding may occur and can produce profound hematemesis and hypovolemic shock. The associated mortality can run as high as 75%.

Treatment for bleeding varices begins with establishing the source of the bleeding. Esophagoscopy is frequently used. Measures are instituted to restore blood volume and control the bleeding. Gastric lavage may be accompanied by the injection of vasopressin (Pitressin) to reduce portal pressure and blood flow. Injection sclerotherapy may be attempted by introducing an endoscopic tube and injecting a sclerosing substance into the bleeding varicosities. Esophagogastric tamponade with a Sengstaken-Blakemore tube may also be used in cases of massive bleeding (see Guidelines box and Figure 11-4).

Surgical portacaval shunting is one of the last measures attempted. Although relatively safe in stable patients, the procedure is associated with a 50% mortality when performed on an emergency basis. A newer approach, the transjugular intrahepatic portosystemic shunt (TIPS), provides a safer and frequently effective alternative. This procedure uses the normal vasculature of the liver to create a shunt between the portal and systemic venous circulation. A connection is established between the portal and hepatic veins, and a stent is inserted. The procedure can be performed in the radiology suite, and early results indicate success in about 90% of patients.

Portal systemic encephalopathy

Hepatic coma is a form of metabolic encephalopathy of the brain associated with liver failure. It is believed to be precipitated by factors that either increase the ammonia level or depress liver function. In liver failure, ammonia (a waste product of the breakdown of protein in the intestine) is not converted to urea by the liver and accumulates in the blood. Ammonia has a toxic effect on the central nervous system and can lead to coma. The effects are enhanced by the multiple other metabolic derangements that occur concurrently, including hy-

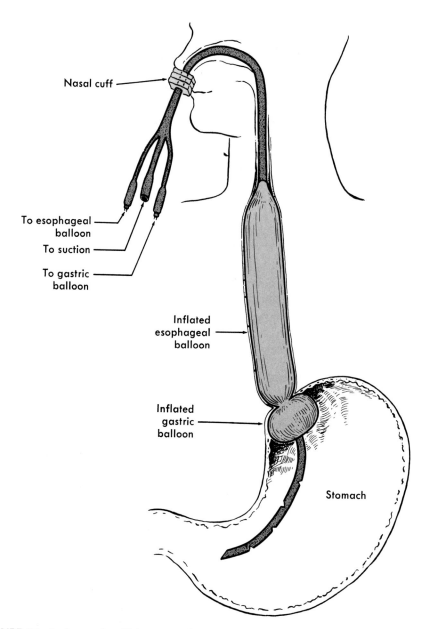

Nasal cuff

To esophageal
balloon

To suction

To gastric
balloon

Inflated
esophageal
balloon

Inflated
gastric
balloon

Stomach

FIGURE 11-4 Sengstaken-Blakemore tube with esophageal and gastric balloons inflated. (Redrawn from *Rubber appliances in surgery and therapeutics,* Providence, RI, Davol, Inc.)

pokalemia and acid-base imbalances. Classic symptoms include the following:

Impaired attention span

Irritability and restlessness

Apathy, loss of interest, lethargy, somnolence

Coma

The serum ammonia may be significantly elevated. The diagnosis is made on the basis of clinical signs.

Treatment centers around identifying and reversing the precipitating cause. Strain on the liver is reduced by severely restricting protein in the diet temporarily, administering antibiotics to reduce ammonia-forming bacteria in the bowel, and administering enemas, cathartics, and/or lactulose to empty the bowel and prevent ammonia formation. General supportive care and moni-

toring are maintained with special attention to the prevention of infection.

DISORDERS OF THE BILIARY SYSTEM
CHOLELITHIASIS, CHOLECYSTITIS, AND CHOLEDOCHOLITHIASIS
Etiology/Epidemiology

Gallstones can occur anywhere in the biliary tree, and cholelithiasis is by far the most common problem of the biliary system. Although it affects 15% of the population, and 1 million new cases are diagnosed each year, its basic etiology remains unknown. Stones are frequently asymptomatic but can trigger acute or chronic episodes of cholecystitis. They represent one of the most common indications for surgery. Stones that are found in the common bile duct are termed *choledoch-olithiasis.*

Cholelithiasis occurs twice as often in females, occurs most frequently in middle-aged and older individuals, and is clearly associated with obesity, elevated triglycerides, pregnancy, and Caucasian race. Other specific clinical states have been found to be associated with increased risk of stones for selected populations. Diet alone has not been found to be an independent risk factor.

Pathophysiology

There are two primary types of gallstones: cholesterol (70% to 80%) and pigmented stones. Any factor that can increase the level of stone components (e.g., bile salts, cholesterol, calcium, bilirubin) or alter the process of cholesterol formation and excretion (e.g., diseases, drugs, and clinical states) can result in stone formation. The bile becomes supersaturated, an insoluble substance forms a nucleus or kernel, and then precipitate forms and grows. Loss of motility in the gallbladder, which leads to stasis, can also increase stone formation. Cholesterol stones are usually contained within the gallbladder, where pigmented stones may also be found in the intrahepatic and extrahepatic ductal system.

Acute cholecystitis results from a blockage of the cystic duct with edema, plus spasms of the ducts and gallbladder itself. The gallbladder becomes very enlarged, thickened, and edematous. A reaction is triggered by retained bile that may impair circulation and produce ischemia. In an acute attack the patient is extremely ill, with nausea, vomiting, and severe abdominal pain. The disease may also follow a chronic pattern, causing permanent scarring and thickening over time.

If a stone lodges in the ductal system, biliary colic can occur. The bile ducts undergo intense spasm as they attempt to move the stone through the system. Colic produces abrupt, severe abdominal pain that begins in the RUQ of the abdomen but also radiates through to the back and up to the right shoulder. The pain is accompanied by tachycardia, diaphoresis, and acute nausea and vomiting. If the obstruction occurs in the common bile duct, bile is prevented from reaching the GI tract and jaundice will occur. Serum bilirubin levels increase and bilirubin is excreted in the urine. Bile fails to reach the intestine, causing impaired absorption of fat and clay-colored stools.

Medical Management

The diagnosis of cholecystitis is typically established by ultrasonography and supplemented by cholecystography if the results are inconclusive. Medical therapy during an acute attack will involve meperidine for pain, IV fluids, antibiotics, and rest of the GI tract. Patients with mild disease, with small stones, or unwilling to consider surgery may be treated with stone dissolution drug therapy (e.g., chenodeoxycholic or ursodeoxycholic acid). Extracorporeal shock wave lithotripsy can also be used in a small select group of patients with a few stones of small size.

Surgery remains the primary treatment for gallbladder disease. Although only introduced in 1988, laparoscopic cholecystectomy (LC) has rapidly become the

Guidelines for Nursing Care of the Patient with a Sengstaken-Blakemore Tube

DESCRIPTION OF TUBE

The esophagogastric tube has three lumens and two balloons:
Nasogastric (NG) suction lumen
Lumen to inflate gastric balloon
Lumen to inflate esophageal balloon
Gastric balloon
Esophageal balloon

PATIENT CARE

Monitoring the Tubes

Measure and record balloon pressures every hour.
Esophageal balloon is left inflated for a maximum of 48 hours.
Gastric balloon must be deflated regularly to prevent erosion and ulceration.
Monitor output from tube. Correct balloon inflation will exceed portal pressure and cause esophageal bleeding to stop.
Monitor patient carefully for respiratory problems.
Any shift in the tube can cause obstruction of the airway.
Patient cannot swallow around the tube and may aspirate secretions.
Provide emesis basin and tissues to handle saliva. Use suction if needed.

Attach NG lumen to suction to remove blood from the stomach.
Stomach may be lavaged to provide vasoconstriction as well as pressure.

Promoting Patient Comfort

Provide comfort measures and support to patient. Carefully explain all interventions.
Provide mouth and nasal care frequently, every 1 to 2 hours.

Preventing Encephalopathy

NOTE: Blood retained in the GI tract will be broken down by protein-digesting enzymes. If the liver cannot convert the ammonia to urea, hepatic coma can result.
Instill saline cathartics or lactulose through the tube as ordered.
Administer enemas as prescribed to cleanse GI tract of blood.
Administer medications as prescribed.
Magnesium sulfate is used to hasten excretion of blood in GI tract.
Antibiotics (Neomycin) are given to reduce bacterial action on blood.
Monitor level of consciousness frequently.

procedure of choice for uncomplicated situations. LC utilizes laser or cautery to remove the gallbladder. It is much less invasive, causes less pain, and results in fewer complications, and patients can usually be discharged within 24 hours and return rapidly to their usual lifestyles. Although effective in most situations the LC approach cannot be used if stones are located within the common bile duct. In these situations a standard abdominal surgical approach is used. A T-tube will be placed for drainage after surgery when the common bile duct is involved (see Guidelines box and Figure 11-5).

NURSING MANAGEMENT

◆ ASSESSMENT
Subjective Data

Knowledge of the problem and expected treatment
History of problem, fat intolerance, dyspepsia
Normal dietary pattern
Patient's complaints
   Mild to severe RUQ abdominal pain and tenderness; referral to scapula or shoulder
   Nausea and vomiting
   Anorexia, bloating, heartburn
   Fever and chills

Objective Data

Presence and degree of jaundice
   Clay-colored stool, dark amber urine
Abdominal distention, tenderness, guarding
Leukocytosis
Abnormal ultrasonogram
The nursing management of the patient undergoing abdominal cholecystectomy is presented in the "Nurs-

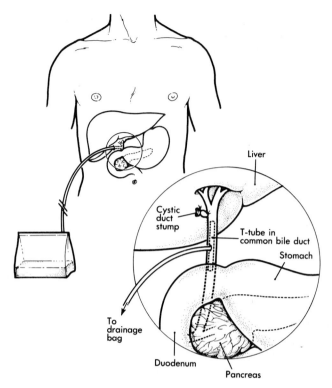

FIGURE 11-5   T-tube insertion into common bile duct.

ing Care Plan." The management of the patient undergoing laparoscopic cholecystectomy is presented in the "Critical Pathway."

DISORDERS OF THE EXOCRINE PANCREAS

ACUTE PANCREATITIS
Etiology/Epidemiology

Pancreatitis is a serious inflammatory disorder of the pancreas that can occur as a single episode or as recurrent attacks. The exact etiology is unknown, but its incidence has been linked to a variety of concurrent conditions including alcoholism (the most common) and biliary disease. Other less definitive conditions include trauma, infections, metabolic imbalances, drug effects, and connective tissue disorders. Many forms are idiopathic.

Pathophysiology

Pancreatitis is theorized to develop from the activation of proteolytic enzymes within the pancreas itself. A process of autodigestion is triggered, creating severe edema, interstitial hemorrhage, coagulation, and fat necrosis. Release of histamine and bradykinin increases vascular permeability and vasodilation. A critical situation involving hypotension, shock, and disseminated intravascular coagulation may result.

Guidelines for Nursing Care of the Patient with a T-Tube

PURPOSE
To ensure patency of the common bile duct after surgical exploration. Edema produced by surgical probing can produce obstruction.

ASSOCIATED NURSING INTERVENTIONS
Attach tube to closed gravity drainage.
Never irrigate or clamp tube without direct order.
Avoid pulling or kinking tube; teach patient not to lie on it.
Monitor and record amount and color of drainage each shift.
   Initial output will be 500 to 1000 ml/day and gradually
      taper off as bile begins to flow again into the duodenum.
   Report presence of blood in drainage.
Change dressings as needed. Cleanse surrounding skin of bile
   to avoid irritation.
Assess patient's response to on and off clamping regimen if
   ordered.
Assess stools and urine for indications of returning bile flow.
   Assess for jaundice.

NURSING CARE PLAN

THE PATIENT UNDERGOING ABDOMINAL CHOLECYSTECTOMY WITH EXPLORATION OF THE COMMON BILE DUCT

■ NURSING DIAGNOSIS
Pain (related to incisional discomfort)

Expected Patient Outcomes	Nursing Interventions
Patient will experience decreasing levels of pain and tenderness.	1. Assess type and quality of pain. 2. Administer medications as prescribed for pain. Assess for effectiveness. Meperidine (Demerol) is usually administered rather than morphine, because it does not cause spasm in sphincter of Oddi. 3. Offer comfort measures. Provide position changes, skin care, fresh linen. 4. Keep patient in low Fowler's position to reduce pressure on diaphragm. 5. If NG tube is present, give mouth and nose care as needed. 6. Encourage activity.

■ NURSING DIAGNOSIS
Breathing patterns, high risk for ineffective (related to pain and splinting of high abdominal incision)

Expected Patient Outcomes	Nursing Interventions
Patient's lungs will be clear to auscultation.	1. Monitor respirations and breath sounds (especially right lower lobe) every 2 to 4 hours for 24 hours, then every 4 hours while awake until patient is ambulating well. 2 Place patient in low Fowler's position, and encourage patient to change position frequently. 3. Encourage deep breathing and coughing exercises at least every 1 to 2 hours for 24 hours, then every 2 to 4 hours while awake until patient is ambulating well. Encourage use of incentive spirometer. 4. Provide adequate pain relief to enable good ventilation. NOTE: High abdominal incision makes respiratory hygiene difficult in postoperative period. 5. Splint incision to encourage deep coughing. 6. Encourage ambulation as permitted.

Continued.

The acute inflammatory process results in a wide range of physiologic alterations that may present as mild or extremely critical. A unique feature of the disease is the fact that, except in alcohol-induced disease, the pancreas returns to normal after successful treatment and rarely is there any residual dysfunction. However, the mortality during the initial episode runs as high as 5% to 10%.

The primary symptom of pancreatitis is pain that can be incapacitating. It may be epigastric or found in other parts of the abdomen and may radiate to the back, flanks, or substernal area. Nausea, vomiting, and distention are also common. A low-grade fever and signs of dehydration are also common.

Medical Management

The diagnosis of pancreatitis is established from the serum enzyme levels. A serum amylase level above 300 Somogyi units in a symptomatic patient usually is considered diagnostic. Serum lipase and urinary amylase

NURSING CARE PLAN—CONT'D

THE PATIENT UNDERGOING ABDOMINAL CHOLECYSTECTOMY WITH EXPLORATION OF THE COMMON BILE DUCT

■ NURSING DIAGNOSIS

Skin integrity, high risk for impaired (related to pruritus or postoperative wound drainage)

Expected Patient Outcomes	Nursing Interventions

Patient will maintain an intact skin.	1. Employ measures to control itching.
	2. Assess skin around incision and stab wound with each dressing change.
	3. Change dressings as needed to maintain a dry dressing, because bile is highly irritating to skin.
	   a. Use Montgomery straps if frequent changes are necessary.
	   b. Use soap and water to remove bile drainage from skin.

■ NURSING DIAGNOSIS

Injury or infection, high risk for (related to obstruction of bile drainage)

Expected Patient Outcomes	Nursing Interventions

Patient will not experience obstruction or dislodgement of T-tube drainage.	1. Maintain patency of T-tube:
	   a. Connect tube to closed gravity drainage.
	   b. Provide sufficient tubing to facilitate patient mobility.
	   c. Explain to patient importance of avoiding kinks, clamping, or pulling of tube.
	2. Monitor amount and color of drainage from T-tube. Initial output may be 500 to 1000 ml.
	3. Monitor color of urine and stool.
	4. Report signs of peritonitis (abdominal pain or rigidity, fever) immediately.
	5. If clamping of T-tube is prescribed before removal, monitor patient for signs of distress; if this occurs, unclamp tube and notify physician.

will also be elevated. Other common findings will include leukocytosis, elevated bilirubin and liver enzymes (particularly if gallstone-induced disease is present), and hyperglycemia. An ultrasound may be used to rule out pseudocyst, and an ERCP (see p. 244) may be ordered if pancreatic duct obstruction is suspected.

Treatment is aimed at resting the pancreas and providing supportive care. Management of pain is a primary consideration, and meperidine is the drug of choice. Fluids are administered to restore the vascular volume. The patient is NPO during the acute period and may require NG suctioning to control nausea and vomiting. TPN may be initiated during this period to ensure an adequate nutritional base for healing. The patient is monitored carefully for the development of complications and may require intensive care.

NURSING MANAGEMENT

◆ ASSESSMENT

Subjective Data

History of biliary disease

Pattern of alcohol use

Patient's complaints of:

Sudden-onset pain: sharp, severe, constant, located in epigastric region or radiating to the back, worsened by ingestion of food or alcohol

Nausea and vomiting

NURSING CARE PLAN—CONT'D

THE PATIENT UNDERGOING ABDOMINAL CHOLECYSTECTOMY WITH EXPLORATION OF THE COMMON BILE DUCT

■ NURSING DIAGNOSIS
Knowledge deficit (related to necessary diet modifications and care after discharge)

Expected Patient Outcomes	Nursing Interventions

Patient will correctly describe diet and self-care requirements after discharge.	1. Give nothing by mouth until peristalsis resumes. Progress to soft, low-fat diet as tolerated.
	 2. Assess patient's response and tolerance.
	 3. Teach patient to avoid excessive fat intake, but no special diet is required.
	 4. Suggest use of smaller, more frequent meals.
	 5. Plan diet for patient to reduce weight if needed.
	 6. Teach patient the following:
	   a. Techniques of dressing change if drainage is still occurring at time of discharge
	   b. Signs to report to physician (excessive drainage, jaundice, light-colored stools)
	   c. Resumption of normal activities by 4 weeks but avoidance of heavy activity until 6 weeks

CRITICAL PATHWAY	Laparoscopic Cholecystectomy Without Complications

DRG #: 195; expected LOS: 2

	Day of Surgery Day of Admission Day 1	Day of Discharge Day 2
Diagnostic Tests	Preoperative: CBC, UA Postoperative: Hgb and HCT	
Medications	POST-PAR: IVs decreased to saline lock after nausea subsides; IV, then PO, analgesic	Discontinue saline lock; PO analgesic
Treatments	POST-PAR: I & O q shift; VS q 4 hr × 4, then q 8 hr; assess bowel sounds q 4 hr; check drainage on bandages q 2 hr	Discontinue I & O; VS q 8 hr; assess bowel sounds q 8 hr; remove bandages and reapply bandages after shower if necessary
Diet	NPO until nausea subsides, then clear liquids; advance to full liquids, low fat	Regular diet, low fat
Activity	Up in room with assistance about 6-10 hr after surgery; T & DB q 2 hr	Up ad lib, OK to shower
Consultations		

NOTE: Acknowledge that patients recover at varying rates; therefore specified daily actions should be based solely on patient need.

Home Care Management of a Person with a T-tube

Many patients are discharged with a T-tube in place to complete their recovery at home. Teaching should include the following:

> Whether to allow the tube to drain continuously or to follow a schedule of intermittent clamping
> How to empty the bag
> How to clamp and unclamp the tubing
> Importance of keeping the bag below the level of the insertion site
> How to convert drainage system from leg bag to overnight drainage if needed
> Skin care
>> Daily shower is adequate
>> Dry sterile dressing over insertion site
>> Skin barriers (e.g., karaya or zinc oxide) if needed
> Symptoms to report
>> Redness, warmth, or swelling at insertion site
>> Purulent drainage or fever
>> Obstructive signs (e.g., recurrence of RUQ pain, nausea and vomiting, jaundice, dark urine, or clay-colored stools)

GERONTOLOGIC PATIENT CONSIDERATIONS FOR GALLBLADDER DISEASE

Gallbladder disease increases in frequency in the elderly population but is treated in the same manner as in a younger population. The symptoms may be more subtle, and the patient may be experiencing severe disease or complications before seeking medical care. There is an increased incidence of associated pancreatic disease. Surgical considerations are the same, but the patient is at greater risk for complications and delayed healing.

Objective Data

General affect: looks ill and distressed
Fluid status
 Intake and output
 Body weight
 Skin turgor, status of mucous membranes
 Vital signs
Fever
Abdominal tenderness and rigidity
Decreased bowel sounds
Tachypnea, dyspnea, decreased breath sounds
Jaundice
Presence of elevated amylase and lipase levels, leukocytosis

◆ NURSING DIAGNOSES

Nursing diagnoses for the person with acute pancreatitis may include, but are not limited to, the following:

Pain, acute (related to inflammation and obstruction within the pancreas)
Fluid volume deficit, actual or potential (related to vomiting and fluid shifts in the abdomen)

Nutrition, altered: less than body requirements (related to nausea, vomiting, or malabsorption)
Knowledge deficit (related to diet and life-style modifications appropriate to support healing)

◆ EXPECTED PATIENT OUTCOMES

Patient will experience decreasing pain.
Patient's fluid and electrolyte balance will be restored to normal limits.
Patient will have basic nutritional needs met and gradually resume oral intake.
Patient will be knowledgeable about diet and life-style modifications appropriate to preventing recurrent attacks of pancreatitis.

◆ NURSING INTERVENTIONS

Promoting Comfort

Administer prescribed pain medication liberally. Meperidine (Demerol) is usually used, because it is not spasmogenic.
Position patient to achieve greatest comfort.
 Suggest sitting with trunk flexed.
 Suggest side-lying position with knees to chest.
 Use noninvasive measures to increase comfort and relaxation.

Maintaining Fluid and Electrolyte Balance

Monitor intake and output accurately.
 Administer IV fluids as ordered.
 Assess patient for dehydration and incipient shock.
Monitor vital signs frequently.
 Weigh patient daily.
 Assess for edema and increasing abdominal girth.
 Observe for signs of hypocalcemia (positive Chvostek's or Trousseau's signs). Administer calcium as ordered.
Assist patient to deep breathe and cough every 2 hours. Auscultate breath sounds.

Promoting Nutrition

Give patient nothing by mouth.
 Offer frequent mouth care.
 Maintain patency of NG tube if present.
Monitor TPN if ordered.
Assess patient for response to oral feedings when initiated. Advance to low-fat, bland diet with five to six meals daily.
Monitor carefully for pain, nausea, and vomiting with refeeding.
Check urine or blood for glucose every 4 to 6 hours.
Teach patient to avoid alcohol and rich foods after discharge.

Teaching for Self-Care

Teach patient signs and symptoms to be reported:
 Recurrence of pain, nausea, or vomiting
 Change in bowel pattern, weight loss

Encourage patient to consider support group or referral for alcohol treatment as indicated.

Encourage weight loss as indicated.

◆ EVALUATION

Successful achievement of expected outcomes for the patient with acute pancreatitis is indicated by the following:

Statements that pain is absent

Balanced intake and output; weight returns to normal and remains stable

Ability to ingest a balanced, low-fat diet without pain or nausea

Appropriate description of signs of complications that need medical management; expressed commitment to modify life-style to reduce risk factors for recurrent disease

CHRONIC PANCREATITIS
Etiology/Epidemiology

Chronic pancreatitis results in permanent and progressive destruction of the pancreas and eventually leads to insufficiency of pancreatic hormones. It is primarily caused by alcoholism in adults but also results from cystic fibrosis. Little else is known about its incidence.

Pathophysiology

The underlying pathologic condition is similar to acute pancreatitis with autodigestion as the primary feature. As the organ is destroyed, the tissue is replaced by fibrous tissue with a loss of functional capacity. The initial symptoms may be quite similar to those described for acute disease, with pain the prominent feature. Nausea and vomiting, weight loss, and malnutrition may also be present. CT of the abdomen may reveal calcification of the organ.

Medical Management

The initial care will be similar to that presented for acute disease. Once this critical period has passed the focus shifts to nutritional management and control of diabetes mellitus. Chronic pain management can be a challenge and may involve antacids, cimetidine, or surgery to remove chronic obstruction. Nutritional problems are primarily managed with the administration of pancreatic extract replacement to control chronic diarrhea, steatorrhea, and malnutrition. The diabetes is usually insulin dependent and requires frequent insulin administration. Most patients are quite brittle in their responses to insulin and difficult to control.

NURSING MANAGEMENT

The focus of nursing care is twofold. During the acute period, care mimics that described for acute pancreatitis. Once this critical period has resolved the focus shifts to the attempt to teach patients the knowledge and skills needed for successful self-management and to encourage them to make the necessary life-style changes to be successful. This frequently involves control of alcohol use and may be the greatest stumbling block to management.

CANCER OF THE PANCREAS
Etiology/Epidemiology

Cancer of the pancreas occurs primarily in elderly persons and in men more often than women. Its incidence is associated with smoking, exposure to chemicals, and high alcohol consumption. It is the fifth leading cause of cancer-related deaths.

Pathophysiology

Most pancreatic tumors appear to begin in the ductal areas, causing eventual blockage. They grow rapidly and are highly invasive. Symptoms are not usually present until late in the course of the disease, and pain is the primary feature. The cancer may mimic the obstructive pattern of chronic pancreatitis. Vague abdominal symptoms and weight loss are also common.

Medical Management

Surgery is the primary treatment modality although the prognosis is usually poor. Conservative procedures may be employed to restore patency of bile flow, or more aggressive procedures may be used to attempt to resect the cancer. Radiation and chemotherapy may also be employed, but there is little evidence of documented positive effects.

NURSING MANAGEMENT

The care of the patient with pancreatic cancer will vary depending on the selected treatment modality. In all cases the patient and family are dealing with a diagnosis that carries a very poor prognosis and the realization that survival time may be limited despite aggressive treatment. Psychosocial care and support are essential. Patients who are treated surgically are often critically ill and will need meticulous monitoring and general surgical care. Pancreatic enzyme replacement will be essential whenever radical surgery is performed. Care will involve monitoring for steatorrhea, management of dumping syndrome, and management of glucose metabolism, which may require insulin therapy.

SELECTED REFERENCES

Adams L, Soulen MC: TIPS: a new alternative for variceal bleeder, *Am J Crit Care* 2(3):196-201, 1993.

Anderson FP: Portal systemic encephalopathy in the chronic alcoholic, *Crit Care Q* 8(4):40-52, 1989.

Clouse ME: Current diagnostic imaging modalities of the liver, *Surg Clin North Am* 69(2):193-234, 1989.

Diehl AK: Laparoscopic cholecystectomy: too much of a good thing? *JAMA* 270(12):1469-1470, 1993.

Doherty MM, Carver DK: Transjugular intrahepatic portosystemic shunt: new relief for esophageal varices, *Am J Nurs* 93(4):58-63, 1993.

Greifzu S, Dest V: When the diagnosis is pancreatic cancer, *RN* 22(9):38-44, 1991.

Gullate MM, Foltz AT: Hepatic chemotherapy via implantable pump, *Am J Nurs* 83:1674-1678, 1983.

Gurevich I: Enterically transmitted viral hepatitis: etiology, epidemiology, and prevention, *Heart Lung* 22(4):370-372, 1993.

Hoofnagle JH: Type D (Delta) hepatitis, *JAMA* 261:1321-1325, 1989.

Jeffres C: Complications of acute pancreatitis, *Crit Care Nurs* 9(4):38-48, 1989.

Krumberger JM: Acute pancreatitis, *Crit Care Nurs Clin North Am* 5(1):185-202, 1993.

Kucharski SA: Fulminant hepatic failure, *Crit Care Nurs Clin North Am* 5(1):141-151, 1993.

McMillan-Jackson M, Rymer TE: Viral hepatitis: anatomy of a diagnosis, *Am J Nurs* 94(1):43-48, 1994.

Mudge C, Carlson L: Hepatorenal syndrome, *AACN Clin Issues Crit Care Nurs* 3(3):614-632, 1992.

Munn NE: When the bile duct is blocked, *RN* 52(2):50-57, 1989.

Renkes J: GI endoscopy: managing the full scope of care, *Nurs 93* 23(6):50-55, 1993.

Rowland GA, Marks DA, Torres W: The new gallstone destroyers and dissolvers, *Am J Nurs* 89:1473-1478, 1989.

Smith A: When the pancreas self-destructs, *Am J Nurs* 91(9):38-48, 1991.

Wilkinson M: Nursing implications after endoscopic retrograde cholangiopancreatography, *Gastroenterol Nurs* 13(2):105-109, 1990.

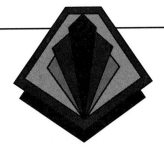

Disorders of the Urinary System

◆ ASSESSMENT

Health history

Past/family history

    Previous or concurrent illnesses (e.g., hypertension, diabetes, renal or urologic infection) or surgery

    Family history of nephritis, nephrosis, polycystic kidney disease

    Medications in use:

        Prescription and over the counter (OTC)

        Antibiotics, analgesics, laxatives, and antacids

Urologic symptoms

    Usual voiding patterns

        Frequency and amount of urine

        Changes in pattern if any, for example, frequency, urgency, hesitancy, dysuria, nocturia, incontinence

        Measures taken to cope with changes

    Presence, location, and severity of pain

        Kidney: in the back between twelfth rib and the iliac crest (costovertebral angle)

        Ureters: pain radiates to front and down into groin or thigh

        Bladder: suprapubic area

        Referred pain also common

Urine output and characteristics

    Presence of:

        Polyuria (greater than 2500 ml/day)

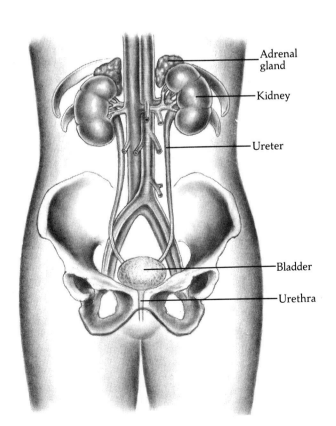

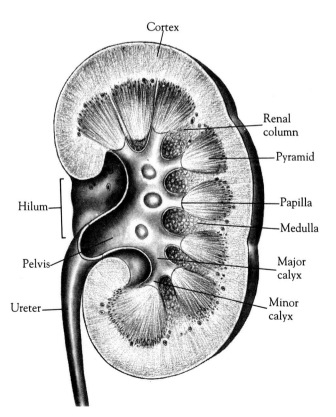

FIGURE 12-1 **A,** The urinary system. **B,** Cross section of kidney. (From Thompson JM et al: *Mosby's clinical nursing,* ed 3, St Louis, 1993, Mosby.)

GERONTOLOGIC PATIENT CONSIDERATIONS: PHYSIOLOGIC CHANGES IN UROLOGIC FUNCTION

Physiologic changes associated with aging create a high incidence of:

Nocturia, frequency, urgency
  Decreased bladder and pelvic muscle tone
  Decreased urine concentrating ability at night
Mobility problems that might contribute to urinary problems
Symptoms of urinary tract infections (UTIs)
  Related to prostatic enlargement in men
  Related to vaginal pH changes in women
NOTE: Urinary incontinence is *not* an expected aspect of aging.

Oliguria (less than 400 ml/day)
Anuria (less than 100 ml/day)
Color
  Normal: pale to deep yellow
  Hematuria (blood in urine)
  Cloudy (phosphate precipitation or bacteria)
Fluid balance (see also Chapter 4)
  Weight changes
  History of fluid retention
  Vital sign changes

PHYSICAL ASSESSMENT

NOTE: Physical assessment techniques do not play a major role in assessment of the urinary system. The following elements may be included:

Skin and mucous membranes: presence and severity of edema
Percussion and palpation of bladder
  Bladder distention causes organ to rise out of the pelvis
  Percussion produces a dull sound
Kidney palpation (requires advanced training)

✍ DIAGNOSTIC TESTING
BLOOD TESTS

Multiple blood tests may be used to evaluate renal function. Major tests are summarized in Table 12-1.

URINE TESTS

Urinalysis is usually the first step in the diagnostic workup. Simple urinalysis gives indications of potential locations and causes of urologic disease. Normal values are summarized in Table 12-2.

Urine culture is used to confirm suspected infection and identify causative organisms and their sensitivities. Urine is obtained by catheterization or clean catch. A normal specimen contains less than 10,000 organisms/ml. UTI is diagnosed when specimen contains greater than 100,000 organisms/ml.

TABLE 12-1 Common Blood Tests of Renal Function

RANGE OF NORMAL VALUES	DESCRIPTION AND PURPOSE
SERUM CREATININE	
Males: 0.85-1.5 mg/dl Females: 0.7-1.25 mg/dl	Tests ability of kidneys to excrete creatinine; not influenced by diet or metabolic rate; provides rough estimate of glomerular filtration rate
BLOOD UREA NITROGEN (BUN)	
5-20 mg/dl	Tests ability of kidneys to excrete nitrogenous waste; affected by protein in diet, fever, and catabolic state

TABLE 12-2 Urinalysis

CHARACTERISTIC	NORMAL FINDINGS	SIGNIFICANCE
Color	Amber-yellow	Alkalinity usually
Clarity	Clear	accompanies
pH	4.6-8.0 (average 6.0)	bacterial infection
Specific gravity	1.010-1.026	Usually reflects fluid intake
Protein	0-8 mg/dl	Proteinuria usually indicates renal disease
Glucose	0	Glycosuria and
Ketones	0	ketonuria may occur with diabetes mellitus; ketonuria present in catabolism
Red blood cells (RBCs)	0-4	Kidney injury
White blood cells (WBCs)	0-5	Urinary tract infection

Clean catch specimens are collected to decrease the likelihood of external bacterial contamination of the urine (see Guidelines box).

Urine tests that assist in the evaluation of renal function are summarized in Table 12-3.

TEST OF BLADDER FUNCTION
Cystometrogram

Description—A cystometrogram evaluates bladder tone as part of an incontinence workup.

Procedure—A Foley catheter is inserted, and the patient is positioned supine. A liter bag of saline or sterile water and a cystometer are attached to the catheter. Fluid is instilled, and measurements are made of the pressure exerted on the fluid by the bladder muscle after each 50 ml. The patient is asked to report the presence and degree of fullness or urge to void. Fluid is instilled until urgency occurs. The effects of cholinergic (Urecholine) and anticholinergic medications on bladder tone may be evaluated.

Guidelines for Collecting a Midstream (Clean Catch) Urine Specimen

PREPARATION

Female
    Separate labia and hold apart until specimen is collected.
    Cleanse meatus with cleansing sponges using a front to
        back motion.
Male
    Retract foreskin if uncircumcised.
    Cleanse glans with cleansing sponges.

COLLECTION

Touch only the outside of the sterile container.
Establish urine stream and then collect 100 ml of urine.

TABLE 12-3   Common Urine Tests of Renal Function

RANGE OF NORMAL VALUES	DESCRIPTION AND PURPOSE
URINE OSMOLALITY	
400-600 mOsm/kg	Represents total concentration of particles in solution; excellent reflection of renal function
CREATININE CLEARANCE	
Males: 100-150 ml/min Females: 85-125 ml/min	Represents rate at which kidneys remove creatinine from plasma and provides an estimate of glomerular filtration; urine collected for exactly 24 hr
PHENOSULFOPHTHALEIN EXCRETION TEST (PSP)	
30%-50% of dye excreted in 15 min	Measures tubular secretion rates; patient drinks 8-10 glasses of water and then is given dye intravenously (IV); urine specimens collected at 15-, 30-, and 60-min intervals
FISHBERG CONCENTRATION TEST	
Urine volume: 300 ml/12 hr Specific gravity of 1.024 or greater Osmolality of 850 mOsm or greater	Tests ability of kidneys to conserve fluid; no fluids administered for 12 hr; urine specimens collected hourly for 3 hr

Patient preparation and aftercare—No special preparation is needed. The patient is instructed about the test and elements that will require his or her participation. No aftercare is required, but fluids are encouraged and patients are instructed to report the development of any symptoms of UTI.

RADIOLOGIC TESTS

Intravenous Pyelogram (IVP)

Description—This test serves as the cornerstone of a urologic workup. It allows visualization of the renal parenchyma, pelvis, and calyces, as well as the ureters and bladder by means of a contrast medium.

Procedure—Contrast medium is injected intravenously, and a series of x-rays are taken at 5-minute intervals as the dye moves through the urinary system. Pressure is applied over the ureters by means of an inflated belt to retain the dye in the upper tract. Pressure is released after 10 minutes, and pictures of the lower tract are completed.

Patient preparation and aftercare—A laxative may be administered the night before the test to remove feces and gas from the gastrointestinal (GI) tract. The patient is kept NPO for 8 hours. The patient is carefully questioned concerning allergies to iodine, shellfish, or contrast media. The dye frequently causes a warm flushing sensation on administration and may create a metallic or salty taste. The patient is encouraged to drink fluids liberally after the test to facilitate excretion of the dye.

Retrograde Urethrography, Cystography, and Ureteropyelography

Description—These tests allow visualization and examination of the urethra (usually performed only in males), bladder, and renal collecting system through the direct injection of contrast material.

Procedure—The patient is catheterized, and contrast medium is inserted into the urethra, bladder, or kidney by means of ureteral catheterization. X-ray films are taken in a variety of positions.

Patient preparation and aftercare—No preparation is required for urethrography or cystography aside from patient teaching and assessment for allergies. Patients generally are NPO before pyelography and are prepared for general or spinal anesthesia. Patients are carefully monitored after each test for adverse reactions to the dye (chills and fever), sepsis, and allergic responses. Urine is assessed for the presence of hematuria. Dysuria is common after pyelography.

Radionuclide Renal Imaging

Description—Radionuclide renal imaging permits the evaluation of structure, blood flow, and function of the kidneys by means of a radionuclide.

Procedure—A radionuclide is administered intravenously, and both perfusion and function are evaluated by means of scintillating probes placed over the kidneys. Multiple photographs are taken of the uptake and movement of the isotope. The entire test takes about 1½ hours.

Patient preparation and aftercare—The patient is instructed and reassured about the safety and brief half-life of the radionuclide. No special precautions are needed. Transient flushing and nausea are experienced by some patients. No special aftercare is needed. The patient may be instructed to drink fluids liberally and double flush the toilet for 24 hours after the test.

SPECIAL TESTS

CT scans and ultrasonography may be used to detect and evaluate renal pathologic conditions such as tumors, stones, and polycystic kidneys by mapping the size, shape, and position of the structures. The procedure and patient care are similar to those used for evaluation of other organs.

Renal Angiography

Description—Renal angiography permits the detailed visualization of the renal vasculature following arterial injection of a contrast medium.

Procedure—The femoral artery is catheterized, and the catheter is advanced up the femoroiliac arteries to the aorta by means of fluoroscopy. Heparinized saline is used to prevent clotting. The contrast medium is injected into the renal arteries, and serial x-rays are taken. The test takes about 1 hour.

Patient preparation and aftercare—The patient is NPO for 8 hours before the test and assessed carefully for allergies to iodine, shellfish, or contrast media. Baseline vital signs and peripheral pulses are assessed and recorded before the test. After the test the patient is kept flat with the leg fully extended for 4 to 6 hours. Vital signs are recorded initially every 15 minutes, gradually moving to hourly. Peripheral pulses are assessed at the same time, and the insertion site is monitored for signs of bleeding. A pressure dressing is usually in place. Fluids are encouraged to facilitate removal of the dye.

Renal Biopsy

Description—Renal biopsy allows for evaluating type and stage of renal pathologic condition, differentiating diagnoses, and establishing prognosis.

Procedure—The biopsy specimen may be obtained percutaneously through a skin puncture or through an incision. Open biopsy reduces the risk of hemorrhage but is more invasive and carries the risks of anesthesia and infection.

Patient preparation and aftercare—Because the kidney is such a vascular organ, the risk of bleeding after biopsy is significant. The patient is carefully evaluated for bleeding disorders and may be typed and cross matched. The lower pole of the kidney is identified and marked on the skin. A local anesthetic is administered, and the patient is asked to hold his or her breath during insertion and removal of the biopsy needle. The patient is informed that pressure pain may be perceived as the needle penetrates the kidney capsule.

A pressure dressing is applied, and the patient is kept flat for 4 hours after the biopsy. Vital signs are recorded every 15 minutes initially and advanced slowly to hourly if stable. Hematuria is common for the first 24 hours.

The patient is kept at rest for 24 hours and discharged with instructions to avoid exertion and heavy lifting for 10 days.

CYSTOSCOPY

Description—Cystoscopy allows for direct examination of the bladder by means of a cystoscope.

Procedure—The cystoscope is slowly inserted into the urethra and bladder. The fiberoptic light source allows for visualization, and the instrument provides a channel for biopsy, excision of small lesions, and stone removal. Local, spinal, or general anesthetic may be utilized. The test takes about 30 minutes. Ureteral catheterization can also be performed through the cystoscope during the procedure.

Patient preparation and aftercare—No special preparation is needed unless a general anesthetic is planned and then the patient will be NPO. If a local anesthetic is planned the patient should anticipate a burning sensation when the cystoscope is passed through the urethra. Instillation of irrigating solution may create a strong urge to urinate.

Vital signs are monitored every 15 minutes immediately after the test. The patient should get out of bed cautiously and with supervision, because the lithotomy position can create dizziness and faintness as blood pools and shifts. The patient is instructed to consume fluids liberally and report any incidence of chills, fever, or flank pain immediately. Temporary mild hematuria and burning on urination are common but should subside promptly. Sitz baths may be comforting. A short course of antibiotics is often prescribed.

URINARY TRACT DISORDERS

The kidneys and other structures of the urinary system play a major role in regulating the body's internal environment. Functions include regulating the fluid and electrolyte balance, excreting metabolic wastes, maintaining the acid-base balance, producing or modifying the level of hormones responsible for regulation of blood pressure, metabolizing calcium, and synthesizing RBCs. Diseases and disorders of the urinary system are a significant cause of morbidity and mortality in the United States.

CONGENITAL DISORDERS

Structural malformations of the urinary system occur in about 10% to 15% of the population. They range from minor and inconsequential conditions to conditions that are incompatible with life. Common congenital problems are outlined in Box 12-1.

Polycystic Kidney Disease
Etiology/epidemiology

Polycystic kidney disease is the most common form of a relatively large group of disorders characterized by the

Duplication of ureters (partial or complete)
   Usually requires no intervention unless complications occur
Hydroureters
   Dilation of ureters
   May require surgical repair
Exstrophy of bladder
   Eversion of bladder on outer abdominal wall
   Requires extensive surgical correction in infancy
Epispadias or hypospadias
   Opening of urethra on dorsum or underside of penis
   Usually necessitates surgical correction

formation of fluid-filled cavities within the kidneys. It follows an autosomal dominant pattern of inheritance and may be recognized early in life or not until young adulthood. It is usually bilateral.

Pathophysiology

The cysts are scattered throughout the renal parenchyma. As they enlarge they compress and destroy the surrounding tissue by ischemia. The disease progresses relentlessly to renal failure by midlife. Dull, aching pain and episodes of hematuria are the most common early clinical manifestations. The risk of infection is increased, and patients may experience hypertension in advance of the classic signs of renal failure (see p. 273).

Medical management

There is no cure for polycystic kidney disease, and management is aimed at alleviating symptoms and slowing progression if possible. Strategies include the control of hypertension, prevention of infection, and management of progressive renal insufficiency.

NURSING MANAGEMENT

The nursing role is largely supportive. Comfort measures are explored for flank pain, and the patient is instructed in measures to prevent or identify infection. Psychosocial support is essential in dealing with the diagnosis, prognosis, and decisions about bearing children. Minimal life-style changes are needed until renal failure develops, but patients should avoid strenuous or contact sports.

URINARY TRACT INFECTIONS AND INFLAMMATIONS
Cystitis/Pyelonephritis
Etiology/epidemiology

Infections within the urinary tract are extremely common health problems, especially in women. They may occur at any point in the urinary system and are commonly associated with urinary retention and stasis, intrusive procedures, obstruction, and the presence of chronic illnesses such as diabetes. *Ascending* infection is the most common cause related to the short urethra in women and frequent contamination resulting from intercourse. Infection may also be spread via the blood, lymph, or direct extension from another organ.

Cystitis involves infection of the bladder or urethra. Pyelonephritis involves infection of the kidney tissue and may occur when bacteria ascend the urinary tract following cystitis. It is also commonly associated with pregnancy, obstruction, and instrumentation. Pyelonephritis, may be acute or chronic. Infection usually starts in the medulla and in chronic forms spreads to the cortex. It can produce kidney fibrosis and scarring and in rare cases may advance to renal failure.

Pathophysiology

Most infections result from gram-negative bacteria that originate in the intestinal tract and ascend to the bladder and urethra. They are most likely to occur when host resistance is compromised and in the presence of stasis plus an alkaline urine, which encourages bacterial growth. Reflux of urine into the ureters may facilitate movement of the organisms upward to the kidney itself. Chronic pyelonephritis can cause permanent destruction of renal tissue from repeated or ongoing inflammation and scarring.

Clinical manifestations of UTI typically include frequency, urgency, dysuria, cloudy or foul-smelling urine, and mild hematuria. Many persons, however, are either asymptomatic or experience minimal symptoms. Pyelonephritis may present with urinary symptoms, but systemic signs of inflammation are more common—chills and fever, malaise, flank pain, and tenderness along the costovertebral angle. Urinalysis and culture serve as the basis for diagnosis.

Medical management

The treatment of cystitis and pyelonephritis revolves around identification of the infecting organism through urine cultures and sterilization of the urine with appropriate antibiotic therapy. Follow-up cultures are indicated in pyelonephritis to identify and treat chronic forms. Medications commonly prescribed include the following:

   Urinary antiseptics—nitrofurantoin (Furadantin)
   Sulfonamides—cotrimoxazole (Bactrim, Septra)
   Urinary analgesics—phenazopyridine (Pyridium)
   These medications work directly on the mucosa of the urethra and bladder to relieve burning and discomfort.

Systemic antibiotics (ampicillin, cephalosporins) are also commonly prescribed and are particularly important in treating pyelonephritis.

Urine acidifiers (methenamine hippurate [Hiprex] or mandelate [Mandelamine]) may be used in chronic situations to reduce the suitability of the urine for bacterial growth.

NURSING MANAGEMENT

◆ ASSESSMENT

Subjective Data

History of urinary tract infection or disease

History of chronic disease

History of renal stones, prostatic enlargement, stasis, or intrusive procedure

Patient's complaints of the following:

Dysuria (painful urination): urgency, frequency, burning sensation

Fatigue or malaise

Flank pain or tenderness (pyelonephritis)

Objective Data

Hematuria (blood in urine)

Urine sample: odor, cloudiness, pH

Chills and fever

Positive laboratory reports from urine culture; elevated WBC count

◆ NURSING DIAGNOSES

Possible nursing diagnoses for the person with a urinary tract infection may include, but are not limited to, the following:

Pain and burning on urination (related to bladder inflammation and irritation)

Knowledge deficit (related to health promotional activities that prevent the recurrence of urinary tract infection)

◆ EXPECTED PATIENT OUTCOMES

Patient's urinary symptoms will gradually decrease.

Patient will be knowledgeable about measures that can help prevent recurrences of UTI.

◆ NURSING INTERVENTIONS

Promoting Comfort

Administer prescribed medication.

Advise patient that use of phenazopyridine (Pyridium) will cause urine to be a bright orange red.

Administer analgesics as needed for flank pain.

Encourage patient to take warm sitz baths for comfort if urethral burning is present.

Maintain high fluid intake during infection. Give 3000 to 4000 ml/day if not contraindicated.

Teaching for Self-Care

Teach patient health promotion activities to decrease chance of recurrence.

Explain importance of scrupulous perineal hygiene to female patients.

Patient should wipe carefully from front to back after urination or defecation.

Patient should empty bladder and cleanse self and partner before and after intercourse.

Patient should avoid use of bubble baths, contraceptive jellies, and other products that may alter vaginal pH.

Explain importance of maintaining high fluid intake (approximately 3 L daily).

Patient should modify diet to ensure urinary acidity (fish and poultry, whole grains) and monitor urine pH regularly. Explore need for urine acidifiers with physician.

Explain importance of responding promptly to urge to void. Patient should empty bladder every 2 to 3 hours.

Teach patient importance of taking full course of antibiotics.

Describe signs and symptoms of reinfection.

◆ EVALUATION

Successful achievement of expected outcomes for the patient with a UTI is indicated by the following:

Absence of symptoms of dysuria

Correct description of:

Optimal fluid intake and voiding pattern

Measures to reduce reinfection risk

Practices to promote hygiene

Signs of reinfection

Glomerulonephritis

Etiology/epidemiology

Glomerulonephritis affects the glomeruli of both kidneys and may be triggered by vascular injury, metabolic disease, or immunologic reactions. The most common form occurs 2 to 3 weeks after a streptococcal infection and primarily affects children. It usually resolves without complications but can progress to renal failure, especially in its chronic form. Adults are more likely to experience problems and complications with the disorder. Chronic disease may follow an acute episode, but most patients present with no history and no evidence for predisposing infection can be found.

NOTE: An acute form of nephritis can be the result of an idiosyncratic reaction to various drugs and chemicals.

GERONTOLOGIC PATIENT CONSIDERATIONS: URINARY TRACT INFECTION

UTIs are common problems in elderly persons. The risk of UTI increases steadily for women throughout their lives. The incidence rate is 1% among school-age girls but is up to 20% in persons over 65 years. The incidence is over 30% in persons over 80 years, particularly those who live in chronic care facilitie. Decreased vaginal secretions and pH changes, lower fluid intake, and decreased activity all play a role. In the older male, the increasing size of the prostate may create problems with retention and provide a breeding ground for infection. Many elderly persons do not have acute signs of dysuria, and the problem may be overlooked.

Solvents, pesticides, heavy metals, and certain antibiotics have all been implicated.

Pathophysiology

Glomerulonephritis is the result of an antigen-antibody reaction in the glomerular tissue. It causes swelling and death of capillary cells, activates the complement pathway, and attacks the glomerular basement membrane, increasing permeability. Obstruction and scarring may interfere with renal function. The chronic form of glomerulonephritis is characterized by progressive glomerular destruction that eventually leads to renal failure.

Clinical manifestations reflect the glomerular damage and include the following:

Leakage of protein and RBCs
Decreased glomerular filtration
Retention of waste products
General signs of systemic illness

Medical management

Glomerulonephritis is diagnosed by its classic signs and urinalysis showing proteinuria and hematuria. Serum values reflect elevations in BUN and creatinine. There is no specific treatment. Patients will be given prophylactic antibiotics and symptomatic therapy with diuretics and antihypertensives as needed. Dietary sodium will also be restricted. No specific treatment exists for the chronic form of the disease either.

NURSING MANAGEMENT

The nursing role is also supportive. The patient is initially on bed rest and fluid balance is carefully assessed through I & O, vital sign assessment, and daily weights. The nurse assesses daily for periorbital, pretibial, pedal, and sacral edema and explains the rationale and importance of the sodium restriction.

Activity may need to be strictly curtailed for weeks if proteinuria and hematuria persist, and the rationale for the restrictions should be reinforced. Maintaining skin integrity and providing for support and diversion will be important. Full recovery, if it occurs, may take months. Ongoing monitoring of urine parameters will take place.

Nephrotic Syndrome

Nephrotic syndrome is not a disease but a group of symptoms involving glomerular damage and losses of large amounts of protein in the urine. Although severe idiopathic forms occur in childhood, adult forms usually accompany identifiable glomerular disease and progress to renal failure. The pattern is similar to that described for glomerulonephritis, but the edema is severe and generalized and the protein losses are significant. Treatment is directed at reducing the protein losses and usually involves administration of corticosteroids. Dietary protein is increased to a level of 1 g/kg of body weight until the protein leakage subsides. Anorexia interferes with the effectiveness of protein replacement.

Diabetic nephropathy

Diabetic nephropathy is the leading cause of end-stage renal disease. It is estimated that 50% of patients with insulin-dependent diabetes mellitus (IDDM) will develop renal insufficiency or failure. Diabetics develop vascular changes more rapidly than nondiabetics. Lipids are theorized to leak into the renal vessels and precipitate, creating both glomerulosclerosis and nephrosclerosis. The most effective treatment is prevention through ongoing long-term metabolic control of the diabetes.

Nephrosclerosis

Hypertension is identified as the second most common cause of kidney failure. It is estimated that as many as 10% of individuals with essential hypertension will develop severe renal damage. Hypertension causes thickening and narrowing of the renal vessel, reducing blood flow and resulting in tubular necrosis and atrophy. The disease cannot be treated once it is established but can be largely prevented through careful screening and effective control of hypertension.

OBSTRUCTIVE DISORDERS
Renal Calculi
Etiology/epidemiology

Urinary stones may develop at any level in the urinary system but are most commonly found within the kidney. It is estimated that at least 1% of the general population will develop a stone. Over half of all cases are idiopathic. The presence of UTI is a major predisposing factor, because infection increases the amount of organic matter around which the mineral can precipitate. Urine alkalinity increases the rate of precipitation of calcium and magnesium phosphate.

Renal calculi produce urinary tract problems that reflect the stones' size and position. Large stones may produce obstruction of urine flow, pressure destruction of kidney tissue, and infection. Small stones may be successfully excreted from the urinary tract but cause severe local pain, spasm, and inflammation in the process. Rough stone edges may cause hematuria.

Pathophysiology

Stones are crystallizations of minerals around an organic base. Calcium stones account for about 75% of the total, and anything that leads to hypercalciuria can trigger the crystallization. Increased intake, immobility, and steroid use are all possibilities, but concentrated urine that directly increases the mineral content of the urine is felt to be more significant. Excesses of uric acid and cystine can also lead to stone formation.

Pain is the classic symptom of a stone. Its severity and location reflect the location of the stone. Pain triggered by movement along the ureter can be excruciating and is frequently accompanied by hematuria. A stone in the kidney may be asymptomatic for months or years.

Medical management

The diagnosis is established from the classic symptoms and may be verified by IVP or ultrasound. After the acute episode has subsided serum mineral levels will be determined to rule out any underlying disease that could influence stone formation. Since about 90% of renal calculi are passed spontaneously, the patient receives symptomatic support with hydration and analgesics. Ureteral catheters may be inserted via cystoscope to dilate the ureter and facilitate stone passage. Stones in the lower ureter may be removed by cystoscopic manipulation. Larger stones may need to be treated with extracorporeal shock wave lithotripsy (Box 12-2). Surgery will be used if other treatment approaches fail or if the kidney itself must be removed.

Common procedures are defined in Box 12-3.

NURSING MANAGEMENT

◆ ASSESSMENT

Subjective Data

Patient's complaint of:
    Pain (classic feature)
    Constant, dull pain if stone is in kidney
    Excruciating pain if stone is in ureter; pain may radiate to genitals or thigh
    Nausea and vomiting
Prior history of stones or urinary tract infection
Family history of stones

Objective Data

Hematuria
Changes in vital signs—fever or mild shock
Positive results from intravenous pyelogram (IVP)
Serum mineral levels

BOX 12-2	Extracorporeal Shock Wave and Ultrasonic Lithotripsy

These procedures have eliminated the need for surgery in most cases of renal calculi. In shock wave lithotripsy the patient is submerged in water in a large tank and shock waves are generated and focused directly on the stone to break it up. Epidural or general anesthesia may be used. The newer machines have eliminated the need for the water immersion, utilize ultrasound to localize the stone, and can be used without anesthesia.

After treatment, small stone particles are passed in the urine for several days and urine output is monitored. Hematuria is present initially but should resolve within a few hours. Redness or bruising may be present on the skin at the impact site for the shock wave, and local pain is expected. Episodes of renal colic may recur as the stone fragments are passed.

BOX 12-3	Surgical Management of Renal Calculi

URETEROLITHOTOMY

Removal of a stone by incision into the ureter, using either a flank (upper) or abdominal (lower) approach (Figure 12-2, *A*)
Ureteral catheter, referred to as a *stent,* placed to prevent stricture as ureter heals; must be carefully anchored to prevent dislodgement

PYELOLITHOTOMY

Removal of stone through or from renal pelvis (Figure 12-2, *B*)
Nephrostomy or pyelostomy tube may be inserted into kidney pelvis
Catheter must be carefully anchored to prevent dislodgement and *must* drain freely; not irrigated without a specific order

NEPHROLITHOTOMY

Removal of a stone through the kidney parenchyma (Figure 12-2, *C*)
May require splitting kidney
Placement of drainage tubes depends on specific procedure

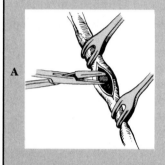
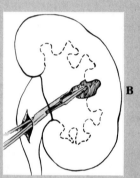
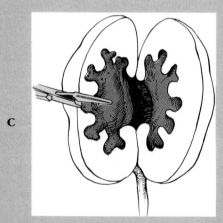

FIGURE 12-2   Location and methods of removing renal calculi from upper urinary tract. **A,** Ureterolithotomy. **B,** Pyelolithotomy. **C,** Nephrolithotomy with kidney split.

◆ NURSING DIAGNOSES

Possible nursing diagnoses for the person with renal calculi may include, but are not limited to, the following:
    Pain, acute (related to spasm and pressure in kidney or ureter)

Knowledge deficit (related to measures to prevent stone recurrence)

◆ EXPECTED PATIENT OUTCOMES

Patient's pain will be reduced to manageable levels; nausea and vomiting will be relieved.

Patient will be knowledgeable concerning measures that can prevent the recurrence of calculi.

◆ NURSING INTERVENTIONS

Promoting Comfort

Administer analgesics liberally as prescribed (morphine is usually ordered).

Assess effectiveness of pain relief.

Administer antispasmodics as ordered (Pro-Banthine).

Instruct patient to strain all urine.

Force fluids orally or administer intravenously to at least 3000 to 4000 ml daily.

Encourage patient to ambulate as tolerated once pain is controlled.

Monitor intake and output.

Assess urine for blood.

Teaching to Prevent Recurrence

Teach patient measures to prevent recurrence of stones.

Patient should maintain high daily fluid intake—approximately 3000 ml daily.

Patient should engage in active exercise and avoid constipation and immobility.

Patient should modify diet if appropriate. Possible modifications include the following:

Restrict calcium, found in milk and milk products, beans, dried fruit, chocolate, and cocoa.

Restrict oxalate, found in coffee, tea, chocolate, spinach, and beans.

Restrict purines, found in organ meats, legumes, sardines, and herring; moderate amounts are present in most meats.

Acidify the urine by eating an acid ash diet (Box 12-4) or taking prescribed urine acidifiers.

Monitor urine pH at regular intervals.

Explain purpose and side effects of prescribed medications.

◆ EVALUATION

Successful achievement of expected outcomes for the patient with renal calculi is indicated by the following:

Absence of pain, nausea, or tenderness

Correct description of:

Optimal fluid intake and activity pattern

Diet modifications and rationale

Proper administration of all medications

Care of the patient undergoing urologic surgery is summarized in the Guidelines box located on p. 272.

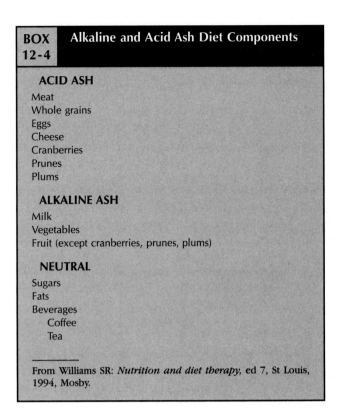

BOX 12-4 Alkaline and Acid Ash Diet Components

ACID ASH
Meat
Whole grains
Eggs
Cheese
Cranberries
Prunes
Plums

ALKALINE ASH
Milk
Vegetables
Fruit (except cranberries, prunes, plums)

NEUTRAL
Sugars
Fats
Beverages
    Coffee
    Tea

From Williams SR: *Nutrition and diet therapy*, ed 7, St Louis, 1994, Mosby.

Hydronephrosis

Hydronephrosis results from dilation of the renal pelvis and calyces with urine. It may be unilateral or bilateral and is caused by obstruction in the urinary system that causes urine to collect behind it. Excess pressure that reaches the renal pelvis leads to tissue destruction. Urine flow is decreased, and the stagnant urine is an excellent medium for infection. The person is asymptomatic as long as kidney function is adequate and the urine is able to drain. Pain results from tissue overdistention and may be dull or colicky in nature. The medical management is directed at the specific cause of the obstruction. Strictures can often be successfully dilated, but other causes may need surgical correction.

Tumors of the Urinary System

Renal tumors

Renal tumors, primarily adenocarcinomas, account for 3% of all cancers. They are most commonly seen in late middle-aged males. They usually develop unilaterally and can be successfully treated surgically if identified early. Nephrectomy is the treatment of choice for renal tumors, and the associated care is similar to that provided for other renal or abdominal surgery.

Tumors of the bladder

Etiology/epidemiology—The bladder is the most common cancer site in the urinary tract. The tumors occur primarily in men in late middle age and frequently with multiple tumor sites. The incidence of bladder cancer is associated with chronic exposure to cigarette smoke, chemicals, dyes, and heavy alcohol use.

Guidelines for Nursing Care of the Patient Following Urologic Surgery

PREOPERATIVE

Reinforce teaching about procedure and aftercare as needed.
Teach coughing and deep breathing methods. Emphasize importance of effective coughing to patients with high flank incision, since the incision's proximity to diaphragm will make coughing difficult.

POSTOPERATIVE

Provide adequate analgesia to facilitate deep breathing and coughing. Utilize patient-controlled analgesia (PCA) if possible.
  Use incentive spirometer every 2 hours.
  Help patient to splint incision.
Change positions frequently.
Monitor urine output every 1 to 2 hours; should be at least 50 ml/hr.
  Record output separately for each drainage tube.
  Estimate urine drainage on dressings.
  Observe urine's color and consistency.
Weigh patient daily.
Encourage patient to ambulate if ureteral catheters are not in place.
Assess patient for return of bowel sounds, passage of flatus.
Ensure IV hydration until patient tolerates food and fluids orally. Ensure intake of 3000 ml/day.
Monitor patient carefully for signs of bleeding.
  Risk is high if parenchyma has been incised.
  Risk is greatest on day of surgery and 8 to 12 days after surgery.
Change dressing aseptically and frequently to keep site of incision dry. Use of Montgomery straps will facilitate dressing changes. Copious drainage is expected.
  Stoma bags may be utilized for large amounts of drainage.
  Keep skin clean and odor free.
Maintain patency of all drainage tubes.
  Position patient so kinking or obstruction does not occur.
  Never clamp or irrigate ureteral catheters or nephrostomy tubes without specific orders.

Pathophysiology—Most bladder tumors begin as benign papillomas and occur in multiple locations. They arise from transitional epithelium cell types. Painless hematuria is a common early sign. Advanced disease may cause infection, fistula development, or ureteral obstruction leading to renal failure.

Medical management—The diagnosis of bladder cancer is established by means of cystoscopic visualization and biopsy. Determination of the invasiveness of the tumor is important in establishing a treatment program. Benign papillomas and small tumors are treated with transurethral fulguration or excision. Segmental resection may be performed if the dome of the bladder is involved. Cystectomy is performed only if the disease appears to be curable. External radiation treatment may be given before surgery to slow tumor growth. Chemotherapy is primarily used for palliation.

If the entire bladder is removed, urinary diversion is required. The ileal conduit has been the most common

choice, but several other options exist (Figure 12-3, *A*). Continent urostomies involve creation of a valve that permits self-catheterization. The Kock pouch is formed from the small intestine, whereas the Indiana pouch consists of portions of large intestine and ileum (Figure 12-3, *B* and *C*). With continent urostomies the ureters are anastomosed to the colon reservoir in a manner to prevent the reflux of urine.

NURSING MANAGEMENT

The nursing care for patients with urinary diversions is similar to that provided after any major abdominal surgery. It may necessitate short-term hemodynamic monitoring. The care is outlined in the Guidelines box.

URINARY RETENTION AND INCONTINENCE
Urinary Retention

Urinary retention is the inability to expel urine from the bladder. The problem can have either mechanical or functional causes. Anatomic obstructions are the most common cause. The bladder becomes distended and may be displaced out of the pelvis. Discomfort results from pressure, and the person may have a strong urge to urinate. Voiding of 25 to 50 ml of urine at frequent intervals often represents retention with overflow. The bladder does not empty.

Retention can create a urologic emergency. Treatment is aimed at reestablishing urine flow and may involve urethral catheterization, stimulation of the detrusor muscle with the cholinergic agent bethanechol (Urecholine), suprapubic catheterization, or immediate surgical intervention. Urethral catheter options are described in Box 12-5.

Urinary Incontinence

Urinary incontinence is the involuntary loss of urine from the lower urinary tract. It produces hygiene, social, and emotional consequences that can be profound for the patient. More than 10 million Americans suffer some degree of incontinence (15% to 30% of the noninstitutionalized population over 60 years). The incidence is greater than 50% in nursing home residents. Women experience twice the incidence of men.

Incontinence may be caused by multiple temporary or permanent anatomic, pathologic, and physiologic factors affecting the urinary tract. The major types of incontinence are outlined in Box 12-6.

The management of incontinence is complex and may involve surgical repair, bladder retraining, and the long-term use of a urine collection device. These options are described in Box 12-7 and the Guidelines box.

Perineal exercises may be an important aspect of gaining control with stress incontinence. All older women should be instructed in the practice (Box 12-8) and encouraged to perform these exercises several times daily.

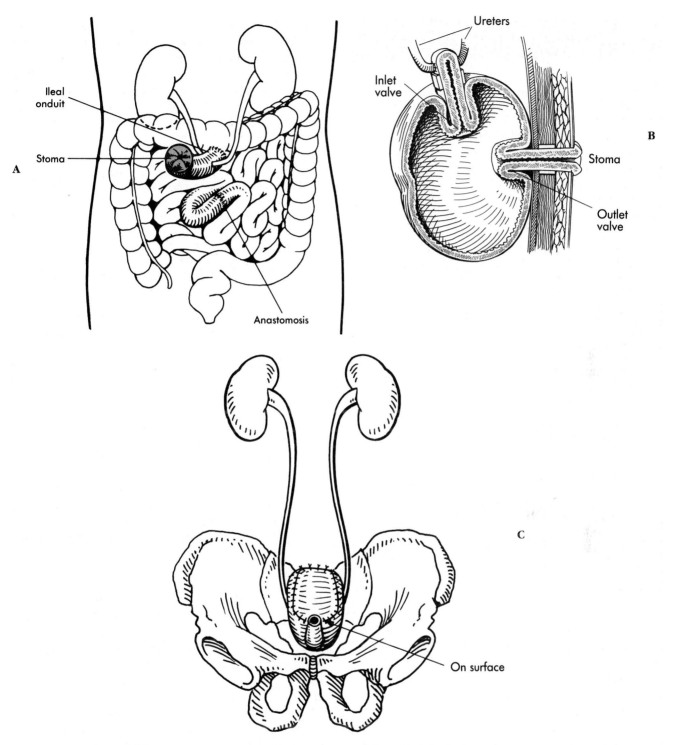

FIGURE 12-3 Options for urinary diversion. **A,** Ileal conduit. **B,** Kock continent urostomy. **C,** Indiana pouch—continent urostomy.

Despite consistent efforts, incontinence may be a persistent problem for many persons. Numerous pads and diaper systems are available, but skin integrity is an ongoing concern. Catheterization may be the best choice for some people. External systems can be easily applied for men. An alternative to commercial products is shown in Figure 12-4. The catheter should be removed at least once daily for soap and water cleansing and skin inspection.

RENAL FAILURE

The kidneys have a tremendous ability to adapt to a decreasing number of functioning nephrons and still maintain adequate function. Renal failure is a state of severe impairment or total lack of renal function, and it does not occur until the number of functioning nephrons falls below 25%. The patient is then unable to maintain the internal equilibrium of the body fluids. The

Guidelines for Nursing Care of the Patient Undergoing Urinary Diversion (Ileal Conduit)

PREOPERATIVE CARE

Provide accurate information about procedure and care.

Provide introduction to self-care materials if patient exhibits readiness.

Introduce enterostomal therapist to begin teaching plan. Select and mark the proposed ostomy site.

Explore patient's openness to visitation by a volunteer from the United Ostomy Association.

Prepare patient for appearance of stoma and provide with written materials if appropriate.

Encourage patient to verbalize feelings about change in body image and function.

Initiate bowel preparation as ordered.

Provide clear liquids.

Administer enemas, intestinal antibiotics, and oral bowel cleansing solutions.

POSTOPERATIVE CARE

Use standard interventions to identify and prevent complications.

Provide TED stockings; encourage patient to do range of motion exercises, make position changes, and ambulate as permitted to prevent thrombophlebitis (risk is high after pelvic surgery).

Assess for Homans' sign every shift.

Maintain patency of nasogastric (NG) tube until peristalsis returns (3 to 5 days). Auscultate abdomen for bowel sounds.

Observe stoma for complications.

Stoma should be healthy bright pink or red.

Observe for bleeding or erosion.

Assess surrounding skin.

Maintain high fluid intake. Teach patient symptoms of urinary tract infection.

Stent tubes will be placed initially to promote drainage (approximately 10 days).

Urine will contain mucus from bowel.

Empty bag every 2 hours; attach to Foley drainage bag at night.

Monitor urine output. Edema in the stoma may obstruct urine outflow. Catheter placement may be required.

Provide meticulous care to surrounding skin.

Ensure proper fit of appliance; remeasure carefully as stoma shrinks.

Maintain an acid pH.

Teach patient skills for self-care of appliance (assembly, application, emptying and changing of the pouch) (see Guidelines box).

Pouches are generally changed every 3-4 days before skin problems occur.

Encourage patient to verbalize feelings about surgery. Discuss impact of surgery on work, leisure, clothing, and sexual activity.

Put patient in touch with support groups and agencies in the community to facilitate adjustment.

Refer for home health assistance as needed. Teach patient to monitor carefully for signs of UTI.

Guidelines for Changing a Urinary Pouch

1. Assemble all supplies.
2. Empty the pouch and gently remove the pouch from the skin.
3. Cleanse the skin surrounding the stoma with mild soap and water. Rinse and pat dry. Mucus secretions should be washed off the stoma gently.
4. Place a rolled piece of gauze or cotton balls over the stomal opening to absorb draining urine while the skin is being cared for.
5. Measure the diameter of the stoma and cut a corresponding opening in the skin barrier and the pouch or select the corresponding size of precut pouch.
6. Apply skin sealant around the stoma if desired. Allow the area to dry completely.
7. Attach the pouch to the skin barrier. The pouch and skin barrier may be applied to the skin separately or together. In the early postoperative period it is easier to attach the pouch to the skin barrier and then to apply the system in one piece to the skin.
8. Apply the pouch and skin barrier around the stoma, keeping the adhesive area free of wrinkles or creases. Press gently but firmly into place. The valve at the bottom of the pouch must be closed or attached to drainage tubing and a collection bag.

BOX 12-5   Bladder Catheterization

Note: Catheterization is a major cause of UTI, and strict aseptic technique should be maintained. Options include the following:

Whistle-tip	Open slant end
Robinson	Closed end, many "eyes"
Foley	Balloon (5 or 30 ml) to secure catheter in bladder, 14 to 18 Fr size
Coudé	Tapered curved end
Malecot	"Bat wing"–shaped tip
Pezzar	Mushroom-shaped tip

Intermittent catheterization is used primarily in the treatment of neurogenic bladder dysfunction. Periodic complete emptying eliminates residual urine, maintains bladder tone, and reduces the incidence of infection, even with clean technique.

BOX 12-6 Incontinence

TYPES

Stress

Related to incompetence of the bladder outlet or urethral closure

Any increase in abdominal pressure (laughing, sneezing, coughing) leads to involuntary loss of less than 50 ml of urine

Related to relaxed pelvic muscles and obesity

Urge

Related to infection, decreased bladder capacity, overdistention of bladder

Unopposed detrusor muscle contractions occur

Involuntary loss of urine occurring soon after a strong sense of urgency to void

Reflex

Related to neurologic impairment such as spinal cord injury or lesion

Involuntary loss of urine when a specific volume is reached

Functional

Related to sensory, cognitive, or mobility deficits

Involuntary unpredictable loss of urine

Total

Related to neurologic dysfunction, spinal nerve disease, or trauma

Continuous and unpredictable loss of urine

COMMON CAUSES OF INCONTINENCE

Cerebral Clouding

Lack of awareness of sensation of full bladder or lack of energy and involvement in self-care to exercise voluntary control

Common cause in institutionalized elderly persons

Disturbance of CNS Pathways

Adequate voluntary control impaired by cerebral damage

May follow trauma, embolus, or cerebrovascular accident (CVA)

Reflex Disturbances

Lesions above S2 do not destroy reflex arc but destroy ability to inhibit reflex

Bladder emptying automatic at low volumes

Damage below sacral segments interrupts reflex arc and creates a flaccid bladder characterized by retention of urine

Relaxed Musculature

Seen primarily in postmenopausal women who have had vaginal deliveries but also occurs in men after perineal prostatectomy

---

 ## Home Bladder Catheterization

Utilize clean technique unless physician orders otherwise.

Wash hands carefully before handling catheter.

Intermittent catheters may be reused with soap and water cleansing after each use.

Indwelling catheters

  Cleanse meatal catheter junction with soap and water twice daily.

  Keep drainage system intact as much as possible. If leg bag is in use during the day:

    Clean connecting sites with alcohol before each disconnection and reconnection.

    Wrap exposed tubing tip in sterile gauze secured with a rubber band.

    Wash bag and tubing with soap and water daily.

    Always keep collecting bag below the level of the pelvis to prevent reflux.

  Shower or tub bathing is permissible. Replace thigh tape after bathing.

  Report any sign of infection to physician promptly.

BOX 12-7 Surgical Correction of Incontinence

Vesicourethropexy (Marshall-Marchetti procedure) involves fixation of the urethra to the fascia of the rectus muscle with support provided to the bladder neck. A catheter is inserted postoperatively for about 1 week.

The Stamey procedure involves suspension of the bladder neck by sutures passed adjacent to the ureterovesical junction. The procedure is less invasive.

Repair of uterine prolapse/rectocele and support of the bladder are often excellent strategies for relieving pressure on the bladder.

With artificial sphincters a hydraulically activated sphincter mechanism is placed around the urethra or bladder neck. It is opened and closed by means of pressure on small implanted bulbs. It has had more success with men than women.

Guidelines for Bladder Retraining

Incontinence that is primarily related to cerebral clouding can often be treated with a persistent retraining program. The person is slowly reconditioned to recognize and respond appropriately to the stimulus to void. A bladder program involves the following:

Establishing a strict voiding schedule, using expected voiding times, such as bedtime, awakening, and before or after meals

Tracking accidental voidings and adjusting schedule as needed

Establishing a 1- to 2-hour planned pattern if longer intervals are ineffective

Utilizing normal toilets or commodes if possible

Ensuring a fluid intake near 3000 ml daily
   Administer at scheduled intervals
   Consider effects of diuretic administration
   Restrict fluids after 4:00 PM

Gaining the patient's attention to voiding and reinforcing successful efforts
   Mobilizing the patient
     Assuming a natural position

Being consistent and allowing adequate time

BOX 12-8   Perineal Exercises

1. Tighten the perineal muscles as if to prevent voiding; hold for 3 seconds, then relax.
2. Inhale through pursed lips while tightening perineal muscles.
3. Bear down as if to have a bowel movement. Relax and then tighten perineal muscles.
4. Hold a pencil in the fold between the buttock and thigh.
5. Sit on the toilet with knees held wide apart. Start and stop the urinary stream.

---

problem may develop abruptly or be the end result of a long-standing, progressive kidney disorder.

Renal insufficiency exists when enough kidney function remains to sustain homeostasis despite extensive loss of renal function. It is usually a stage in a progressive problem.

Acute Renal Failure

Etiology/epidemiology

Acute renal failure is a sudden and potentially reversible decrease or cessation in kidney function. The potential for recovery depends on the nature of the underlying problem, treatment received, and the patient's underlying health status. There are multiple potential causes (Box 12-9), which are commonly categorized as prerenal, renal, and postrenal.

Pathophysiology

Renal ischemia occurs when blood flow to the kidneys is decreased. The kidney responds with vasoconstric-

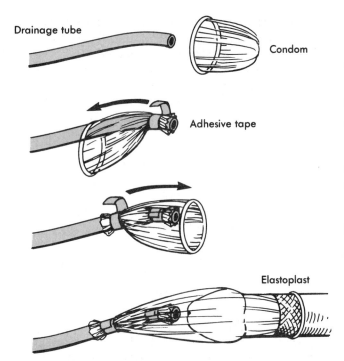

FIGURE 12-4 An alternative to commercial external drainage systems.

BOX 12-9   Common Causes of Acute Renal Failure

PRERENAL

Hypovolemic or septic shock
Anaphylaxis
Massive GI losses
Cardiac failure, dysrhythmia
Trauma, burns, hemorrhage

RENAL

Toxic chemicals, metals, dyes, pesticides
Drug and transfusion reactions
Drug overdoses
Neoplasms
Lupus, malignant hypertension

POSTRENAL

Kidney stones
Urethral obstruction
Prostatic hypertrophy
Stricture or stenosis

---

tion, which further reduces blood flow and worsens ischemia. Prolonged ischemia produces death of renal tubular tissue and triggers the failure. The kidneys are then unable to excrete fluid loads, regulate electrolytes, or excrete metabolic wastes. Acute failure commonly occurs in three phases:

Oliguric phase—Outputs falls to 400 ml or less per day, reflecting damage to nephrons. Urine may also be dilute because of the tubules' loss of concentrating ability. Fluid is retained, which leads to volume overload. Sodium is diluted by the excess fluid, but potassium accumulates rapidly. The serum BUN and creatinine elevate as waste products of metabolism collect.

Diuretic phase—Second phase begins in days or weeks. Increasing output indicates healing of the nephrons. Inability to excrete proportional amounts of wastes or concentrate urine reflects continued tubular damage. Large amounts of fluids and electrolytes are lost. Metabolic wastes are gradually excreted as healing occurs, and BUN and creatinine return slowly to baseline.

Recovery phase—Recovery may take months as kidneys gradually return to normal or near normal levels of functioning. Fluid and electrolyte levels are at or near normal levels.

Table 12-4 summarizes the major clinical manifestations of acute renal failure.

Medical management

The treatment of acute renal failure is specific to the cause of the problem and the unique needs of each stage. In the oliguric phase, the goals are to control fluids and electrolytes and promote the excretion of metabolic wastes. In milder cases these goals are met through fluid restriction; dietary restriction of sodium, potassium, and protein; and drug therapy. In more severe cases, dialysis is required. Peritoneal dialysis, hemodialysis, or continuous renal replacement therapy may be utilized (Box 12-10).

During the diuretic phase the goals remain to balance fluids and electrolytes, but fluid replacement may be necessary. Dialysis is often continued to balance electrolytes and excrete wastes, and dietary restrictions are maintained until the blood values normalize.

BOX 12-10	Continuous Renal Replacement Therapy (CRRT)

CRRT provides for almost continuous ultrafiltration of the extracellular fluid. Both arterial access and venous access are established and often use the femoral artery. The patient's blood pressure powers the system. Water, electrolytes, and other solutes are removed as blood passes over a semipermeable membrane in the hemofilter. The transfer utilizes both convection forces (supplied by the blood pressure) and diffusion forces (supplied by creating a concentration gradient in the filter with dialysate solution).

The process is gradual and prevents rapid fluctuations in fluid and electrolyte status. It is appropriate for unstable and critically ill patients. Three basic variations are in current use:

1. Slow continuous ultrafiltration (SCUF) slowly removes water and some solutes. It focuses on fluid balance and is useful in extreme CHF. It is ineffective for severe azotemia.
2. Continuous arteriovenous hemofiltration (CAVH) continuously removes larger volumes of water and solutes. Ultrafiltrate losses are replaced intravenously as indicated to establish normal balance.
3. Continuous arteriovenous hemodialysis (CAVHD) combines the filtration of CAVH with diffusion dialysis. Solute removal is significantly increased. It can be used as primary dialysis therapy for a wide range of patients.

NURSING MANAGEMENT

Monitor and record all hemodynamic and fluid balance parameters.
Maintain patency of ultrafiltration system.
Maintain patency of arterial and venous access sites.
Monitor for signs of infection.

NURSING MANAGEMENT

◆ ASSESSMENT
Subjective Data

History of precipitating factors
Use of drugs—prescription or recreational
Patient's complaints of the following:
    Change in voiding pattern
    Abrupt weight gain, edema
    Weakness, fatigue, nausea
    Confusion or drowsiness

Objective Data

Signs of fluid overload
    CHF, pulmonary edema
    Hypertension
    Peripheral edema
    Distended neck veins
Accurate intake and output records; low specific gravity of urine, urine output below 400 ml/24 hr
Daily weights
Level of consciousness
Laboratory reports demonstrating hyperkalemia, elevated creatinine and BUN (blood urea nitrogen), metabolic acidosis, hyponatremia

■ ■ ■

TABLE 12-4	Clinical Manifestations of Acute Renal Failure	
PHYSIOLOGIC CHANGE	**CLINICAL MANIFESTATIONS**	
OLIGURIC PHASE		
Inability to excrete fluid	Edema, low specific gravity, low urine output	
	Neck vein distention	
	Hypertension, congestive heart failure (CHF)	
	Pulmonary edema	
Inability to regulate electrolytes: hyperkalemia, hyponatremia, acidosis	Anorexia, nausea, vomiting	
	Kussmaul breathing	
	Drowsiness, confusion, coma	
	Cardiac arrhythmias	
Inability to excrete metabolic wastes: increased serum BUN, creatinine	Nausea and vomiting	
	GI bleeding	
	Drowsiness, confusion	
	Pericarditis	
DIURETIC PHASE		
Inability to reabsorb filtered fluid in tubules	Urine output of 4-5 L/day	
	Tachycardia, postural hypotension	
	Weight loss	
	Thirst, decreased skin turgor	

Nursing management during the oliguric phase of acute renal failure is summarized in the "Nursing care plan." Interventions during the diuretic phase include the following:

Maintain interventions outlined in the Nursing Care Plan on pp. 279 to 281.

Monitor patient for fluid and electrolyte depletion.
 Monitor output hourly.
 Assess skin turgor and mucous membranes.
 Assess mental status every 8 hours.

Provide replacement fluid as prescribed.

Teach patient rationale for ongoing dialysis in face of rising urine output.

Teach patient about diet restrictions and medications for long-term rehabilitation, and explain importance of avoiding infection.

Chronic Renal Failure

Etiology/epidemiology

Chronic renal failure is a significant health care problem, causing nearly 60,000 deaths each year and leaving an additional 200,000 persons dependent on lifelong dialysis. Chronic failure exists when the kidneys are unable to maintain the body's internal environment and recovery is not expected. The development of chronic failure is usually a slow process, occurring over a period of years. Recurrent infections, obstruction, and blood vessel destruction from diabetes and hypertension are common predisposing causes. Prevention efforts therefore focus on the diagnosis and control of hypertension and effective metabolic management of diabetes mellitus. Repeated episodes of tissue death and scarring may trigger insufficiency and finally total failure.

Pathophysiology

In chronic failure the nephrons are selectively affected. The exact pathologic process depends on the underlying disease process, but the net result is loss of functioning nephrons. Intact nephron units hypertrophy and allow the kidney to compensate until about 75% of the nephrons are destroyed. Initially, the heavy solute load may trigger an osmotic diuresis, but eventually, with the loss of more nephrons, oliguria and retention of waste products occur.

Although the process varies substantially from person to person, there are some common features. The specific clinical manifestations are the result of fluid and electrolyte disturbances, altered regulatory mechanisms, and waste product retention and are summarized in Box 12-11.

Medical management

In early stages, chronic renal failure may be managed conservatively through control of fluid intake, diet restrictions, and treatment of concurrent disorders. This approach is usually short term and involves the following:

Fluid: intake proportional to output

| BOX 12-11 | Organ Changes and Clinical Manifestations of Chronic Renal Failure |

FLUID AND ELECTROLYTE IMBALANCES

Hypertension
Congestive heart failure
Atherosclerotic heart disease secondary to hypertension
Bone pain, osteodystrophy secondary to decreased calcium absorption and phosphate retention
Seizures secondary to electrolyte imbalance

RETENTION OF WASTE PRODUCTS

Halitosis secondary to ammonia accumulation
Anorexia, nausea and vomiting
Gastritis, GI bleeding secondary to mucosal irritation by ammonia
Fatigue, headache, sleep disturbances
Pericarditis
Dry scaly skin, pruritus, brittle nails

ALTERED REGULATORY MECHANISMS

Anemia secondary to dialysis, RBC destruction, and decreased secretion of erythropoietin
Decreased platelet activity, bleeding tendencies
Glucose intolerance
Sexual dysfunction, infertility, impotence
Protein wasting
Hyperpigmentation of skin

Diet
 Low potassium, sodium, phosphorus
 Protein restricted to less than 40 g/day from high biologic value sources
 High complex carbohydrates and fat to prevent catabolism

Medications
 Exchange resins (Kayexalate) to reduce serum potassium
 Phosphate binders (Amphogel, Basaljel) to facilitate phosphorus excretion
 Vitamin D (Calcitriol) to support calcium absorption
 Epoetin alpha (EPO) recombinant erythropoietin to stimulate RBC production
 Iron to support blood cell production
 Folate and vitamin B_{12} for red cell production
 Antihypertensive agents (calcium channel blockers or ACE inhibitors)
 Androgens (nandrolone decanoate) to stimulate renal and extrarenal erythropoietin production

NURSING MANAGEMENT

◆ ASSESSMENT
Subjective Data

History/duration of disease and its treatment
Knowledge of disease and treatment
Medications in use and patient's knowledge of their purpose

NURSING CARE PLAN

PERSON WITH ACUTE RENAL FAILURE

■ NURSING DIAGNOSIS
Fluid volume excess (related to failure of renal regulatory mechanism)

Expected Patient Outcome	Nursing Interventions

Patient will maintain a fluid and electrolyte balance that is within an acceptable range. Body weight will be stable.	1. Maintain accurate intake and output records.
	   a. Record hourly during acute stage.
	   b. Measure urine specific gravity.
	2. Weigh patient daily.
	3. Restrict fluids as prescribed (usually 500 ml daily plus output).
	   a. Utilize controller for all IV fluids.
	   b. Plan with patient to distribute fluids effectively throughout the day.
	   c. Teach the rationale and importance of fluid restrictions.
	   d. Employ comfort measures for thirst (mouth care, ice chips, moist cloth for mouth).
	4. Assess status of edema.
	   a. Monitor vital signs frequently. Monitor for CHF and pulmonary edema.
	   b. Assess neck veins, skin turgor, and mucous membrane; note peripheral edema. Assess dependent areas (periorbital, presacral, feet and legs).
	5. Monitor for and report signs of hyperkalemia, hyponatremia, or acidosis during oliguric phase.

■ NURSING DIAGNOSIS
Nutrition, altered: high risk for less than body requirements (related to diet restrictions, anorexia, and nausea)

Expected Patient Outcome	Nursing Interventions
Patient will ingest a diet that conforms to needed restrictions yet meets all nutritional needs.	1. Administer antiemetics if prescribed. 2. Explore food preferences and encourage adequate intake. Ginger ale is often well tolerated. 3. Give good mouth care before oral feedings. 4. Provide patient with a moist cloth to keep lips moist. Offer ice chips if allowed. 5. Plan with patient to distribute allowed fluid intake effectively throughout the day. 6. Restrict protein content as prescribed—ensure high biologic value. 7. Encourage a high-carbohydrate, high-fat diet as tolerated. 8. Assess nutrient intake. Perform calorie counts.

Continued.

NURSING CARE PLAN—CONT'D

PERSON WITH ACUTE RENAL FAILURE

■ NURSING DIAGNOSIS
Skin integrity, high risk for impaired (related to alterations in skin turgor associated with edema)

Expected Patient Outcome	Nursing Interventions
Patient will maintain an intact skin.	1. Assess skin each shift. 2. Keep skin clean and dry. 3. Put pressure devices on bed—special attention to heels and sacrum. 4. Turn every 2 hours. 5. Avoid shearing force when moving patient. 6. Bathe patient frequently, using bland, super-fat soap and tepid water. 7. Administer prescribed antipruritics as needed.

■ NURSING DIAGNOSIS
Fatigue (related to waste product accumulation)

Expected Patient Outcome	Nursing Interventions
Patient will gradually resume self-care activities and activities of daily living (ADL).	1. Promote maximal rest to lower metabolic load. 2. Assist with ADL as needed. 3. Employ active nursing measures to prevent complications related to immobility. 4. Encourage ambulation as condition stabilizes. 5. Avoid exposing patient to persons with infections.

Usual dietary patterns, adherence to restrictions

Impact of disease and treatment on preferred life-style

Effect of disease on relationships, sexual functioning

Patient's complaints of the following:

Lethargy, fatigue, irritability, or depression

Headaches, anorexia, nausea

Paresthesias, muscle twitching, pruritus

Weight loss

Bone pain with ambulation, neuropathies

Objective Data

Skin changes—sallow, brownish, pale, dry

Evidence of petechiae, bruising

Edema

Hypertension, signs of CHF

Intake and output—oliguria or anuria

Daily weights

Dry hair and brittle nails

Evidence of calcium deposits in skin

Ammonia odor to breath

Laboratory reports showing hyperkalemia and elevated BUN, creatinine, and phosphate levels; metabolic acidosis; anemia

◆ NURSING DIAGNOSES

Nursing diagnoses for the person with chronic renal failure may include, but are not limited to, the following:

Fluid volume excess (related to the failure of renal regulatory mechanisms)

Nutrition, altered: high risk for less than body requirements (related to multiple restrictions, anorexia, and nausea)

Fatigue (related to anemia and decreased nutrition)

Pain (bone, muscle cramping, pruritus) (related to uremia and electrolyte imbalance)

Knowledge deficit (related to the treatment protocol necessary to sustain healthy functioning)

Coping, high risk for ineffective individual or family (related to life-style restrictions and dependence on dialysis for sustaining life)

◆ EXPECTED PATIENT OUTCOMES

Patient will maintain an acceptable fluid and electrolyte balance on dialysis.

Patient will plan and consume a daily food intake that meets the body's nutritional needs and stays within prescribed restrictions.

NURSING CARE PLAN—CONT'D

PERSON WITH ACUTE RENAL FAILURE

■ NURSING DIAGNOSIS
Alteration in thought processes (related to the accumulation of waste products)

Expected Patient Outcome	Nursing Interventions
Patient will be fully oriented and able to problem solve effectively.	1. Assess mental status for changes (confusion, somnolence). 2. Orient to person, place, and time as necessary. 3. Provide simple explanations, and repeat instructions as necessary. 4. Ensure a safe environment. Keep side rails up, and supervise ambulation. 5. Reassure patient that mental capacities will return with recovery. 6. Explain reasons for behavior to family and friends.

■ NURSING DIAGNOSIS
Knowledge deficit (related to treatment and progression of disease process)

Expected Patient Outcome	
Patient will understand nature of disorder and therapeutic regimen.	1. Teach patient the following: a. Basis of symptoms and therapy b. Avoidance of preventable factors, if appropriate c. Prescribed medications and dietary regimens d. Rationale for dialysis and mechanisms of action e. Signs of returning renal problems or infections f. Need for follow-up care

Patient's energy level will improve to the point where patient can complete normal daily activities.

Patient will have less pruritus, anorexia, and nausea as condition stabilizes with dialysis. Patient's pain will not interfere with normal activities.

Patient will be knowledgeable about all aspects of treatment protocol: medications, diet, dialysis.

Patient and family will make adequate adjustments to the life-style changes caused by dialysis.

◆ NURSING INTERVENTIONS
Maintaining Fluid Balance

Maintain accurate intake and output records. Monitor for imbalances.

Weigh patient daily.

Restrict fluids as prescribed. Plan with patient to distribute fluids effectively throughout the day. Offer fluids in small amounts.

Monitor patient for edema; assess thirst.

Assess vital signs for signs of fluid overload.

Monitor skin integrity, and promote excellent hygiene.

Promoting an Adequate Diet

Provide frequent gentle oral hygiene, especially before meals.

Make meals and environment as pleasant as possible.
Explore food preferences with patient and incorporate where possible.
Use herbs for seasoning.
Offer small frequent meals.
Utilize antiemetics as ordered.
Reinforce importance of sufficient nutrients and calories to prevent catabolism.
Initiate calorie counts if intake is low.

Use stool softeners as needed to avoid constipation.

Administer aluminum hydroxide with meals to bind excess phosphorus.

Administer vitamin D and calcium as prescribed to combat bone demineralization.

Conserving Energy

Help patient plan and space activities to conserve energy.
Plan for adequate rest.
Assist patient with ADL as needed.

Assess patient for dyspnea and tachycardia, peripheral perfusion, and other symptoms of activity intolerance.

Provide adequate warmth.

Encourage patient to remain involved in self-care activities.

Promoting Comfort

Attempt to relieve muscle cramps with use of heat and massage. Quinine sulfate may be used at bedtime.

Ensure environmental safety.

Institute measures to control pruritus.

Teach patient importance of maintaining skin integrity. Administer antipruritics.

Control heat and humidity in environment.

Use oils and lotions to keep skin soft.

Assess regularly for bleeding or bruising. Avoid use of aspirin.

Use artificial tears to combat eye dryness.

Teaching for Self-Care

Teach patient about diet restrictions and rationale.

Protein

Ensure use of high biologic value protein.

Restriction usually is not below 40 g daily.

Ensure adequate intake of carbohydrates and fats for energy.

Sodium

Teach patient principles of sodium-restricted diet.

Encourage patient to read product labels carefully.

Caution patient that most salt substitutes are high in potassium and should not be used.

Potassium

Teach patient importance of restricting potassium in diet. Explain which foods are high in potassium.

Teach patient to avoid trauma and infection, because tissue breakdown liberates potassium.

Help patient develop effective strategies for taking medications as prescribed. Teach patient importance of general hygiene and avoidance of infection. Ensure that patient has a detailed plan for follow-up care.

Promoting Active Coping

Encourage patient to verbalize feelings about restrictions and treatment regimen.

Help patient maintain open communication with family and sexual partner.

Help patient explore financial and social resources in community.

Support all positive coping strategies employed by patient and family.

Support maintenance of family structure and desired roles.

Provide patient with opportunities to discuss issues involving sexuality and reproduction. Provide patient with accurate information.

Encourage patient to maintain hope and positive feelings about dialysis.

Identify all available community resources.

Refer for vocational guidance and reimbursement assistance for care needs.

♦ EVALUATION

Successful achievement of expected outcomes for the patient with chronic renal failure is indicated by the following:

Balanced intake and output; absence of hypertension or evidence of edema

Consumption of a diet that meets baseline nutritional needs and follows prescribed restrictions; positive nitrogen balance maintained

Participation in normal ADL

Hemoglobin and hematocrit levels stable

Muscle cramping, bone pain, and pruritus absent or controlled; skin intact

Accurate discussion of components of treatment plan; medications taken on schedule

Participation as informed decision maker in all aspects of care planning and is consulted about proposed changes in treatment regimen

Dialysis

Dialysis involves the movement of fluid and particles across a semipermeable membrane. It can help restore normal fluid and electrolyte balance, control acid-base balance, and remove waste and toxic material from the body through the processes of diffusion, osmosis, and ultrafiltration. It is used temporarily in acute failure and as a permanent substitute for the loss of renal function in patients with chronic end-stage disease. There are two main types: hemodialysis and peritoneal dialysis.

Dialysis technology has improved dramatically over the last decade, allowing for an improved range of choices in treatment approach, as well as more comfortable and efficient treatments. Outpatient renal centers are a significant health care industry.

All forms of dialysis utilize the basic principles of diffusion, osmosis, and ultrafiltration (Figure 12-5). Ultrafiltration is the most efficient process and is the basis of hemodialysis.

Hemodialysis—Hemodialysis shunts the patient's blood from the body through a dialyzer in which diffusion and ultrafiltration occur. Hemodialysis requires access to the patient's blood. The primary methods of vascular access include the following:

The external cannula or shunt, in which a Silastic cannula is implanted into an artery and adjacent vein in the forearm or elsewhere; the two ends are connected by a U-shaped external connector (Figure 12-6).

The internal arteriovenous fistula, in which a subcutaneous anastomosis is made between an artery and a vein. Fistulas may also be created using bovine or synthetic grafts.

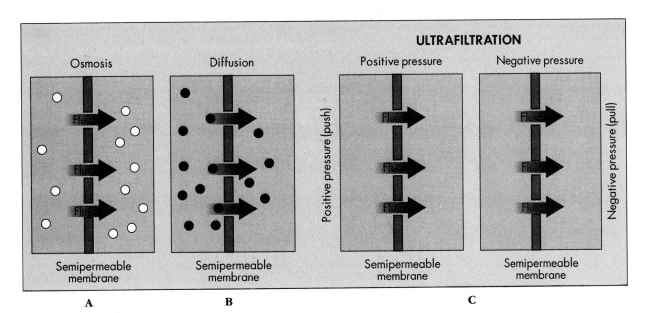

FIGURE 12-5 Principles of dialysis. **A,** Osmosis. **B,** Diffusion. **C,** Ultrafiltration.

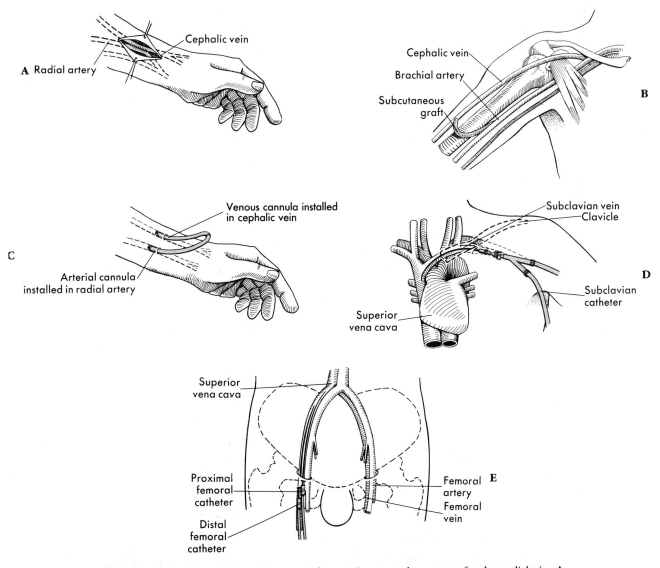

FIGURE 12-6 Frequently used means for gaining vascular access for hemodialysis. **A,** Arteriovenous fistula. **B,** Arteriovenous graft. **C,** External arteriovenous shunt. **D,** Subclavian catheterization. **E,** Femoral vein catheterization.

TABLE 12-5   Indications and Nursing Interventions Associated With Vascular Access for Hemodialysis

INDICATION FOR USE	ADVANTAGES	NURSING INTERVENTIONS
EXTERNAL SHUNT		
Long-term access Need for immediate access	Ease of access Can be used immediately	Do not start IV lines or take blood pressure on affected arm or leg. Assess for bleeding from insertion sites, tubing connections. Assess patency by observing color of blood flow through shunt. Listen for bruit. Assess adequacy of perfusion to extremity. Assess for infection; change dressing frequently, using institution's protocol. Keep clamps or tourniquet at bedside.
ARTERIOVENOUS FISTULA/GRAFT		
Permanent access needed	Easy access once graft has matured Least likely to develop infection or dislodge	Assess for patency by palpating for thrill or auscultating bruit. Teach patient to avoid compression caused by tight clothing or positioning with arm bent. Assess adequacy of perfusion to extremity. Teach patient to assess site for signs of infection. Do not start IVs or take blood pressure on affected arm.
SUBCLAVIAN OR FEMORAL VEIN CATHETER		
Femoral: immediate short-term access Subclavian: immediate short- or long-term access	Ease of access Immediate use Subclavian does not restrict activity	Assess for bleeding from insertion site. Requires heparin irrigation to maintain patency. Sterile technique is essential; monitor for infection.

Femoral or subclavian vein catheterization, in which a catheter is inserted into a major venous vessel such as the femoral or subclavian vein. This access is likely to be short term.

BOX 12-12   Dialysis Disequilibrium

The disequilibrium syndrome typically occurs near the end of or after dialysis. It is theorized to occur from clearance of excess solutes from the blood more rapidly than they can diffuse from inside body cells, creating an imbalance. Since particle content is greater *inside* the cell, the cells take on water and swell.

SYMPTOMS

Headache
Hypertension
Restlessness and confusion
Nausea and vomiting
Severe disequilibrium, possibly resulting in convulsions

TREATMENT

Treatment is aimed at preventing wide swings in metabolic values so the degree of shift is lessened.
If major disarray is present patients may undergo partial dialysis several days in a row.
Patients are monitored carefully, and environmental stimuli and lights are kept low.
Instruct patients to anticipate mild headache and nausea after dialysis. Well-being is improved the day *after* the treatment.

Hemodialysis nursing is a specialty area of practice. The major nursing responsibilities for nondialysis nurses include the following:

Protecting and monitoring the vascular access site (Table 12-5)

Teaching the patient and family ways to manage the disease effectively

Helping the patient plan a work and activity schedule that is minimally disrupted by dialysis routine

Peritoneal dialysis—The dialyzing fluid is instilled into the peritoneal cavity, and the peritoneum becomes the dialyzing membrane. It may take up to 36 hours to complete the treatment. Dialysis may be done intermittently or on a continuous daily ambulatory basis with the insertion of a permanent peritoneal catheter (Figure 12-7).

Continuous cyclic dialysis uses a machine with a series of timers that control the instillation and drainage of the fluid. It can be connected at bedtime for dialysis during sleep. It is relatively simple and allows the patient more control over daily life. Fewer medications and dietary restrictions are usually necessary. The placement of a permanent catheter, however, presents a continual potential route for organisms to enter the peritoneum, and strict asepsis and careful monitoring for infection are essential. Nursing interventions are summarized in the Guidelines box.

Kidney transplantation

Successful kidney transplantation allows for the restoration of normal kidney function. It eliminates depen-

Guidelines for Nursing Care for Patients Receiving Peritoneal Dialysis

PREDIALYSIS

Take baseline weight and vital signs.
Have patient empty bladder before catheter insertion.
Provide meticulous skin and catheter prep per institution's protocol before connecting dialysis fluid line.

DURING DIALYSIS

To initiate each cycle:
    Run prescribed amount of solution (usually 2 L) into peritoneal cavity over about 10 minutes.
    Solution is warmed to body temperature before infusion.
Clamp tubing for prescribed time (usually 20 to 30 minutes).
Drain cavity by gravity (usually takes 20 minutes).
    First drainage may be pink tinged from trauma of catheter insertion. Fluid should never be grossly bloody.
Check dialysate drainage for signs of infection, for example, cloudy, yellow, particles, mucus.
Repeat procedure with fresh dialysate solution as many times as prescribed.

Maintain sterility during bottle changes.
Monitor patient continuously for the following:
    Changes in vital signs indicating hypotension (common) or hypovolemia
    Pain (pressure pain quite common)
    Respiratory distress
    Signs of peritonitis
Turn patient side to side to facilitate drainage of fluid.
Firm pressure may be applied to the abdomen with both hands and the head of bed adjusted.
Maintain accurate intake and output records.
    Record amount of fluid instilled.
    Record amount of fluid drained.
    Note net gains or losses of fluid.
Discontinue dialysis following institution's protocol, keeping strict asepsis.
Send fluid cultures as ordered.

---

dence on dialysis and the multiple life-style restrictions of chronic renal failure. Current success rates make transplant a fairly cost-effective procedure, especially considering the typical annual cost of $40,000 for hemodialysis. Transplant is presented in Chapter 17.

SELECTED REFERENCES

Andreesen G: A fresh look at assessing the elderly, *RN* 52(6):28-40, 1989.

Baer C, Lancaster L: Acute renal failure, *Crit Care Q* 14(1):1-21, 1992.

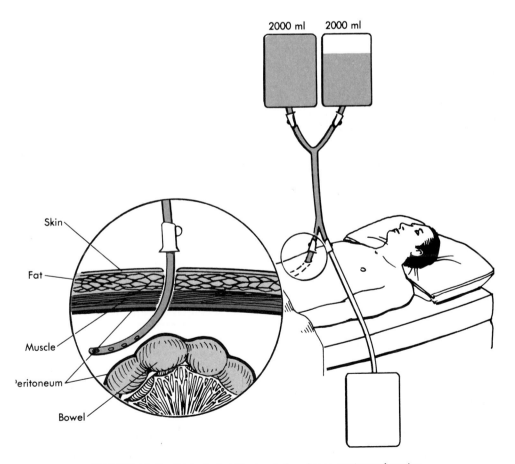

FIGURE 12-7 Dialysis fluid being infused into peritoneal cavity.

Bosworth C: SCUF/CAVH/CAVD: critical differences, *Crit Care Nurs Q* 14(4):45-55, 1992.

Coe FL, Parks JH, Asplin JR: The pathogenesis and treatment of kidney stones, *N Engl J Med* 327(16):1141-1152, 1992.

Counts C: Potential complications of the internal vascular access: implications for nursing, *Dialysis Transpl* 22(2):75-87, 105, 1993.

Dunn SA: How to care for the dialysis patient, *Am J Nurs* 93(6):26-33, 1993.

Faller NA, Lawrence KG: Obtaining a urine specimen from a conduit urostomy, *Am J Nurs* 94(1):97, 1994.

Flaherty JM, O'Brien ME: Family styles in coping in end-stage renal disease, *ANNA J* 19(4):345-349, 1992.

Graham-Macaluso MM: Complications of peritoneal dialysis: nursing care plans to document teaching, *ANNA J* 18(3):479-483, 1991.

Heneghan GM et al: The Indiana pouch: a continent urinary diversion, *J Enterostom Ther* 17:231-236, 1990.

Licklinder D, Mauffray D: Conventional urostomy vs continent urostomy, *Ostomy/Wound Management* 34:26-29, 1991.

Moon S et al: Treating bladder cancer: new methods and new management, *Am J Nurs* 93(5):32-39, 1993.

Newman DK et al: Restoring urinary continence, *Am J Nurs* 91(12):44-45, 1991.

Powers I, William D: Urinary incontinence, *Nurs 92* 22(12):46-47, 1992.

Price C: Continuous renal replacement therapy: the treatment of choice for acute renal failure, *ANNA J* 18(3):239-244, 1991.

Resnick B: Retraining the bladder after catheterization, *Am J Nurs* 93(11):46-49, 1993.

Smith DB, Babaian RJ: Patient adjustment to an ileal conduit after cystectomy, *J Enterostom Ther* 16:244-246, 1989.

Tootla J, Easterling AD: Current options in bladder cancer management, *RN* 55(4):42-49, 1992.

Wiseman KC: Nephrotic syndrome: pathophysiology and treatment, *ANNA J* 18(5):469-478, 1991.

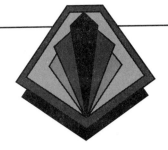

Disorders of the Nervous System

◆ ASSESSMENT

Health history
Past/family history
    History of neurologic disease, trauma, surgery; related diseases, for example, hypertension, diabetes
    Neurologic problems in nuclear or extended family; congenital and related disease processes
    Prescription and over the counter (OTC) medications in use
        Use of alcohol and other drugs
Neurologic symptoms
    Onset, pattern, and progression; measures used to treat
    Headache, vertigo, visual changes
    Pain or weakness in muscles
    Behavioral changes
        Irritability, personality changes
        Memory or attention loss
        Cognitive, thought process changes
        Sleep pattern changes
    Effect of symptoms on activities of daily living (ADL), work, leisure activities
    Language, speech
    Sensory disturbance; numbness, paresthesia

PHYSICAL ASSESSMENT

Mental status examination
    General behavior, speech, and appearance
        Appropriateness, fluidity
    General affect and responsiveness, emotional lability
Level of consciousness
    Alertness, responsiveness (describe specific behavior if not fully alert)
    Orientation to person, place, and time
Attention
    Responsiveness to questions, appropriateness of responses
    Ability to repeat back words or number series
    Serial subtraction: "count back from 100 by. . ."
Memory
    Test remote, recent, and new memory*

Cognition
    Elicit data concerning hobbies, current events, and so on
    Abstract reasoning and judgment, for example, meaning of proverbs, rational decision making concerning symptoms
Language and speech
    Dysarthria: speech problems related to muscle weakness or impairment (tested with cranial nerves)
    Aphasia/dysphasia: speech problems related to the use or understanding of symbolic language
        Ability to follow directions, comprehend (sensory, receptive)
        Ability to name items, speak fluidly
        Reading comprehension
        Writing or copying ability
Sensory function (tested with patient's eyes closed)
    Pain†: pinprick perception against hands, feet, and so on, moving proximally from extremities
        Sharp versus dull discrimination
        Deep pain: nail-bed or supraorbital pressure, sternal rub
    Touch: cotton ball perception against foot, ankle, wrist, or hand
    Temperature‡: warm/hot versus cool/cold
    Proprioception (motion and position sense): move patient's great toe or thumb up and down and ask patient to indicate direction of movement
    Romberg test: ability to stand erect with feet together and eyes closed and maintain a stable position
    Vibration: tuning fork perception
    Object recognition, praxis, and gnosis: ability to recognize objects through special senses; tested by visual recognition and identification by touch (stereognosis)

---

*Note: Loss or impairment of recent memory is a common *early* sign of neurologic impairment. Elderly persons also commonly have difficulties with recent or new memory.

†Note: Deep pain assessment is necessary *only* when a person has a decreased level of consciousness.

‡Note: Temperature is transmitted via the same pathways as pain and is usually not tested if pain perception is intact.

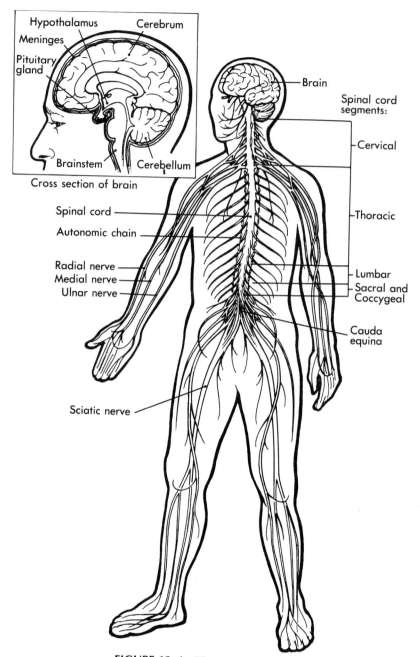

FIGURE 13-1 The nervous system.

Graphesthesia: recognition of letters or numbers traced in palm of hand

Motor function

Strength, movement, symmetry, presence of involuntary movements (intentional and unintentional)

Hand grips (a common grading scale ranges from 0 to 5)

Strength against resistance (arm or leg)

Voluntary movement

Muscle tone: hypertonia (rigidity), hypotonia

Cerebellar function

Finger tip to nose touch repetition (eyes closed)

Gait and balance

Walking, heel toe, stand on one foot

Ataxia: lack of coordination

Reflex activity

See Box 13-2 for commonly tested reflexes

Deep tendon (Figure 13-2)

Strike tendon quickly and lightly with hammer

Evaluate response: normal, hypoactive, hyperactive

Compare both sides for symmetry of response

Record on stick figure

Cranial nerves

I: Olfactory

Test one nostril at a time with familiar odors, such as coffee, mint, tobacco

Anosmia (absence of smell); hyposmia (decreased smell sensitivity)

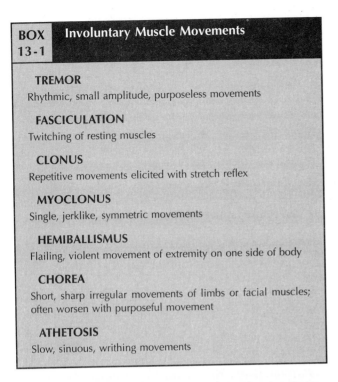

BOX 13-1 Involuntary Muscle Movements

TREMOR
Rhythmic, small amplitude, purposeless movements

FASCICULATION
Twitching of resting muscles

CLONUS
Repetitive movements elicited with stretch reflex

MYOCLONUS
Single, jerklike, symmetric movements

HEMIBALLISMUS
Flailing, violent movement of extremity on one side of body

CHOREA
Short, sharp irregular movements of limbs or facial muscles; often worsen with purposeful movement

ATHETOSIS
Slow, sinuous, writhing movements

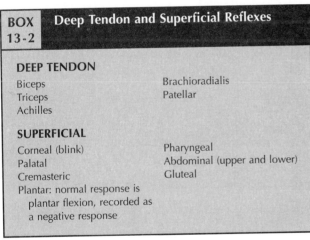

BOX 13-2 Deep Tendon and Superficial Reflexes

DEEP TENDON
Biceps   Brachioradialis
Triceps   Patellar
Achilles

SUPERFICIAL
Corneal (blink)   Pharyngeal
Palatal   Abdominal (upper and lower)
Cremasteric   Gluteal
Plantar: normal response is
  plantar flexion, recorded as
  a negative response

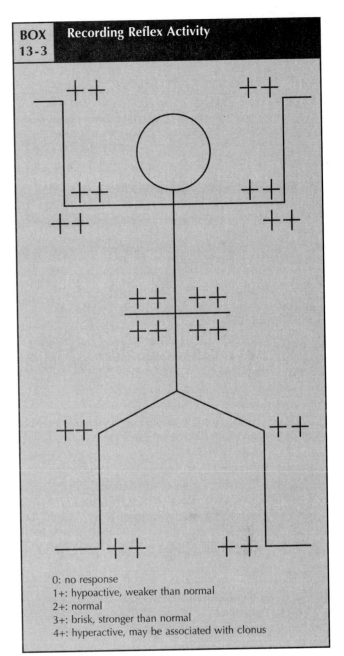

BOX 13-3 Recording Reflex Activity

0: no response
1+: hypoactive, weaker than normal
2+: normal
3+: brisk, stronger than normal
4+: hyperactive, may be associated with clonus

II: Optic
    Each eye tested alone
    Snellen chart for acuity, visual fields
    Funduscopic examination
III: Oculomotor; IV: Trochlear; VI: Abducens
    Motor nerves that innervate extraocular muscles
    Pupil response: light brought from side
    PERRLA: *p*upils *e*qual, *r*ound, *r*eactive to *l*ight and *a*ccommodation
    Consensual response of nontested eye (Box 13-4)
    Six cardinal fields of gaze
    Track finger through the following positions: straight, up and down, left and right (Figure 13-3)

Conjugate movement (working together), diplopia (double vision), strabismus (squint), or nystagmus (rapid, involuntary eye movements)
V: Trigeminal (motor)
    Corneal reflex: touch with a wisp of cotton or make threatening gesture toward face
VII: Facial
    Ability to frown, smile, wrinkle forehead, puff out cheeks
    Symmetry of response

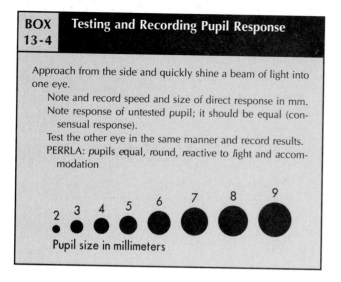

BOX 13-4 | **Testing and Recording Pupil Response**

Approach from the side and quickly shine a beam of light into one eye.

Note and record speed and size of direct response in mm.
Note response of untested pupil; it should be equal (consensual response).
Test the other eye in the same manner and record results.
PERRLA: *p*upils *e*qual, *r*ound, *r*eactive to *l*ight and *a*ccommodation

Pupil size in millimeters

VIII: Acoustic
    Hearing
    Ticking watch, rubbing finger and thumb
    Weber and Rinne tests: see Chapter 14
    Equilibrium: Romberg test
IX: Glossopharyngeal; X: vogus
    Taste
    Usually not tested unless problems reported
    Posterior third of tongue: sweet, sour, bitter, salty
    Motor
    Vocalizing "ah" sound should cause uvula and palate to rise bilaterally and equally
    Gag and swallow reflexes
XI: Spinal accessory
    Strength of trapezius and sternocleidomastoid muscle
    Head turn against resistance and shoulder shrug: strength and symmetry
XII: Hypoglossal
    Tongue movement, deviation from midline at rest

✍ DIAGNOSTIC TESTS

BLOOD AND URINE TESTS

Blood and urine testing will be included in any neurologic workup, but few of these tests are definitive for neurologic diseases.

CEREBROSPINAL FLUID TESTS

Cerebrospinal fluid (CSF) is normally clear and colorless. Specimens are typically obtained via lumbar puncture and examined for increases or decreases in its normal constituents and for the presence of foreign or pathogenic substances. CSF circulates under pressure, which may also be measured during the puncture. Normal and abnormal values for CSF components are summarized in Table 13-1.

RADIOLOGIC TESTS

X-Ray Films

X-ray films are usually the first step of a workup to rule out traumatic skeletal injury to the nervous system or degenerative bone abnormalities.

Computed Tomography Scan

Description—Computed tomography (CT) scan provides a computerized image that reproduces sections of the brain or spinal column sliced front to back on the coronal or sagittal planes. It is noninvasive but may be enhanced by the use of a contrast medium. The scan provides detailed information about tissue structure but not functional status.

Procedure—The patient lies supine with the head immobilized by straps. The scanner rotates around the head taking pictures at 1-degree intervals. A contrast medium may be injected and another series of films taken. The test takes 15 to 30 minutes.

Patient preparation and aftercare—No special preparation is required. The patient is instructed about the equipment and the need for lying still during the test and is assessed for any history of allergy to iodine or shellfish. No posttest care is required.

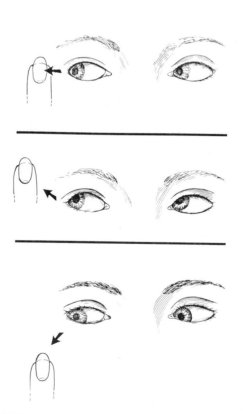

FIGURE 13-3 Testing cardinal fields of gaze.

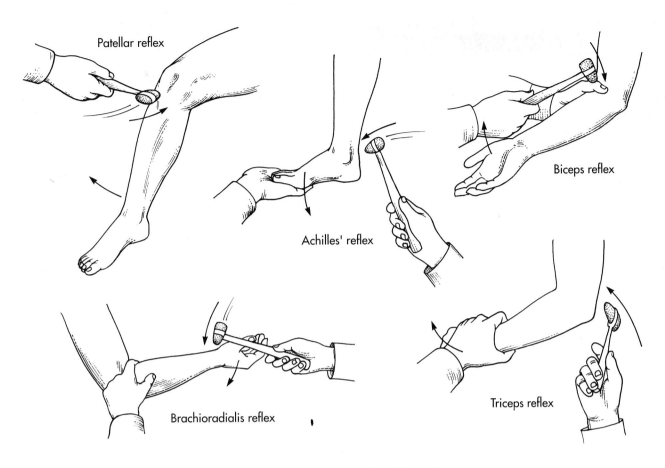

FIGURE 13-2   Deep tendon reflex testing.

Magnetic Resonance Imaging

Description—Magnetic resonance imaging (MRI) uses radiofrequency energy and a powerful magnetic field to generate multiplane images of the brain and spine. It provides detailed images of anatomic details by "seeing through" bone and delineating fluid-filled tissues.

Procedure—The patient lies supine on a narrow bed that slides into the scanner. Radiofrequency energy is directed at the head. The images created are displayed on a monitor and recorded on tape. The test takes about 90 minutes.

Patient preparation and aftercare—No special preparation is indicated. The patient is instructed about the equipment and procedure length. The scanner and very narrow bed can induce claustrophobic responses. The machine noises are significant, and ear plugs may be provided. All metallic objects such as jewelry or hair pins are removed. Patients with pacemakers, metal joint structures, or other metal implants cannot undergo the test. No special aftercare is required.

GERONTOLOGIC PATIENT CONSIDERATIONS: PHYSIOLOGIC CHANGES IN THE NEUROLOGIC SYSTEM

MEMORY
Recent and new memory frequently impaired

SLEEP PATTERNS
Difficulty falling asleep and frequent nighttime awakenings

TOUCH
Sensation diminished, fewer pain receptors

REFLEXES
Slowed; reaction time prolonged

BALANCE AND COORDINATION
Affected by musculoskeletal changes rather than neurologic

TEMPERATURE
Slowed metabolism, decreased ability to sustain body temperature

TABLE 13-1	Normal and Abnormal Values for Components of CSF
NORMAL VALUES	**MEANING OF ABNORMAL FINDINGS**
COLOR	
Clear, colorless	Cloudy: WBCs or bacteria Straw color: RBCs
PRESSURE	
70-180 mm H₂O	Elevated: cerebral edema, tumor, hematoma, hydrocephalus Decreased: dehydration, CSF blockage
GLUCOSE	
50-75 mg/dl	Elevated: not significant neurologically Decreased: presence of bacteria
PROTEIN	
14-45 mg/dl	Elevated: demyelinating or degenerative disease, infection, or tumor Decreased; not significant neurologically
CHLORIDE	
126-130 mEq/L	Elevated: not significant neurologically Decreased: associated with meningitis
WHITE BLOOD CELLS (WBCS)	
0-5/mm³, mononuclear	Elevated: associated with tumor, abscess, meningitis, hemorrhage Decreased: not significant neurologically
RED BLOOD CELLS (RBCS)	
None	Presence associated with traumatic lumbar puncture or subarachnoid hemorrhage

Positron Emission Tomography

Description—Positron emission tomography (PET) scan combines the elements of CT scanning and radionuclide imaging. It details brain function and biochemical processes as well as brain structure. Computer reconstructions create tomographic images of the brain. At present the cost of the test is prohibitive.

Procedure—The patient either inhales a radioactive gas or is injected with one. A gamma scanner measures the uptake of the substance by tissues, and the computer creates images of the areas of cellular metabolism.

Patient preparation and aftercare—No special preparation is required. The patient is informed that the test may take several hours, and he or she must remain still throughout. Reassurance is offered about the safety and brief half-life of the radionuclide. No aftercare is required.

Transcranial Doppler Sonography

Description—Doppler studies provide information about the presence, quality, and changing nature of the brain's circulation by measuring the velocity of blood flow through the arteries. The speed of blood flow is an indication of the size of the vascular channel and degree of resistance.

Procedure—The patient is positioned comfortably, and a probe is directed toward specific vessels. The ultrasonic energy creates reflected sound waves that are analyzed. Waveforms may be recorded for future comparison. The test takes 30 to 60 minutes and can be performed at the bedside.

Patient preparation and aftercare—No special preparation is required except patient education about the test, which is noninvasive. There are no known adverse effects and no required aftercare.

Myelography

Description—A myelogram combines fluoroscopy and radiography to evaluate the subarachnoid space of the spine through the use of a contrast medium. It can reveal partial or complete obstruction, spinal cord compression, and disk herniation.

Procedure—A lumbar puncture is performed, and the patient is then positioned prone and secured to the examining table. A contrast medium is injected, and the table is tilted to move the medium along the spinal canal. The flow is monitored fluoroscopically and recorded on x-rays. Either an oil-based (Pantopaque) or a water-based (metrizamide) medium may be used. The test takes about 2 hours to complete.

Patient preparation and aftercare—No special preparation is required, but some centers restrict food and fluid for 8 hours. The patient is instructed about the test, assessed for allergies, and informed that the dye may produce a flushed warm feeling, salty taste, headache, or nausea. Aftercare is based on the contrast medium in use. With oil-based dyes the patient is kept on bed rest, flat in bed for up to 24 hours. With metrizamide the patient is on bed rest with the head elevated 30 to 50 degrees for at least 8 hours. Fluids are encouraged, and the patient is monitored for headache, nausea, and back spasms after the test.

Cerebral Angiography

Description—The test allows for radiographic examination of the cerebral vessels after injection of a contrast medium. The vessels are examined for patency, narrowing, occlusion, and structural abnormalities.

Procedure—The patient is positioned supine on the x-ray table. After a local anesthetic is administered, a catheter is inserted into the femoral or possibly the carotid artery and advanced. A contrast medium is injected into each common carotid and each vertebral artery, and x-rays are taken. The test takes 2 to 4 hours.

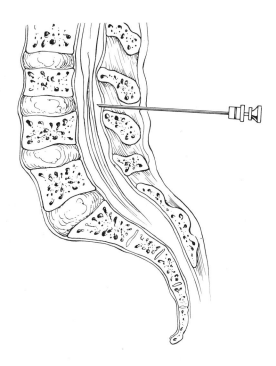

FIGURE 13-4 Lumbar puncture at fourth lumbar interspace.

Patient preparation and aftercare—The patient is NPO for 8 hours before the test and receives detailed teaching about the test and posttest procedures. Careful assessment for allergies is performed. Vital signs, baseline neurologic status, and peripheral pulses are assessed before the test. The need to lie still on a hard surface is emphasized, and the patient is prepared for the flushing, salty taste and nausea that may accompany injection of the dye. The patient is placed on bed rest for 12 to 24 hours. Vital signs and neurologic status are carefully monitored, and the puncture site is assessed for bleeding or swelling. The leg is kept straight for 8 to 12 hours, and peripheral pulses are monitored to assess patency of the circulation distal to the puncture site. Fluids are encouraged to assist in dye excretion.

Digital Subtraction Angiography

Description—Digital subtraction angiography is a sophisticated radiographic technique that allows for examination of the extracranial and intracranial circulation to detect cerebrovascular abnormalities. It utilizes the venous rather than the arterial system and is safer and somewhat more comfortable for the patient.

Procedure—The patient is positioned supine on an x-ray table, and fluoroscopic x-rays of the head are taken. A catheter is inserted through the antecubital fossa and advanced to the vena cava where the contrast medium is injected. A second set of x-rays is taken, and the computer converts both sets of images into digital

form and "subtracts" the data from the plain films from the contrast ones. An enhanced image results. The test takes 30 to 45 minutes.

Patient preparation and aftercare—The patient typically fasts for about 4 hours before the test and is taught about the procedure and the importance of lying still. A feeling of warmth, flushing, and nausea and a salty taste may accompany injection of the dye, and the patient is carefully assessed for allergies. The venipuncture site is monitored after the test, and fluids are encouraged to facilitate dye excretion. No special activity restrictions are required.

SPECIAL TESTS
Lumbar Puncture

Description—A lumbar puncture is performed to obtain CSF for analysis. It is not performed in the presence of elevated intracranial pressure (ICP) because of the risk of brainstem herniation through the foramen magnum. In special situations punctures may be made directly into the ventricles or through the cisterna magna.

Procedure—The patient is positioned on the side in a fetal, spine-flexed position. A sitting position may be used if preferred. Following a local anesthetic, a needle is inserted in the L4-5 or L5-6 interspace (Figure 13-4). Pressure is measured, and CSF specimens are collected. A dressing is applied. The test takes about 15 minutes.

Patient preparation and aftercare—No special preparation is required. The patient is instructed about the test and the need to lie still during the test. A feeling of pressure or pain is common as the needle penetrates the dura. The patient is instructed to lie flat after the test, but recommendations for the duration of bed rest vary from minutes to 8 hours. Posttest headache is fairly common. The insertion site is monitored for redness or leakage.

Electroencephalogram

Description—Electrodes record a portion of the brain's electrical activity as brain waves on moving paper. The test helps detect and localize abnormal activity, aids in detection of seizure foci and the diagnosis of metabolic imbalances or sleep disturbances, and provides data for determination of brain death.

Procedure—The patient is positioned comfortably in a bed or reclining chair, and electrodes are attached to the scalp. Recordings are taken at rest, after hyperventilation, and in response to visual stimulation. The test takes about 1 hour.

Patient preparation and aftercare—The patient is instructed to avoid caffeine, but no other preparation is required. The patient is reassured that the electrodes can only record brain activity and cannot deliver shocks. The hair should be clean for optimal recording and is washed again after the test to remove the collodion adhesive.

Electromyography

Description—Electromyography measures and records the electrical activity of selected skeletal muscle groups at rest and during voluntary contraction. It provides direct evidence of motor dysfunction and aids in the diagnosis of neuromuscular disorders.

Procedure—The patient is positioned sitting or lying so the targeted muscles are at rest. Needle electrodes are inserted into the muscle, and the electrical signal is recorded both at rest and during contraction. Nerve conduction studies may also be performed with electrical stimulation. The test takes about 1 hour.

Patient preparation and aftercare—No special preparation is needed except teaching about the procedure. The patient is informed that insertion of the needle electrodes does cause discomfort. No specific aftercare is needed except monitoring the insertion sites. The tested muscles may also ache after the test, and warm compresses or mild analgesics may be used.

Evoked Potentials

Description—Evoked potential tests evaluate the integrity of the visual, auditory, and somatosensory pathways by measuring the brain's electrical response to stimulation of the sense organs.

Procedure—The patient is comfortably positioned, and electrodes are attached to the scalp or over peripheral nerve pathways. A stimulus is provided either by TV image to the eye or painless electrical shocks to the peripheral nerve, and recordings are made for computer interpretation. The test takes 45 to 60 minutes.

Patient preparation and aftercare—The patient's education is the only preparation. The patient needs to be relaxed and at rest and reassured that the test is not painful. There is no postcare.

NEUROLOGIC DISORDERS

Neurologic problems and disorders can arise from a wide variety of causes including trauma, infection, vascular impairment, neoplasm, and degenerative processes. The nervous system functions as the primary coordinator and regulator of body activity, collecting and processing sensory data and transmitting impulses along the motor pathways to effector muscles and organs for action. The effects of neurologic disease are frequently devastating and may involve voluntary and reflex movement, muscle tone, posture, and sensation. Disturbances in motor function may be classified by their impairment of either upper motor neuron (UMN) or lower motor neuron (LMN) structures. Characteristics of each structure are presented in Box 13-5. Occasionally a pathologic condition may involve both the UMN and LMN.

BOX 13-5	**Upper and Lower Motor Neuron Lesions**

UPPER MOTOR NEURON (UMN) PYRAMIDAL SYSTEM

Originates in the motor strip of the cerebral cortex and in brainstem nuclei

Axons pass through internal capsule and brainstem and decussate in medulla

Descends spinal cord via corticospinal tract and synapse with LMNs

Pathologic Conditions Involving UMNs

Birth injuries
Trauma
Degenerative disease
Neoplasms
Inflammation or infection
Vascular lesions: embolism, hemorrhage, thrombosis

Classic Signs of UMN Disorders

Weakness or paralysis of voluntary muscle tone, progressing to spasticity
Hyperreflexia
Late atrophy from disuse
Increased muscle tone

LOWER MOTOR NEURON (LMN) EXTRAPYRAMIDAL SYSTEM

Originates in anterior gray column of spinal cord
Contains both a sensory (afferent) and a motor (efferent) component
Terminates in motor end-plates

Pathologic Conditions Involving LMNs

Infection (poliomyelitis)
Inflammation (polyneuritis)
Degenerative processes (muscular dystrophies, myasthenia gravis)

Classic Signs of LMN Disorders

Flaccid muscle weakness or paralysis
Loss of reflex activity
Loss of muscle tone
Atrophy of involved muscle(s)

CHRONIC NEUROLOGIC DISORDERS
Parkinson's Disease
Etiology/epidemiology

Parkinson's disease is one of the more common diseases of the nervous system and typically affects individuals in the late middle years (50 to 60 years of age). It involves a classic cluster of symptoms whose cause is usually unknown, but it can be induced by certain drugs, arteriosclerosis, and viral diseases. It is estimated to affect 100 to 150 persons per 100,000 population, and at present there is no known cure.

Pathophysiology

The pathophysiologic process involves depigmentation of the substantia nigra of the basal ganglia with substantial loss of neurons. Selective depletion of dopamine occurs that can be correlated with striatal degeneration. Without dopamine (a neurotransmitter essential for proper muscle movement) there is a loss of inhibiting influence and excitatory mechanisms are unopposed. The result is impairment in the centers of coordination, in control of muscle tone, and in the control of the initiation and inhibition of movements.

Parkinson's disease often begins with a faint tremor and initially progresses so slowly that it is usually unnoticed. The classic tremor is the most outstanding feature of the disease. Muscle weakness, rigidity, and loss of postural reflexes are also classic. The disease is progressive, and the number and severity of symptoms increase with time.

Medical management

No definitive diagnostic test exists. Parkinson's is typically diagnosed from its classic symptom pattern. Care is basically palliative and directed toward controlling symptoms. Drug therapy is the cornerstone of medical care and may include the following:

Anticholinergic drugs (Artane, Cogentin, Akineton) lessen muscle rigidity and have been in use for more than a century. They have little effect on tremor, and their use is accompanied by significant side effects (dry mouth, urinary retention, constipation).

Antiviral agents (Symmetrol) exert antiparkinsonian activity from the drugs' blockage of the reuptake of catecholamines, which allows for the accumulation of dopamine at synaptic sites.

Dopamine precursor drugs (levodopa) assist in restoring striatal dopamine. The improvement is often dramatic. With prolonged use a decrease in effectiveness with a corresponding increase in side effects is often experienced. A hospitalized "drug holiday" may restore some sensitivity to the drug's action. Side effects such as nausea and vomiting, orthostatic hypotension, agitation and confusion, and insomnia occur frequently.

Combination agents (Sinemet [carbidopa/levodopa]) limit the peripheral metabolism of levodopa, making more available to the brain. This allows for the administration of lower doses of the drug and minimizes side effects.

Transplantation of tissue from the adrenal medulla to the substantia nigra is used experimentally to attempt to restore the balance of dopamine and acetylcholine. The procedure is technically difficult and still in the research stage.

Drug therapy is supplemented by appropriate diet and exercise prescriptions. In certain cases medical management may be supplemented by stereotactic surgery that involves local destruction of portions of the globus pallidus or thalamus to relieve rigidity and tremor.

NURSING MANAGEMENT

◆ ASSESSMENT
Subjective Data

History and course of the disease

Patient's knowledge of the disease process, medications, and side effects

Patient's awareness that symptoms worsen with stress or fatigue

Patient's complaints of fatigue, incoordination

Defects in judgment and emotional instability (intelligence not affected)

Objective Data

Presence of "classic triad" of symptoms
Tremor (pill-rolling type; more prominent at rest)
Rigidity (jerky movements)
Muscle weakness with bradykinesia (slow or retarded movements)
Loss of postural reflexes
Absence of automatic associated body movements: stooped posture, deadpan expression, shuffling gait (may be propulsive), difficulty initiating movement, drooling saliva
Signs of complications: dysphagia, constipation, movement "freezing," incontinence, general debilitation, depression
General nutritional status
Elimination patterns and control over micturition and defecation

◆ NURSING DIAGNOSES

Nursing diagnoses for the person with Parkinson's disease may include, but are not limited to, the following:
Mobility, impaired physical (related to muscle rigidity and bradykinesia)
Nutrition, altered: less than body requirements (related to dysphagia)

Communication, impaired verbal (related to rigid facial muscles and decreased voice volume)

Injury, high risk for (related to posture defects, muscle rigidity, and propulsive gait)

◆ EXPECTED PATIENT OUTCOMES

Patient will maintain sufficient muscle strength and flexibility to remain independent in ADL.

Patient will eat a diet that maintains appropriate weight and meets body's baseline nutritional needs.

Patient will be able to communicate verbally and maintain active social interaction.

Patient will not experience injury related to disease symptoms.

◆ NURSING INTERVENTIONS

Promoting Optimal Mobility and Self-Care

Administer medications as prescribed; teach about side effects (nausea, hypotension, palpitations, arrhythmias, confusion, and hallucinations are all common side effects of dopaminergic drugs).

Encourage family to allow sufficient time for all activities so patient can remain independent and not feel rushed.

Encourage active or passive range of motion every 4 hours.

Explore use of hot packs and massage to relieve stiffness.

Suggest that patient modify clothing with wide zippers or Velcro closures as needed to remain independent.

Encourage patient to hold hands behind back to improve gait and posture.

Encourage patient to rest on firm mattress and lie prone at intervals to support full extension of all joints.

Supporting Adequate Nutrition

Plan nutritious meals high in roughage, easily chewed.

Cut all foods into safe sizes.

Keep fluid intake high.

Provide smaller, more frequent meals to prevent exhaustion.

Allow sufficient time for eating. Do not attempt to hurry patient.

Monitor weight.

Keep patient upright for meals; monitor effectiveness of swallowing efforts.

Encourage patient to keep an adequate supply of soft cloths or tissues to control excess saliva and drooling. Small towels may be used to protect linens and clothes during naps or sleep.

Facilitating Effective Communication

Allow enough time and be patient.

Listen carefully. Encourage patient to speak aloud.

Encourage patient to do breathing and vocal exercises to strengthen diaphragm and increase voice volume and strength.

Preventing Injury

Encourage use of cane or walker if gait is disturbed, particularly if forward or backward propulsion occurs.

Teach patient to use upright straight chair; raising back chair legs on blocks makes it easier to get up.

Remove scatter rugs and clutter furniture; encourage family to install hand rails and other safety devices.

Encourage patient to change positions frequently and remain active to avoid freeze ups and prevent immobility-related complications.

◆ EVALUATION

Successful achievement of expected outcomes for the patient with Parkinson's disease is indicated by the following:

1. Engages in regular exercise
   Maintains muscle flexibility and joint range of motion
   Accomplishes ADL with minimal assistance
2. Ingests a balanced diet
   Maintains stable weight
   Does not experience aspiration
3. Modifies home environment to promote safety
   Does not experience falls or "freeze ups"

Multiple Sclerosis

Etiology/epidemiology

Multiple sclerosis (MS) is a degenerative disease that occurs primarily in northern temperate climates and typically affects young adults between the ages of 20 and 40 years. Women are affected more often than men. It follows a variable course but usually progresses slowly toward progressive disability over a period of about 20 years.

The exact etiology remains elusive, but the role of viruses and autoimmunity is increasingly supported by research. There is also some evidence of a familial pattern.

Pathophysiology

MS causes random patches of demyelination of the white matter of the spinal cord and brain, which causes interruption or distortion of the nerve impulses so that they are slowed or blocked. When the destruction is confined to the myelin sheath in the early stages of the disease, partial healing is possible. This helps to explain the transitory nature of the early symptoms. In later stages the degeneration often extends into the gray matter, and the effects are irreversible. The disease follows a pattern of exacerbation and remission, and most persons recover from the early episodes. Since the degenerative patterns may occur throughout the nervous system, MS produces a wider range of symptoms than any other neurologic disease. Early symptoms frequently include visual problems (diplopia, spots before the eyes), muscle weakness, tremor, or numbness.

Medical management

No definitive diagnostic test exists for MS, and the diagnosis is often a matter of clinical judgment. A workup will include analysis of the CSF for evidence of increased IgG and oligoclonal bands, and visual evoked potentials to assess the integrity of the optic nerve. The classic demyelinization plaques can be clearly visualized with MRI scanning, and this test is now considered the gold standard for the diagnosis of MS. No medical treatment has been proven to alter the course of the disease.

Treatment is directed at symptom management and often includes short-course, high-dose IV steroid therapy followed by a slow taper with oral steroids over about 1 month. Immunosuppressive agents and plasma exchanges are also being employed, but their effectiveness is unclear. Symptomatic treatment includes physical therapy and medications to relieve spasticity, bladder dysfunction, and gastrointestinal (GI) symptoms. Patient and family education efforts are directed at the maintenance of optimal health and supporting effective coping.

NURSING MANAGEMENT

◆ ASSESSMENT
Subjective Data

History and course of the disease (early symptoms are usually transitory)

Patient's knowledge of disease process, treatment, and medication

Complaints of weakness, numbness, or fatigue

Eye problems
Double vision
Diplopia
Scotomas (spots)

Emotional response to diagnosis or symptoms

Objective Data

Bowel or bladder problems: frequency, urgency, incontinence

Presence of tremor, muscle spasm, spastic ataxia, loss of coordination

Nystagmus (rapid oscillation of eyeballs), speech disorders (scanning speech)

Behavior patterns, including euphoria or depression and crying spells

◆ NURSING DIAGNOSES

Nursing diagnoses for the person with MS may include, but are not limited to, the following:

Mobility, impaired physical (related to tremor, muscle spasticity, and incoordination)

Incontinence, stress (related to interrupted nervous stimulation)

Constipation (related to interruption of motor impulses to the bowel)

Coping, high risk for ineffective individual or family (related to the chronic progressive nature of the disease)

Knowledge deficit (related to life-style modifications to control or limit disease exacerbations)

◆ EXPECTED PATIENT OUTCOMES

Patient will maintain sufficient muscular function and control to remain independent in ADL.

Patient will maintain control over bowel and bladder function.

Patient and family will work together to cope effectively with condition and plan for the future.

Patient will remain involved in usual occupational, family, and recreational activities.

Patient will describe life-style modifications to follow to promote health and prevent exacerbations of the disease.

◆ NURSING INTERVENTIONS
Promoting Optimal Mobility

Refer to physical therapy for stretching exercises and gait training.

Encourage patient to perform active range of motion exercises at least three times daily.

Encourage ambulation; teach use of assistive devices as indicated. Suggest use of eye patch if diplopia exists.

Encourage activity, but avoid overfatigue.

Teach patient and family the importance of frequent position changes, use of foam mattresses, and other general measures to prevent immobility-related complications.

Promoting Urinary and Bowel Elimination

Teach patient the symptoms of urinary tract infection (UTI).

Teach patient to acidify the urine and keep the daily fluid intake high.

Explore the use of antispasmodics if urinary urgency occurs (propantheline bromide [Pro-Banthine], oxybutynin [Ditropan]).

If UTIs occur, explore the use of prophylactic doses of nitrofurantoin (Macrodantin) or trimethoprim and sulfamethoxazole (Bactrim).

Follow intermittent catheterization program or bladder retraining program if incontinent.

Protect patient against soiling, leaking, and skin breakdown.

Teach patient to inspect skin for signs of redness or breakdown during routine hygiene, especially when sensory impairments exist.

Initiate bowel program with stool softeners and suppositories.

Encourage the use of a fiber-rich diet. Avoid the use of enemas and laxatives if possible.

Supporting Individual and Family Coping

Encourage patient to verbalize feelings and concerns.
Calmly assist patient and family to control and deal with mood swings.
Refer patient to support groups in community and services of the National Multiple Sclerosis Society.
Encourage patient to pace daily activities to remain successfully involved in family and social activities.
Encourage family to provide needed assistance but support the patient's self-care efforts.

Teaching for Successful Self-Care

Administer prescribed medications; teach patient and family about drugs and side effects.
Teach patient to follow a health-promoting life-style that helps to limit the frequency of disease exacerbations.
Teach patient to eat nutritious high-protein diet and take supplemental vitamins.
Encourage patient to balance rest and activity and avoid fatigue.
Encourage patient to avoid hot baths and extremes of heat and cold, which increase weakness.
Teach patient to avoid exposure to infection and treat all infection immediately.
Encourage patient to utilize an eye patch for safety when diplopia is present.
Explore home modifications with patient and family to reduce physical demands and increase environmental safety.
Provide occupational therapy referral for energy conservation techniques for daily activities.

♦ EVALUATION

Successful achievement of expected outcomes for the patient with MS is indicated by the following:
1. Ability to ambulate, transfer, and participate in ADL
   Presence of full range of motion in all joints
2. Absence of bladder incontinence
   Regular bowel elimination
   Absence of skin irritation or breakdown
3. Verbalization of fears and concerns over the disease and prognosis
   A workable plan for future care and support needs
   A positive attitude about the future
   Involvement with patient and family support groups
4. Correct description of prescribed medications, management of side effects, and symptoms to report
   Modification of home environment to improve safety and conserve energy
   Ingestion of nutritious diet and maintenance of stable weight
   Verbalization of importance of avoiding fatigue, promoting rest, avoiding extremes of heat and cold, and avoiding stress

Myasthenia Gravis

Etiology/epidemiology

Myasthenia gravis is a relatively rare disease that primarily occurs in young adults, women more often than men. Its etiology is unknown, although autoimmunity is clearly implicated. An initial viral etiology is being researched. Antiacetylcholine antibodies are isolated in 60% to 90% of affected persons. These antibodies may be produced by thymic lymphocytes, but the links have not been clearly drawn. The disease is usually progressive, although it may follow a variable course.

Pathophysiology

No observable structural changes can be identified in either the muscles or nerves in patients with myasthenia gravis and yet the nerve impulses fail to pass to the muscles at the myoneural junction. Causative theories include (1) failure of the motor end-plate to secrete adequate acetylcholine, (2) excessive quantities of cholinesterase (an enzyme that inactivates acetylcholine) at the nerve ending, or (3) nonresponse of the muscle fibers to the acetylcholine. Current therapies focus on reducing the amount of cholinesterase at the myoneural junction.

Twenty-five percent of myasthenia gravis patients are found to have thymomas, and 80% exhibit cellular changes in the thymus gland, although the significance of these abnormalities is not fully understood. The characteristic features of myasthenia gravis are muscle weakness and fatigue that initially dissipate rapidly with rest. The weakness primarily affects the facial, arm, and hand muscles but may extend to the trunk and lower limbs as the disease progresses. Respiratory and bulbar cranial nerves may also be involved, which can create a life-threatening situation.

Medical management

Primary medical management revolves around the administration of anticholinesterase medications, primarily pyridostigmine (Mestinon) and neostigmine (Prostigmin). These drugs block the action of cholinesterase and allow acetylcholine to act as a neurotransmitter at the myoneural junction. The drug dosage is highly individualized and must be administered at specific intervals throughout the day to support normal daily activities. Except during disease exacerbations or crises, the remaining medical interventions are basically supportive in nature. High-dose steroids, plasmapheresis, and surgical thymectomy are being employed in research medical centers.

Once the disease is suspected from the clinical picture, myasthenia gravis can be diagnosed through a combination of antibody titers, electromyography (EMG), and the use of the Tensilon test. Edrophonium chloride (Tensilon) is a very short-acting anticholinesterase that can be administered intravenously. Its administration in myasthenia gravis causes an immediate increase in muscle strength.

NURSING MANAGEMENT

◆ ASSESSMENT

Subjective Data

Pattern and severity of muscle fatigue and weakness
Presence of diplopia
Perceived difficulties in chewing and swallowing
Patient's understanding of the disease and its management

Objective Data

Presence and severity of ptosis
Documented muscle weakness, facial "snarl"
Presence of dysphonia (leaking air while speaking), soft weak voice
Presence and quality of breath sounds, muffled cough

◆ NURSING DIAGNOSES

Nursing diagnoses for the person with myasthenia gravis may include, but are not limited to, the following:

Activity intolerance (related to generalized muscle weakness)

Aspiration, high risk for (related to chewing and swallowing difficulties, respiratory muscle weakness)

Nutrition, altered: less than body requirements (related to difficulties in ingesting sufficient calories and nutrients)

Home maintenance management, high risk for impaired (related to inadequate knowledge about the disease process, medications and side effects, and symptoms of crises)

◆ EXPECTED PATIENT OUTCOMES

Patient will experience sufficient muscle strength and energy to carry out self-care activities and engage in preferred life-style.

Patient will maintain clear breath sounds and not experience aspiration.

Patient will adapt daily diet to successfully ingest adequate nutrients and calories to maintain a stable body weight.

Patient will be knowledgeable about the disease process, take medications on an optimal schedule, manage drug-related side effects, and be able to identify the symptoms of myasthenic and cholinergic crisis.

◆ NURSING INTERVENTIONS

Promoting Activity and Self-Care

Work with patient to establish patterns of weakness.
Encourage planned rest periods and balancing activity with rest.
Plan medication administration to meet daily activity needs.
Explore energy conservation techniques and self-help devices.
Refer to occupational therapy for assistance as needed.

Provide assistance as needed during times of weakness.
Perform or assist patient to perform range of motion exercises every 4 hours while patient is awake.

Preventing Aspiration

Monitor for signs of respiratory distress, dyspnea.
Monitor respiratory rate and depth every 4 hours, and auscultate lungs.
Encourage frequent position changes, diaphragmatic breathing, and use of incentive spirometer every 2 hours.
Measure and record tidal volume/vital capacity as ordered.
Monitor O_2 saturation by pulse oximetry.
Teach patient to cough effectively.
Utilize postural drainage or chest physical therapy as indicated.
Place suction equipment at the bedside if indicated.
Position patient with the head of bed elevated.
  Always put patient upright for meals.
  Assess intactness of swallowing before administering any food or fluid.
Utilize nasogastric (NG) tube if swallowing is severely compromised.

Promoting Adequate Nutrition

Provide small frequent meals and nutritious snacks that are easily chewed and swallowed.
Administer medications 45 to 60 minutes before meals for maximum effectiveness.
Remind patient to eat slowly and take small bites. Do not attempt to speak while eating.
Administer fluids in small quantities and monitor carefully for choking or nasal regurgitation.
Keep suction equipment available for use at bedside.
Remind patient to always remain upright for meals.
Monitor patient for constipation or diarrhea, and adjust diet as needed or seek dosage adjustment for medications.

Teaching for Effective Home Management

Assess patient and family's knowledge about the disease process and reinforce as needed.
Emphasize the importance of taking medications on schedule and parameters for making dosage adjustments.
Teach patient the importance of seeking prompt medical care for any upper respiratory infection.
Reinforce the importance of balancing activity and rest to support muscle strength and endurance.
Teach patient to avoid the use of drugs that may increase muscle weakness:
  Tranquilizers or muscle relaxants
  Barbiturates or morphine sulfate
  Neomycin (affects myoneural junction)
  Quinine and quinidine
  Procainamide

Encourage patient to avoid infection, stress, or excess exercise that may exacerbate the disease process.

Teach patient the signs of myasthenic and cholinergic crisis (Box 13-6).

Refer patient to the Myasthenia Gravis Foundation for information and support services.

◆ EVALUATION

Successful achievement of expected outcomes for the patient with myasthenia gravis is indicated by the following:

Successful participation in self-care and social activities

No evidence of immobility-related complications

Clear breath sounds, regular respiratory rate and depth

Ingestion of nutritious diet without aspiration or need for suctioning

Maintenance of stable body weight

Correctly describes administration and side effects of all medications

States importance of balancing rest and activity, avoiding respiratory infection and physical and emotional stress

States correct parameters for self-adjustment of medication dosages

Correctly states principal features of myasthenic and cholinergic crisis and actions to be taken if symptoms develop

Amyotrophic Lateral Sclerosis

Amyotrophic lateral sclerosis (ALS), also called Lou Gehrig's disease, is a fatal degenerative disease affecting upper and lower motor neurons in the brain and spinal cord. It is a rare disease that usually develops in early middle age and affects males more often than females. Its etiology is unknown. Both heredity and the effects of slow viral infection are theories under investigation. The disease destroys the myelin sheaths of the motor nerves and replaces them with scar tissue. Nerve impulses are distorted or blocked. The disease may affect a wide variety of nerves but usually begins with progressive muscle weakness, muscle atrophy, and fasciculations. Complications develop as respiratory, swallowing, and speech muscles become involved. There is no sensory involvement, and intelligence is not affected.

The medical management of ALS is largely symptomatic, supporting ventilation, nutrition, and mobility. Death usually occurs within 5 to 10 years. Nursing management focuses on supporting mobility and self-care skills and assisting the patient and family to deal with the progressive and ultimately fatal nature of the disease.

Alzheimer's Disease
Etiology/epidemiology

Alzheimer's disease is a degenerative disorder affecting the cells of the brain that causes progressive and irreversible impairment of intellectual functioning. It is estimated to affect 4 million persons per year and is the fourth leading cause of death in elderly persons. Its incidence is clearly related to aging, but the disease shows no pattern of involvement for any particular race, sex, or cultural group. The specific cause of the disease remains unknown. Research is exploring the role of viral agents, environmental toxins, and deficiencies in neurotransmitters.

Pathophysiology

The normal effects of aging on the brain are dramatically accelerated with Alzheimer's disease. The brain is small with narrowed gyri and enlarged sulci and ventricles. The classic feature is the presence of microscopic plaques composed of degenerating nerve terminals, particularly in the hippocampus region. These plaques interfere with nerve cell functioning. In addition, the concentrations of acetylcholine, norepinephrine, and

---

BOX 13-6	Myasthenic versus Cholinergic Crisis

MYASTHENIC CRISIS

Triggered by inadequate medication, disease exacerbation or stress

Symptoms

Respiratory distress
Extreme weakness and fatigue
Tachycardia and increased blood pressure
Speech impairment
Facial weakness, ptosis
Anxiety

Treatment

Diagnosis with the Tensilon test
Ventilatory support if needed
Cautious adjustment of medications with continuous monitoring

CHOLINERGIC CRISIS

Triggered by an overdose of anticholinesterase medication

Symptoms

Increased secretions: salivation, lacrimation, perspiration
Nausea and vomiting
Diarrhea
Severe dysphagia
Severe muscle weakness

Treatment

Reduction or withdrawal of medications
Ventilatory monitoring and assistance
Administration of atropine (reverses drug effects)

dopamine in the brain are all significantly reduced. The exact meaning of these deficiencies has not yet been accurately determined.

Alzheimer's disease is classified by severity. Early stages are characterized by memory lapses, short attention span, and a loss of interest in the environment or personal affairs. Memory and cognitive losses progress steadily and incorporate disintegration of the personality, disorientation, and gradual physical impairments with complete loss of self-care ability and sense of self.

Medical management

Few treatment options exist. Traditional medications typically worsen the symptoms. A number of new drugs are being utilized experimentally, and some show early promise. Most research is focusing on altering the balance and metabolism of neurotransmitters in the brain.

NURSING MANAGEMENT

Nursing management focuses on preventing patient injury and assisting the family to cope with the deterioration in the patient. Approaches vary by the stage of the disease. The implementation of a structured environment with multiple memory aids is useful for some families in enabling them to postpone any decision concerning nursing home placement. Prevention of falls, injury, harm to others through forgetfulness, and wandering is an ongoing challenge. Support for the patient is also critical, since in the early stages of the disease the person is often aware of deteriorating mental state and is naturally prone to depression, low self-esteem, and powerlessness, as well as anger and aggression. In the later stages the focus of care becomes largely custodial. Families should be strongly encouraged to utilize the services of the Alzheimer's Disease Association for peer support and respite care.

HEADACHE

Headache is a common symptom experienced by most individuals at some point. It has many potential causes, some based in neurologic disease and others related to eye, ear, sinus, or psychologic factors. The three most common categories are as follows:

1. Migraine headache
   a. Episodic; lasts hours to days
   b. Strong hereditary component; more common in women
   c. Evolves slowly; pain usually affects one side of the head more severely than the other
   d. May have prodromal symptoms; often associated with nausea, vomiting, irritability
   e. Treated with ergotamine, propranolol, nonsteroidal antiinflammatory drugs (NSAIDs), and relaxation techniques

2. Cluster headache
   a. Episodes clustered together in rapid succession for a few days or weeks followed by prolonged remission; lasts minutes to hours
   b. Develops in early adulthood, precipitated by use of alcohol or nitrites
   c. Intense, deep pain that is often unilateral; begins in infraorbital region and spreads to head and neck
   d. Narcotic relief may be necessary

3. Tension headache
   a. Episodic and of variable duration
   b. Common onset in adolescence, usually directly attributable to tension or anxiety
   c. Constant, dull pain; variable intensity; usually bilateral and may involve neck and shoulders
   d. Treated with NSAIDs, amitriptyline, and relaxation techniques

The pathophysiology of headache is poorly understood since the brain tissue is not capable of sensing pain. Pain is theorized to arise from the scalp, blood vessels, muscles, and dura mater. The blood vessels may dilate and become congested both intracranially and extracranially, initiating stretch pain. Most headaches are self-managed by the patient. Prescription medications may be utilized in selective situations as indicated above. Any headache that persists, recurs, or is outside of the person's normal experience should receive prompt medical workup as a potential warning of a serious neurologic problem.

CONVULSIVE DISORDERS: EPILEPSY

Etiology/epidemiology

Seizures may be defined as transitory disturbances in motor, sensory, or autonomic functions with or without loss of consciousness, resulting from uncontrolled electrical discharges in the brain. Seizures may be triggered by a wide variety of causes including the following:

Cerebral anoxia
Hypoglycemia
Infections accompanied by high temperature
Neoplasms
Trauma and scar tissue
Metabolic disturbances
Electrolyte imbalances
Drugs and poisons
Inflammation and abscess
Increased intracranial pressure

In idiopathic epilepsy the actual cause of the seizures may remain unknown; the role of heredity remains unclear.

More than 1 million persons in the United States are subject to seizures, and there is no identifiable racial, sexual, cultural, or geographic pattern. Seizure activity may begin at any point in the life span depending on the cause, but most cases of idiopathic epilepsy begin before 20 years of age. Box 13-7 presents one common classification for seizures.

BOX 13-7 **Common Types of Seizures**

GENERALIZED

Bilaterally symmetric, with no local onset

Grand Mal

Most common and dramatic type of seizure
Progression:
1. Aura—change in sensation or affect that precedes seizure and occurs in about 50% of all patients; may include numbness, odors, lights, dizziness
2. Cry—caused by spasms of thorax expelling air through glottis or abrupt inspiratory effort
3. Loss of consciousness—sudden, profound, and variable in duration (usually several minutes)
4. Fixed dilated pupils
5. Tonic clonic contractions—immediate bilateral tonic contraction with cessation of respiration and cyanosis, followed by clonic rhythmic contractions of increasing strength and return of shallow respiration; urinary and fecal incontinence may occur
6. Postictal condition—patient experiences partial return of consciousness to a groggy confused state; headache, muscle pain, and need for deep sleep frequently follow, and general fatigue may persist for 1 to 2 days

Petit Mal

Most common during childhood
Progression:
1. Sudden impairment of or loss of consciousness with little or no motor movement
2. Sudden vacant facial expression with eyes focused straight ahead
3. Duration is usually not more than 10-20 seconds but may occur many times in a day

Status Epilepticus (Box 13-9)

When recurrent generalized seizure activity occurs at such frequency that full consciousness is not regained between episodes:

1. It can lead to death from brain damage secondary to hypoxia and requires intensive care
2. Patient usually in a coma for 12-24 hours or more

PARTIAL SEIZURES

Have a localized onset

Psychomotor: Temporal Lobe, Complex Partial

Complex seizures may occur at any age
1. Sudden change in awareness or consciousness—patient may have complex hallucination aura
2. Patient may behave as if partially conscious or intoxicated and engage in antisocial behavior such as exposing self or perform repetitive meaningless acts such as buttoning and unbuttoning
3. Patient may have autonomic complaints—chest pain, dyspnea, etc.
4. End of seizure—patient may be confused, amnesic, and groggy
5. Duration of seizure much longer than petit mal

Focal Seizures: Jacksonian

Arise in any localized motor or sensory portion of cortex
1. Symptoms depend on site of occurrence; limited almost exclusively to patients with structural brain disease
2. Progressive involvement of adjacent motor or sensory areas possible
3. Consciousness usually maintained unless seizure progresses to full grand mal seizure

Myoclonic

May be mild or cause rapid forceful movements
1. Sudden involuntary contraction of a muscle group, usually in the extremities or trunk
2. No loss of consciousness
3. May precede grand mal seizures by months or years

Pathophysiology

Seizures represent sudden, excessive, disorderly discharges of the neurons of the brain. The process may last from a few seconds to as long as 5 minutes. Fatigue of the precipitating neurons is believed to help end the seizure. The seizure may involve only a minute focal spot in the brain or virtually all of it at once.

A seizure is typically followed by a period of inhibition of cerebral function. The inhibition is usually incomplete and variable depending on the area of the brain involved. It often lasts longer than the seizure itself.

Medical management

The electroencephalogram (EEG) is the most common diagnostic tool used in the diagnosis of seizures. It may be supplemented by the CT scan, MRI, or another more invasive diagnostic tool. The treatment of seizures almost always involves the use of anticonvulsant medication, especially if no correctable cause can be uncovered. Dosages of anticonvulsant medications are difficult

to establish and regulate because of the high incidence of side effects and the toxicity of the drugs. Drugs are usually introduced in an average therapeutic dose and then increased or decreased until adequate control of the seizures is obtained and side effects are maintained in an acceptable range. Blood levels are monitored at intervals to prevent toxicity. Common medications used to control seizures are presented in Table 13-2. Surgical excision of the irritable focus may be attempted in cases in which seizure activity cannot be controlled by more conventional means.

NURSING MANAGEMENT

◆ ASSESSMENT
Subjective Data

History of seizure disorder and manifestations
Patient's knowledge of seizure disorder
Patient's knowledge of prescribed medications, side effects; degree of compliance

TABLE 13-2   Drugs Used to Prevent Seizures

DRUG	SEIZURE TYPE	TOXIC EFFECTS
Phenytoin sodium (Dilantin)	Grand mal, focal, psychomotor	Ataxia, vomiting, nystagmus, drowsiness, rash, fever, gum hypertrophy, lymphadenopathy
Phenobarbital (Luminal)	Grand mal, focal, psychomotor	Drowsiness, rash
Primidone (Mysoline)	Grand mal, focal, psychomotor	Drowsiness, ataxia
Mephenytoin (Mesantoin)	Grand mal, focal, psychomotor	Ataxia, nystagmus, pancytopenia, rash
Ethosuximide (Zarontin)	Petit mal, psychomotor, myoclonic, akinetic	Drowsiness, nausea, agranulocytosis
Trimethadione (Tridione)	Petit mal	Rash, photophobia, agranulocytosis, nephrosis
Diazepam (Valium)	Status epilepticus, mixed	Drowsiness, ataxia
Carbamazepine (Tegretol)	Grand mal, psychomotor	Rash, drowsiness, ataxia
Valproic acid (Depakene)	Petit mal	Nausea, vomiting, indigestion, sedation, emotional disturbance, weakness, altered blood coagulation
Clonazepam (Clonopin)	Petit mal	Drowsiness, ataxia, hypotension, respiratory depression

Patient's description of aura experience, if any, and postictal feelings

Patient's social adjustment to seizure disorder

Objective Data

Character of seizure (see Box 13-8 for observations to be made about a person having a seizure)

Duration, pattern, and severity of involvement

Number observed if multiple

Observed behavior before seizure: signs of stress or fatigue

Side effects of medications

The nursing management of the patient experiencing a seizure is summarized in the "Nursing Care Plan."

BOX 13-8   Observations to be Made About a Person Having a Seizure

AURA

Presence or absence; nature if present; ability of patient to describe it (somatic, visceral, psychic)

CRY

Presence or absence

ONSET

Site of initial body movements; deviation of head and eyes; chewing and salivation; posture of body; sensory changes

TONIC AND CLONIC PHASES

Movements of body as to progression; skin color and airway; pupillary changes; incontinence; duration of each phase

RELAXATION (SLEEP)

Duration and behavior

POSTICTAL PHASE

Duration; general behavior; ability to remember anything about the seizure; orientation; pupillary changes; headache; injuries present

DURATION OF ENTIRE SEIZURE

Measure by clock

LEVEL OF CONSCIOUSNESS

Length of unconsciousness if present

BOX 13-9   Status Epilepticus

Status epilepticus involves a condition in which one seizure follows another with little or no recovery time. The condition can be life threatening, and vigorous therapy is aimed at controlling the seizures. Drug therapy is given intravenously and may include phenobarbital, diazepam (Valium), phenytoin (Dilantin), and paraldehyde.

GUIDELINES FOR CARE

Ensure a patent airway.

Provide supplemental oxygen.

Assess respiratory adequacy, and prepare for potential need for intubation.

Monitor vital signs and neurologic status frequently.

Maintain a safe environment and protect patient from injury.

Continue to monitor and record type and duration of seizure activity.

NOTE: When phenytoin is given IV it must be given by direct injection, not added to an existing infusion, because precipitation may occur. The rate of injection should never exceed 50 mg/min (50 mg/2-3 min for elderly persons). The drug is very irritating to the veins, and the vein should be flushed with sterile saline after administration. Monitor for adverse effects, which may include CNS depression and cardiovascular collapse. Drug effects are dose related.

NERVOUS SYSTEM INFECTIONS AND INFLAMMATIONS

The nervous system may be attacked by a variety of organisms and viruses as well as suffer from toxic reactions to bacterial and viral disease. The meninges or the brain itself may be affected. If an infection becomes walled off, it may cause an abscess.

Meningitis

Etiology/epidemiology

Meningitis is an acute infection of the meninges that may be caused by a wide variety of bacteria and viruses including pneumococci, meningococci, or *Haemophilus influenzae*. Any pathogenic organism that gains access to the subarachnoid space can cause meningitis.

THE PERSON WITH A SEIZURE DISORDER

■ NURSING DIAGNOSIS

Injury/aspiration, high risk for (related to loss of consciousness and tonic clonic muscle movements)

Expected Patient Outcomes	Nursing Interventions

Patient will not experience injury during seizures.
Patient will maintain a patent airway and not experience aspiration.
	1. Institute seizure precautions:
	  a. Keep padded tongue blade or oral airway at bedside.
	  b. Use padded side rails. Avoid use of soft pillows because of risk of suffocation.
	  c. Supervise ambulation.
	  d. Ensure prompt access to oxygen, suction, and anticonvulsant medications.
	2. In the event of a seizure:
	  a. Never leave the patient alone during seizure.
	  b. If patient is upright, lower to bed or floor and clear immediate environment to prevent injury.
	  c. Loosen constrictive clothing, especially around the neck.
	  d. Position patient: turn head to side if feasible to help keep airway open.
	  e. Cushion head.
	  f. Provide privacy.
	  g. *No effort should be made to restrain the individual during the seizure.*
	  h. A padded tongue blade or oral airway may be inserted between the back teeth to protect tongue and mouth if jaws are not already clenched. *Never attempt to pry open the mouth once jaws are clenched.*
	  i. Record sequence and progression of seizure accurately.
	  j. Gently reorient patient at end of seizure, and provide for postictal rest and sleep.

■ NURSING DIAGNOSIS

Coping, high risk for impaired individual (related to diagnosis, activity, and life-style restrictions)

Expected Patient Outcome	Nursing Interventions
Patient will successfully incorporate treatment limitations into preferred life-style.	1. Encourage patient to verbalize feelings about diagnosis and problems encountered in social settings. 2. Discuss restrictions on employment, driving, and leisure mandated by seizure activity. Driver's license may usually be obtained after one seizure-free year. 3. Encourage the patient to live as normal a life-style as possible. 4. Encourage patient and family to make contact with local epilepsy society for support. 5. Assist patient to identify pleasurable and nonhazardous activities. 6. Encourage patient to share diagnosis with family, friends, and co-workers.

NURSING CARE PLAN—CONT'D

THE PERSON WITH A SEIZURE DISORDER

■ NURSING DIAGNOSIS

Health maintenance, high risk for altered (related to lack of knowledge concerning diagnosis, drug therapy, life-style management)

Expected Patient Outcome	Nursing Interventions
Patient will be knowledgeable about the disease, medications, and life-style adaptations related to seizure management.	1. Teach patient about prescribed medications and expected side effects.
	2. Encourage good mouth care, particularly if patient is receiving phenytoin (Dilantin).
	3. Encourage patient to follow guidelines for a healthy life-style:
	a. Nutritious diet
	b. Balance of rest and activity
	c. Avoidance of alcohol and acute stress, which frequently trigger seizures
	d. Avoidance of ingestion of excessive caffeine
	4. Stress the importance of ongoing adherence to the medication regimen.
	5. Stress importance of regular follow-up to assess effectiveness of drug therapy and monitor for toxicities.

The disease occurs more frequently in fall and winter when upper respiratory infections are common. Children are affected more often than adults.

Pathophysiology

Organisms that reach the brain disseminate quickly through the meninges and into the ventricles. This dissemination produces the following:

Congestion of the meningeal vessels

Edema of brain tissue

Increased intracranial pressure

Generalized inflammation with WBC exudate formation

Hydrocephalus if exudate blocks ventricular passages

Diagnosis is confirmed by the identification of the organism from the cerebrospinal fluid (CSF).

Medical management

Medical management consists of the following:

Massive doses of antibiotic specific for the causative organism

Steroids and osmotic diuretics if necessary to reduce cerebral edema

Anticonvulsants may be administered to prevent or control seizures

Respiratory isolation for 24 to 48 hours after antibiotics begin

Although the disease presentation is variable, classic symptoms include severe headache, acute neck stiffness, fever, malaise, nausea, and vomiting. Kernig's and Brudzinski's signs, which indicate acute meningeal irritation (Figure 13-5), are usually present. The patient may recover without sequelae or experience residual damage in the form of deafness, blindness, mental impairment, hydrocephalus, or paralysis.

NURSING MANAGEMENT

Nursing care for the patient with meningitis is largely supportive and directed at increasing comfort and relieving symptoms. The room is kept darkened and quiet, and the patient is offered tepid baths and frequent linen changes if high fever is present. The nurse monitors intake and output, vital signs, and level of consciousness frequently. Fluids and antibiotics are administered IV. Isolation precautions are maintained until therapy has been administered for about 48 hours. The patient is monitored for complications such as diabetes insipidus or inappropriate secretion of antidiuretic hormone (SIADH).

Encephalitis

Encephalitis is an inflammation of the brain tissues that may be caused by viruses such as herpes simplex or may

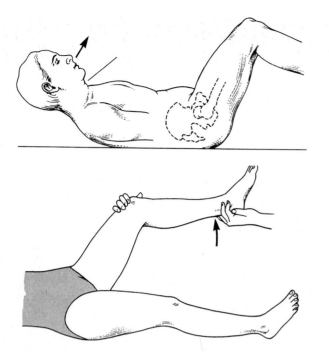

FIGURE 13-5 Signs of acute meningeal irritation. **A,** Brudzinski's sign. **B,** Kernig's sign.

follow other generalized infections such as measles, chickenpox, and syphilis or the ingestion of toxins such as lead, arsenic, or carbon monoxide. It has occurred worldwide in epidemic form following widespread epidemics of influenza. The death rate is quite high, and patients who survive the disease may suffer a wide range of residual neurologic effects including the symptoms of Parkinson's disease.

The disease is characterized by abrupt onset, high fever, and rapid neurologic deterioration into stupor or coma. Generalized seizures are common. Medical management revolves around the administration of drugs to eradicate the virus and measures to control seizures or rising intracranial pressure (ICP). Nursing care involves careful monitoring, supportive care, and the prevention of complications.

Guillain-Barré Syndrome

Etiology/epidemiology

Guillain-Barré syndrome is an acute polyneuritis that typically follows an upper respiratory infection, trauma, surgery, or immunization by about 2 weeks. Its basic etiology is unknown, but it is attributed to a cell-mediated immunologic reaction. It is theorized that the prodromal infection or stressor produces a limited malfunction of the immune system, sensitizing the T cells to the person's own myelin. The condition achieved notoriety when its incidence increased dramatically following population-wide efforts to immunize for swine flu. It occurs most commonly in persons between 30 and 50 years of age and may be mild or assume life-threatening proportions.

Pathophysiology

The syndrome produces patchy demyelination of peripheral nerves, nerve roots, and the spinal cord. When the process affects the seventh, ninth, and tenth cranial nerves, the patient has difficulty speaking and swallowing and may experience respiratory failure. The syndrome produces symmetric muscle weakness and flaccid paralysis, which begins in the lower extremities and ascends up the body. The progression may stop at any point and may also involve the sensory system, creating paresthesias and hyperesthesias. The bowel and bladder are rarely affected, but autonomic symptoms such as unstable vital signs may occur. The patient may recover quickly, recover slowly, or experience chronic residual effects.

Medical management

Medical care primarily revolves around maintaining patency of the ventilatory system. Intubation and mechanical ventilation may be required. High-dose steroid therapy may be employed in severe cases, and plasmapheresis is being utilized with encouraging results in limiting symptoms.

NURSING MANAGEMENT

Nursing management provides supportive care and monitoring and is directed at preventing complications. The priority in the acute stage is monitoring tidal volume/vital capacity. Patients are often intubated when their vital capacity drops below 15 to 20 ml/kg, especially if the cough is weak. Nursing also focuses on providing routine skin care, range of motion exercise, turning and positioning, nutrition via tube feedings, and bowel and bladder management, plus comfort measures for extremity pain and hyperesthesia. Psychosocial support and reassurance are critical as the patient and family attempt to cope with this frightening experience. Reassurance is offered that extensive recovery is expected as the nerves begin to remyelinate, but that full recovery will take time and rehabilitation effort.

CENTRAL NERVOUS SYSTEM TRAUMA
Head Injury
Etiology/epidemiology

Trauma to the head may result in injury to the scalp, skull, and/or brain tissues. It affects an estimated 70,000 people yearly and is the major cause of death in persons aged 1 to 35 years, although head injury affects people of all ages. Morbidity and mortality are slightly higher in males. It is estimated that 70% of motor vehicle accidents result in head injury, and the incidence is directly related to the passage and enforcement of helmet and seat belt legislation. The degree of external damage is not necessarily indicative of the extent of brain injury,

TABLE 13-3 Damage of Brain Tissue Caused by Trauma

CHARACTERISTICS	STRUCTURAL ALTERATION	EFFECTS
CONCUSSION		
Immediate and transitory impairment of neurologic function caused by the mechanical force	No	Possible loss of consciousness that may be instantaneous or delayed and usually is reversible
CONTUSION		
Likened to bruising with extravasation of blood cells	Yes	Injury may be at site of impact or at opposite site; cortex often damaged
LACERATION		
Tearing of tissues caused by sharp fragment or shearing force	Yes	Hemorrhage is serious complication
INTRACRANIAL HEMORRHAGE		
Bleeding into epidural, subdural, subarachnoid spaces or into brain or ventricles	Yes	Effects depend on site of injury and degree of bleeding
Epidural hemorrhage		
Rupture of large vessel that lies above dura mater; tear is usually in an artery (middle meningeal is most common site)		Signs of rising ICP develop rapidly with rapid deterioration into full coma
Subdural hemorrhage		
Usually results from venous bleeding below dura mater; bleeding may produce acute, subacute, or chronic hematoma formation		Signs of rising ICP may develop within days, weeks, or even months after injury

but compound and depressed skull fractures are associated with serious damage. Table 13-3 summarizes the common types of injuries produced.

Pathophysiology

When the head receives a direct blow or injury, the brain moves in the skull and suffers damage of varying degrees, not all of which occurs at the site of direct injury. All head injuries create concern over rising ICP, since the brain swells abruptly and often severely after injury. The rigid skull leaves little room for expansion. Changes in ICP can create severe hypoxia in brain tissue. The pathologic sequence that occurs as ICP rises is outlined in Box 13-10. Symptoms of head injury will depend on the exact nature and severity of the injury and whether the injury is open or closed. A change in level of consciousness is by far the most common sign. Classic signs of rising ICP are outlined in Box 13-11.

Medical management

The diagnosis of head injury is made based on the patient's history and presenting symptoms. Skull x-rays may be used to rule out skeletal injury, and CT scans may be ordered to verify the presence and severity of elevated ICP. Treatment measures may include repair of lacerations, or surgery to place burr holes to release hematomas or to repair cranial defects. In most situations, control of ICP will be the primary concern. Drug therapy may include the following:

- Corticosteroids (dexamethasone) to reduce inflammation and edema

> ### BOX 13-10 Pathologic Sequence of Increasing Intracranial Pressure
>
> An increase in brain tissue, vascular tissue and volume, or CSF volume from any cause increases pressure within the cranial cavity. After the brain's compensatory mechanisms have been utilized, the following sequence occurs:
> 1. Cerebral blood flow decreases, resulting in inadequate perfusion.
> 2. Inadequate perfusion leads to increasing pCO_2 and decreasing pO_2 values.
> 3. Oxygenation changes trigger vasodilation and cerebral edema.
> 4. Edema further increases ICP, resulting in a downward spiral of tissue compression and displacement that may be irreversible and fatal.
> 5. Life-sustaining mechanisms for consciousness, blood pressure, pulse, respiration, and temperature regulation fail.

- Osmotic diuretics (mannitol or urea) to reduce cerebral edema
- Anticonvulsants (phenytoin) to control seizures
- Hypertonic glucose solutions (25% to 50%) to promote diuresis
- Barbiturate coma (pentobarbital) to reduce brain metabolism and activity
- Loop diuretics (furosemide) to reduce circulating volume

Rapidly rising or unresponsive ICP may require ventricular puncture or drainage via ventriculostomy tube or removal of a portion of skull to allow for the brain to expand. Unstable ICP may necessitate the insertion of

---

BOX 13-11 **Signs of Increasing Intracranial Pressure**

1. Change in level of consciousness
   NOTE: One of the earliest and most sensitive signs of rising ICP is restlessness.
2. Pupillary signs
   Result from pressure on the oculomotor nerve (III)
   Slower response, pupil inequality, or fixed dilated pupils
3. Blood pressure and pulse
   Increasing systolic pressure with stable or falling diastolic pressure
   Widening pulse pressure
   Slowing of pulse rate from pressure on vagus nerve
4. Respirations
   Changes usually quite late
   Slowing of rate and irregular breathing pattern
   NOTE: Hypoxia worsens ICP.
5. Temperature
   Failure of thermoregulatory center occurs late
   High uncontrolled temperature (increases metabolic needs of brain tissue)
6. Focal signs
   Muscle weakness or paralysis
   Decreasing response to pain stimulus in comatose patients
   Positive Babinski's sign
   Decerebrate or decorticate posture
7. Decreasing visual acuity; papilledema
8. Headache and vomiting (projectile)

BOX 13-12 **ICP Monitoring Devices**

One of three types of devices is standardly used:

1. **Intraventricular catheter:** a small tube is inserted into the anterior horn of the lateral ventricle in the patient's nondominant hemisphere. Device allows for draining CSF and taking fluid specimens as well as monitoring pressure.
2. **Subarachnoid screw or bolt:** a hollow device is placed into the subarachnoid space for direct pressure measurement. Fluid cannot be drained from this system.
3. **Epidural monitor:** a sensor is placed between the skull and the dura without penetrating the dura. Its major advantage is the decreased risk of infection. Fluid cannot be drained from this system.

Burr holes are required for the first two types of monitors. In each case the catheter is connected to a transducer that must be maintained at the level of the ventricle. Continuous waveform printouts of the pressure patterns are drawn by the monitor.

---

an ICP monitoring device. These tools allow for the continuous monitoring of a patient's pressure status. They are described in Box 13-12 and illustrated in Figure 13-6.

NURSING MANAGEMENT

♦ ASSESSMENT

Subjective Data

History of the trauma and sequence of symptoms
Patient's complaints of headache, double vision, nausea
History of loss of consciousness
Patient's ability to understand, reason

Objective Data

Vital signs
Level of consciousness, alertness, orientation
Motor strength and equality
Speech difficulties
Bleeding or CSF drainage from ears or nose
Vomiting
Pupils: size, equality, reactivity

♦ NURSING DIAGNOSES

Nursing diagnoses for the person with a head injury may include, but are not limited to, the following:

Cerebral tissue perfusion, altered (related to increased ICP)
Injury and infection, potential for (related to decreasing level of consciousness and head trauma)
Mobility, impaired physical (related to decreasing level of consciousness and interruption of motor impulses)
Ineffective family coping, high risk for (related to the crisis of injury and uncertain outcomes)

♦ EXPECTED PATIENT OUTCOMES

Patient will maintain adequate cerebral perfusion as indicated by the absence of undetected increases in ICP.
Patient will not experience environmental injury or develop preventable infection.
Patient will not experience common complications of immobility during period of bed rest and treatment.
Family will verbalize adequate coping and make realistic plans for ongoing rehabilitation and care.

♦ NURSING INTERVENTIONS

Monitoring Cerebral Perfusion

Perform accurate neurologic checks at frequent intervals including the following:
Vital signs
Level of consciousness using Glasgow Coma Scale, Rancho Los Amigos Scale, or other standardized hospital-approved tool (Boxes 13-13 to 13-15)
Pupil size, equality, and reaction to light
Motor and sensory status—hand grips, voluntary movement, sensation
Monitor ICP readings and blood gases.

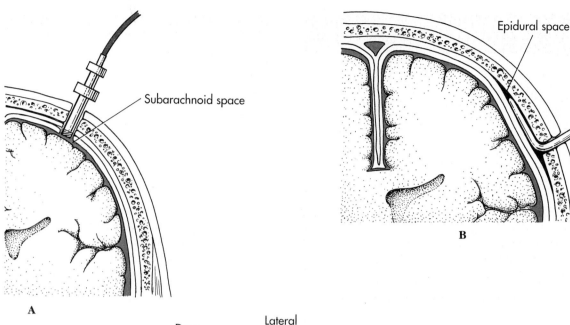

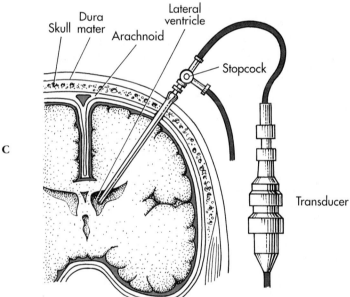

FIGURE 13-6 Intracranial pressure monitoring. **A,** Subarachnoid bolt. **B,** Epidural monitor. **C,** Intraventricular catheter.

<table>
<tr><td>**BOX 13-13**</td><td>**Five-Point Level of Consciousness Rating Scale**</td></tr>
</table>

1 Alert—normal mental activity, aware, mentally functional
2 Obtunded/drowsy—sleepy, very short attention span, can respond appropriately if aroused
3 Stupor—apathetic, slow moving, expression blank, staring; aroused only by vigorous stimuli
4 Light coma—not oriented to time, place, or person; aroused only by painful stimuli—response is only grunt or grimace or withdrawal from pain
5 Deep coma—no response except decerebrate or decorticate posture to even the most painful stimuli

Assess for signs of hypoxia: cyanosis, color changes in nail beds and mucous membranes, restlessness, altered respiratory rate.

Follow institutional guidelines for hyperventilation if pressure rises.

Administer medications as ordered to reduce or stabilize ICP.

Maintain bed rest with head of bed slightly elevated as ordered (15 to 30 degrees). Keep environmental stimuli to a minimum. Space nursing care activities.

Administer codeine or other mild analgesic as needed for discomfort and restlessness. NOTE: Morphine is not used, because it depresses responsiveness and alters pupillary responses.

Preventing Injury and Infection

Avoid head rotation, plantar flexion, or any Valsalva type of movements.

BOX 13-14	**Glasgow Coma Scale Scoring**

EYES OPEN

4 Spontaneously
3 On request
2 To pain stimuli (supraorbital or digital)
1 No opening

BEST VERBAL RESPONSE

5 Oriented to time, place, person
4 Engages in conversation, confused in content
3 Words spoken but conversation not sustained
2 Groans evoked by pain
1 No response

BEST MOTOR RESPONSE

5 Obeys a command ("Hold out three fingers.")
4 Localizes a painful stimulus
3 Flexes either arm
2 Extends arm to painful stimulus
1 No response

Use side rails and seizure precautions; avoid neck flexion or sudden movements.

Institute nursing measures or cooling blanket to control temperature. NOTE: Increased temperature dramatically increases brain's metabolic demands.

Observe for bloody or serous drainage from nose or ears.

NOTE: Drainage may indicate tearing of meninges and escape of CSF and precede meningitis. If present:

Do not clean, pack, or obstruct in any way.

Promote gravity drainage onto sterile towel or dressing.

Determine whether serous fluid is CSF or mucus (CSF tests positive for sugar and produces a halo when blotted and dried on gauze).

Administer antibiotics as ordered.

Do not suction through the nose.

Monitor intake and output carefully. Fluid intake may be restricted. Check specific gravity hourly. Diabetes insipidus increases urine output, whereas inappropriate antidiuretic hormone (ADH) syndrome decreases it.

Urine output should remain above 45 to 60 ml/hr and be greater if osmotic diuretics are used. A Foley catheter is usually needed to track output.

Monitor serum electrolytes, particularly for imbalances in sodium that may accompany diabetes insipidus or SIADH.

Test all secretions for blood. Administer antacids and cimetidine as ordered to prevent stress ulcers.

Teach patient to avoid coughing and sneezing if possible. Avoid all isometric contraction.

Preventing the Complications of Immobility

Institute standard nursing measures for passive range of motion, turning, skin care, and TED stockings to prevent complications of immobility.

Employ bulk cathartics and stool softeners to prevent straining at elimination.

Supporting Effective Family Coping

Offer support to patient and family to deal with high-anxiety situation with uncertain outcome.

Provide family with liberal opportunities to visit, and explain all treatments and equipment.

Involve family members in care where feasible. Encourage them to talk with and encourage the patient. Remind them that even semiconscious or comatose patients may hear what is said at the bedside.

Provide referral to social services as indicated to assist with planning for postdischarge care as needed.

Reassure family that improvement in neurologic status frequently continues for months after discharge. Foster hope.

NOTE: Many individuals who experience minor head injury are sent home after the initial evaluation. The Guidelines box lists specific teaching instructions that should be provided to patients and families.

◆ EVALUATION

Successful achievement of expected outcomes for the patient with a head injury is indicated by the following:

Adequate cerebral perfusion as indicated by stable ICP and blood gases within normal range

BOX 13-15	**Levels of Cognitive Functioning (Rancho Los Amigos Scale)**	
I	No response	Patient is completely unresponsive to any stimuli.
II	Generalized response	Patient reacts inconsistently and nonpurposefully to stimuli in nonspecific manner.
III	Localized response	Patient reacts specifically but inconsistently to stimuli.
IV	Confused, agitated	Patient is in heightened state of activity with severely decreased ability to process information.
V	Confused, inappropriate	Patient appears alert and is able to respond to simple commands fairly consistently.
VI	Confused, appropriate	Patient shows goal-directed behavior but depends on external input for direction.
VII	Automatic, appropriate	Patient appears appropriate and oriented within hospital and home setting, goes through daily routine automatically, with minimal to absent confusion and has shallow recall of actions.
VIII	Purposeful, appropriate	Patient is alert and oriented, is able to recall and integrate past and recent events, and is aware of and responsive to culture.

Guidelines for Teaching Head Injury Patients and Families

Patient should be awakened periodically through the first 24 hours to ensure patient is arousable.

During first 24 to 48 hours, patient and family should watch carefully for the following warning signs:

Vomiting—often with force behind it

Unusual sleepiness, dizziness, loss of balance, or falling

Complaint of double vision, blurring, or jerky eye movements

A slight headache is expected—worsening headache or complaints of feeling worse when moving about should be reported

Bleeding or discharge from nose or ears

Seizures—any twitching or movement of arms or legs that patient cannot stop

Any behavior or symptom not normal for the individual

A physician should be called at once if any of these signs are observed. If a physician is unavailable, emergency services should be contacted immediately.

BOX 13-16 **Spinal Shock**

A period immediately following spinal cord injury in which the spinal cord ceases to function. Spinal shock may persist for days or weeks. During this time the patient exhibits:
1. Flaccid paralysis and loss of sensation
2. Urinary and bowel retention
3. Inability to perspire to cool the body
4. Vascular instability with bradycardia and hypotension from loss of sympathetic stimulation

The gradual return of reflexes signals the resolution of spinal shock.

Absence of physical injury or infection

Presence of full range of motion, intact skin, normal bilateral muscle strength, and regular patterns of elimination

Family involvement

Statements of adequate coping by family members

Involvement in and stated understanding of care regimen

Utilization of resources to plan for postdischarge care

Spinal Cord Injury

Etiology/epidemiology

The spinal cord may be damaged by the effects of tumors, by protrusion of intervertebral disks, or from trauma and fracture of the spinal vertebrae with resultant compression or tearing of the underlying cord. Approximately 10,000 to 12,000 new cases occur annually in the United States, creating a catastrophic health crisis of enormous economic cost for the involved patients and families. Spinal cord injury (SCI) primarily affects young males and is caused by motor vehicle accidents, falls, diving accidents, and wounds from guns or knives.

Pathophysiology

The spinal cord is very tough and is rarely torn or transected by direct trauma. However, even relatively minor compression can have serious results. Significant cord edema occurs, which can extend the level of injury. Actual spinal cord destruction in severe trauma is related to autodestruction. This complex process involves hemorrhage into the gray matter, inflammation, edema, vasospasm, and ischemia, which can lead to irreversible spinal cord necrosis in a matter of hours after the injury.

A complete cord injury is accompanied by total loss of voluntary movement and sensation below the level of the injury. An incomplete injury involves partial destruction of the cord with variable patterns of sensory or motor function loss.

In *Brown-Séquard syndrome* a half cord lesion produces loss of pain, temperature, and touch sensation on one side of the body and loss of motor function, position, and vibration sense on the other side of the body.

In *central cord syndrome* a compression injury to the center of the cord produces complete motor loss in the upper extremity, partial loss in the trunk, and retained function in the lower body.

In *anterior cord syndrome* an injury to the anterior portion of the cord produces loss of motor function below the level of the injury with preservation of touch, position, and vibration sense.

Immediately following an SCI a period of flaccid paralysis with complete absence of reflexes occurs. This period is termed *spinal shock*. Its duration is variable, but it typically persists to some degree for 4 to 6 weeks. The major features of spinal shock are outlined in Box 13-16. The distribution of muscle losses and residual muscle function remaining after spinal cord injury is outlined in Table 13-4.

TABLE 13-4	Muscle Function After Spinal Cord Injury	
SPINAL CORD INJURY	**MUSCLE FUNCTION REMAINING**	**MUSCLE FUNCTION LOST**
Cervical		
Above C4	None	All including respiration
C5	Neck	Arms
	Scapular elevation	Chest
		All below chest
C6-C7	Neck	Some arm, fingers
	Some chest movement	Some chest
	Some arm movement	All below chest
Thoracic	Neck	Trunk
	Arms (full)	All below chest
	Some chest	
Lumbosacral	Neck	Legs
	Arms	
	Chest	
	Trunk	

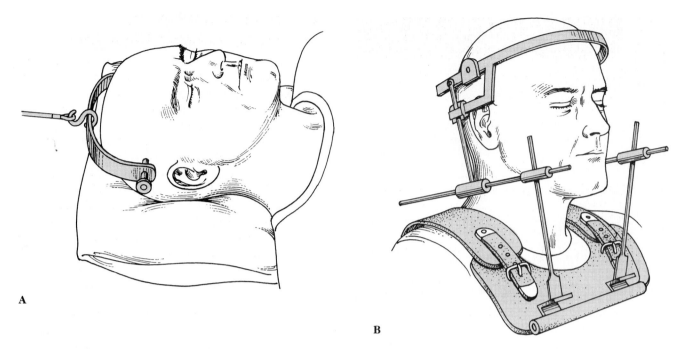

A

B

FIGURE 13-7 Options for cervical traction. **A,** Gardner-Wells tongs. **B,** Halo fixation device.

Medical management

SCI can be readily diagnosed through the history of the injury and pattern of symptoms. When the diagnosis is unclear, spinal x-rays are usually sufficient to confirm or rule out the injury. CT scanning may also be employed.

Initial medical interventions are aimed at supporting vital functions and preventing further cord damage through stabilization and realignment. Early surgery may be indicated to decompress or fuse the spinal column, insert rods to stabilize the spine, and correct deformities.

Initial management may involve skeletal traction with the use of Crutchfield or Gardner-Wells tongs (Figure 13-7, *A*) and special beds such as the Stryker frame or kinetic treatment table.

Surgical decompression or repair may not be scheduled until after an initial period of stabilization with skeletal traction. This allows for resolution of some of the cord edema and stabilization of the patient, particularly if mechanical ventilation is required and spinal shock with vascular instability is severe (Box 13-16). The development of anterior approaches to the cervical spine has allowed earlier and safer surgical intervention to be accomplished.

The application of halo traction vests (Figure 13-7, *B*) allows the patient with a cervical injury to be treated without prolonged immobilization. Fluids and vasoconstrictors may be needed during the period of spinal shock. The use of high-dose steroids to reduce cord edema is still under investigation.

NURSING MANAGEMENT

NOTE: The following discussion is directed at the rehabilitation phase following SCI. Interventions for the immediate acute phase are summarized in the Guidelines box.

◆ ASSESSMENT
Subjective Data

Description of the accident or injury
History of loss of consciousness
Absence of sensation—sensory level
Sensory disturbances: pain, paresthesias
Presence of dyspnea

Objective Data

Respiratory status and quality of respirations
Level of consciousness
Degree and level of motor ability and strength
Baseline vital signs
Body position and alignment
Bowel and bladder status, presence of distention, time of last voiding
Methodical systems assessment for other injuries

◆ NURSING DIAGNOSES

Nursing diagnoses for the person with a spinal cord injury may include, but are not limited to, the following:
Breathing pattern, ineffective, or airway clearance, ineffective (related to weakness or paralysis of intercostal muscles and diaphragm)

Guidelines for Nursing Care During the Immediate Phase Following SCI

Maintain alignment of head, neck, and spinal column.
 Log roll patient if movement is needed.
 Avoid any neck flexion.
 Maintain patency of skeletal traction.
Assess tidal volume and degree of dyspnea every 30 minutes.
 Provide assistance (quad cough) to the patient to clear the airway.
 Provide appropriate care to intubated patient; suction as needed.
Record vital signs regularly; assess for signs of spinal shock.
 Provide vasopressors or other medications as ordered.
 Apply TED stockings or Ace wraps to legs to support venous return.
 Monitor body temperature, and add blankets or cool patient as needed. NOTE: During spinal shock the patient is unable to adjust core body temperature and is very vulnerable to environmental shifts.
 Initiate intermittent catheterization routine, or insert Foley catheter if ordered.
 Record intake and output accurately.
 Initiate bowel program.
 Monitor for changes in motor or sensory status frequently.
 Initiate therapy to prevent stress ulcer: antacids, cimetidine.
 Assess all excretions for signs of bleeding.
 Assess bowel sounds.
Gradually resume oral diet when peristalsis is well established.
Initiate skin care protocol, turning regimen, and range of motion exercise.
Provide support and reassurance for patient and family.
Explain rationale for all needed care.

Mobility, impaired physical (related to loss of spinal nerve innervation)

Feeding, bathing/hygiene, dressing/grooming, or toileting self-care deficit, (related to loss of voluntary muscle control)

Skin integrity, high risk for impaired (related to decreased sensory perception and immobility)

Dysreflexia (related to massive sympathetic response to visceral stimuli)

Sexuality patterns, altered (related to effects of spinal cord injury)

◆ EXPECTED PATIENT OUTCOMES

Patient will maintain adequate oxygen and carbon dioxide exchange and not develop atelectasis or pneumonia.

Patient will not develop complications related to decreased mobility.

Patient will be independent in ADL to the extent possible with level of injury, using appropriate assistive devices.

Patient will not experience skin breakdown.

Patient will maintain a stable blood pressure without incidence of dysreflexia.

Patient will receive counseling concerning sexual gratification within limitations of the injury.

◆ NURSING INTERVENTIONS

Supporting Ventilation and Airway Clearance

Encourage deep breathing; use incentive spirometer for patients with thoracic and cervical injuries. Assist with coughing.

Teach patient to use shoulder girdle muscles to support ventilation.

Assess degree of dyspnea, respiratory adequacy, and breath sounds every 4 hours.

 Lesions below C5 may involve the abdominal muscles and weaken coughing efforts.

 Lesions at C5 paralyze the intercostal muscles.

 Lesions above C5 paralyze the diaphragm and phrenic nerves and may require permanent ventilatory support.

Incorporate chest physical therapy techniques and quad coughing into daily care routines.

Preventing Immobility-Related Complications

Maintain good body alignment, and perform range of motion exercises to all limbs every shift.

Turn patient according to protocol for type of bed and degree of stability of injury.

Utilize TED stockings or Ace bandages to support venous return.

 Assess for signs of deep vein thrombosis (DVT).

 Slowly increase the angle toward a sitting posture.

Monitor for hypotension.

Use of a reclining wheelchair may allow the patient to get out of bed while the blood pressure remains unstable.

Utilize a brace or shell if ordered. Apply before getting the patient out of bed.

Focus on transfer techniques and wheelchair mobility.

Encourage participation in physical therapy exercise program.

Institute bowel program.

 Provide adequate or increased fluid and roughage in diet.

 Use stool softeners, suppositories, digital stimulation. Avoid regular use of laxatives.

Maintain schedule and keep accurate records.

Promoting Self-Care Abilities

Institute bladder retraining if possible.

 Teach patient signs of urinary tract infection (UTI).

 Teach catheterization techniques to patient or family member.

 Teach importance of maintaining an acid urine, high fluid intake and acting promptly if appearance or smell of urine changes. UTI is the most common complication of spinal cord injury.

Assist patient to improve self-care capacities.

 Teach use of appropriate assistive devices.

Teach transfer techniques and wheelchair safety.
Encourage family involvement in techniques of care.

Maintaining an Intact Skin

Teach patient the importance of frequent skin inspection.

Use mirrors to visualize skin on sacrum and buttocks.

Employ appropriate pressure-relieving devices on the bed and in the wheelchair.

Use sufficient staff for transfers to avoid shearing factors on the skin.

Teach the importance and technique of pressure release exercises (wheelchair push-ups) every 20 minutes when out of bed.

Preventing Autonomic Dysreflexia (Box 13-17)

Be alert for dysrelexia episodes in patients with injuries above T6.

NOTE: Dysreflexia is not a concern until the period of spinal shock is resolved. The spontaneous spasmodic movements may induce false hope in the patient and family. Careful teaching about the nature of dysreflexia is important. The condition can be life threatening.

Maintain the bladder-emptying protocol and prevent constipation.

Be aware of the symptoms, and initiate the standard protocol if they appear.

Supporting Sexual Function

Provide patient with accurate information about sexual capacities and fertility specific to the level of injury.

Males typically lose the ability to have psychogenic erections but are capable of reflexogenic erections.

Stroking the inner thigh, stimulating the rectum, or manipulating the catheter may produce reflex erection.

The experience of orgasm is possible, but the sensations are different than before the injury.

Males with sacral injuries lose the ability to both have an erection and ejaculate.

Ejaculation is usually not possible with complete cord injuries.

Females can participate fully in sexual activity although they may not experience orgasm.

Fertility is usually preserved, and birth control should be considered.

Most males have decreased sperm counts and are infertile, even if ejaculation is possible.

Teach patient to ensure that the bowel is empty before sexual activity.

Teach patient to catheterize before sexual activity.

Patients with Foley catheters may remove the catheter or secure it folded back onto the penis.

Women may leave the catheter in place if desired.

Refer for community support in coping.

Encourage partner openness in discussing sexual issues and needs.

◆ EVALUATION

Successful achievement of expected outcomes for the patient with spinal cord injury is indicated by the following:

1. Practices deep breathing and clears airway effectively
   Clear breath sounds, no evidence of atelectasis or pneumonia
2. Full range of motion in all joints
   Regular pattern of bowel elimination
   Stable vital signs, no evidence of orthostatic hypotension or DVT
3. Self-catheterizes successfully, no evidence of UTI
   Able to transfer self
   Wheelchair mobility established
4. Skin intact
   Utilizes pressure-relieving devices and techniques daily
5. Recognizes symptoms of dysreflexia and prevention and treatment strategies
6. Correctly states impact of injury on sexuality
   Working with partner to establish mutually satisfying sexual practices

---

BOX 13-17	Autonomic Dysreflexia

Autonomic dysreflexia occurs in patients with injuries above T6, most commonly with cervical damage. It represents a condition in which there are grossly exaggerated autonomic responses to simple visceral stimuli.

SIGNS AND SYMPTOMS

Paroxysmal hypertension to malignant levels
Bradycardia
Severe throbbing headache
Diaphoresis
Gooseflesh

INTERVENTIONS

The most effective intervention is to decrease the stimuli.
A full bowel or bladder is the most common stimulus.
   Place patient in sitting position if permitted.
   Check catheter for patency.
   Catheterize if a prolonged interval since last emptying bladder.
   Check rectum for impaction. (Use dibucaine ointment to anesthetize before treatment.)
If interventions are ineffective, it may be necessary to administer potent vasodilator or ganglionic blocking agent to reduce blood pressure, which can result in cerebrovascular accident (CVA) or blindness.

CEREBROVASCULAR ACCIDENT

Etiology/epidemiology

Cerebrovascular accident, also known as a CVA or stroke, is the most common problem of the nervous system. Over 500,000 persons experience stroke each year. CVA is the third leading cause of death, although there has been a steady decline in stroke deaths over the last decades. This decline is attributed to improved control of hypertension and increased emphasis on decreasing cigarette smoking and heart disease. The major causes of CVAs include thrombus, embolus, and hemorrhage. Common conditions that contribute to the development of strokes are identified in Box 13-18. The term CVA is used clinically to refer to that sudden interruption of the blood supply to the brain the causes the sudden and dramatic development of neurologic defects. Hemiparesis or hemiplegia is considered to be the defining symptom.

Thrombi and emboli are by far the most common causes, accounting for greater than 90% of all cases. Thrombotic strokes tend to occur in persons over 60 years and are usually related to cerebral atherosclerosis. Hypertension and diabetes are other common risk factors. Embolic strokes tend to occur in younger individuals and are usually associated with an embolus that originates in the heart. Rheumatic heart disease presents a classic scenario. Intracranial hemorrhages may be caused by bleeding from a vessel on the surface of the brain or a vessel in the brain substance itself. Aneurysms and arteriovenous malformations may bleed at any age.

BOX 13-18 — **Conditions Causing CVA**

THROMBUS

Atherosclerosis in intracranial and extracranial arteries
Adjacency to intracerebral hemorrhage
Arteritis caused by collagen (autoimmune) disease or bacterial arteritis
Hypercoagulability such as in polycythemia
Cerebral venous thromboses

EMBOLI

Valves damaged by rheumatic heart disease
Myocardial infarction
Atrial fibrillation (This arrhythmia causes variable emptying of left ventricle. Blood pools and small clots form, and then at times the ventricle will be emptied completely with release of small emboli.)
Bacterial endocarditis and nonbacterial endocarditis causing clots to form on endocardium

HEMORRHAGE

Hypertensive intracerebral hemorrhage
Subarachnoid hemorrhage
Rupture of aneurysm
Arteriovenous malformation
Hypocoagulation (as in patients with blood dyscrasias)

GENERALIZED HYPOXIA

Severe hypotension, cardiopulmonary arrest, or severe depression in cardiac output caused by arrhythmias

LOCALIZED HYPOXIA

Cerebral artery spasms associated with subarachnoid hemorrhage
Cerebral artery vasoconstriction associated with migraine headaches

---

Bleeding related to hypertension and arteriosclerosis tends to occur at a later age.

Pathophysiology

The brain has no reserve oxygen supply. Therefore any condition that alters perfusion can lead to cerebral hypoxia and rapid cell death (Box 13-18). Hypoxia promptly alters the cerebral metabolism. Cell death and permanent damage can occur within 3 to 10 minutes. Ischemia triggers cerebral edema, which can worsen the neurologic effects. Unlike cerebral thrombosis or embolism, intracranial hemorrhage also causes damage to the brain by destroying and displacing adjacent brain tissue. As the blood is hemolyzed, it acts as a noxious agent, irritating the blood vessels, meninges, and brain tissue. Vasoactive substances are released that promote arterial spasm, further decreasing cerebral perfusion.

The neurologic effects of any type of CVA depend on which cerebral vessels are involved, which hemisphere and areas of the brain are affected, and the adequacy of the collateral circulation to the area. Specific symptoms may vary widely. The two vessels affected most frequently are the middle cerebral and the internal carotid arteries.

Thrombotic strokes tend to occur during sleep, just after arising, or when the person is at rest. This pattern may be related to postural hypotension and decreased sympathetic activity during sleep. Symptoms may worsen progressively during the first 24 to 48 hours. Intracranial hemorrhages are frequently accompanied by sudden explosive headache and loss of consciousness.

Transient ischemic attacks (TIAs) occur when transient cerebral ischemia produces temporary episodes of neurologic dysfunction. They are a frequent precursor of thrombotic CVAs and are a warning of an underlying pathologic condition. At least one third of the patients who have TIAs will experience a CVA within 5 years. Appropriate treatment remains controversial, however. Additional information about TIAs is presented in Box 13-18.

Medical management

CVAs are initially diagnosed by their classic presenting symptoms. A CT scan will typically be performed to differentiate thrombotic from hemorrhagic strokes. A lumbar puncture may be performed to measure pressure and assess for blood in the CSF, which would indicate subarachnoid hemorrhage. A lumbar puncture is not performed in the presence of severe elevations in intracranial pressure, since it may precipitate brainstem herniation. A cerebral arteriogram is typically performed in cases of hemorrhage to isolate and evaluate the bleeding vessel.

Patients with thrombotic strokes may be given anticoagulants or vasodilators in the effort to prevent further damage. Both of these interventions are controversial, and their effectiveness is unclear. Surgical intervention through carotid endarterectomy may be indicated in selected patients. Research protocols are

BOX 13-19	Left Versus Right Cerebrovascular Accident

Each cerebral hemisphere controls some unique functions and abilities. Injury to a single hemisphere typically produces unique deficits and behaviors that need to be considered in planning interventions.

LEFT HEMISPHERE

Sensory input and motor control of the right side of the body
Speech and language skills (writing, reading, symbols) if dominant hemisphere affected
Arithmetic and calculation abilities
Reasoning, logic, ordering and processing information
Injury to left hemisphere frequently causes the following:
    Slow cautious behavior
    Distress and depression in response to losses
NOTE: Patient's abilities are often underestimated because of loss of speech abilities.

RIGHT HEMISPHERE

Sensory input and motor control of left side of body
Visual ideation, spatial relationships, spatial perceptual ability
Nonverbal ideation, emotionality
Musicality, creativity
Injury to right hemisphere frequently causes the following:
    Quick impulsive responses
    Distractability
    Seeming indifference to disabilities
NOTE: Patient's abilities may be overestimated because of a positive affect.

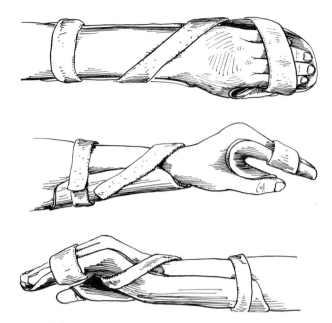

FIGURE 13-8 Resting hand splits provide support to wrist, thumb, and fingers. (From Dittmar SS: *Rehabilitation nursing*, St Louis, 1989, Mosby.)

testing reperfusion techniques using tissue plasminogen activator in a few settings. After a brief initial period of bed rest and stabilization the patient moves to active rehabilitation.

Patients with hemorrhagic strokes are initially placed on absolute bed rest to prevent additional bleeding. Meticulous monitoring of vital functions is necessary until their condition stabilizes.

Dexamethasone is administered to reduce cerebral edema, and aminocaproic acid (Amicar) may be administered in an effort to seal the clot. Surgery may be attempted if an aneurysm is the cause of the bleeding. If a hematoma has formed, it may be evacuated to relieve pressure. Surgical options include ligation of the affected artery with a clip, wrapping, coating with a liquid plastic that reinforces the weakened area of the artery, or serial embolization to wall off the damaged vessel. If surgery is not feasible, the common carotid artery may be partially or completely obliterated to reduce the blood flow through the affected vessel. This procedure is performed over several days to ensure that an adequate collateral circulation exists to meet the brain's metabolic needs.

NURSING MANAGEMENT

◆ ASSESSMENT
Subjective Data

Onset and sequence of symptoms

BOX 13-20	Transient Ischemic Attacks (TIAs)

DEFINITION
Transient episodes of reversible cerebral ischemia accompanied by temporary occurrences of neurologic dysfunction

CAUSE
May be produced by any of the conditions that cause CVA. Most commonly they precede a thrombotic stroke and may result from vessel spasm. Attacks may occur many times over the course of weeks, months or years. They warn of an underlying pathologic condition.

SYMPTOMS
Focal deficits are quite varied depending on the site of ischemia. The more common deficits include the following:
    One-sided weakness of the lower face, hands and fingers, arm, or leg
    Transient dysphasia
    Some sensory impairment
    Moment of clumsiness or incoordination

TREATMENT
Resolve associated risk factors and health conditions.
Vasodilators, anticoagulants, and aspirin may be used to decrease platelet aggregation and prevent clotting.
Surgical correction may be needed if cause is an isolated extracranial lesion.

Coexisting health problems
History of TIAs
Patient's complaints of headaches and sensory disturbances: visual, touch, hearing
Emotional response of patient and family
Patient's and family's understanding of symptoms and diagnosis

---

BOX 13-21   Bobath Principles in Stroke Rehabilitation

Bobath rehabilitation techniques are based on the premise that stroke patients have the potential to relearn movement and function on the affected side. They focus on involving the affected side in care activities and facilitating normal muscle tone and posture.

APPLYING BOBATH TECHNIQUES

Transfer toward the affected side to force weight bearing on the affected leg.

Dress patient in a sitting or standing position. Dress the affected side first.

Position patient on the affected side; bring the shoulder forward.

Establish normal positions and posture from head to toe.

Utilize bilateral movements for rolling, scooting, or position changes. Incorporate both sides in all activities.

BOX 13-22   Sensory/Perceptual Alterations

PROPRIORECEPTION

Ability to know position of body and its parts without looking

DYSESTHESIA/PARESTHESIA

Abnormalities of touch sensation

APRAXIA

Inability to perform skilled purposeful movements in absence of motor problems

AGNOSIA

Inability to recognize objects through use of special senses

HEMIANOPSIA

Loss of selected portions of visual fields

BOX 13-23   Types of Aphasia

MOTOR (EXPRESSIVE)

Patient unable to use symbols of speech to speak or write words; muscles of speech not paralyzed

SENSORY (RECEPTIVE)

Patient unable to comprehend spoken or written word

GLOBAL APHASIA

Both motor and sensory problems present at same time

DYSARTHRIA

Weakness in muscles of speech creates difficulties in pronouncing words or swallowing

---

 Guidelines for Nursing Care for Persons With Aphasia

GENERAL

Establish a relaxed environment.
Encourage persistence and the desire to communicate.
Control and limit the amount of stimuli in environment.

SENSORY (RECEPTIVE)

Sit down and establish eye contact. Keep distractions to a minimum.
Face patient and speak simply and slowly.
Reword the message if misunderstood.
Use appropriate gestures to supplement words.
Allow sufficient time for patient to process words.
Use a normal tone of voice.

MOTOR (EXPRESSIVE)

Avoid interrupting and rushing patient.
Emphasize simple concrete words used for daily care.
Discuss topics of interest to patient.
Encourage use of other means of communication.
Convey acceptance and encourage patient to talk.
Do not speak for the patient.
Keep practice sessions short. Avoid fatigue.
Offer praise and encouragement.

 Guidelines for Nursing Care for Persons With Sensory/Perceptual Alterations

Keep familiar objects in the patient's environment.
Approach patient from the side of intact vision.
Teach patient to scan to increase visual field.
Provide full mirror to assist patient with posture and balance.
Remind patient to care for, inspect, and protect affected side.
Be alert for incidences of impulsive behavior.

Presence of expressive or receptive aphasia or dysarthria

Bowel and bladder function

Signs of increased ICP (see Box 13-11)

Seizure activity

The nursing management of the patient with a CVA is summarized in the "Nursing Care Plan."

THE UNCONSCIOUS PATIENT

Etiology/epidemiology

Consciousness can be impaired by a variety of causes, many of which are not primarily neurologic. They range from cerebral trauma, vascular disease, infection, and neoplasm to hypoglycemia/ketoacidosis, hepatic encephalopathy, uremia, hypoxia, and toxicity from drugs or toxins. Consciousness is a wide spectrum, and multiple levels exist between consciousness and coma, which represent the ends of the continuum. Although the two end points can be recognized fairly easily, it is not as easy to classify the intervening stages.

Objective Data

Level of consciousness—general thinking ability
Vital signs
Presence of motor deficits—hemiparesis or hemiplegia

NURSING CARE PLAN

THE PATIENT WITH A CEREBROVASCULAR ACCIDENT

■ NURSING DIAGNOSIS

Injury, high risk for (related to decreased reflexes and altered sensory input)

Expected Patient Outcome	Nursing Interventions

Patient will not experience aspiration, corneal abrasion, or environmental injury.	1. Maintain an open airway.
	  a. Keep patient in side-lying position.
	  b. Keep the head of bed elevated 30 degrees unless ordered to keep patient flat.
	  c. Administer prescribed oxygen.
	  d. Use oral airway and have suction ready for use if needed.
	  e. Initiate regular deep breathing. Encourage gentle coughing only as needed to keep airway clear.
	2. Assess vital signs and level of consciousness at frequent intervals during first 2 days; be alert to signs of rising ICP.
	3. Monitor fluid balance accurately.
	  a. Keep careful records of intake and output.
	  b. Regulate IV line carefully. Do not overhydrate.
	  c. Maintain fluid intake at 1000 ml/day if ordered.
	4. Give prescribed medications to prevent further cerebral thrombosis, hemorrhage, or edema or to prevent seizures.
	5. Assess for intactness of blink reflex and adequacy of lid closure.
	  a. If needed, keep eyes moist with artificial tears and covered with eye patch.
	  b. Inspect eyes for infection or irritation every 2 to 4 hours.
	6. Assess intactness of swallowing and gag reflexes.
	  a. Avoid oral food or fluid if not intact.
	  b. Position to support drainage of saliva.
	  c. Keep suction apparatus at bedside.
	  d. Monitor swallowing competence with 5-10 ml of fluid several times daily.

Pathophysiology

Many different parts of the nervous system must work together to support consciousness. Cerebral function is most commonly affected by lack of oxygen or glucose. The brain is extremely sensitive to hypoxia, and only a few seconds of anoxia can cause unconsciousness. The brain must also receive a constant supply of glucose to support its function, and a drastic fall in blood sugar can have profound negative consequences on consciousness and brain function.

Unconsciousness implies that the person is unaware of the environment and is not responding to sensory stimuli. Pathologic motor responses may also be present, but these are more common when a neurologic cause is present. Decorticate posturing (sustained flexion of the arms, wrists, and fingers) indicates damage to

NURSING CARE PLAN—CONT'D

THE PATIENT WITH A CEREBROVASCULAR ACCIDENT

■ NURSING DIAGNOSIS
Mobility, impaired physical (related to hemiplegia or hemiparesis)

Expected Patient Outcome	Nursing Interventions

Patient will maintain adequate muscle tone and achieve maximal independence in ambulation.	1. Turn and position every 2 hours.
	2. Implement range of motion exercises.
	   a. Administer passive range of motion exercises each shift.
	   b. Encourage patient to get involved with active range of motion exercises as soon as possible.
	   c. Passive exercise may help reestablish neuromuscular pathways.
	3. Implement exercise program designed by physical therapy department.
	   a. Emphasize full extension of joints and good alignment.
	   b. Build strength in gluteal and quadriceps muscles to support ambulation.
	   NOTE: Spasticity will worsen during the recovery phase.
	4. Initiate balance exercise at bedside.
	   a. Anticipate dizziness, diplopia, and spatial perceptual deficits. Promote safety.
	5. Ensure adequate rest periods.
	6. Teach technique for safe transfer to wheelchair or toilet.
	   a. Chair is placed toward unaffected side, and strong leg leads on the transfer.
	7. Teach use of assistive device for ambulation.
	   a. Crutch or cane is held on strong side.
	   b. Consider the use of resting splints (Figure 13-8).
	8. Explore need for sling to prevent shoulder subluxation.
	9. Provide good shoe support for transfer and ambulation.

■ NURSING DIAGNOSIS
Skin integrity, high risk for impaired (related to decreased mobility and impaired sensation)

Expected Patient Outcome	Nursing Interventions
Patient's skin will remain intact.	1. Examine and massage skin every 2 hours. 2. Keep skin clean and dry. a. If patient is incontinent, monitor frequently and keep bed pads clean and dry at all times; wash and dry perineal area as needed. 3. Use foam mattresses, heel protectors, or other devices to prevent pressure sores. 4. Use turning sheet when changing patient's position every 2 hours to prevent shearing effect on skin.

Continued.

NURSING CARE PLAN—CONT'D

THE PATIENT WITH A CEREBROVASCULAR ACCIDENT

■ NURSING DIAGNOSIS

Nutrition, altered: less than body requirements (related to decreased swallowing and self-care abilities)

Expected Patient Outcome	Nursing Interventions
Patient will consume an adequate amount of balanced oral nutrients to maintain a stable body weight.	1. Administer IV fluids and/or nasogastric (NG) tube feedings until swallowing is reestablished and patient is alert.
	2. Always position the patient upright for meals.
	3. Provide foods initially that are easier to swallow (soft or pureed foods, except for mashed potatoes). Avoid clear liquids.
	4. Place food in unaffected side of mouth.
	5. Be patient when feeding patient and provide directions for swallowing, as needed.
	a. Encourage patient to chew food thoroughly. Remind patient to tilt head forward to facilitate swallowing.
	6. Ensure adequate hydration if patient is having swallowing difficulties.
	a. Utilize supplemental IV lines if oral intake is insufficient.
	7. Cleanse mouth after eating to remove retained food particles. Teach patient to use tongue to clear food from paralyzed side of mouth.
	8. Encourage patient to begin feeding self as soon as possible. Provide self-help devices such as rocker knife and plate guards.

■ NURSING DIAGNOSIS

Feeding, bathing/hygiene, dressing/grooming, or toileting self care decifit (related to hemiplegia and altered thought processes)

Expected Patient Outcome	Nursing Interventions
Patient will regain independence in ADL.	1. Assist patient to shift self-care activities to unaffected side.
	2. Provide basic needs for ADL as necessary during initial period, but encourage patient to begin to participate at ability level.
	3. Provide sufficient time for ADL.
	4. Meet with physical therapist and occupational therapist to optimize patient's learning needs.
	5. Facilitate use of self-help devices, as needed.
	6. Explore use of Bobath techniques in rehabilitation, such as encouraging weight bearing and use of affected limbs during activities (see Box 13-21).

NURSING CARE PLAN—CONT'D

THE PATIENT WITH A CEREBROVASCULAR ACCIDENT

■ NURSING DIAGNOSIS
Incontinence, functional (related to disruption of normal voluntary control)

Expected Patient Outcome	Nursing Interventions
Patient will reestablish a normal pattern of urinary elimination and be free of incontinence.	1. Monitor urinary output and signs of retention or incontinence. 2. Reassure patient that reestablishing continence is a reasonable goal. 3. Avoid prolonged use of Foley catheter. a. Provide catheter care if Foley catheter is used. 4. Offer bedpan or urinal after meals and at regular intervals. 5. Provide fluids to maximum amount prescribed; provide greater amounts before 4:00 PM. 6. Use disposable pads or external urinary drainage system as indicated.

■ NURSING DIAGNOSIS
Constipation or bowel incontinence (related to interruption of voluntary motor control)

Expected Patient Outcome	Nursing Interventions
Patient will establish a regular pattern of bowel elimination and not experience incontinence, constipation, or impaction.	1. Record bowel elimination. 2. Reassure patient that bowel continence is an achievable goal. 3. Institute use of stool softeners and suppositories as needed. 4. Get patient out of bed to commode or toilet at regular times to attempt defecation. 5. Caution patient to avoid straining at stool. Repeat suppositories if no results.

the sensorimotor cortex. Decerebrate posturing (rigid extension of all four extremities) indicates a lesion at the level of the brainstem. It carries a very grave prognosis. Both neurologic postures are illustrated in Figure 13-9.

The respiratory rate and pattern are also helpful in localizing and evaluating the severity of the damage. Classic respiratory patterns are summarized in Box 13-24. Reflex eye movements may also be used to evaluate brainstem functioning in unconscious patients. The oculocephalic reflex (doll's eyes) is elicited by holding the patient's eyelids open and moving the head from side to side. When nerve pathways are intact, the eyes move left as the head is rotated to the right. When a neurologic pathologic condition is present, the eyes either do not turn or do not move in a conjugate manner. The oculovestibular reflex is elicited by irrigating the ear with ice water. This "caloric" test causes nystagmus (rapid horizontal eye movements).

Medical management
The medical management of the unconscious patient is primarily aimed at correcting the underlying cause if possible. The patient's metabolic imbalances are corrected, and treatment for neurologic injury or disease is begun. Treatment of elevations of ICP may be needed. The medical plan also establishes the parameters for supporting ventilation, circulation, and nutrition.

NURSING MANAGEMENT

Ongoing neurologic assessment is a primary nursing responsibility. There are numerous assessment tools, but all are vulnerable to variations in interpretation of terms by staff. It is vital that all persons involved in the patient's care use a single technique and record all clues that support the use of a specific term for a level of consciousness. The Glasgow Coma Scale is frequently used (see Box 13-14). It is simple to use, and the numeric responses can be graphed to present a visual

NURSING CARE PLAN—CONT'D

THE PATIENT WITH A CEREBROVASCULAR ACCIDENT

■ NURSING DIAGNOSIS
Communication, impaired verbal (related to expressive or receptive aphasia [see Box 13-23 and Guidelines box])

Expected Patient Outcome	Nursing Interventions

Patient will successfully communicate needs to family and staff.	1. Establish nature, extent of communication disorder.
	2. Work with speech therapy department to plan appropriate therapy.
	3. Speak slowly and distinctly.
	4. Try to anticipate patient needs. Reassure patient that improvement is possible.
	5. Provide call signal within reach of unaffected hand.
	6. Apply basic principles for aphasic patients (see Guidelines box).
	7. Encourage patient to verbalize and practice speech.
	   a. Allow sufficient time for patient to respond.
	8. Phrase questions that can be answered by yes or no (or by appropriate signals).
	   a. Provide communication aids such as picture boards as needed.
	9. Teach family about disorder and the importance of not "speaking for" the patient.
	   a. Share appropriate techniques with family.

■ NURSING DIAGNOSIS
Sensory/perceptual alteration (visual or kinesthetic; related to cerebral hypoxia)

Expected Patient Outcome	Nursing Interventions
Patient will learn to compensate for sensory/perceptual deficits and function safely in the environment.	1. Be alert to spatial perceptual difficulties associated with right hemisphere stroke. Patient may have trouble judging position and distance and with vision (see Box 13-22, Guidelines box, and Figure 13-12). 2. Avoid private room. Patient will need sensory input from environment. 3. Suggest family bring some familiar objects, such as pictures. 4. Keep objects within patient's visual field. 5. Place patient's bed so that people approach from side of intact vision. 6. Teach patient to scan the environment to increase visual field. 7. Use mirror to teach posture corrections.

NURSING CARE PLAN—CONT'D

THE PATIENT WITH A CEREBROVASCULAR ACCIDENT

■ NURSING DIAGNOSIS

High risk for ineffective individual and family coping (related to the physical and mental changes resulting from the CVA)

Expected Patient Outcomes	Nursing Interventions
Patient and family will adjust to nature of residual disabilities and plan appropriately for postdischarge care. Patient will not experience significant mood disorder.	1. Provide information about condition and probable progress toward increased function. 2. Assist patient to reestablish control over emotion and behavior and set limits. a. Anticipate behavior associated with left- and right-sided CVA (see Box 13-20). b. Explain that emotional lability is part of the disorder and that improvement will be noted. c. Explain patient's behavior to family and friends and encourage them to visit and interact with patient. 3. Assist family to assess patient's capabilities and plan for postdischarge care. a. Initiate referrals to appropriate community agencies. 4. Teach family to support patient's efforts at independence and encourage involvement in outside world. 5. Encourage family to maintain previous role relationships, as possible.

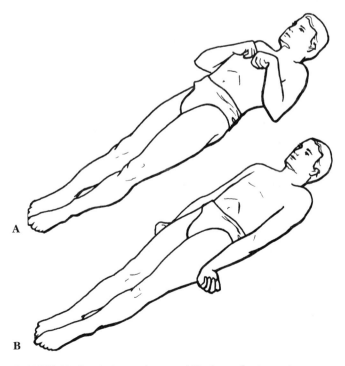

FIGURE 13-9 **A,** Decorticate and **B,** decerebrate postures.

BOX 13-24	Respiratory Patterns in Coma

CHEYNE-STOKES

Cycles of hyperventilation that gradually diminish to apnea; period of apnea variable and followed by resumption of respiration

CENTRAL NEUROGENIC HYPERVENTILATION

Continuous rapid and deep respirations at a rate of 25/min or greater

APNEUSTIC BREATHING

Prolonged inspiration followed by a period of apnea of variable duration

CLUSTER BREATHING

Closely grouped respirations followed by a period of apnea

ATAXIC BREATHING

Chaotic respirations

GASPING BREATHING

Gasp breaths followed by variable periods of apnea; may precede respiratory arrest

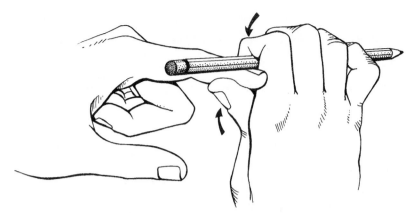

FIGURE 13-10 Nail-bed pressure stimulation using pencil.

picture of the patient over time. A combined score of 7 or less on the scale represents coma.

The patient who is not responsive to voluntary commands may be tested for response to painful stimuli. There are multiple potential techniques, but all those involving pinching or pricking should be avoided. The two preferred methods are nail-bed pressure (Figure 13-10) and supraorbital pressure. Responses range from purposeful withdrawal or avoidance to no response. Brainstem function is assessed through evaluation of the corneal reflex, which tests the integrity of the pons, and the gag reflex, which tests the integrity of the medulla.

The balance of nursing management focuses on active prevention of the complications of immobility, maintaining a safe environment, supporting ventilation and circulation, meeting nutritional and elimination needs, and supporting the family. These basic interventions are summarized in the Guidelines box.

CENTRAL NERVOUS SYSTEM TUMORS
Brain Tumors
Etiology/epidemiology

Brain tumors may be primary, arising from the brain tissue itself, or secondary metastatic tumors that develop from a primary cancer source elsewhere in the body. Primary tumors in the lung, breast, and colon frequently metastasize to the brain. Interestingly, primary brain tumors rarely metastasize to other organs. There is a wide range of intracranial tumors that vary significantly based on their specific size, location, and invasive qualities. The major types of brain tumors are outlined in Box 13-25.

Pathophysiology

Brain tumors create both local and systemic effects. The local effects arise from the infiltration, invasion, and destruction of brain tissue at a specific site. Local edema typically results, which worsens the symptoms. Because of the tightly encased cranial vault, any tumor in the brain can cause an increase in ICP that is transmitted throughout the brain. Eventually the ventricular system becomes distorted or blocked, obstructing the flow of

Guidelines for Nursing Care for the Unconscious Patient

SUPPORTING VENTILATION
Maintain a patent airway with positioning, suctioning as needed.
Monitor O_2 saturation regularly.
Provide supplemental oxygen as indicated.
Implement mechanical ventilation if needed.

PREVENTING IMMOBILITY COMPLICATIONS
Turn and position every 2 hours. Use a side-lying or prone position if tolerated (Figure 13-11).
Provide passive range of motion to all joints each shift.
Use high-top sneakers to prevent footdrop.
Cleanse and inspect skin each shift.
Use pressure-relieving devices and mattresses.
Have sufficient help to move patient to avoid shearing effect.

PROMOTING ENVIRONMENTAL SAFETY
Keep side rails up, and pad if patient is restless.
Patch eyes if blink reflex is compromised. Cleanse eyes daily, and administer moisture drops.
Maintain normothermia.

SUPPORTING NUTRITION
Administer appropriate tube feedings. Ensure adequate volumes of fiber and free water.
Provide mouth and nasal care at least once per shift, particularly if patient is mouth breathing.
Explore need for G tube for long-term nutrition management.

MAINTAINING REGULAR ELIMINATION
Establish regimen of stool softeners and suppositories.
Ensure adequate fluids and fiber.
Utilize external catheter for males and Foley catheter for females.
Keep perianal skin clean and dry.

PROVIDING MEANINGFUL STIMULATION
Follow care patterns that mimic a normal daily routine.
Assume patient can hear what is said at the bedside. Speak to patient to explain all needed care.
Encourage family to interact verbally with the patient.
Use touch therapeutically for communication.
  Speak to patient before touching.
  Handle the patient gently.
  Encourage touching by family members.
Keep the environment low key, eliminating needless noise.

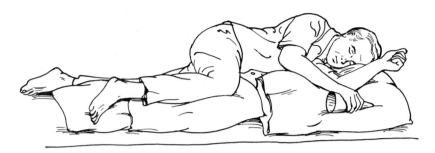

FIGURE 13-11 Lateral position with hand cone to prevent flexion contracture of hand.

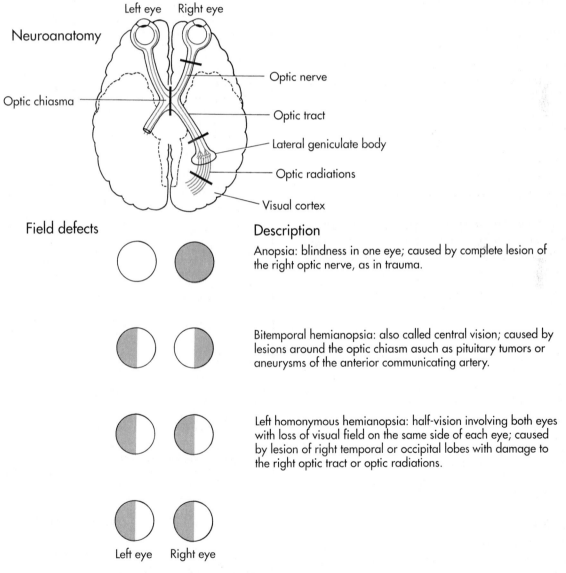

FIGURE 13-12 Visual field deficits and neuroanatomic correlates.

BOX 13-25 Types of Brain Tumors

GLIOMAS

Gliomas, which account for about one half of all brain tumors, arise from the brain connective tissue. They tend to be infiltrative, are difficult to excise completely, and grow rapidly. Glioblastomas and medulloblastomas are the most highly malignant and are usually fatal within a matter of months. Astrocytomas and oligodendrogliomas are slower growing, but still frequently fatal in less than a year.

MENINGIOMAS

Meningiomas, which account for 13% to 18% of all primary intracranial tumors, arise from the meningeal coverings of the brain. They vary widely in histologic features and size and are usually benign. They are frequently encapsulated, and surgical cure is possible.

ACOUSTIC NEUROMAS

Acoustic neuromas account for about 8% of all primary intracranial tumors. Neuromas may arise from any of the cranial nerves. When the acoustic nerve is affected, the tumor grows from nerve sheath but usually extends to affect the nerve fibers. They are slow growing.

PITUITARY ADENOMAS

Pituitary adenomas may arise from a variety of pituitary tissue types. They are successfully treated by surgery, using either the standard craniotomy or the transsphenoidal approach. Recurrence is possible.

BOX 13-26 Symptoms Associated with Tumors in Specific Brain Regions

Note: Headache is an early symptom in about one third of patients with brain tumors. It is often present on first awakening and is described as a deep pain. It may be slight or severe, dull or sharp, on one side or both, and localized or generalized. Late headache is related to elevated ICP and is usually bilateral.

FRONTAL LOBE

Personality changes
Inappropriate affect
Lack of interest in self-care

OCCIPITAL LOBE

Visual disturbances

TEMPORAL LOBE

Olfactory, visual, or gustatory hallucinations
Psychomotor seizures

PARIETAL LOBE

Loss of right and left discrimination

Guidelines for Nursing Care of the Craniotomy Patient

PREOPERATIVE PERIOD

Assess baseline neurologic and physiologic status.
Encourage patient and family to verbalize fears and concerns.
Provide detailed teaching about procedures, postoperative care, movement and activity restrictions, and equipment to be used.
If the head is shaved, it is usually done in the operating room. Shampoo hair.
Prepare family for patient's appearance after the operation:
Head dressing, shaved scalp
Edema and bruising
Temporary decrease in mental status

POSTOPERATIVE PERIOD

Complete or perform nursing interventions for monitoring neurologic status, dealing with rising ICP, and preventing complications related to immobility.

Positioning

Position patient as follows:
Supratentorial surgery—head of bed elevated 45 degrees. Turn patient only between back and unaffected side if tumor was large, to prevent shift of brain tissue.
Infratentorial surgery—head of bed flat. Avoid positioning patient on back, to prevent shift of brain tissue downward. Avoid neck flexion.

Preventing Elevations in Intracranial Pressure

Prevent vomiting. Avoid coughing after deep breathing. Do not perform nasal suctioning. All of these measures are aimed at preventing rises in ICP.
Monitor drainage onto head dressing. Call surgeon for a dressing change if it appears soaked.
Administer stool softeners or laxatives as necessary to prevent straining at stool.

Monitoring for Complications

Check urinary output and specific gravity for the following:
Diabetes insipidus—increased output; decreased specific gravity
Inappropriate ADH syndrome—decreased output
Diabetes in response to high-dose steroids—urine sugar and acetone

Promoting Comfort

Use acetaminophen (Tylenol) or codeine to deal with postoperative discomfort.
Avoid use of narcotics and other CNS depressants.
Apply ice packs to head for pain and to reduce swelling.

Supporting the Patient and Family

Assist and support patient and family in dealing with residual effects of the tumor or surgery.

CSF. General cerebral edema worsens, which may compromise circulation to the brain. At this stage a descending spiral of worsening pressure and hypoxia may be initiated. Common symptoms related to tumors in specific regions of the brain are summarized in Box 13-26.

Medical management

Brain tumors are frequently diagnosed initially by CT scan. MRI and angiography may also be used to gather specific data about the precise size, location, and perfusion of the tumor before treatment. Surgical management is the treatment approach of choice. Typically a craniotomy is performed with the bone replaced following the surgery. The outcome is frequently the result of the accessibility of the tumor. Portions of the frontal lobes may often be removed with little residual damage, whereas limitations in functions may be an inevitable result of surgery in more vital deep structures. Radiotherapy and occasionally chemotherapy may be used as adjuncts to surgery or as primary therapy when the tumor cannot be treated surgically.

NURSING MANAGEMENT

The nursing management of the patient with a brain tumor is primarily surgical care. This care is summarized in the Guidelines box.

Intravertebral Tumors

Both primary and secondary tumors occur in the spinal cord, its coverings, and the vertebrae. They may present with nerve root pain or motor and sensory deficits related to spinal cord compression. The loss of function is gradual and progressive. Treatment options include surgery, radiotherapy, and adjunct chemotherapy. Spinal decompression is frequently performed even if the tumor cannot be completely excised. Although palliative in nature, the decompression may significantly relieve symptoms, particularly back pain. Nursing care follows the guidelines established for SCI (see p. 313).

SELECTED REFERENCES

Andrus C: Intracranial pressure: diagnosis and nursing management, *Neurosci Nurs* 23:85-92, 1991.
Aumick J: Head trauma: guidelines for care, *RN* 54(4):27-31, 1991.
Baggerly J: Sensory perceptual problems following stroke: the invisible deficits, *Nurs Clin North Am* 26(4):997-1005, 1991.
Barker E: Cranial nerve assessment, *RN* 55(5):62-69, 1992.
Barker E, Higgins R: Managing a suspected SCI, *Nurs 89* 19(3):52-59, 1989.
Barker E, Moore E: Neurological assessment, *RN* 55(4):28-35, 1992.
Borgman M, Passarella P: Nursing care of the stroke patient using Bobath principles: an approach to altered movement, *Nurs Clin North Am* 26(4):1019-1035, 1991.
Chadwick A, Oesting H: Not for specialists only: caring for patients with spinal cord injuries, *Nurs 89* 19(11):52-56, 1989.
Chicano L: Humanistic aspects of sexuality as related to spinal cord injury, *J Neurosci Nurs* 21:326-329, 337, 1989.
Delgado J, Billo J: Care of the patient with Parkinson's disease: surgical and nursing interventions, *J Neurosci Nurs* 20:142-150, 1988.
Dykes P: Minding the five P's of neurovascular assessment, *Am J Nurs* 93(6):38-39, 1993.
Finocchiaro D, Hersfeld S: Understanding Alzheimer's disease, *Am J Nurs* 90(9):56-60, 1990.
Goddard L: Sexuality and spinal cord injury, *J Neurosci Nurs* 20:240-244, 1988.
Hickey J: Myasthenic crisis—your assessment counts, *RN* 54(5):54-59, 1991.
Hodges K, Root L: Surgical management of intractable seizure disorder, *J Neurosci Nurs* 23:93-100, 1991.
Holt J: How to help confused patients, *Am J Nurs* 93(8):32-36, 1993.
Jess L: Investigating impaired mental status: an assessment guide you can use, *Nurs 88* 18(6):42-50, 1988.
Kalbach L: Unilateral neglect: mechanism and nursing care, *J Neurosci Nurs* 23:125-129, 1991.
Kim T: Hope as a mode of coping in amyotrophic lateral sclerosis, *J Neurosci Nurs* 21:342-347, 1989.
Larsen P: Psychosocial adjustment in MS, *Rehabil Nurs* 15:242-247, 1990.
Litchfield M, Noroian E: Changes in selected pulmonary functions in patients diagnosed with myasthenia gravis, *J Neurosci Nurs* 12:375-381, 1989.
Lord-Feroli K, Maguire-McGinley M: Toward a more objective approach to pupil assessment, *J Neurosci Nurs* 17:309-312, 1990.
Lower J: Rapid neuro assessment, *Am J Nurs* 92(6):38-45, 1992.
Luchka S: Working with ICP monitors, *RN* 54(3):34-37, 1991.
Morgan S: A passage through paralysis, *Am J Nurs* 91(10):70-74, 1991.
North B et al: Living in a halo, *Am J Nurs* 92(4):54-58, 1992.
Olson E: Perceptual deficits affecting the stroke patient, *Rehabil Nurs* 16(4):212-213, 1991.
Pettibone K: Management of spasticity in spinal cord injury: nursing concerns, *J Neurosci Nurs* 19:269-299, 1988.
Phipps MA: Assessment of neurologic deficits in stroke: acute-care and rehabilitation implications, *Nurs Clin North Am* 26(4):957-970, 1991.
Rhynsburger J: How to fight myasthenia's fatigue, *Am J Nurs* 89:337-341, 1989.
Sherman D: Managing an acute head injury, *Nurs 90* 20(4):44-51, 1990.
Sullivan J: Neurologic assessment, *Nurs Clin North Am* 25(4):795-809, 1990.
Vernon G: Parkinson's disease, *J Neurosci Nurs* 21:273-284, 1989.
Zasler N: Sexuality in neurologic disability: an overview, *Sexuality Disability* 9(1):11-27, 1991.

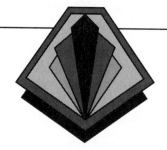

Disorders of the Visual and Auditory Systems

◆ ASSESSMENT

Health history
  Past/family history
    Family history of the following:
      Cataracts, glaucoma, diabetes, uncorrectable poor vision
      Hearing loss, use of hearing aid
    Past history of the following:
      Ocular problems, diabetes, hypertension, multiple sclerosis (MS), lupus, trauma, surgery
      Use of glasses, contact lenses
      Auditory problems, ear infections, trauma
      Use of hearing aid
  Medication use
    Prescription and over the counter (OTC), such as antihistamines, ototoxic drugs (aminoglycosides, aspirin, diuretics)
    Occupational risks and exposures to eyes and ears

Visual symptoms (presence, severity, self-treatment)
  Changes in acuity: unilateral or bilateral
  Burning, tearing, itching, or blurred vision
  Halos, problems with night vision
  Loss of peripheral vision
Auditory symptoms
  Changes in hearing or tinnitus (buzzing or ringing)
    Volume or discrimination
    Unilateral or bilateral
  Dizziness or vertigo
  Ear pain or discharge, itching, fullness, or pressure
  Wax problems
Physical assessment
  Eyes
    Appearance and symmetry
    Presence and severity of exophthalmos (protrusion) or ptosis (drooping of eyelid)
    Presence and severity of redness, swelling, or tenderness

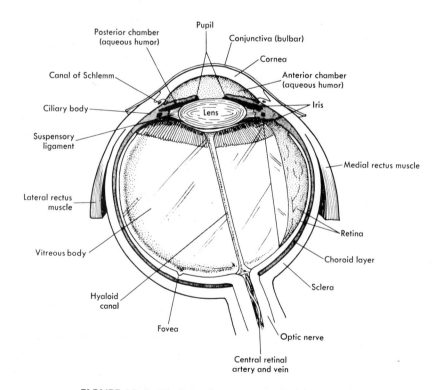

FIGURE 14-1   Horizontal section through left eyeball.

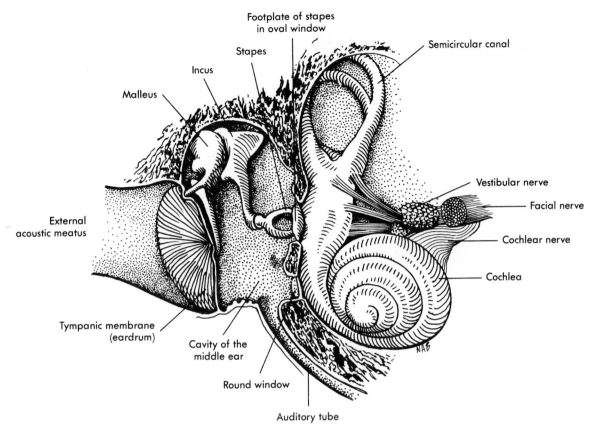

FIGURE 14-2 Structures of the ear.

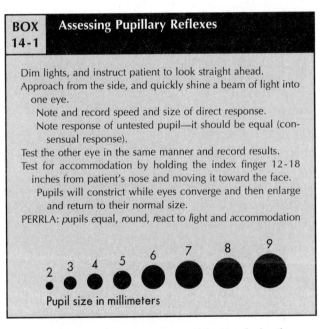

BOX 14-1 Assessing Pupillary Reflexes

Dim lights, and instruct patient to look straight ahead.
Approach from the side, and quickly shine a beam of light into one eye.
   Note and record speed and size of direct response.
   Note response of untested pupil—it should be equal (consensual response).
Test the other eye in the same manner and record results.
Test for accommodation by holding the index finger 12-18 inches from patient's nose and moving it toward the face.
   Pupils will constrict while eyes converge and then enlarge and return to their normal size.
PERRLA: *p*upils *e*qual, *r*ound, *r*eact to *l*ight and *a*ccommodation

2   3   4   5   6   7   8   9
Pupil size in millimeters

Condition of conjunctiva and lacrimal gland
Color of sclera, clarity of cornea
Roundness, size, and equality of pupils
Color, pattern, and shape of iris
Presence of lens opacity
Intactness of blink and pupillary reflexes (Box 14-1)
Ears
   Inspection
      Ear size, configuration, angle of attachment

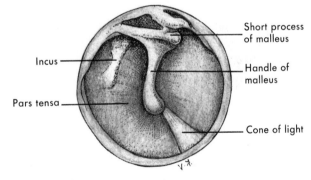

FIGURE 14-3 Normal tympanic membrane. (From Perry AG, Potter PA: *Clinical nursing skills and techniques,* ed 3, St Louis, 1994, Mosby.)

Presence of lumps, skin lesions
Redness or swelling along mastoid process
Redness, drainage, or scaling along external ear canal
Condition of ear canal and tympanic membrane (Figure 14-3 and Box 14-2)

✍ DIAGNOSTIC TESTING
ASSESSMENT OF VISION

Numerous simple and technologically complex visual assessment tools exist. Tests of visual acuity should be part of all routine health assessments (Box 14-3).

BOX 14-2 Otoscopic Assessment

Instruct patient to tip head slightly toward the opposite side.
Gently pull the pinna up, back, and out.
Hold the otoscope upside down in the dominant hand with the hand resting against the patient's head.
Insert the speculum gently. Move it in a circular fashion to visualize the entire ear canal.
Inspect the eardrum for shape and color.
  Color: normal is pearly gray, opaque, shiny, and smooth.
  Shape: slightly concave or conical. Note any bulging, retraction, or perforation.
  Mobility: moves gently in response to puff of air.

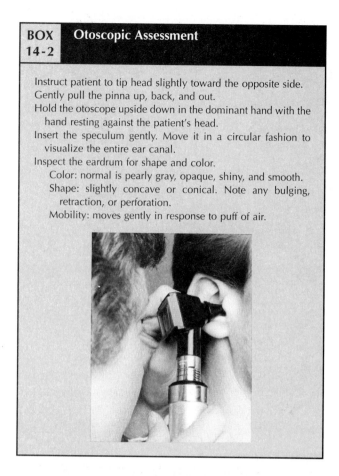

BOX 14-3 Terms Describing Refractive Errors

EMMETROPIA
Normal eye
Light focuses on retina

MYOPIA
Nearsightedness
Light focuses in front of retina

HYPEROPIA
Farsightedness
Light focuses behind retina

PRESBYOPIA
Hyperopia resulting from aging-related loss of lens elasticity

ASTIGMATISM
Irregular curvature of cornea
Light does not focus at same point

Acuity
Distance vision

With the Snellen chart, the person stands 20 feet away from a chart that has rows of letters, numbers, and characters of decreasing size. Each eye is tested separately, and results are recorded as a fraction in comparison with established normal values.

Finger counts, motion, or light perception may be used with persons whose acuity is too poor to test with a chart.

Near vision

A Jaeger chart is a card with rows of letters, numbers, or characters that is held 14 inches away from the person's eyes. Eyes are tested both separately and together. Results are recorded as fractions of established normal values.

Visual Fields

Visual fields represent that portion of the environment that the eye can perceive. Rough assessments can be made by asking the person to look directly ahead but indicate where the examiner's finger comes into view. Tangent screens, Amsler grids, and computer programs may be used for more accurate assessment.

NOTE: More accurate and detailed measures of visual acuity and refractive error will be made when problems exist and corrective lenses are prescribed.

Color Vision

Color vision is assessed with color plates on which numbers are outlined in primary colors and surrounded by confusion colors. Hue discrimination may also be tested. Hereditary color defects are present in 7% of men and 0.5% of women.

Extraocular Muscle Function

To test the six cardinal positions of gaze the person is asked to look straight ahead and then follow a pen or penlight that moves the eye to the extremes of left and right in the upward, lateral, and down positions.

AUDITORY ASSESSMENT

Sound is transmitted by both air conduction and bone conduction.

Voice or Watch Test

The person blocks one ear at a time. The examiner stands 1 to 2 feet away and whispers quietly or holds a ticking watch 5 inches from the ear. A gross assessment can be made for each ear.

Tuning Fork Tests (Table 14-1)

In the Weber test the vibrating tuning fork is placed at midline on the forehead and the person assesses its loudness and equality for both ears.

In the Rinne test the tuning fork is first placed on the mastoid process behind the ear and then is moved in front of but not touching the pinna when it can no longer be "heard." A positive test occurs when the person continues to hear the sound with air conduction after bone conduction has ceased.

VESTIBULAR ASSESSMENT

In the *Romberg test* the person stands with feet together and eyes open. The same test is performed with the eyes closed. Only a minimal amount of swaying should exist.

TABLE 14-1   Tuning Fork Tests for Auditory Acuity

SITE OF PROBLEM	WEBER TEST	RINNE TEST
NORMAL HEARING		
No problem	Tone heard in center of head	Air conduction lasts longer than bone conduction
CONDUCTIVE LOSS		
External or middle ear	Tone heard in poorer ear because ear not distracted by room noise	Bone conduction lasts longer than air conduction
SENSORINEURAL LOSS		
Inner ear	Tone heard in better ear because inner ear less able to receive vibrations	Air conduction lasts longer than bone conduction

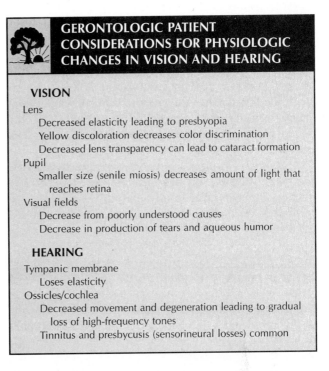

GERONTOLOGIC PATIENT CONSIDERATIONS FOR PHYSIOLOGIC CHANGES IN VISION AND HEARING

VISION

Lens
  Decreased elasticity leading to presbyopia
  Yellow discoloration decreases color discrimination
  Decreased lens transparency can lead to cataract formation
Pupil
  Smaller size (senile miosis) decreases amount of light that reaches retina
Visual fields
  Decrease from poorly understood causes
  Decrease in production of tears and aqueous humor

HEARING

Tympanic membrane
  Loses elasticity
Ossicles/cochlea
  Decreased movement and degeneration leading to gradual loss of high-frequency tones
  Tinnitus and presbycusis (sensorineural losses) common

To test gaze nystagmus the person is asked to follow the examiner's fingers and the eyes are observed for jerky movements. Nystagmus (rapid involuntary movements) may be horizontal or vertical.

To test gait the person walks naturally while posture, balance, arm swing, and coordination are assessed.

Ophthalmoscopy allows for visualization of the retina, optic disc, macula, and blood vessels. The disc is creamy yellow or white in color with clear margins. The vessels are observed for size, color, and light reflection. Veins are larger and darker (Figure 14-4). The retina is creamy pink and regular.

RADIOLOGIC TESTS
Fluorescein Angiography

Description—Fluorescein angiography provides a detailed imaging and record of the ocular circulation through use of a contrast medium.

Procedure—Venous access is established, and fluorescein dye is injected. Photographs are taken as the dye moves through the vessels.

Patient preparation and aftercare—Mydriatic eye drops are instilled 1 hour before the test. The patient is upright with the chin supported while the pictures are taken. Some patients experience nausea and weakness after the test. Fair-skinned persons may note yellow staining of the skin for several hours, and the urine is fluorescent green. The person should drink fluids liberally to aid in excretion of the dye and avoid sunlight until pupil response is restored.

Computed Tomography Scans, Magnetic Resonance Imaging, and Ultrasonography

CT scans, MRI, and ultrasonography may be used as part of a diagnostic workup for visual or auditory problems to provide outlines of organs, structures, nerves, and blood vessels.

OTHER TESTS

Tonometry is used to measure intraocular pressure. Both noncontact (air puff) and contact techniques are

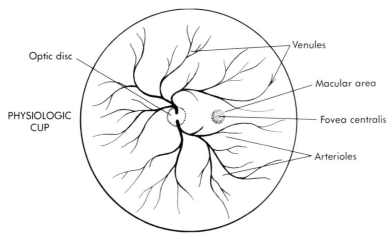

FIGURE 14-4 Structures of the left eye as visualized through the funduscope.

available. The latter measures the amount of force required to flatten the cornea with a flattened cone. It is performed as part of a complete eye examination.

Electroretinography is a process of graphing the retina's response to light stimulation. A contact lens electrode is applied to the anesthetized cornea, lights at various speeds and intensities are flashed, and the neural response is graphed. Electroretinography tests the function of the rods and cones.

Audiometry utilizes mechanical devices to increase the sophistication of hearing loss assessment. Frequency, intensity, and tones may all be varied, and responses are plotted. Soundproof booths are required for testing.

DISORDERS OF THE EYE

Eye disease and blindness remain significant worldwide health problems. The incidence of blindness continues to rise as the U.S. population ages, and at least some of these cases are preventable. Primary health care screening and teaching concerning prevention are important nursing roles in all health care settings.

EYE INFECTION AND INFLAMMATION

Infection and inflammation can occur in any of the eye structures and may be caused by microorganisms, mechanical irritation, or sensitivity to some substance. More than 1 million cases of eye inflammation occur annually in the U.S., two thirds of which are conjunctivitis. Most eye inflammations are relatively benign, self-limiting disorders that respond promptly to local therapy and antibiotics. They create discomfort and minor interruption of function from the inflammatory response but resolve without permanent effect. Standard medical interventions include the application of warm, moist compresses, topical or systemic antibiotics, and patching if eye rest is needed. Table 14-2 summarizes the major features and medical management of the

TABLE 14-2 Infections and Inflammations of the Eye

DESCRIPTION	SIGNS AND SYMPTOMS	MEDICAL THERAPY
HORDEOLUM (STYE)		
Staphylococcus infection of gland at eyelid margin	Localized abscess at base of eyelash, edema of lid, pain	Warm moist compresses to hasten pointing of abscess, topical antibiotic
CHALAZION		
Cyst from obstruction of sebaceous gland at eyelid margin	Initially, edema and discomfort; later, painless mass in lid	Warm compresses and topical antibiotic initially; surgical removal if cyst becomes large and presses on cornea
BLEPHARITIS		
Inflammation of lid margins, usually by staphylococci Seborrheic forms may persist for years	Itching, redness, pain of lid, lacrimation, photophobia; crusting ulceration; lids become glued together during sleep	Warm compresses followed by topical antibiotics; steroid eye drops may be prescribed
CONJUNCTIVITIS (PINK EYE)		
Inflammation of conjunctiva by viruses, bacteria (highly infectious), allergy, trauma (sunburn)	Redness of conjunctiva, lid edema, crusting discharge on lids and cornea of eye; itching with allergies	Cleansing of lids and lashes, warm compresses; topical antibiotics; steroid eye drops for allergies (contraindicated for herpes simplex virus); careful asepsis
KERATITIS		
Inflammation of cornea by bacteria, herpes simplex virus, allergies, vitamin A deficiency	Severe eye pain, photophobia, tearing, blepharospasm, loss of vision if uncontrolled	Warm compresses; topical antibiotics for bacterial infections; atropine sulfate; idoxuridine for herpes simplex; eye patch, rest; corneal transplant if cornea is injured
CORNEAL ULCER		
Necrosis of corneal tissue from trauma, inflammation; may be superficial or may penetrate deeper tissue	Pain and blepharospasm may occur; ulcer may be outlined by fluorescein dye	Superficial ulcer; antibiotic eye drops, eye patch; deep ulcer; topical and systemic antibiotics, atropine sulfate, warm compresses, eye patch; cautery; corneal transplant if necessary
UVEITIS		
Inflammation of the uvea; may involve choroid, ciliary body, iris, or all three; infection, allergy, and trauma are all potential causes	Pain radiating to forehead and temple, photophobia, tearing, and poor vision, pupil contracted and irregular	Often self-limited; atropine eye drops for comfort; moist, warm compresses and dark glasses; corticosteroids to relieve inflammation

Home Care Guidelines for Eye Irrigations

1. Place patient lying toward one side to prevent fluid from flowing into other eye.
2. Direct the irrigating fluid along the conjunctiva from the *inner* to the outer canthus.
3. Avoid directing a forceful stream onto eyeball or touching any eye structure with the irrigating equipment.
4. A piece of gauze may be wrapped around index finger to raise upper lid for better cleaning if heavy discharge exists.

Home Care Guidelines for Application of Moist Eye Compresses

GENERAL PRINCIPLES
Use aseptic technique if infection is present.
If bilateral infection, use separate equipment for each eye.
Wash hands thoroughly before and after soaks.
If bilateral infection, wash hands between treatments of eyes.
Do not exert any pressure on the eye during treatment.

WARM COMPRESSES
Temperature should not exceed 120° F (49° C).
A clean, fresh washcloth is effective for use in the home.
Change compresses frequently over the 10- to 20-minute treatment period.
Never reuse washcloth for a second treatment.
Carefully handle and dispose of infected materials.

COLD COMPRESSES
A rubber glove or plastic bag packed with ice chips may be used as a disposable compress.

Home Care Guidelines for Instilling Eye Medications

EYE DROPS
1. Wash hands before touching eyes.
2. Clean eyes before instilling eye drops if crusting or discharge is present.
3. Ask patient to tilt head back and look up.
4. Evert lower lid by pulling down gently on skin below eye.
5. Approach eye by bringing dropper tip in from side, not directly from front.
6. Place drops on *center* of conjunctival sac of lower lid. Avoid touching eye with dropper.
7. Ask patient to close eyes but not tightly squeeze them shut (to prevent loss of medication down cheek).
8. Provide patient with a tissue or cotton ball to absorb excess moisture.

OINTMENT
1. Follow steps 1 through 4 above.
2. Place the ointment from tube directly onto exposed conjunctival sac from the inner to the outer canthus.
3. Avoid touching eye with tube.

most common eye infections and inflammations. Management frequently involves the use of eye drops or ointments, warm compresses, and irrigations; these principles are summarized in the Home Care boxes.

GLAUCOMA
Etiology/Epidemiology

The term *glaucoma* refers to an eye disease characterized by increased intraocular pressure associated with progressive loss of peripheral visual fields. It is responsible for 12% to 15% of all cases of blindness in the United States, and perhaps as many as 1 million adults have undiagnosed disease. It occurs in middle-aged and older adults, and the prevalence is 15 times greater in the African-American population. Permanent vision loss is preventable with early detection. Although glaucoma may occur secondary to other problems, the basic etiology of primary glaucoma remains unknown.

Pathophysiology

In the normal eye there is a balance between the production and drainage of aqueous humor, permitting a stable intraocular pressure. In glaucoma, obstruction to the drainage of aqueous humor increases the intraocular pressure and produces damage to the optic nerve.

Chronic simple (wide-angle) glaucoma is the primary form of the disease. It takes a slow and insidious course and appears to result from degenerative changes.

Acute (narrow-angle) glaucoma is the result of a change in the angle of the iris against the anterior chamber and causes dramatic symptoms and rapid loss of vision.

A congenital form of glaucoma also exists.

Persons with wide-angle glaucoma are usually asymptomatic until the disease is well advanced. Narrow-angle glaucoma presents with acute eye pain.

Medical Management

Glaucoma is usually diagnosed through routine screening tonometry that measures intraocular pressure. Biennial screening is strongly suggested for all adults over 40 years of age. Ophthalmoscopy is used to evaluate pressure effects on the optic nerve.

Medical management is aimed at providing better drainage of aqueous humor or decreasing the amount produced. This controls the level of intraocular pressure and helps prevent irreversible vision loss.

Pharmacologic treatment is the cornerstone of therapy and includes the following:

Miotics such as pilocarpine to constrict the pupil and facilitate drainage

Beta-adrenergic blockers such as timolol, which decrease intraocular pressure by poorly understood mechanisms without causing pupil constriction

Carbonic anhydrase inhibitors such as acetazolamide to decrease the production of aqueous humor

Commonly used ophthalmic drugs are summarized in Table 14-3.

TABLE 14-3 Commonly Used Ophthalmic Drugs

DRUG	ACTION	USES
MYDRIATICS		
Phenylephrine (Neo-Synephrine, Mydfrin) Hydroxyamphetamine (Paredrine)	Dilate pupil	Examination of interior of eye Prevent adhesions of iris with cornea in eye inflammations
CYCLOPLEGICS		
Atropine sulfate (Atropisol, Isopto-Atropine) Cyclopentolate (Cyclogyl) Homatropine (Isopto-Homatropine) Scopolamine hydrobromide Tropicamide (Mydriacyl)	Dilate pupil Paralyze ciliary muscle and iris	Decrease pain and photophobia and provide rest for inflammations of iris and ciliary body, and for diseases of cornea Eye examinations
MIOTICS (CHOLINERGICS)		
Pilocarpine (Pilocel, Ocusert) Carbachol (Carbacel) Physostigmine (Eserine) Demecarium bromide (Humorsol) Isofluorophate (Fluoropryl)	Constrict pupil Permit better drainage of intraocular fluid	Treat glaucoma
OSMOTIC AGENTS		
Mannitol (Osmitrol) Glycerine (Glyrol, Osmoglyn) Isosorbide (Ismotic)	Decrease intraocular pressure	Treat acute glaucoma Eye surgery
CARBONIC ANHYDRASE INHIBITORS		
Acetazolamide (Diamox) Ethoxzolamide (Cardrase) Dichlorphenamide (Daranide) Methazolamide (Neptazane)	Decrease production of aqueous humor	Treat glaucoma
ADRENERGIC AGENTS		
Epinephryl Borate (EPPY) Epinephrine hydrochloride (Glaucon) Epinephrine bitartrate (Epitrate) Dipivefrin (Propine)	Reduce aqueous humor formation and increase outflow	Treat glaucoma
BETA-ADRENERGIC BLOCKERS		
Timolol maleate (Timoptic) Betaxolol (Betoptic) Levobunolol (Betagen)	Reduce intraocular pressure (mechanism unclear)	Treat glaucoma
TOPICAL ANESTHETICS		
Proparacaine (Ophthaine, Ophthetic, Alcaine) Lidocaine (Xylocaine)	Decrease sensation (pain)	Surgery, treatments Treat eye inflammations
TOPICAL ANTIBIOTICS		
Polymyxin B, bacitracin (Polysporin) Polymyxin B, neomycin, bacitracin (Neosporin) Bacitracin Idoxuridine (IDU) Gentamicin sulfate (Garamycin) Chloramphenicol (Chloromycetin, Chloroptic)	Antiinfective	Treat eye inflammations
STEROIDS		
Prednisone Prednisolone (Pred Forte) Methylprednisolone (Depo-Medrol) Triamcinolone (Aristocort) Dexamethasone (Decadron, Maxidex) Fluorometholone (FML)	Antiinflammatory	Treat eye inflammations and allergic reactions

Surgery may be indicated if conservative management fails. Trabeculoplasty and trabeculectomy are procedures aimed at improving the outflow and drainage from the anterior chamber.

A new surgical option involves implanting a plate of polymethylmethacrylate against the sclera. A tube is then surgically implanted into the anterior chamber to allow drainage of aqueous humor. Acute narrow-angle glaucoma can present as an ocular emergency. Pharmacologic treatment may be used, but surgical correction of the position of the iris through iridotomy or iridectomy is frequently required.

NURSING MANAGEMENT

Nursing interventions are focused on patient education. Most mild cases of glaucoma are asymptomatic and do not require symptom management. It is critical that the patient understand the chronic and incurable nature of glaucoma, and the importance of regular follow-up and adherence to the medication regimen. The nurse focuses on the correct and safe administration of all eye medications and the need to have reserve medication available for travel or times away from home. The patient is cautioned about the effects of miotics on night vision, especially for driving, and the importance of extra home lighting for safety. At least one family member or friend should be instructed on aseptic eye drop administration if possible to provide a backup for the patient.

CATARACT

Etiology/Epidemiology

A cataract is a clouding or opacity of the lens that leads to gradual painless blurring of vision and eventual loss of sight. The most common cause of cataracts is aging; 85% of persons over 80 years of age have some lens clouding. Senile cataracts are identified as the most common cause of blindness despite the ready availability of effective surgical treatment. Cataracts are also associated with injury, can be present at birth, and can be secondary to other eye disease. The etiology of cataracts remains poorly explained.

Pathophysiology

Cataracts develop as the result of alterations in the metabolism and movement of nutrients within the lens. A reduction in oxygen intake and imbalances in water content and electrolyte proportion are all felt to play a role. Persons with diabetes tend to develop cataracts at an earlier age because of an accumulation of sorbitol. As the nuclear portion of the lens becomes increasingly dense, light rays are unable to pass through the opaque lens to the retina.

The predominant symptom is a progressive loss, blurring, or distortion of vision. Cataracts develop

---

BOX 14-4	Approaches to Cataract Removal

TYPES

Intracapsular extraction—removal of the entire lens
Extracapsular extraction—removal of lens material without disturbing the membrane capsule

TECHNIQUES

Phacoemulsification—insertion of an instrument that uses ultrasonic vibration to break up lens material for removal by irrigation
Cryoextraction—cataract lifted out by adhering lens to a subzero probe

---

slowly and, if present in both eyes, frequently mature at an uneven rate.

Medical Management

Operative treatment is the only effective management of cataracts, and vision loss can be restored with surgery. Surgeons no longer wait for cataracts to ripen but intervene when visual loss interferes with activities of daily living (ADL). Box 14-4 summarizes approaches to cataract removal. Virtually all surgical procedures can be done with the patient under local anesthesia on an outpatient basis.

Corrective lenses

The focusing function of the lens is replaced after surgery by the use of cataract glasses, contact lenses, or intraocular lens implants. A lens implant is used whenever possible and usually is inserted at the time of surgery. Near normal vision can be achieved.

An anterior chamber lens is placed in front of the iris and is supported by it. It is used after intracapsular extraction.

A posterior chamber lens is placed behind the iris and is supported by the remnant of the lens capsule. It is used after extracapsular extraction. A posterior chamber lens is used most frequently and has a low incidence of complications.

Cataract glasses are the least desirable option. Loss of depth perception and some peripheral vision make adjustment difficult. Glasses also tend to magnify objects and make them appear closer. Contact lenses correct some of these problems but not in their entirety. Interruption of the nerve supply may enable the person to adapt to the use of extended wear lenses.

NURSING MANAGEMENT

PREOPERATIVE CARE

Ensure that patient understands nature of procedure, use of local anesthesia, and all postoperative care routines.

Encourage patient to discuss fears related to eye surgery.

Explore plans for transportation home and supports available to meet early care needs.

Complete preparation as ordered:
Face scrubs
Clipping eyelashes
Eye medications, for example, mydriatics and cycloplegics
Sedatives

POSTOPERATIVE CARE
Preventing Intraocular Pressure Increases

Avoid activities that increase intraocular pressure:
Squeezing shut the eyelids
Bending over at the waist
Straining for sneezing, coughing, vomiting, defecation

NOTE: Surgeons vary on strictness of activity restrictions.

Maintaining a Safe Environment

Encourage patient to lie on back or unaffected side.
Use eye shield at night to protect the eye.
Organize self-care articles on unaffected side.
Be alert to complaints of severe pain or pressure that may indicate complications.
Keep side rails up to prevent falls and injury.

Preparing for Discharge

Encourage patient to return to normal activities as tolerated. No bending below waist level or heavy lifting is permitted during recovery. Patient should sleep on unoperative side for 3 to 4 weeks.

Teach patient about the corrective lenses to be used during rehabilitation.

Ensure that patient has assistance available for ADL as needed.

Instruct patient to wear metal eye shield at night as instructed.

Review orders for all medications and dressing changes as ordered. Provide written copies of all instructions.

Instruct patient to use caution with face and hair washing to prevent soapy water from contaminating operative field.

RETINAL DETACHMENT
Etiology/Epidemiology

Retinal detachment occurs when the two retinal layers separate because of a full-thickness break in the sensory retina, fluid accumulation, or contraction of the vitreous body. Usually there is no apparent cause, but detachment can be caused by trauma, severe physical exertion, lens loss (as after cataract surgery), degenerative changes of myopia, hemorrhage, or tumor.

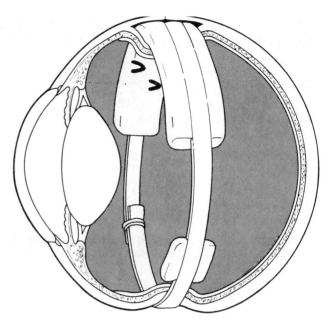

FIGURE 14-5 Scleral buckle.

Pathophysiology

Retinal detachment may occur abruptly or evolve slowly. Detachment interrupts the transmission of visual images from the retina to the optic nerve, and, as the detachment extends and becomes complete, blindness occurs in the eye because the macula separates. The area of visual loss depends on the location of the detachment. Clinical manifestations include floaters, flashes of light, and progressive visual loss. If the detachment is extensive and occurs rapidly, the person may report a feeling that a curtain has been drawn before the eyes.

Medical Management

The diagnosis is made from the symptoms and confirmed by ophthalmoscopic examination. Early surgical intervention is the treatment of choice. Accumulated fluid is drained from the subretinal space, and inflammation is induced by diathermy, photocoagulation, laser beam, or subfreezing temperatures to cause adhesion formation, which closes the retinal break. Scleral buckling is also used in most cases to push the choroid into contact with the retinal tear during healing (Figure 14-5).

NURSING MANAGEMENT

◆ ASSESSMENT
Subjective Data

Patient's complaints of the following:
Floating spots or flashing lights
Progressive constriction of vision in one area
Sensation of "curtain being drawn" across the eye (if tear is acute and extensive)

NURSING CARE PLAN

PERSON WITH A RETINAL DETACHMENT

■ NURSING DIAGNOSIS

Sensory/perceptual alteration (visual) (related to decreased vision or eye patching)

Expected Patient Outcome	Nursing Interventions

Patient's vision will be restored to pre-detachment level.	1. Maintain prescribed activity restrictions.
	2. Position patient's head during initial period so that retinal tear is at lowest portion of eye.
	3. Assist patient with ADL within the ordered restrictions.
	4. If one eye has decreased vision and patient is restricted in movement:
	  a. Place personal objects within easy reach.
	  b. Provide diversion with radio or conversation.
	5. If total vision is limited by eye patches or blurred vision:
	  a. Orient patient to physical surroundings, time, weather, and news events.
	  b. Speak to patient when approaching and identify yourself.
	  c. Explain activities occurring in room.
	  d. Tell patient when you are leaving.

■ NURSING DIAGNOSIS

Injury, high risk for (related to decreased vision)

Expected Patient Outcome	Nursing Interventions
Patient will not experience injury during period of decreased vision.	1. Keep side rails up if binocular patches are used postoperatively or vision is markedly reduced. 2. Keep call button within reach when patient is on bed rest. Orient to immediate physical environment. 3. Assist patient as necessary when ambulating after surgery if vision is still restricted, such as by eye patches. 4. Instruct patient to wear eye shield for sleeping.

Continued.

Objective Data

Ophthalmoscopic evidence of detachment

Nursing management of retinal detachment is summarized in the "Nursing Care Plan" located above and continued on p. 338.

DIABETIC RETINOPATHY

Diabetic retinopathy is a disorder of the blood vessels of the retina that appears 10 or more years after the onset of diabetes mellitus. It is present in 60% to 65% of patients with both insulin-dependent diabetes mellitus (IDDM) and non–insulin-dependent diabetes mellitus (NIDDM). The capillary walls thicken and develop microaneurysms, and the veins widen. Retinal edema and small hemorrhages occur, and neovascularization develops in response to the ischemia. These new vessels bleed easily, and the continuing process leads to substantial visual loss.

The process is identified by ophthalmoscopic examination, and the patient notes both multiple floaters and visual loss. Ongoing monitoring is essential. The neovascularization may be treated by laser photocoagulation, which is reported to have reduced the incidence of blindness by as much as 60%. Proper longer term diabetic glucose control appears to prevent or delay disease development.

NURSING CARE PLAN—CONT'D

PERSON WITH A RETINAL DETACHMENT

■ NURSING DIAGNOSIS
Anxiety (related to possible loss of vision)

Expected Patient Outcome	Nursing Interventions
Patient will experience manageable levels of anxiety and verbalize concerns about possible visual losses.	1. Give patient opportunities to explore concerns about possible decreased vision. 2. Answer questions honestly. 3. Encourage realistic hope about maintaining vision as described by physician. 4. Explore patient's knowledge of disorder and planned therapy, and correct misunderstandings.

■ NURSING DIAGNOSIS
Knowledge deficit (related to surgery and postoperative care routines)

Expected Patient Outcome	Nursing Interventions
Patient accurately describes surgical procedure and postoperative regimen.	1. Teach patient to avoid jerking head (sneezing, coughing, vomiting). 2. Apply cold compresses to reduce swelling. 3. Administer antiemetics or cough suppressants if necessary. 4. Teach patient about temporary activity restrictions. Patient may resume normal activities but should restrict active exercise and heavy lifting. Activity should be sedentary for 1 to 2 weeks. 5. Teach patient to report signs of further retinal detachment—eye pain, floaters, or spots. 6. Teach patient to wear eye shield at night and while resting until healing is complete. 7. Teach patient to safely administer any needed eye medication.

MACULAR DEGENERATION

Macular degeneration is a disease of the aging retina and the leading cause of blindness in elderly persons. The underlying cause is unknown. It causes a central visual loss of varying degree and decreased color discrimination. At present no treatment has proved effective. Persons with macular degeneration need emotional support, because fear of blindness is an overriding concern. Reassurance can be provided that peripheral vision is not usually affected.

DISORDERS OF THE EARS
HEARING LOSS

Hearing loss is the most common disability in the United States, affecting over 13 million persons, most of whom are over 65 years of age. The range of disability is from difficulty understanding particular words and sounds to complete deafness. Hearing loss may be classified as follows:

Conductive: any interference with conduction of sound impulses through the external auditory canal, eardrum, or middle ear, for example, wax, foreign body, infection, or scarring or perforation of the tympanic membrane

Sensorineural: disease or trauma to the inner ear, neural structures, or nerve pathways to the brain stem, for example, infectious diseases (mumps, meningitis), arteriosclerosis, cranial neuromas on cranial nerve VIII, trauma, degeneration of the organ of Corti, and the effects of ototoxic drugs (Box 14-5)

Central deafness: a rare form in which the central nervous system cannot interpret normal auditory signals because of tumor, trauma, or cerebrovascular accident (CVA)

BOX 14-6	Hearing Aids

Hearing aids amplify sound in a controlled manner. They make sound *louder* but do not improve the person's ability to discriminate sounds. The devices amplify all sound, including background noise, which may make crowded or noisy situations extremely confusing, especially for elderly persons. Types of hearing aids include the following:

In the ear: worn in ear concha; for losses of 25-65 dB
In the canal: worn in ear canal; for losses of 25-50 dB
Postauricular: worn behind the ear; for losses of 25-80 dB

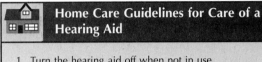

Home Care Guidelines for Care of a Hearing Aid

1. Turn the hearing aid off when not in use.
2. Open the battery compartment at night to avoid accidental drainage of the battery.
3. Keep an extra battery available at all times.
4. Wash the ear mold frequently (daily if necessary) with mild soap and warm water, using a pipe cleaner to cleanse the cannula.
5. Do not wear the hearing aid during an ear infection.

Although some problems can be helped by medicine or surgery, most cannot be effectively treated. Eighty percent of all impairments are caused by sensorineural problems for which there is no known cure. Prevention of hearing loss is an important consideration that should be included in all health promotion and screening activities. Interventions include the following:

Avoiding inserting hard objects into the ear or obstructing the ear canal

Preventing occupational noise-induced hearing loss (The U.S. Occupational Safety and Health Administration [OSHA] demands yearly audiometric testing in high-noise jobs.)

Preventing nonoccupational noise-induced hearing loss (e.g., firearms, high-intensity music) (NOTE: Noise-induced hearing loss is caused by progressive destruction of sensory cells and cannot be medically or surgically repaired. If exposure cannot be avoided, ear plugs should be worn.)

EAR INFECTIONS AND INFLAMMATION
Etiology/Epidemiology

Ear infections may occur at any age and in any portion of the ear. They are common health problems, particularly in children. The possibility of serious complications following ear infection makes prompt identification and treatment important. Table 14-4 lists common infections of the ear.

Pathophysiology

The pathophysiology of ear infections is related to the specific structures involved and basically results from local tissue inflammatory responses to bacteria or viruses. Pain is a common symptom. External and middle ear infections may cause drainage, itching, and redness. Repeated infection may result in tympanosclerosis, or deposits of collagen and calcium within the middle ear that can harden around the ossicles. Because the middle ear transmits sound waves from the tympanic membrane to the inner ear, a hearing loss usually accompanies infections of the middle ear. Inner ear problems may affect balance by disturbing the vestibular system.

Medical Management

Standard medical interventions include systemic antibiotics and topical ear drops. Surgical intervention includes myringotomy to remove fluid through an incision in the tympanic membrane. Tubes are often inserted to keep the incision open and prevent a recurrence of fluid. Other complex and delicate procedures are used in the attempt to repair damage to the delicate structures of the middle ear.

TABLE 14-4 Inflammations of the Ear

DESCRIPTION	SIGNS AND SYMPTOMS	MEDICAL THERAPY
EXTERNAL OTITIS (SWIMMER'S EAR)		
Inflammation of external ear; may be acute or chronic	Pain with movement of auricle, redness, scaling, itching, swelling, watery discharge, crusting of external ear	Cleaning to remove debris; antibiotic drops or ointment; systemic antibiotic if necessary
SEROUS OTITIS MEDIA		
Collection of sterile fluid in middle ear; may be acute or chronic	Sense of fullness in ear, hearing loss, low-pitched tinnitus, earache	Removal of eustachian obstruction by aspiration or insertion of tubes for drainage
ACUTE PURULENT OTITIS MEDIA		
Infection of middle ear, usually by pneumococci, streptococci, staphylococci, or *Haemophilus influenzae*	Sense of fullness in ear, severe throbbing pain, hearing loss, tinnitus, fever	Antibiotics; if severe, bed rest, analgesics, nasal vasoconstrictors; myringotomy if necessary
CHRONIC OTITIS MEDIA		
Chronic inflammation of middle ear; sequela of acute otitis media	Deafness, occasional pain, dizziness, chronic discharge from ear	Local debridement, topical and systemic antibiotics; mastoidectomy and tympanoplasty may be necessary
CHRONIC MASTOIDITIS		
Spread of infection into mastoid from repeated otitis media	Middle ear drainage, tenderness over mastoid cavity	Mastoid irrigation; antibiotics; may need mastoidectomy
LABYRINTHITIS		
Inflammation of inner ear	Severe and sudden vertigo, nausea and vomiting, nystagmus, photophobia, headache, ataxic gait	No specific treatment; antibiotics; dimenhydrinate for vertigo; parenteral fluids if nausea and vomiting persist

NURSING MANAGEMENT

◆ ASSESSMENT
Subjective Data

Patient complaints of the following:
  Pain or itching in ear
  Acute tenderness when pinna pulled or moved
  Sense of fullness in ear, blocked ear
  Tinnitus (ringing in the ear) or roaring sound
  Vertigo

Objective Data

  Decreased hearing
  Fever
  Redness, drainage, scaling

◆ NURSING DIAGNOSES

Possible nursing diagnoses for the person with an ear infection or inflammation may include, but are not limited to, the following:
  Pain and itching (related to pressure and inflammation in the ear)
  Knowledge deficit (related to ear infection prevention and management)

◆ EXPECTED PATIENT OUTCOMES

  Patient will experience decreased pain and irritation.
  Patient will correctly describe measures to prevent and treat ear infection.

◆ NURSING INTERVENTIONS
Relieving Discomfort

  Administer medications as ordered.
  Augment pain relief with nonpharmacologic measures.
  If patient experiences vertigo, keep side rails up and supervise ambulation.
  Experiment with the use of heat and cold for pain relief.

Teaching for Self-Care

  Teach patient how to correctly instill ear drops (see Home Care box).
  Teach patient or family member how to safely irrigate the ear, if ordered (see Home Care box and Figure 14-6).

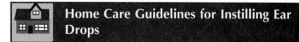

Home Care Guidelines for Instilling Ear Drops

Wash hands before and after the procedure.
Warm solution to body temperature—no more than 100° F (38° C).
Have patient tilt head so ear to be treated is up.
Straighten ear canal by pulling pinna up and back.
Instill drops to run along auditory canal wall.
Have patient hold position for 2 to 5 minutes.
Gently insert cotton into external auditory canal if desired.
Wipe external ear to prevent skin irritation.

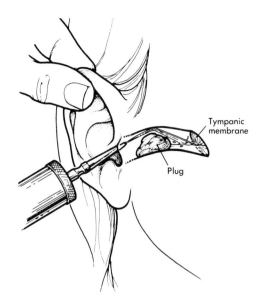

Tympanic
membrane

Plug

FIGURE 14-6 Irrigation of the external auditory canal.

Home Care Guidelines for Ear Irrigation

NOTE: Avoid ear irrigation if ear drum is punctured (increases inflammation) or when attempting to remove foreign body (moisture may swell object).
1. Use tap water or normal saline; peroxide may be added to remove wax.
2. Warm solution to body temperature. Dizziness can result from solutions that are too hot or too cold.
3. Straighten ear by pulling pinna up and back.
4. Use a steady stream of solution against roof of auditory canal.
5. Use gentle pressure; do not obstruct outflow with equipment.
6. Have patient lie on affected side after irrigation to promote drainage. Be alert to possibility of vertigo following irrigation.

Teach patient to take all prescribed medications and the importance of completing the entire prescription.
Instruct patient in measures to prevent reinfection.
Avoid letting water stand in the ear.
Wash hands frequently during episodes of upper respiratory infection (URI).
Ask physician about routine use of decongestants during colds and flu.
Sneeze with mouth open, and blow both sides of the nose together.

◆ EVALUATION

Successful achievement of expected outcomes for the patient with an ear infection or inflammation is indicated by the following:
Free of pain and other symptoms
Able to state purpose and schedule for all medications, administer ear drops correctly, and describe prevention strategies

MENIERE'S DISEASE
Etiology/Epidemiology

Meniere's disease is a disorder of the inner ear that occurs most commonly in women between 50 and 60 years of age. Its cause is unknown. It is characterized by a triad of symptoms that includes vertigo, tinnitus, and unilateral sensorineural hearing loss. Several attacks may occur yearly, and the person is virtually incapacitated during an attack. The initial hearing loss is reversible but usually becomes permanent as the disease persists.

Pathophysiology

A disturbance in the fluid physiology in the ear, resulting from either increased production or decreased absorption, raises the pressure within the labyrinth of the

Guidelines for Nursing Care of the Patient After Ear Surgery

Position the patient per physician's order.
Teach patient to sneeze or cough with the mouth open and avoid use of straws.
Teach patient to anticipate the following:
Decreased hearing initially
Noises in the ear, for example, cracking, popping
Minor earache or discomfort
Protect patient from injury.
Assess regularly for dizziness.
Assist with position changes and ambulation.
Teach patient to keep ear dry.
Protect ear from shampoo, soapy water.
Check with physician before air travel.
Report excessive ear drainage to physician.

inner ear. This pressure produces attacks of severe vertigo, tinnitus, and progressive hearing loss. Usually only one ear is involved. The cause is unknown.

Medical Management

No medical treatment is entirely successful. The major goal is to preserve hearing. During the acute phase atropine or diazepam (Valium) may be given to decrease autonomic nervous system function. Benadryl is given for its antihistamine effect in addition to vasodilators.

During remission the patient may receive diuretics to reduce fluid, antihistamines (Benadryl, Dramamine), and vasodilators (nicotinic acid) and be instructed to follow a low-salt diet and restrict fluids. Most patients respond to this regimen, although acute attacks may still occur at unpredictable times. Complete remission usually occurs over 1 to 2 years as a gradual loss of responsiveness occurs from sensory organ degeneration. Some degree of hearing loss is usually permanent. Surgical decompression procedures may also be attempted to preserve hearing.

NURSING MANAGEMENT

◆ ASSESSMENT
Subjective Data

Patient complaints of the following:
  Episodes of vertigo (described as whirling sensation or room spinning; patient must lie down to keep from falling); attacks often preceded by a feeling of fullness or tinnitus in ear
  Nausea associated with vertigo
  Tinnitus (buzzing sounds to painful loud roaring)
  Headache
History of and patient's knowledge about disorder
Knowledge of circumstances that precipitate attack
Actions taken during attacks and degree of relief they provide

Objective Data

Unilateral or bilateral hearing loss (initially low frequency tones)
Vomiting, diaphoresis, or nystagmus during observed attack
Uncoordinated gait

◆ NURSING DIAGNOSES

Possible nursing diagnoses for the person with Meniere's disease may include, but are not limited to, the following:
  Injury, risk for (related to severe vertigo)
  Sensory/perceptual alteration (auditory) (related to progressive hearing loss)
  Knowledge deficit (related to course of disease and management of attacks)

◆ EXPECTED PATIENT OUTCOMES

Patient will not experience injury during vertigo attacks.
Patient's hearing loss will be minimized.
Patient will be knowledgeable concerning factors that precipitate or control attacks.

◆ NURSING INTERVENTIONS
Preventing Injury

Keep side rails up while vertigo persists.
Supervise position changes and all ambulation.
Encourage regular, slow position changes—do not turn head abruptly.
Try positioning on unaffected side.
Avoid use of bright or glaring lights.
Adjust diet to compensate for nausea or anorexia.
Assist patient to meet hygiene needs as required.
  Keep emesis basin available at bedside.

Minimizing Hearing Loss

Stand in front of patient to foster hearing and prevent head turning.
If tinnitus is severe, increase background sounds with music.
Encourage realistic hope about maintenance of hearing.
Use appropriate measures to communicate with hearing impaired person.
Refer to audiologist or other support services as indicated.

Teaching for Self-Care

Explore patient's knowledge of the disorder and correct misunderstandings.
Teach use of low-salt diet and fluid limitations.
Help patient to identify avoidable actions that precipitate dizziness attacks.
  Identify factors related to attacks, if possible.
  Patient should avoid reading when any vertigo or tinnitus is present.
Patient should avoid smoking.
Teach patient ways to protect self from injury.
  If driving, patient should pull over and stop immediately.
  If standing, patient should sit or lie down immediately.
  Keep medications available at all time.
Reassure patient that disease symptoms are controllable and self-limiting.

◆ EVALUATION

Successful achievement of expected outcomes for the patient with Meniere's disease is indicated by the following:
  Successfully avoids injury during attacks
  Suffers minimal hearing loss and compensates appropriately for decreased perception
  Achieves sufficient disease control to maintain independence in ADL

SELECTED REFERENCES

Allen MN: Adjusting to visual impairment, *J Ophthalmic Nurs Technol* 9:47-51, 1990.
Allen MN, Birse E: Stigma and blindness, *J Ophthalmic Nurs Technol* 10:147-152, 1991.
Anand R: Fluorescein angiography. I. Technique and normal study, *J Ophthalmic Nurs Technol* 8:48-52, 1989.
Burlew JA: Preventing eye injuries: the nurse's role, *Insight* 16(6):24-28, 1991.
Carver JA: Cataract care made plain, *Am J Nurs* 87:626-630, 1987.
DeBlase R et al: Postintraocular lens implant, *Geriatr Nurs* 9:342-344, 1988.
Gallagher CM: The young adult with recent vision loss: a pilot case study, *Insight* 16(6):8-14, 1991.

Hanson CM et al: Glaucoma screening: an important role for N.P.'s, *Nurse Pract* 12(12):14, 18-21, 1987.

Jairath N et al: Effective discharge preparation of elderly cataract day surgery patients, *J Ophthalmic Nurs Technol* 9:157-160, 1990.

Lawlor MC: Common ocular injuries and disorders, *J Emerg Nurs* 15(1):36-43, 1989.

Nodol JB, Jr: Hearing loss, *N Engl J Med* 329(15):1092-1102, 1993.

Okimi PH et al: Effects of caffeinated coffee on intraocular pressure, *Appl Nurs Res* 4(2):72-76, 1991.

Roach VG: What you should know about diabetic retinopathy, *J Ophthalmic Nurs Technol* 7:166-169, 1988.

Smith S: Diabetic retinopathy, *Insight* 17(2):20-25, 1992.

Woods S: Macular degeneration, *Nurs Clin North Am* 27:761-775, 1992.

Zavon B, Slater N: A surgical counseling plan for patients undergoing cataract surgery, *J Ophthalmic Nurs Technol* 7(2):68-71, 1988.

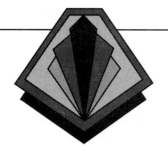

Disorders of the Musculoskeletal System

◆ ASSESSMENT

SUBJECTIVE DATA

Health history

Illness and trauma affecting the musculoskeletal system

Developmental abnormalities

Family history of genetic disorders, congenital abnormalities, rheumatic or other autoimmune diseases

Medication use: note use of acetylsalicylic acid (ASA), nonsteroidal antiinflammatory drugs (NSAIDs), estrogen

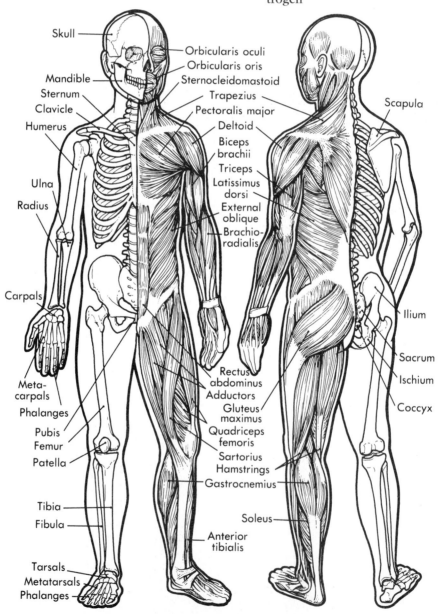

FIGURE 15-1 Musculoskeletal system.

Age, sex, height/weight balance
History of metabolic or other chronic illness
Activities of daily living (ADL) assessment
  Self-care abilities
    Use of assistive devices
  Ambulation and transfer abilities
  Exercise pattern, if any
  Occupation
    Physical demands of work
  Leisure time activities
  Nutrition
    Who shops for and prepares food
    Calcium intake, use of supplements
  Physical layout of the home
    Steps, size, accessibility
  Family and community support services available
Current health problem
  Onset and duration of symptoms
    Circumstances surrounding onset
  Clinical manifestations
  Factors that exacerbate or relieve symptoms

Reasons for seeking treatment
Perception of the problem and its impact on preferred life-style
Pain
  Nature, location, duration, reference to other areas
  Self-treatment measures utilized and effectiveness
Paresthesias, muscle weakness, or paralysis

OBJECTIVE DATA

Inspection
  Posture, balance, and gait
    Limp, ataxic gait, rigidity
  Symmetry and gross deformities
    Scoliosis, lordosis, and kyphosis
    Genu valgus, genu varum
    Arthritic deformities, such as hammertoes, ulnar deviation, boutonniere, Heberden's nodes (Box 15-1)
  Muscle mass
    Size, symmetry
  Presence of swelling or enlargement

BOX 15-1 Common Musculoskeletal System Deformities

ULNAR DEVIATION OR DRIFT
Fingers deviate at metacarpophalangeal joints toward ulnar aspect of hand

SWAN-NECK DEFORMITY
Flexion contracture of metacarpophalangeal joint, hyperextension of proximal interphalangeal joint, and flexion of distal interphalangeal joint; found in advanced rheumatoid arthritis

BOUTONNIERE DEFORMITY
Flexion contracture of proximal interphalangeal joint and hyperextension of distal interphalangeal joint; found in advanced rheumatoid arthritis

Z DEFORMITY
Flexion contracture of metacarpophalangeal joint and hyperextension of interphalangeal joint of thumb; found in advanced rheumatoid arthritis

VALGUS DEFORMITIES
Distal arm of joint angle points away from midline of body

Hallux Valgus
Great toe turns toward other toes

Genu Valgum
"Knock knees"

Talipes Valgus
Eversion of foot

VARUS DEFORMITIES
Distal arm of joint angle points toward midline of body

Genu Varum
Bowing of knees

Talipes Varus
Inversion of foot

HAMMERTOE
Dorsiflexion of any metatarsophalangeal joint, with plantar flexion of adjacent proximal interphalangeal joint of foot

SCOLIOSIS
Lateral spinal curvature

KYPHOSIS
Thoracic spinal curvature

LORDOSIS
Lumbar spinal curvature

BONY ENLARGEMENTS

Heberden's Nodes
Hard, irregular swellings over distal interphalangeal joints of fingers

Bouchard's Nodes
Hard, irregular swellings over proximal interphalangeal joints of fingers

SUBCUTANEOUS NODULES
Hard mobile swellings commonly found in subolecranon area; indicative of rheumatoid arthritis

TOPHACEOUS DEPOSITS
Hard, translucent swellings over joints or in cartilage such as ear; indicative of gout

GERONTOLOGIC PATIENT CONSIDERATIONS: PHYSIOLOGIC CHANGES IN THE MUSCULOSKELETAL SYSTEM

BONE

Decrease in total bone mass
Impaired osteoblastic activity
Increased bone resorption
Erosion of haversian systems
Change of cancellous bone to cortical bone
Cortical bone becomes increasingly porous
Effects of above changes: osteoporosis, delayed bone healing, potential for pathologic fracture

MUSCLES

Decline in strength after 70 years
Decline in number of muscle fibers
Decrease in muscle mass
Atrophy of muscle cells
Effects of above changes: weakness, disuse atrophy, slowed gait

JOINTS

Decreased cartilage elasticity
Increased susceptibility to cartilage tears
Cartilage degeneration
Development of bony spurs or roughening of joint surface
Effects of above changes: arthritis, decreased range of motion, contractures

---

BOX 15-2   Terms Used to Describe Extremity Movements

Adduction   Movement toward the midline of the body.
Abduction   Movement away from the midline of the body.
Flexion   Joint movement that decreases the angle between the two bones.
Extension   Joint movement that widens the angle between the two bones.
Internal rotation   Movement along the longitudinal axis in the direction of the midline of the body.
External rotation   Movement along the longitudinal axis away from the midline of the body.

Palpation
    Head-to-toe gentle palpation of all joints for temperature, swelling, tenderness, pain, or masses
Deep tendon reflexes
Joint range of motion (Box 15-2)
    Active or passive
    Presence of joint subluxation, contracture, crepitus
Muscle strength
    Contraction of a muscle group against an opposing force
    Presence of spasms, flaccidity, hypertonicity
    Atrophy or hypertrophy
NOTE: During assessment, joints or muscles are never moved beyond the point of pain.

✍ DIAGNOSTIC TESTS

LABORATORY TESTS

Blood and urine tests involving the musculoskeletal system are summarized in Table 15-1.

RADIOLOGIC TESTS

Bone and Joint X-Rays

Purpose—Radiologic examination is essential in the diagnosis of fractures and is by far the most commonly utilized test of the musculoskeletal system. X-rays may be employed for virtually any bone or joint in the body. They also present evidence of disease effects such as arthritis or tumors.

Procedure—The procedure varies based on the bones being examined. The patient must be able to assume the necessary position for appropriate visualization of the structure and hold still during the x-ray exposure. Each x-ray will take only a few minutes, but the actual duration will depend on the number of x-rays required.

Patient preparation and aftercare—No specific preparation is needed. Patients are often in pain during this time and should be adequately medicated with analgesics if possible. Patients with arthritis may have difficulty lying flat on hard surfaces or reaching desired positions for x-ray. Additional time and gentleness are required, and additional help may be indicated. No specific aftercare is needed.

Arthrography

Purpose—Arthrography involves radiographic examination of a joint after the injection of dye or air. It outlines soft tissue structures and identifies acute or chronic tears in the joint capsule or ligaments and the presence of cysts.

Procedure—The joint is cleansed, and the surface tissue is anesthetized. Fluid may be aspirated from the joint, and then dye is inserted into the joint space. A series of x-ray films is taken with the joint in various positions. If a tear is present, the dye will leak out of the joint.

Patient preparation and aftercare—Teaching is the primary pretest preparation. The patient is reassured that the joint is anesthetized, but a feeling of pressure or a tingling sensation may be experienced as the dye is injected. It is important to assess for a history of hypersensitivity to dyes, iodine, local anesthetics, or seafood. The patient is instructed to rest the joint for at least 12 hours after the test, and it may be wrapped in an Ace bandage. Some swelling and discomfort may be present for the first 2 days. Ice and analgesics should be sufficient to ensure comfort.

Bone Scan

Purpose—A bone scan permits imaging of the skeleton after the injection of a radioactive compound. The

TABLE 15-1   Blood and Urine Tests for Diagnosis of the Musculoskeletal System

NORMAL RANGE	SIGNIFICANCE OF RESULTS
BLOOD TESTS	
Calcium	
8.0-10.5 mg/dl or 4.5-5.5 mEq/L	Hypercalcemia
	Immobility and bone demineralization cause elevated serum levels as calcium is drawn out of bone; metastatic bone cancer, hyperparathyroidism, Addison's disease
	Hypocalcemia
	Rickets, vitamin D deficiency, osteomalacia, renal failure, hypoparathyroidism, pancreatitis
Phosphorus	
2.5-4.0 mg/dl	Hyperphosphatemia
	Inverse relationship between calcium and phosporus levels; examples: hypocalcemia, renal failure, hypoparathyroidism, and bony metastasis
	Hypophosphatemia
	Inadequate ingestion, chronic antacid ingestion (phosphate binders, e.g., Amphogel, Basaljel), hypercalcemia, hyperparathyroidism, osteomalacia, rickets
Alkaline Phosphatase	
30-90 IU/L	Elevated
	Metastatic bone cancer, osteomalacia, Paget's disease, rickets
	Decreased
	Hypophosphatemia
Serum Muscle Enzymes	
Aspartate aminotransferase (AST; formerly serum glutamic oxaloacetic transaminase [SGOT]) 10-50 mU/ml	Elevated
	Skeletal muscle trauma, primary myopathic diseases
Aldolase 1.3-8.2 U/dl	Elevated
	Polymyositis, muscular dystrophy
Creatine kinase (CK_3) 15-150 IU/L	Elevated
	Muscle trauma, progressive muscular dystrophy
Lactic dehydrogenase (LDH) 60-150 IU/L	Elevated
	Skeletal muscle necrosis, extensive cancer, muscular dystrophy
Erythrocyte Sedimentation Rate	
Men: 0-15 mm/hr	Elevated
Women: 0-20 mm/hr	Inflammation, infection, or cancer (Westergren's method)
Antinuclear Antibody (ANA)	
No ANA detected	Presence
	Helpful in diagnosis of connective tissue diseases, such as systemic lupus erythematosus (SLE), scleroderma
Rheumatoid Factor	
Negative: <60 U/ml	Presence
	Titrations of these antibodies of 1:40 usually accompany rheumatoid arthritis or SLE
URINE TEST	
24-Hour Uric Acid	
250-750 ml/24 hr	Elevated
	Gout

isotope collects at sites of abnormal metabolism and can identify cancerous and metastatic disease and inflammatory and degenerative disorders.

Procedure—The patient receives an injection of radioactive technetium or gallium, and then after an interval of about 2 to 3 hours, the body is passed through a scanner that detects the low-level radiation from the skeleton and translates it into a film or chart. The scan itself takes about 1 hour. "Hot" spots on the scan indicate areas of increased bone activity, and "cold" spots indicate areas with no bone metabolic activity.

Patient preparation and aftercare—Careful pretest teaching includes reassurance that the brief half-life of the isotope presents no danger from radioactivity. A signed consent is usually obtained. No special pretest preparation is required, but the patient is encouraged to drink four to six glasses of water in the interval after injection of the isotope before the scan. The patient must remain still during the scan. No special aftercare is required, but the injection site is monitored for redness or hematoma.

Myelography

Purpose—Myelography involves the injection of a radiopaque solution into the arachnoid space of the spine and allows for visualization of the structures of the spinal canal. It is used to identify lesions such as herniated disks, nerve root involvement, spinal stenosis, and tumors.

Procedure—A local anesthetic is injected before the needle is inserted. Approximately 10 ml of cerebrospinal fluid (CSF) is drawn off, and the contrast medium is injected. Either an oil-based (Pantopaque) or a water-based (metrizamide, Omnipaque) contrast medium is used. The viscosity of the oil-based solutions creates excellent contrast, but they must be removed after the test and they can trigger arachnoiditis and severe headache. Water-based solutions are absorbed into the CSF and do not need to be removed. They cause fewer adverse effects. The x-ray table is moved and tilted to allow the dye to completely fill the spinal canal as films are taken. The test takes about 1 hour to complete.

Patient preparation and aftercare—Thorough patient education is essential before the test. The patient is usually limited to a clear liquid breakfast and assessed carefully for allergies to dyes, iodine, and shellfish. The patient is placed in a prone position. Fluids are encouraged after the test to aid in the excretion of the dye. If an oil-based dye was used the patient is kept flat in bed for approximately 8 hours. Following metrizamide use the patient is positioned with the head of bed elevated at least 30 degrees for 8 to 16 hours according to institutional policy to prevent ascension of the dye into the cranial structures. The patient is monitored for headache, nausea, vomiting, or the development of seizures. Strenuous activity is avoided for at least 24 hours. The puncture wound is monitored for edema, drainage, or other signs of infection.

Computed Tomography

Purpose—Computed tomography (CT) scanning is used in the diagnosis of the musculoskeletal system to determine the existence of primary bone and soft tissue tumors and to diagnose joint abnormalities. It may be used to evaluate the hip before joint replacement.

Procedure—The patient is placed on the radiographic table in a supine position. The table slides into the scanner, which then revolves around the patient and takes x-rays at preselected intervals. Contrast dye

may be used and a second set of x-rays taken. The images are computer integrated into a detailed mapping of the targeted tissue. The full test takes about 30 to 60 minutes.

Patient preparation and aftercare—No special pretest preparation is required beyond careful teaching about the procedure. If contrast is planned the patient is carefully assessed for allergies to dye, iodine, and shellfish. A flushed feeling and salty taste may accompany the injection of the dye. The patient must lie still during the test, and patients with claustrophobic tendencies must be warned about the confined nature of the scanner. No special posttest care is required.

Magnetic Resonance Imaging

Purpose—Magnetic resonance imaging (MRI) is used in diagnosis of the musculoskeletal system to evaluate bony and soft tissue tumors, identify changes in bone marrow composition, and identify spinal disorders. Since bone contains little hydrogen it cannot be visualized well, but bone marrow has an extremely bright signal and visualizes very well.

Procedure—The patient is placed on a narrow table that is moved into the scanner tunnel. While the patient lies within the strong magnetic field, the targeted area is stimulated with high-frequency radio waves. The resulting energy changes in the sites are measured and transformed by the computer into images that provide clear tomographic views through the tissue. The test takes about 90 minutes.

Patient preparation and aftercare—No special pretest preparation is required except careful patient teaching. The patient is reassured that the test is painless and involves no radiation exposure. The patient is informed that the opening into the scanner is deep and narrow, and the patient should be assessed for claustrophobic tendencies. The noises of the scanner can be quite loud from the inside, and earplugs are generally available. All metallic objects must be removed, and patients with artificial joints, valves, or pacemakers cannot have the test. The patient must lie still during the test. No posttest care is needed.

BIOPSIES

Biopsies of tissues from a variety of organs may be helpful in diagnosing diseases and disorders of the musculoskeletal system. Examples of common biopsies are summarized in Box 15-3.

Joint Aspiration

Purpose—A joint may be aspirated to obtain a sample of synovial fluid for analysis to aid in the differential diagnosis of arthritis, identify the cause of joint effusion, relieve pain, or administer local therapy such as corticosteroids.

Procedure—The skin is carefully cleansed over the planned puncture site, and a local anesthetic is admin-

BOX
15-3
Musculoskeletal System Biopsies

SKIN (PUNCH BIOPSY)
Used for immunofluorescent staining indicating the presence of rheumatic disease, e.g., scleroderma, SLE

MUSCLE
Used for histochemical staining indicating lower motor neuron disease, degeneration, inflammatory reaction, or primary myopathic disease

SYNOVIUM
Used for histologic examination to differentiate various forms of arthritis

BONE
Used for microscopic analysis to confirm presence of neoplasm or infection

istered. The needle is inserted into the joint space, and as much fluid as possible is aspirated from it.

Patient preparation and aftercare—The procedure is carefully explained to the patient. There is usually no special pretest preparation. The patient is informed that despite the anesthetic, pain is commonly experienced when the needle is inserted. Ice packs may be used after the test to control swelling and discomfort. The joint is supported with pillows, and an elastic wrap may be applied. Normal activity may be resumed after the test, but the patient should avoid strenuous activity for several days. The joint should be monitored carefully for pain, swelling, drainage, or the development of fever that could indicate infection.

ARTHROSCOPY

Purpose—Arthroscopy involves the visual examination of the interior of a joint with an endoscope. It is used to diagnose structural problems, monitor the progress of disease, and perform joint surgery. The knee is the joint examined most often.

Procedure—Arthroscopic techniques vary, but patients are generally placed in a supine position. The joint is carefully prepped and then positioned with the aid of pneumatic wraps and tourniquets to drain as much blood from the area as possible. Local anesthetic is administered. The arthroscope is inserted through a 3 to 5 mm incision, and the examination and/or surgery is performed.

Patient preparation and aftercare—Patient teaching about the procedure is the key component of patient preparation. The patient is generally instructed to fast after midnight before the test. The patient may begin to walk immediately after the test but should avoid any excess use of the joint. The duration and extent of immobilization depend completely on the nature of the treatment performed. The incision is monitored for swelling, increased pain, and inflamma-

tion. Analgesics are provided for routine posttest discomfort.

MUSCULOSKELETAL SYSTEM TRAUMA
FRACTURES
Etiology/Epidemiology

Bone fractures are one of the most common problems of the musculoskeletal system, and trauma is the most common cause. It is estimated that 1 in 10 persons experiences an acute injury to the musculoskeletal system. In addition to fracture these injuries may include damage to soft tissues, muscles, ligaments, tendons, or joints. Although fracture can and does occur at any age the highest incidence occurs in the 15- to 24-year-old group and then again in persons over 65 years. Fractures in elderly persons typically involve normal activity or minimal trauma in a bone weakened by osteoporosis or other disease. Some of the many ways to classify fractures are described in Box 15-4.

Pathophysiology

A bone is fractured when there is a complete or partial interruption of the osseous tissue. Any force significant enough to cause a bone fracture may also injure the surrounding muscles, nerves, ligaments, tendons, blood vessels, and soft tissues. The immobilization necessary for bone healing may produce additional problems. Immobilization of a fractured bone is essential for proper healing to take place.

Bone healing occurs by a process known as callus, or new bone, formation. This is a multistage process that begins with hematoma formation at the fractured bone ends. Gradually this hematoma transforms into a fibrous

BOX
15-4
Types of Fractures

Complete Bone is completely separated, producing two fragments.
Incomplete There is a partial break in the bone without separation.
Simple or closed Bone is broken; skin is intact.
Compound or open Fracture parts extend through the skin.
Fracture without displacement Bone is broken; bone fragments are in alignment in normal position.
Fracture with displacement Bone fragments have separated at the point of fracture.
Comminuted Bone has broken into several fragments.
Impacted (telescoped) One bone fragment is forcibly driven into another.
Greenstick Fracture is limited to splintering of one side of the bone (occurs most often in children with soft bones).
Transverse Break is across the bone.
Oblique Line of fracture is at an oblique angle to the bone shaft.
Spiral Line of fracture encircles the bone.

BOX 15-5	Fat Emboli

Fat embolism syndrome is a potentially fatal complication of fracture. It occurs most commonly following fracture of the long bones (femur and tibia) and the pelvis. It occurs within 24 to 48 hours in most cases. The incidence is 0.5% to 2% after long bone fracture and 5% to 10% after multiple fractures.

PATHOPHYSIOLOGY

Fat globules are released from the bone marrow into the circulation and travel to the lungs where they can embolize the small capillaries and arterioles. Lipase is released to break down the globules into fatty acids, but the chemical action is irritating and causes edema, interstitial hemorrhage, and an increase in alveolar capillary membrane permeability. Adult respiratory distress syndrome may result.

SYMPTOMS

Dyspnea, tachypnea, and hypoxemia
Petechiae: considered to be a "classic" symptom but only occurs in 50% to 60%; appear on chest, neck, axilla, and conjunctiva possibly from capillary occlusion
Altered mental status: critical indicator, occurs in over 75% of patients; restlessness, confusion, lethargy, and coma possible
Fever
Chest pain

MANAGEMENT

Critical care monitoring
Oxygen therapy
Mechanical ventilation with positive end-expiratory pressure (PEEP)
Steroid administration (controversial)

BOX 15-6	Compartment Syndrome

Compartment syndrome occurs after fracture when pressure increases within a tissue to the point where it compromises circulation and viability of the tissue. If unrecognized and untreated, it can lead to loss of function, deformity, or even amputation. Pressure can increase from anything that causes either an increase in mass of the contents or a decrease in size. Restrictive dressings or casts are possible causes, but following fracture the syndrome develops most often in a fascia compartment.

PATHOPHYSIOLOGY

The body contains 46 compartments: regions of muscles, nerves, and blood vessels surrounded by a nonelastic covering (Figure 15-2). Thirty-eight of these compartments are found in the extremities, including four in the lower leg and two in the forearm. When edema occurs after trauma, the inelastic fascia cannot expand sufficiently to accommodate it, and pressure within the compartment rises. The blood flow is decreased, and hypoxia occurs. Histamine is released to promote vasodilation, and the ischemia worsens. Ischemic changes can occur within 4-12 hours and neuropathic changes within 12-24 hours.

SYMPTOMS

Pain
  Severe and unrelenting
  Unrelieved by analgesics
  Worsened by movement or elevation of the part
  Greater than expected for the injury
Hypesthesia or paresthesias
Muscular weakness or paralysis
NOTE: Skin color, capillary refill, coolness, and quality of peripheral pulses are unreliable parameters. They are typically present only when extensive and possibly irreversible damage is present.

MANAGEMENT

Prompt diagnosis is the key, and monitoring is critical in high-risk patients. If the patient's mental status is compromised, invasive pressure monitoring may be initiated. Early compartment syndrome may be relieved by splitting dressings or bivalving casts, but more severe cases will require surgical intervention with fasciotomy to open the affected compartments. Secondary closure is performed later in the healing process.

---

network with calcium deposits, new bone formation, and destruction of dead bone. Optimal bone healing may be impeded by poor approximation of the fracture fragments, excessive edema at the site, infection, or necrosis of the bone. Delayed union or nonunion occurs in about 5% of all fractures. Nonunion represents a condition where healing does not occur after 6 to 9 months.

The clinical manifestations of fracture depend on the bones involved and the degree of accompanying tissue damage. Classic symptoms include pain, loss of function, edema, presence of obvious deformity, and crepitus or a grating sound with movement.

Bone fractures may be complicated by the development of fat emboli or compartment syndrome. These acute problems are described in Boxes 15-5 and 15-6.

Medical Management

The diagnosis of fracture is established from the presenting symptoms and confirmed by x-ray. The cornerstone of medical treatment of fractures is the realignment of the bony fragments of the fracture plus immobilization to allow healing to occur. Depending on the severity and the location of the fracture, medical management may involve reduction and realignment with either a cast or traction.

Reduction and fixation may be either external or internal. External fixation (closed reduction) involves manual realignment of the fractured bone parts, which is verified by x-ray. Internal fixation (open reduction) employs direct operative visualization and realignment of the bone parts. It frequently involves the use of pins, plates, screws, wires, or prostheses, as well as surgical debridement of the wound.

Immobilization of the repaired fracture may be accomplished with a splint, cast, or traction device.

Traction involves the application of a continuous pull on a bone and surrounding tissue to reduce and immobilize the fracture, overcome muscle spasm, and correct deformities. There are numerous forms of traction. Most fit into one of the categories in Box 15-7.

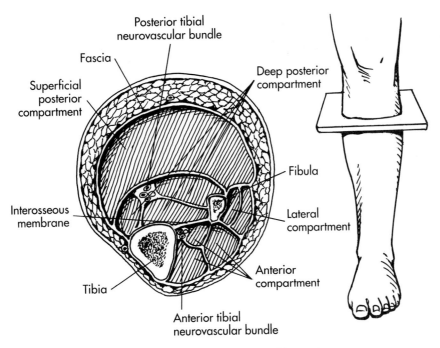

FIGURE 15-2 Compartments of lower leg.

BOX 15-7	**Types of Traction**

Skin traction   Traction is applied to the skin through moleskin or adhesive, and the traction weight is applied indirectly to the bone through the skin (examples: Buck's, Russell, pelvic).
Skeletal traction   Traction is applied directly to the bone through the insertion of wires or pins usually positioned distally to the fracture site (examples: overhead arm, balanced suspension).
Running traction   Direct pull is applied without support of the part (examples: Buck's, cervical).
Balanced traction   Direct pull on the part is applied with the extremity supported in a splint and held in place with balanced counterweights (examples: Thomas splint with Pearson attachment).

External fixation devices consisting of metal struts attached to pins inserted into bone (Box 15-8) may be used to provide rigid fixation of a complex fracture while still allowing the patient some degree of mobility. Patients with external fixators can be out of bed and even ambulate without weight bearing.

NURSING MANAGEMENT

◆ ASSESSMENT
Subjective Data

History of trauma
Health history for conditions that may influence healing and treatment
Degree of pain, weakness
Loss of sensation or movement

BOX 15-8	**External Fixation Devices**

ADVANTAGES

Enhances fracture healing by ensuring excellent stability at the fracture site
Allows for improved visibility of injury and access for assessment and wound care
Permits greatly increased patient mobility
Particularly valuable with extremely complex fractures

DISADVANTAGES

Pins can dislodge with excessive use of part
Risk of refracture with weak bone once apparatus is removed

POSSIBLE COMPLICATIONS

Neurovascular or muscular damage from pins
Infection at pin sites
Body image disturbance from visibility of device

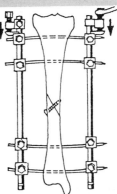

FIGURE 15-3 External fixation device on tibial fracture.

BOX 15-9	Cast Options

PLASTER OF PARIS

Dries slowly
Heavy
Loses strength and integrity if it gets wet
Removed and reapplied if revision needed
Inexpensive to use

FIBERGLASS OR PLASTIC

Dries quickly
Lightweight
Maintains strength when wet
Can be reheated and remolded for revision
Expensive to use
   All three types of cast materials are available as rolled bandages and are applied over the part in much the same way as an Ace bandage. Plaster is immersed in water before application.

Objective Data

Loss of function, obvious deformity
Swelling and discoloration
Presence of bleeding or tissue damage
Baseline vital signs, neurocirculatory data
Crepitus (grating sound) with movement

◆ NURSING DIAGNOSES

Nursing diagnoses for the person with a fracture may include, but are not limited to, the following:
Pain (related to bone displacement and muscle spasm)
Altered peripheral tissue perfusion, high risk for (related to edema and cast constriction)
Mobility, impaired physical (related to presence of cast or traction)
Impairment of skin integrity, high risk for (related to trauma, cast irritation, skeletal traction, or immobility)
Knowledge deficit (related to the correct use of ambulatory assistive devices)

◆ EXPECTED PATIENT OUTCOMES

Patient will experience minimal discomfort from fracture once reduction and realignment have been completed.
Patient will maintain adequate circulation and nerve conduction to areas distal to cast or traction setup.
Patient will continue maximal activity level permitted by treatment.
Patient's skin will remain intact; tissue injuries will heal without infection or complications.
Patient will demonstrate the correct use of canes, crutches, walkers, or other self-help devices.

◆ NURSING INTERVENTIONS
Promoting Comfort

Administer narcotic analgesics as prescribed.
   Assess frequently for effectiveness.
   Explore the use of patient-controlled analgesia (PCA) or epidural catheter, because orthopedic pain is severe.
   NOTE: Pain should decrease after fracture is realigned and tissue damage resolves.
Administer ice compresses as ordered.
   Protect cast (if present) from moisture.
Reposition patient frequently for comfort.

Monitoring Peripheral Tissue Perfusion

Perform and record neurovascular checks hourly after the fracture repair for at least 24 hours and then each shift unless a more frequent schedule is ordered (Table 15-2):
Circulatory status:
   Palpate for warmth
   Observe color
   Assess capillary refill
   Palpate accessible pulses
   Evaluate severity of swelling

TABLE 15-2	Observations* for Signs and Symptoms of Neurocirculatory Impairment
OBSERVATION	**INTERPRETATION**
Tissue color white	Decreased arterial blood supply
Tissue color blue	Venous stasis and poorly oxygenated tissue
Color slow to return to nail bed after application of moderate pressure	Decreased arterial blood supply
Edema	Fluid accumulating in tissues; poor venous return
Tissue cold or cool to touch	Decreased arterial blood supply
Patient unable to move parts distal to injury or external fixation device	Pressure on nerves innervating parts distal to injury or underlying external fixation device
Patient complaint of extreme pain unrelieved by elevation, analgesic, or repositioning	Pressure on nerves innervating parts distal to injury or underlying external fixation device
Patient complaint of heightened or decreased sensation or paresthesia in part distal to injury or underlying external fixation device	Pressure on nerves innervating parts distal to injury or underlying external fixation device

*Comparison of tissue should be made with uninvolved limb to determine extent of deviation from normal.

Neurologic status:

    Assess degree and character of pain

    Assess sensation, presence of paresthesias

    Assess ability to move parts distal to the fracture

Elevate affected extremity above the level of the heart

Preventing Complications of Immobility

Prepare bed with firm mattress and overbed trapeze.

    Teach patient to transfer safely and move comfortably in bed.

Ensure a daily fluid intake of 2500 to 3000 ml.

Adjust diet.

    Reduce calories.

    Ensure enriched protein and limited calcium.

    Increase fiber content.

    Administer stool softeners or bulk-forming laxatives.

Encourage hourly deep breathing and coughing as needed.

Assess for signs of deep vein thrombosis.

    Check for positive Homans' sign.

    Administer one aspirin twice daily if ordered or low-dose subcutaneous heparin.

    Check for calf and thigh circumference changes.

Encourage patient to remain active within the limits of the cast or traction apparatus.

Teach range of motion and isometric exercises to uninvolved extremities.

Provide patient with age-appropriate diversions and assess for sleep or sensory disturbances.

Maintaining Skin Integrity

Prepare bed with 3-inch foam mattress.

Inspect skin at least once per shift for signs of irritation.

Turn and reposition patient frequently within the limits of activity restrictions.

Avoid shearing forces when assisting patient to change positions.

    Provide additional protection for elbows and heels as needed.

Assist patient to keep skin clean and dry.

Provide routine back care and massage each shift.

Clean cast application debris from skin, and petal cast margins with stockinette to prevent abrasion (Box 15-10).

    A nail file can be used to smooth edges of fiberglass casts.

Provide pin care as ordered:

    Inspect pin insertion sites each shift.

    Cleanse sites with saline, peroxide, or povidone-iodine (Betadine) solution if ordered.

    Use antibiotic ointments and dry sterile dressings if ordered.

Promoting Safe Ambulation

Teach patient techniques for safe transfers.

Ensure proper fit of crutches:

BOX 15-10   Cast Care

Support fresh cast on pillows until dry. Place absorbent material beneath cast until dry.

Use flat of hand to move cast if necessary—do not embed fingers. Support at normal joint positions.

Allow free air circulation for drying; do not use heat lamps or hot hair dryers. Drying plaster casts generate heat.

Change patient's position frequently to aid drying process.

Do not tightly cover cast with any substance (cloth, paint, varnish). Skin breathes through porous plaster.

Inspect skin at margins of cast for redness and irritation.

Use creams and lotions sparingly.

Protect casts exposed to body excretions with waterproof material around perineal area. Remove soiling with scouring powder on a damp cloth.

Teach patient to report any symptoms of burning beneath the cast.

Note any odor that may indicate necrotic tissue or infection.

Teach patient to keep cast clean and dry and not put foreign objects into the cast for scratching.

BOX 15-11   Common Crutch-Walking Gaits

WEIGHT BEARING

Two-point gait—crutch on one side moves forward simultaneously with opposite leg; same motion is repeated on other side.

Four-point gait—two-point gait is broken down and performed more slowly. Crutch is placed and then followed by the opposite leg. Both motions are then repeated with the opposite side.

Swing-through gait—both crutches are moved forward together, then both legs are swung past the crutches by lifting both lower limbs.

NON–WEIGHT BEARING

Three-point gait—both crutches are moved forward together. Then the body swings forward to that position by lifting placed leg. Second limb is held off the ground at all times.

Two to three finger widths between the axilla and top of the crutch when crutch is in a normal support position

Padded hand grips and axillary bars

Rubber tips on the crutches

Hand grip positioned so elbow is flexed no more than 30 degrees

Teach safe use of crutches (Box 15-11):

    Flat-heeled, rubber-soled shoes at all times

    Home preparation:

        Removal of scatter rugs

        Furniture repositioning to allow clear pathways

        Safety devices in bathroom as needed, such as raised toilet seat, grab bars

    Avoid "hopping."

> ### Guidelines for Nursing Care of the Person in Traction
>
> Inspect traction apparatus frequently:
> Ropes are running straight and through the middle of the pulleys.
> Weights are hanging freely.
> Sheets, blankets, and bed are not interfering with traction line.
> Do not release or alter traction weights.
> Avoid bumping or jarring bed.
> Encourage patient to use trapeze to alter position and relieve pressure on skin of sacrum and scapulae.
> Check for irritation around groin or heels if balanced skeletal traction is in use.

> ### BOX 15-12 Sequential Compression Device
>
> The sequential compression device (SCD) is an important adjunct to routine measures for preventing deep vein thrombosis. Its components include the following:
> Plastic leg sleeves with air chambers
> Plastic tubing
> Electric motor
> The leg sleeves are wrapped around the patient's legs and secured with a Velcro closure. Air is pumped into the air chambers at controlled pressure gradients—greater at the ankle and decreasing toward the top of the thigh. The device substitutes for the normal muscle pump of active movement by alternately filling and then decompressing, thereby supporting venous return. The therapy is continued until the patient is ambulatory.

Exercise the quadriceps, gluteal, and triceps muscles for needed strength for walking.

Ensure correct use of cane: held in hand *opposite* the weak part.

♦ EVALUATION

Successful achievement of expected outcomes for the patient with a fracture is indicated by the following:
Statements that pain is minimal or absent
Evidence of adequate circulation and nerve conduction to affected areas
Maintenance of allowable activity and self-care activities without evidence of complications
Presence of an intact skin
Safe ambulation with assistive devices as ordered

HIP FRACTURE
Etiology/Epidemiology

Fractures of the hip are one of the most common fractures treated in the hospital. Over 200,000 hip fractures occur annually, and the number is expected to increase dramatically as the number of elderly persons continues to rise. Repair of hip fracture is the most common surgical procedure performed in elderly persons. Aging and the incidence of osteoporosis are the most significant factors, and the incidence is much greater in women. The hospital stay is often complicated by concurrent chronic illnesses and complications. Up to 30% of patients die within the year, and 30% to 50% never regain their preinjury level of functioning.

Pathophysiology

Fractures of the hip generally fall into two categories. Intracapsular fractures occur within the hip joint and capsule. Extracapsular fractures occur outside the capsule to an area 2 inches below the lesser trochanter. The fracture is rarely the result of significant trauma. Patients typically report fracture following simple movements such as stepping off a curb or stairs.

Blood is supplied to the femoral head through the neck of the femur and may be disrupted in an intracapsular fracture. Avascular necrosis of the head can result.

Classic symptoms of hip fracture include pain at the fracture site, inability to move the affected leg, and shortening with external rotation of the affected leg.

Medical Management

Hip fracture is generally diagnosed from the presenting symptoms and confirmed by x-ray. The treatment of choice is surgical repair, which allows for early mobilization of the patient. Either pinning with screws, nails, and pins or prosthetic replacement of the femoral head and neck is the usual approach. The site of the fracture, condition of the bone, and adequacy of the blood supply to the hip will dictate the approach and device used. Patient management for both treatments is similar. Surgery may be delayed while the patient's overall health status is evaluated. Buck's traction is frequently employed to relieve pain and muscle spasm before surgery (Box 15-13).

NURSING MANAGEMENT

♦ ASSESSMENT
Subjective Data

Circumstances of the injury
Current general health and chronic illnesses
Mental status
Severity of pain and muscle spasm
Understanding of injury and proposed treatment

Objective Data

Presence of classic symptoms
Affected leg shortened, externally rotated

BOX 15-13   **Buck's Traction**

Buck's traction is commonly used in the preoperative period after a hip fracture. The displaced femur triggers severe flexion spasms in the quadriceps and other muscles of the leg, which are extremely painful. Buck's traction stabilizes the fracture and provides for some countertraction to the flexion pull of the muscles, reducing spasm (Figure 15-4).

Commercial foam rubber extension splints are widely available and easy to use. The affected leg is placed in the splint and secured with Velcro straps. A foot plate is attached for connection to the traction weight, which should not exceed 8 pounds. As with all forms of traction, the weight should hang freely and in alignment, and the affected extremity should be checked regularly for signs of neurovascular or skin impairment.

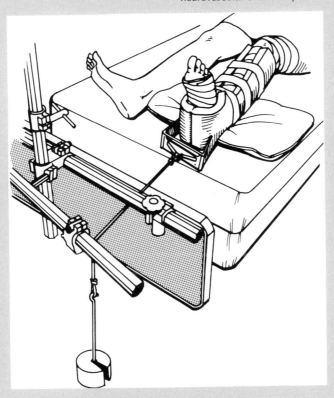

FIGURE 15-4   Buck's traction

Ability to move extremity, if any
   Presence of crepitus
Ability to urinate
Baseline systems review

The remainder of the nursing management for the patient undergoing surgical repair for a fractured hip is presented in the "Nursing Care Plan." A "Critical Pathway" for the same treatment is provided.

SOFT TISSUE TRAUMA

Trauma frequently involves the soft tissue structures as well as the bones. Injuries to ligaments and tendons occur most frequently in the knee, especially in active and contact sports. Blows, twisting, and severe stretching are the most common predisposing events. Pain, swelling, and loss of function are the most identifiable features. Strains involve the muscles and usually occur from overuse of the muscle beyond its intended or functional ability. The back is a particularly vulnerable location. Sprains involve the joint, usually as a result of a twisting force that may tear the joint capsule, and can result in dislocation or subluxation. The ankle is by far the most common site and is associated with running or contact sports. Pain, swelling, and loss of function are again the primary symptoms of strains and sprains.

Most soft tissue injuries can be adequately treated with first aid measures. The RICE approach is widely accepted; it includes *r*est of the injured part; *i*ce for at least 48 to 72 hours to control edema; *c*ompression through elastic bandages, splints, or casts; and *e*levation of the part to a level slightly above the heart. More definitive corrective measures, including surgical repair, may be needed if the injury does not promptly respond to this standard regimen.

NURSING CARE PLAN

THE PATIENT WITH A HIP FRACTURE REPAIRED BY OPEN REDUCTION AND INTERNAL FIXATION BY PROSTHETIC IMPLANT

■ NURSING DIAGNOSIS

Pain (related to displaced fracture, muscle spasm, or surgical procedure)

Expected Patient Outcome	Nursing Interventions
Patient will report decrease or absence of pain and spasm after administration of analgesics or other pain relief measures.	1. Assess and record patient's pain level hourly until controlled effectively. 2. Administer analgesics as ordered and evaluate response to comfort measures provided. a. NOTE: Elderly patients are frequently undermedicated, especially in the preoperative period. 3. Apply Buck's traction in the preoperative period to control muscle spasm. 4. Use other pain-relieving techniques as appropriate, for example, back rubs, repositioning. 5. Teach relaxation techniques as appropriate.

■ NURSING DIAGNOSIS

Mobility, impaired physical (related to fracture, traction, and non–weight bearing status in the postoperative period)

Expected Patient Outcomes	Nursing Interventions

Patient will demonstrate optimal level of mobility with adaptive devices within prescribed limitations of activity by time of discharge.
Patient will be free from complications associated with immobility.
	1. Preoperative: elevate the head of the bed no more than 45 degrees.
	2. Determine from physician the limits of movement and weight bearing permitted in the postoperative period. General guidelines include the following:
	  a. Maintain abduction of affected leg with splints or pillows at all times (Figure 15-5). Avoid any adduction beyond midline.
	  b. Turn patient from back to unoperated side every 2 hours and PRN.
	    (1) Avoid positioning patient on operative side, and observe flexion restrictions when elevating the head of the bed.
	    (2) Avoid flexion beyond 60 degrees during hospitalization.
	    (3) Elevate sitting surface with pillows to keep angle of hip within prescribed limits.
	  c. When turning the patient, hold the operative leg in abduction; use pillows to maintain 30-degree abduction when turning is accomplished.
	  d. Use trochanter rolls to prevent external rotation. Avoid any extreme internal or external rotation.
	  e. Assist patient to walk using the appropriate ambulatory aid. Be-

NURSING CARE PLAN—CONT'D

THE PATIENT WITH A HIP FRACTURE REPAIRED BY OPEN REDUCTION AND INTERNAL FIXATION BY PROSTHETIC IMPLANT

Expected Patient Outcomes	Nursing Interventions
	gin walking the first or second postoperative day, and increase the frequency and distance of ambulation as tolerated.

    (1) Restrict to partial weight bearing on affected side for 2-3 months.

    (2) Teach patient quadriceps and gluteal set exercises for strengthening the muscles of ambulation.

    (3) Work with physical therapy plan to teach safe ambulation, transfer techniques, and range of motion.

    (4) Always transfer patient toward the strong side and support the strong side. Be sure that sufficient help is available.

3. Utilize aggressive general measures to prevent the complications of immobility. Monitor patient for signs of atelectasis, wound infection, skin breakdown, DVT (deep vein thrombosis), or pulmonary embolus.

    a. Encourage hourly deep breathing and coughing.

    b. Apply TED stocking or sequential compression device (See Box 15-12) to unaffected leg.

    c. Assess for urinary retention or stasis.

    d. Use fracture pan for voiding or insert Foley catheter if patient is unable to void.

    e. Provide raised toilet seat when patient is ambulatory.

    f. Monitor back and sacrum for signs of pressure.

    g. Use deep foam mattresses or other device as appropriate.

    h. Use heel pads and other protective pads as necessary.

    i. Monitor bowel elimination pattern. Give prescribed stool softeners, suppositories, or laxatives.

        (1) Encourage high-fiber foods in diet.

        (2) Encourage fluid intake of 2000-3000 ml/day.

    j. Encourage patient to remain active in self-care.

    k. Provide meaningful stimuli to keep patient oriented and hopeful about the future.

Continued.

NURSING CARE PLAN—CONT'D

THE PATIENT WITH A HIP FRACTURE REPAIRED BY OPEN REDUCTION AND INTERNAL FIXATION BY PROSTHETIC IMPLANT

■ NURSING DIAGNOSIS

Injury or infection, risk for (related to surgical procedure and decreased mobility)

Expected Patient Outcome	Nursing Interventions
Patient will not experience neurocirculatory complications. Wound will heal without infection. Hip will remain in alignment.	1. Perform neurocirculatory checks every 2 hours for the first 24-48 hours. Notify physician of any changes from preoperative status. 2. Notify physician if patient complains of sudden onset of increased pain, especially groin pain, particularly if accompanied by deformity or external rotation. 3. Assess incision for signs or symptoms of infection or excessive drainage. a. Maintain patency of Hemovac or other wound drainage system.

■ NURSING DIAGNOSIS

Impaired home maintenance management, risk of (related to lack of knowledge of postdischarge regimen or lack of adequate support systems)

Expected Patient Outcomes	Nursing Interventions

Patient will correctly describe all positioning and weight-bearing restrictions.
Patient will demonstrate the correct use of a walker or crutches.
Patient and family will make safe and mutually satisfactory plans for care after discharge.
	1. Teach patient rationale for activity restrictions as prescribed by physician.
	   a. Restrict hip flexion to no more than 90 degree for 2-3 months.
	   b. Partial weight bearing.
	   c. No severe adduction, internal or external rotation.
	2. Use chairs with firm, nonreclining seats and arms.
	3. Assist patient and family to acquire equipment and supplies needed for safe self-care at home.
	4. Assist patient and family to explore resources available in community for postdischarge care.
	   a. Refer for community home health assistance or physical therapy as needed.

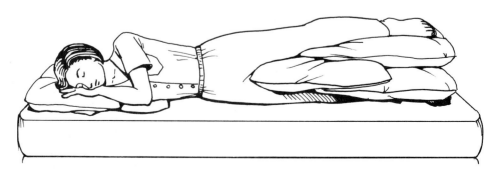

FIGURE 15-5   Pillows are staggered in a wedge-shaped arrangement to maintain abduction of the hip.

DRG #: 236; expected LOS: 7+

	Day of Admission Day 1	Day 2	Day of Surgery Day 3	Day 4	Day 5	Day 6	Day of Discharge Day 7
Diagnostic Tests	Hip and chest x-rays, CBC, UA, SMA/18,‡ T & X match, PT/PTT, ECG		Preoperative: CBC, SMA/8,§ ECG Postoperative: CBC, electrolytes, PT/PTT daily until discharge if sodium warfarin (Coumadin) prescribed	PT/PTT	PT/PTT	CBC, PT/PTT	PT/PTT
Medications	IVs; IV/IM analgesic; IV antibiotic	IVs; IV/IM analgesic; IV antibiotic	IVs; IV analgesic; anticoagulant	IV to saline lock if tolerating PO fluids, IV/IM analgesic; IV antibiotic; anticoagulant; stool softener	IV saline lock; IM/PO analgesic; discontinue antibiotic and anticoagulant; stool softener	Discontinue saline lock; analgesic; discontinue antibiotic; stool softener	PO analgesic; stool softener
Treatments	I & O q 8 hr; VS q 4 hr; Buck's traction to affected leg; neurocirculatory checks to both legs q 2 hr; skin assessment and special care q 2 hr; elastic leg stocking (ELS) to unaffected leg; pneumatic intermittent (ICD) compression devices to both lower extremities	I & O q 8 hrs; VS q 4 hr; neurocirculatory checks to both legs q 2 hr; skin assessment and special care q 2 hr; ELS; ICD	I & O and drain q 8 hr, including Foley; VS q 4 hr; discontinue traction postoperatively; neurocirculatory checks to both legs q 2 hr; check drainage on dressing q 2 hr; ELS; ICD	I & O and drain q 8 hr including Foley; VS q 6 hr; neurocirculatory checks to both legs q 4 hr; check drainage on dressing q 4 hr; ELS; ICD	DC drain at 48 degrees; I&O q 8 hr; disk; Foley, VS q 8 hr; neurocirculatory checks to both legs; ELS; ICD	I & O q 8 hr; VS q 8 hr; ELS; disc; ICD	Disc; I & O; VS q 12 hr; ELS
Diet	As tolerated	NPO p MN for morning of surgery; diet as tolerated	NPO; clear liquids postnausea or on return of bowel sounds	Advance diet as tolerated	Regular diet	Regular diet	Regular diet
Activity	Bed rest; pillow splint; trapeze on bed; C-DB q 2 hr	Bed rest; pillow splint; trapeze on bed; C-DB q 2 hr	Bed rest; trapeze with abductor pillow; C-DB q 2 hr; hip flexion limited to 90 degrees; no adduction beyond midline, minimal internal/external rotation	Bed rest, up with help and walker × 1; minimal weight bearing; ROM to unaffected side	Up with help and walker × 3, minimal weight bearing; ROM to unaffected side; up in chair as tolerated	Up with help and walker × 4, minimal weight bearing; ROM to unaffected side	Up with walker × 4, minimal weight bearing; ROM to unaffected side
Consultations	PT; social service; other specialists as needed for other medical problems; medical clearance for surgery		PT‖	PT¶; dietary	Rehabilitation/SNU/home health PT	PT	

NOTE: Acknowledge that patients recover at varying rates; therefore specified daily actions should be based solely on patient need.

*Type of prosthesis will affect postoperative course. Critical pathway is based on bipolar type of prosthesis.

†Some patients may be admitted to hospital and undergo surgery the same day, which will decrease LOS to 5 days.

‡Serum calcium, phosphorus, triglycerides, uric acid, creatinine, BUN, total bilirubin, alkaline phosphatase, aspartate aminotransferase (AST) (formerly serum glutamic oxaloacetic transaminase [SGOT]), alanine aminotransferase (ALT) (formerly serum glutamic pyruvic transaminase [SGPT]), lactic dehydrogenase (LDH), total protein, albumin, sodium, potassium, chloride, total CO_2, glucose.

§Serum sodium, potassium, chloride, total CO_2, glucose, BUN.

‖ORIF (open reduction, internal fixation) with nail, plate does not require abduction pillow or positioning restrictions.

¶Weight-bearing status depends on type of implant and use of methylmethacrylate.

THE DISEASES OF ARTHRITIS
RHEUMATOID ARTHRITIS/OSTEOARTHRITIS
Etiology/Epidemiology

The term *arthritis* literally means "problems with the joint" and can be used to describe over 100 separate forms of rheumatic diseases. It is estimated that arthritis affects over 20 million people in the United States at an annual cost of billions of dollars. Rheumatoid arthritis and osteoarthritis are by far the most frequently occurring forms of the disease.

Rheumatoid arthritis is a chronic, systemic inflammatory disease characterized by recurrent inflammation in joints and related structures that can result in crippling deformities. It is more prevalent in women than men by a 2:1 to 3:1 ratio and usually appears during the young adult years. Rheumatoid arthritis primarily affects proximal joints, although virtually any joint can become involved. Involvement is usually bilaterally symmetric. Lesions of the vasculature, lungs, and other major organs also occur.

The etiology of the disease remains unknown, but it is theorized to be an autoimmune process involving an altered immune response to an unknown antigen. Prolonged exposure to the antigen causes normal antibodies to become autoantibodies that attack host tissues and form immune complexes in the blood and synovial membrane.

Osteoarthritis or degenerative joint disease is a slow, progressive, noninflammatory, chronic disease primarily affecting the weight-bearing joints. It is characterized by pain, stiffness, and limitation of motion. Most prevalent in the 50- to 70-year-old group, it is believed to be a degenerative process that accompanies aging but can occur secondary to trauma or excess strain. Osteoarthritis is estimated to affect over 17 million individuals seriously enough to cause pain.

Table 15-3 compares the major characteristics of the two disease processes.

Pathophysiology

The disease process of rheumatoid arthritis begins with synovial inflammation with edema, congestion, and fibrin exudate. Continued inflammation produces synovial thickening and formation of pannus where it joins the articular cartilage, interfering with the nutrition of the cartilage, which may become necrotic. Pannus also invades the subchondral bone and soft tissue structures and may destroy them. The destruction of cartilage and bone and the weakening of tendons and ligaments can lead to dislocation, subluxation, and ankylosis. The destructive process can progress to joint deformities, including subluxation, varus and valgus deformities, ulnar drift, swan neck, boutonniere, and Z deformities (described on p. 346).

Early disease manifestations may include low-grade fever, fatigue, and generalized aching. Early morning

TABLE 15-3 Differential Characteristics Between Rheumatoid Arthritis and Osteoarthritis	
RHEUMATOID ARTHRITIS	**OSTEOARTHRITIS**
Systemic disease; people are sick with malaise, fever, fatigue	Local joint disease; no systemic symptoms
Signs of inflammation present both locally in joints and systemically as pain, fever, soreness, malaise	Inflammatory signs less prominent and local (not systemic) when present
Fingers and proximal interphalangeal joints involved more commonly	Distal interphalangeal joints involved more commonly
Subcutaneous, extraarticular (rheumatoid) nodules present in tissues around (not in) the joints in 20% of patients	No periarticular or subcutaneous nodes are present; Heberden's nodes are bony enlargements within joints
Bony ankylosis and osteoporosis common	Ankylosis and osteoporosis uncommon
Elevated sedimentation rate; elevated serum rheumatoid factors	Normal sedimentation rate and blood chemistries
Young adults to older adults are affected (25-50 yr)	Adults affected during later years (from 45 yr of age)

From Mourad L: *Nursing care of adults with orthopedic conditions,* ed 2, New York, 1988, Wiley.

joint stiffness is classic. Specific joint symptoms such as gross inflammation with joint swelling, warmth, redness, and pain may appear at the onset or later in the process. Virtually all joints can be involved, but the most common are the joints of the hands, wrists, feet, ankles, elbows, and knees. The pattern of involvement is usually bilaterally symmetric and follows a course of exacerbation and remission. Rheumatoid arthritis is accompanied by an elevated erythrocyte sedimentation rate, decreased red blood cell count, and mild elevation in white blood cell count; 50% to 90% of patients exhibit a positive rheumatoid factor. Painless subcutaneous nodules may develop near joints and along extensor surfaces of the bones.

In osteoarthritis the normally white, translucent, and smooth cartilage becomes yellow and opaque. It softens, and the surfaces become roughened, frayed, or cracked. The cartilage may be destroyed, and the underlying bone goes through a remodeling process in which osteophytes, or spurs of new bone, appear at the joint margins and the sites of attachment of supporting structures. Serologic and synovial fluid examinations have essentially normal outcomes. The disease is not systemic and creates only mild local inflammation.

Classic clinical manifestations include pain that worsens with activity and improves with rest, joint stiffness that is worst in the morning and recurs after rest periods, joint enlargement, and decreased range of motion and strength. Heberden's and Bouchard's nodes

TABLE 15-4 Surgical Interventions for Arthritis

DESCRIPTION	EXPECTED OUTCOME
SYNOVECTOMY	
Removal of synovial tissue to arrest the arthritic process in a particular joint	Maintains joint function Prevents recurrent inflammation
ARTHROTOMY	
Exploration of a joint	Drains Removes damaged tissue
ARTHROPLASTY	
Joint reconstruction by reshaping bones, replacement of all or part of a joint with prosthetic parts	Restores motion and function Relieves pain Corrects deformity
ARTHRODESIS	
Surgical fusion of joint performed to eliminate pain and provide stability	Relieves pain Improves stability Restores function
OSTEOTOMY	
Cutting a bone to change its alignment	Corrects deformity Alters weight-bearing surface to relieve pain

(see p. 346) are classic finger deformities resulting from osteophyte activity. Table 15-3 compares the major features of these two disorders.

Medical Management

The diagnosis of rheumatoid arthritis is made from the history, physical examination, x-rays, and laboratory tests. The diagnosis is confirmed by the presence of at least five specific criteria, including the pattern of pain, stiffness, and joint swelling; x-ray changes showing narrowing of joint spaces or erosion; and the presence of subcutaneous nodules, a positive rheumatoid factor, and histologic changes in the synovium. Most patients will also exhibit anemia, mild leukocytosis, and an elevated erythrocyte sedimentation rate. Osteoarthritis is diagnosed from the pattern of symptoms and x-ray evidence of narrowed joint spaces, osteophyte formation, and sclerosis of the subchondral bone.

Treatment for arthritis involves a balanced program of exercise and rest, patient education, joint protection, and control of inflammation through the use of salicylates and nonsteroidal antiinflammatory drugs. Additional medications may be needed in rheumatoid arthritis to achieve disease remission. Adjunctive therapy may include analgesics, intraarticular steroids, antidepressants, and surgery. Occupational and physical therapy may be ordered. Common surgical interventions for arthritis are described in Table 15-4. Medications that may be used in the management of arthritis are summarized in Table 15-5.

NURSING MANAGEMENT

◆ ASSESSMENT

Subjective Data

Current health status
History and management of disorder
Diet and medication history
Pain pattern and severity
Patient and family coping patterns
Complaints of fatigue, weakness, and stiffness, especially early morning and following periods of inactivity
Effects of disease on usual patterns of activities—work and recreation

Objective Data

Joint range of motion, muscle strength/atrophy, swelling
Presence of obvious joint deformities
Functional abilities for self-care—gait and ambulation, bathing, feeding, toileting activities
Presence of bony protuberance, such as Heberden's or Bouchard's nodes (osteoarthritis only)
Systemic symptoms of fever, tachycardia, weight loss, subcutaneous nodules, anemia (rheumatoid arthritis only)
Crepitus with joint movement
Presence of limp or gait alterations

◆ NURSING DIAGNOSES

Nursing diagnoses for the person with arthritis may include, but are not limited to, the following:
Pain (related to joint inflammation or degeneration)
Mobility, impaired physical (related to joint destruction and decreased muscle strength)
Self-care deficit in feeding, bathing/hygiene, dressing/grooming or toileting (related to pain and limitation of movement)
Fatigue (related to weakened muscles, chronic pain, and anemia)
Ineffective individual coping, high risk for (related to chronic illness, loss of functional abilities, and chronic pain)

◆ EXPECTED PATIENT OUTCOMES

Patient will experience a decrease in pain and stiffness.
Patient will maintain joint range of motion and improve muscle tone and strength through planned exercise.
Patient will adapt self-care activities and utilize assistive devices to remain independent in self-care.
Patient will balance activity and rest and incorporate energy conservation techniques to increase energy level and decrease fatigue.

TABLE 15-5 Medications Prescribed in the Treatment of Rheumatoid Arthritis

MEDICATION	ACTION	SIDE EFFECTS/TOXIC EFFECTS	PRECAUTIONS
SALICYLATES			
Examples: acetylsalicylic acid, choline salicylates	Analgesic; antipyretic; antiinflammatory	Gastric irritation; dose-related tinnitus; skin rash; hypersensitivity; decreased platelet aggregation	Take with food, milk, or antacid; space every 4-6 hr to maintain antiinflammatory effect; report incidence of bleeding or hearing changes
NONSTEROIDAL ANTIINFLAMMATORY AGENTS			
Indomethacin (Indocin)	Analgesic; antiinflammatory	Headache; dizziness; insomnia; confusion; gastrointestinal (GI) irritation	Take with food, milk, or antacid; discontinue if central nervous system (CNS) symptoms develop and notify physician
Ibuprofen (Motrin)	Same as indomethacin	Same as indomethacin but believed less irritating to GI tract	Delayed absorption if taken with food
Tolmetin sodium (Tolectin)	Same as ibuprofen	Same as ibuprofen	Take with food or milk
Naproxen (Naprosyn)	Same as ibuprofen	Same as indomethacin; also drowsiness	Take with food, milk, or antacid; avoid driving until dosage effect is established
Fenoprofen calcium (Nalfon)	Same as ibuprofen	Same as naproxen	Delayed absorption if taken with food; avoid driving until dosage effect is established
Sulindac (Clinoril)	Same as ibuprofen	Same as ibuprofen; plus skin rash	Take with food, milk, or antacid; do not use with acetylsalicylic acid
Diflunisal (Dolobid)	Analgesic; antiinflammatory	Gastric irritation; headache; dizziness; skin rash; tinnitus; fluid retention	Take with food or milk; do not use with salicylates or other antiinflammatory medications
Piroxicam (Feldene)	Analgesic; antiinflammatory	Gastric irritation; anemia; skin rash; fluid retention; dizziness; headache	Take with food or antacid
Diclofenac sodium (Volteran)	Analgesic; antiinflammatory	Possible intestinal irritation; headache; drowsiness; fatigue	Enteric coated; may be taken with food or milk
Ketorolac (Toradol)	Analgesic; antiinflammatory	Diarrhea/constipation; indigestion; nausea; skin rash	May give with food or antacid but absorption decreased; monitor bowel elimination

Patient will accept the chronic nature of the disease and remain involved in family and social activities.

◆ NURSING INTERVENTIONS

Relieving Pain

Teach patient to balance rest and activity.

Teach patient about medications and their side effects.

Caution about GI effects of drugs and importance of buffering with food or antacid.

Tell patient to maintain adequate blood levels of antiinflammatories and avoid PRN use.

Evaluate effectiveness of pain relief measures.

Teach relaxation techniques and alternate methods of pain control.

Promote frequent changes of position. Assist if needed.

Apply heat or cold to joints for comfort and muscle relaxation (Table 15-6).

During acute attack, rheumatoid arthritis patient should be on bed rest with joints held in position of function.

Encourage use of resting splints.

Explore patient knowledge and use of unproven remedies and "quack" therapies.

Refer to local support groups and the services of the Arthritis Foundation.

Promoting Mobility

Encourage patient to perform prescribed exercises. Use heat to reduce stiffness before exercise.

Patient should avoid morning exercise when stiffness is acute.

Teach patient to exercise only to the point of pain.

Assist patient with range of motion exercises as needed.

Focus on exercise directed at increasing functional capacities.

Avoid positioning in a way to encourage contracture, such as pillows under knees and head when supine.

Avoid positions of flexion.

TABLE 15-5   Medications Prescribed in the Treatment of Rheumatoid Arthritis—Cont'd

MEDICATION	ACTION	SIDE EFFECTS/TOXIC EFFECTS	PRECAUTIONS
SLOW-ACTING ANTIINFLAMMATORY AGENTS			
Antimalarials Hydroxychloroquine (Plaquenil)	Antiinflammatory (mechanism unknown); effect not expected to be noted for 6-12 mo after beginning therapy	GI disturbances; retinal edema that may result in blindness	Eye examination before beginning therapy and every 6 mo thereafter
Chloroquine (Aralen)	Same as hydroxychloroquine	Same as hydroxychloroquine	Same as hydroxychloroquine
Quinacrine (Atabrine)	Same as hydroxychloroquine	Same as hydroxychloroquine but may be better tolerated; yellow discoloration of skin	May be stopped periodically to prevent deepening of skin discoloration
Gold salts IM: gold sodium thiomalate (Myochrysine), gold thioglucose (Solganol) Oral: auranofin (Ridaura)	Antiinflammatory; effect not noted for 3-6 mo after beginning therapy	Renal and hepatic damage; corneal deposits; dermatitis; ulcerations in mouth; hematologic changes	Urinalysis and complete blood count (CBC) before each injection; report dermatitis, metallic taste in mouth, or lesions in mouth to physician Oral gold may produce fewer side effects than injectable, but periodic laboratory tests are required
Penicillamine (Cuprimine)	Antiinflammatory (mechanism unclear); effect not expected to be noted until several months after beginning treatment	Fever; rash; nephrotic syndrome; hematologic changes; GI irritation; lupuslike syndromes; allergic reactions (33% probability if allergic to penicillin); retarded wound healing	Urinalysis, CBC, differential, hemoglobin and platelet count at least weekly for 3 mo, then monthly; report skin rash, fever to physician; food interferes with absorption— take on empty stomach between meals
POTENT ANTIINFLAMMATORY AGENTS			
Adrenocorticosteroids (e.g., prednisone)	Interfere with body's normal inflammatory response	Fluid retention; sodium retention; potassium depletion; hypertension; decreased healing potential; increased susceptibility to infection; GI irritation; hirsutism, osteoporosis, fat deposits; diabetes mellitus; myopathy; adrenal insufficiency or adrenal crisis if abruptly withdrawn	Take with food, milk, or antacid; dosage not to be increased or decreased without physician's supervision; take in morning if taken on once-a-day basis
Phenylbutazone (Butazolidin)	Antiinflammatory; analgesic at subcortical site in brain	GI irritation; hematologic toxicity; hypertension, impaired renal function	Used for a short term (7-10 days); take with food or milk

NOTE: It should also be noted that the immunosuppressive agents azathioprine (Imuran), cyclophosphamide (Cytoxan), and chlorambucil (Leukeran) have been used on an investigational basis in patients with severe disease that has not responded to the conventional medications. These agents are used with great care because of their severe side effects and the attendant risks of the development of neoplasms. The drug methotrexate has received U.S. Food and Drug Administration (FDA) approval for use in rheumatoid arthritis.

Explore use of splints, braces, and assistive devices with physical therapy (Table 15-7).

Encourage isometric exercise when joints are inflamed.

Provide appropriate ambulatory assistive devices.

Encourage use of supportive shoes rather than slippers when ambulating.

Promoting Self-Care

Help patient utilize joint protection principles in planning daily activities (See Table 15-6).

Assist patient to analyze home arrangements and explore alternatives for reducing energy demands for routine activities.

Explore the use of assistive devices for ADL and daily activities, for example, kitchen tools, adapted silverware and plates, buttonholers, and sock and shoe aids (Table 15-8).

Involve family in planning and design of changes.

Reducing Fatigue

Encourage patient to consider and discuss factors that increase fatigue.

TABLE 15-6 Joint Protection and Energy Conservation Techniques

TECHNIQUE	EXAMPLES
Avoid positions of possible joint deformity	Avoid keeping joints in positions of flexion for prolonged periods of time
	Avoid twisting motions such as turning a jar lid with small joints
Avoid holding muscles or joints in one position for a long time	When working at a desk, stand up and walk about for a few minutes every half hour
Use the strongest joints for all activities	Use the knees, not the back, when lifting heavy objects
	Push a door open with the shoulder, not the wrist
	Use a shoulder strap, not a hand-held strap, to carry a heavy purse
Use joints in their best position, maintaining good standing and sitting posture	Avoid reaching or bending when another approach would work as well
	Work at a comfortable height
Conserve energy	Avoid trying to accomplish difficult tasks in a single time period
	Take breaks during work periods
	Slide rather than lift objects
	Use a wheeled cart to move objects from one place to another

TABLE 15-7 Types of Splints and Braces and Their Function

TYPE	FUNCTION
Spring-loaded braces	Oppose the action of unparalyzed muscles and act as partial functional substitutes for paralyzed muscles
Resting splints	Maintain a limb or joint in a functional position while permitting the muscles around the joint to relax
Functional splints	Maintain the joint or limb in a usable position to enable the body part to be used correctly
Dynamic splints	Permit assisted exercise to joints, particularly following surgery to finger joints

Assess for periods of greatest fatigue, and restructure activities accordingly.

Encourage patient to pace activities and provide for rests or naps during the day.

Incorporate energy conservation techniques into daily activities.

Assess adequacy of pain relief for night rest and sleep.

Assess adequacy of diet and degree of anemia.

Promoting Effective Coping

Explore usual coping patterns and support effective techniques.

TABLE 15-8 Assistive Devices for Persons With Motor Impairments

ASSISTIVE DEVICE	PATIENT LIMITATION
Utensil with built-up handle	Cannot adequately close hand
Utensil with cuffed handle	Loss of opposition of thumb
Combination knife-fork	Loss of only one hand
Mug with special handle	Unable to grasp regular cup handle
Long-handled shoehorn	Unable to bend to reach feet
Long-handled reacher (to reach for or pick up objects)	Unable to stoop or reach
Stocking guide	Inability to reach feet

Encourage patient to express fears and frustration about chronic progressive nature of the disease.

Encourage use of basic nutritious diet to foster optimal general health.

Encourage weight loss if indicated.

Provide patient with opportunities to discuss feelings about body changes and need for increased dependence on others.

Teach environmental modifications for safety and comfort such as supportive shoes, hand rails in bathtub, and raised toilet seats.

Explore use of self-help devices to foster independence in ADL.

Teach patient and family to maintain regular medical supervision and avoid quack therapies.

◆ EVALUATION

Successful achievement of expected outcomes for the patient with arthritis is indicated by the following:

Statements that pain is consistently decreased or absent

Increased joint range of motion and muscle strength and absence of deformity

Ability to accomplish self-care and participate in social ADL

Improved energy level and ability to participate in daily activities

Involvement with support groups, increased optimism about self and the future

GOUTY ARTHRITIS
Etiology/Epidemiology

Gouty arthritis is a metabolic disorder of purine metabolism in which excess uric acid leads to the formation of urate crystals in the synovial tissue, producing intense inflammation. It is an inherited disorder affecting men eight to nine times more often than women. The peak age of onset is the fifth decade, but it can occur at any age. The great toe is most commonly involved. Patients may develop tophi, deposits of monosodium urate, in the tissues.

Home Care Guidelines for Using Heat and Cold

HEAT

Used for relieving stiffness and relaxing muscles and for its analgesic effects. It may be applied as follows:

Dry heat
- Electric heating pad
- Warm towels
- Aqua k-pads

Moist heat
- Hydrocollator packs
- Paraffin baths
- Warm soaks, tub baths, showers

COLD

Used to reduce or prevent swelling, relieve pain and stiffness. It may be applied as follows:
- Plastic bags with ice
- Commercial gel packs that can be refrozen
- Bags of frozen vegetables

GUIDELINES FOR USE

Use for 15-20 minutes for maximum effect.
Wrap in protective towels to prevent skin damage.
Check skin 5 minutes after application for any evidence of tissue damage.
Heat and cold should be applied with caution to any patient with decreased sensation or circulation.

GERONTOLOGIC PATIENT CONSIDERATIONS FOR ARTHRITIS

Arthritis, particularly degenerative arthritis, is so commonly associated with aging that it is easy to think of it as an expected finding. Patients may not receive coordinated care for the disease and may largely engage in self-management. Although the basic care parameters are the same at any age, elderly persons are more vulnerable to the negative effects of chronic pain on sleep patterns, which are already problematic for many elderly persons, as well as depression and social isolation as their physical capacities diminish.

OSTEOPOROSIS

Osteoporosis complicates the management of arthritis in elderly persons, particularly in women. Joint stiffness and muscle weakness can predispose patients to falls and injury, particularly when they get up at night to urinate. Concerns over injury and the presence of chronic pain can combine to encourage the elderly person to limit active exercise, a move that will rapidly escalate the osteoporosis process. Patients need to be encouraged to remain active, especially to ambulate, but to take measures to improve their safety, such as reducing environmental hazards, for example, cluttered surroundings and scatter rugs, and to utilize assistive devices as indicated, particularly standard and quad canes.

DRUG EFFECTS

The chronic use of NSAIDs is clearly associated with the breakdown of the mucous barrier of the stomach and the development of gastric ulcers in elderly persons. The effect is systemic rather than just related to direct irritation and cannot be prevented by buffering drugs with food or antacid. Patients taking NSAIDs need to be taught and carefully monitored for the symptoms of ulceration and minor GI bleeding, and the use of drugs to support the mucous barrier such as sucralfate and misoprostol should be considered for this population.

Pathophysiology

In gouty arthritis uric acid deposits trigger intense inflammation and pain in the joint and surrounding tissue. Deposits and tophi cause gradual destruction of joints and bone. If unchecked, the disease can also produce renal damage. It is accompanied by elevated serum uric acid levels and by urate crystals in the synovial fluid.

Medical Management

Acute gouty arthritis attacks can be controlled and recurrent attacks can be prevented through administration of antiinflammatory drugs and reduction of the body pool of urates and uric acid. Colchicine is the drug of choice for treatment of acute attacks. Allopurinol (Zyloprim), probenicid (Benemid), and sulfinpyrazone (Anturane) are used to decrease uric acid levels. Dietary restriction of purine intake (found in red meats and legumes) may also be recommended. Increasing fluid intake helps to prevent crystal formation in the urine.

NURSING MANAGEMENT

The nursing role is primarily supportive and follows the general principles of arthritis management. During acute attacks the focus is on managing pain and inflammation through analgesics, ice, and immobilization. Ongoing management focuses on adherence to the drug regimen, management of side effects, and maintaining joint function through appropriate exercise.

OTHER RHEUMATIC AND CONNECTIVE TISSUE DISORDERS

The broad category of the diseases of arthritis contains over 100 distinct disorders that may include articular, nonarticular, and connective tissue disorders. Although systemic lupus erythematosus is by far the most widely recognized of these disease processes, a variety of other examples are summarized in Tables 15-9 and 15-10.

Systemic Lupus Erythematosus (SLE)

Etiology/epidemiology

SLE is a chronic inflammatory disease of autoimmune origin that primarily affects the skin, joints, and kidneys, although it can eventually involve virtually any organ of the body. It affects women, particularly adolescents and young adults, 8 to 10 times more often than men and is particularly common in African-American women. The disease was named for the characteristic erosive rash that accompanies it. Research into the etiology of SLE is primarily exploring genetic factors, environmental factors (viruses, drug exposure), and alterations in immune response.

TABLE 15-9 Nonarticular Rheumatic Diseases

DESCRIPTION	SIGNS AND SYMPTOMS	MEDICAL MANAGEMENT
BURSITIS		
Inflammation of the bursa, acute or chronic, caused by trauma, strain, or overuse of joint; shoulder bursa most commonly affected	Severe pain; limitations in joint movement	Rest for involved area Antiinflammatory analgesic agents Application of cold during acute period
CARPAL TUNNEL SYNDROME		
Pressure exerted by flexion tendon sheaths on median nerve at wrist; condition usually localized	Disorders in sensation (burning, tingling) in thumb, index, and middle fingers—especially during prolonged flexion Referred pain to upper extremity	Rest Splinting of wrist Surgical release of transverse carpal ligament
FIBROSITIS AND FIBROMYOSITIS		
Commonly occurring self-limiting symptom complex	Pain and stiffness in neck, shoulder girdle, and extremities Pain worsens with activity and subsides with rest	Management directed at specific symptoms Rest, analgesics, and physical therapy

TABLE 15-10 Collagen Disorders

DEFINITION	PATHOPHYSIOLOGY	SIGNS AND SYMPTOMS	MEDICAL MANAGEMENT
POLYMYOSITIS (DERMATOMYOSITIS)			
Inflammatory disease involving striated, voluntary muscle	Primary degeneration of muscle fibers Necrosis of parts or entire groups of muscle fibers Interstitial fibrosis	Muscle weakness and fatigue, especially in pelvic and shoulder muscles Muscle pain or tenderness Eventual contractures and atrophy if weakness persists Dusky red skin rash if dermatomyositis form Electromyography (EMG), muscle biopsy results Elevated serum enzymes	High-dose glucocorticosteroids or other immunosuppressive agents to effect remission Physical therapy and occupational therapy for exercise regimen; rest
PROGRESSIVE SYSTEMIC SCLEROSIS (PSS, SCLERODERMA)			
Sclerosis involving connective tissue throughout the body	Involved tissue becomes fibrotic Changes may be accompanied by vascular lesions	Gradual thickening and tightening of skin on face and body Telangiectasis on lips, tongue, face Pain and stiffness; muscle weakness Local effects produced by fibrosis of vital organs	Glucocorticosteroids for those with myositis symptoms Salicylates Range of motion exercise
NECROTIZING ARTERITIS			
Inflammation of blood vessels	Inflammation and necrosis of arterial wall Fibrosis and intimal proliferation result from body's attempts to clear necrosis Partial or complete vessel occlusion, infarction, or aneurysm	Involvement of vessels anywhere in body—angina, myocardial infarction, hypertension, peripheral neuropathy, intractable headaches Elevated white blood count (WBC) and erythrocyte sedimentation rate (ESR); angiography results show vessel destruction	High-dose glucocorticosteroids to effect remission Rest
SJÖGREN'S SYNDROME			
Chronic inflammation of lacrimal and parotid glands	Infiltration of lacrimal and parotid glands by lymphocytes and plasma cells Decrease in flow of tears and saliva	Dry gritty sensation in eyes—redness and itching Difficulty in chewing or swallowing or with speech Corneal, tongue, and lip ulceration	Symptomatic care with eye drops, increased fluids, and hard candy to stimulate saliva
ANKYLOSING SPONDYLITIS			
Inflammatory disease affecting sacroiliac joints and spine; primarily affects men	Inflammation causes bones of spine to grow together and ankylose (fuse) Vertebral bodies lose contour, and entire spine deforms	Low back pain Gradual loss of motion in back Loss of normal lordotic curve with severe kyphosis in cervical region Can compromise chest expansion	Antiinflammatories and analgesics Physical therapy Braces and traction Surgical osteotomy and fusion

Pathophysiology

Numerous cellular antibodies have been identified in persons with SLE in addition to abnormalities in both B and T cells. Immune complexes containing antibodies are deposited in tissue, causing tissue damage. Most lesions are found in the blood vessels, kidney, connective tissue, and skin. Common pathologic manifestations include the following:

Severe vasculitis with necrosis of small arterial walls

Thickening of glomerular basement membrane and necrosis of glomerular capillaries

Lymph node necrosis

Fibrous villous synovitis

Glomerulonephritis

Pleuritis or pericarditis

Multisystem involvement can cause an overwhelming clinical picture. Arthritis accompanied by weakness, fatigue, and weight loss is often the first symptom. Sun sensitivity and an erythematous rash, usually in a butterfly pattern, may appear over the cheeks and bridge of the nose. The rash lesions do not ulcerate but can cause degeneration and tissue atrophy. The renal and neurologic problems are among the more serious aspects of the disease.

Medical management

The diagnosis of SLE is made from the history and physical findings supplemented by laboratory studies. A positive LE test, positive anti-DNA antibody, abnormal titer of antinuclear antibody, and other findings such as hemolytic anemia, leukopenia, lymphopenia, and thrombocytopenia all lend support to the presumptive diagnosis.

The use of adrenocorticosteroids is the cornerstone of therapy and is often successful in controlling the course of the disease. Aspirin or NSAIDs may be given for arthritic pain, along with ointments for rash. Cytotoxic agents may be employed if other drug therapies fail to control disease exacerbations. Advanced disease may require kidney dialysis, transplant or joint replacement.

NURSING MANAGEMENT

The nursing role is largely supportive. During exacerbations the patient may be given high-dose steroids. The nurse will assist the patient to understand their action and manage common drug-related side effects through diet and fluid balance modification. Arthritic symptoms are managed with analgesics, comfort measures, and a balanced plan of rest and exercise as discussed previously. The patient is encouraged to avoid sun exposure through the use of sunscreens and protective clothing. The presence of the visible rash and the side effects of steroid use can cause profound changes in the patient's body image. The nurse encourages the patient to verbalize feelings and concerns and helps the patient minimize these effects when possible.

 Guidelines for Nursing Care of the Person with Total Hip Replacement

PREOPERATIVE CARE

Scrupulously cleanse and prepare skin per surgeon's routine.

Administer prophylactic antibiotics as ordered.

Verify patient's understanding of surgical procedure and mobility restrictions to be followed in postoperative period.

POSTOPERATIVE CARE

Positioning

Follow surgeon's protocol.

Operative hip is maintained in abduction with slings or pillows (see Figure 15-5).

Avoid external rotation with sandbags or trochanter rolls.

Keep head of bed elevated less than 45 degrees except for meals.

Do not position on operative side; turn to unaffected side with operative leg maintained in abduction.

Mobility

Ensure patient comfort with adequate analgesia.

Instruct patient in use of overhead trapeze to assist with position changes.

Encourage active foot and ankle exercises plus isometric bed exercises for the quadriceps and gluteal muscles to support venous return and strengthen the muscles needed for ambulation.

Administer aspirin or subcutaneous heparin as ordered to prevent thrombus formation.

Begin ambulation as ordered by surgeon.

Maintain flexion, adduction, and weight-bearing precautions as ordered.

Instruct in safe use of assistive devices, namely, walker, crutches.

Increase amount of ambulation daily.

Wound Care

Maintain patency of wound drainage system.

Monitor and record the amount and type of drainage.

Keep operative area free of contamination.

Assess site regularly.

Change dressings as needed.

Administer antibiotics as ordered.

Discharge Teaching

Mobility restrictions

Flexion is restricted to 90 degrees for 2-3 months.

No adduction beyond midline is allowed for 2-3 months.

Sleeping on operative side is not permitted.

Progressive weight bearing is as ordered by surgeon.

Ensure that patient has supplies needed for home care:

Crutches or walker for ambulation

Raised toilet seat

Self-help devices to avoid bending and stooping

Teach patient importance of lifelong prevention of urinary tract and other systemic bacterial infections that could migrate to prosthesis:

Liberal fluid intake and regular voiding

Prophylactic antibiotics before routine procedures such as dental extractions

NURSING CARE PLAN

THE PATIENT WITH A TOTAL KNEE REPLACEMENT

■ NURSING DIAGNOSIS
Pain (related to tissue trauma and edema)

Expected Patient Outcomes	Nursing Interventions
Patient will report that incisional pain is effectively controlled. Patient will actively participate in rehabilitation exercises.	1. Administer narcotic analgesics as ordered. a. Implement PCA if desired. 2. Monitor pain level and assess the effectiveness of analgesics. 3. Utilize relaxation, positioning, and other nonpharmacologic comfort measures.

■ NURSING DIAGNOSIS
Mobility, impaired physical (related to pain, stiffness, and activity restrictions)

Expected Patient Outcome	Nursing Interventions

Patient will gradually increase activity and utilize adaptive devices.	1. Change position every 2 hours while in bed.
	2. Elevate operative leg on pillows when in bed and chair for first 24-48 hours.
	   a. Avoid passive flexion of the knee when positioning leg (Box 15-14).
	3. Utilize continuous passive motion at degree of flexion ordered.
	   a. Use a minimum of 8-12 hr/day.
	   b. Advance flexion as ordered.
	4. Assist patient out of bed to ambulate on first postoperative day.
	   a. Light weight bearing with crutches or walker is usually permitted.
	   b. Encourage steady increase in duration of ambulation.
	5. Begin active flexion exercise of knee as ordered, usually second postoperative day after removal of bulky dressing.
	   a. Exercise four times daily.
	6. Encourage active foot and ankle exercise and isometric exercise of gluteals and quadriceps to support venous return.
	   a. Begin quadriceps exercise after drain is removed.
	7. Initiate straight leg raises as ordered.
	   a. Repeat every 2 hours until fully ambulatory.

TOTAL JOINT REPLACEMENT SURGERY

Total joint replacement surgery is increasingly being used to correct deformities and maintain functional capacities in patients with severe arthritis. The objectives of such surgery include relief of chronic pain, restoration of joint function if possible, and prevention of further disability or disease progression in the affected joint. Surgery to the hip and knee is by far the most common, although other joints are being treated with increasing frequency. The care of the patient undergoing total hip replacement is summarized in the Guidelines box on p. 367. The principles are similar to those discussed for fractures of the hip. The care of the patient undergoing total knee replacement is presented in the "Nursing Care Plan" and corresponding "Critical Pathway." The prevention of infection and adherence to mobility restrictions are the most important concerns of total joint replacement.

THE PATIENT WITH A TOTAL KNEE REPLACEMENT

Expected Patient Outcome	Nursing Interventions
	8. Utilize a knee immobilizer at night as a resting splint to prevent excessive flexion or hyperextension of joint.

■ NURSING DIAGNOSIS

Impaired home maintenance management, risk of (related to insufficient knowledge of complications and postdischarge care)

Expected Patient Outcomes	Nursing Interventions

Patient will describe activity restrictions.
Patient will state signs and symptoms of complications.
	1. Discharge instructions:
	  a. Observe partial weight bearing and use assistive device for about 2 months.
	  b. Continue active flexion and straight leg-raising exercises.
	  c. Apply ice to knee for 20 minutes before and after exercise.
	  d. Continue to monitor wound healing. Report any evidence of the following:
	    (1) Redness and swelling
	    (2) Incisional drainage
	    (3) Fever
	2. Ensure that patient has access to assistive and self-help devices for home use.
	3. Instruct patient in the lifelong need for antibiotic prophylaxis before surgery or dental work.

BOX 15-14   **Continuous Passive Motion Machine**

Guidelines for use
  Keep the leg in a neutral aligned position.
  Position the knee at the hinged joint of the machine.
  Encourage the patient to keep the leg in the machine for 20 hours or more daily unless otherwise ordered by the physician.

Monitor for pressure areas at the knee and groin.
Follow physician's orders concerning speed and degrees of flexion and extension.
Assess patient's tolerance to any ordered changes.

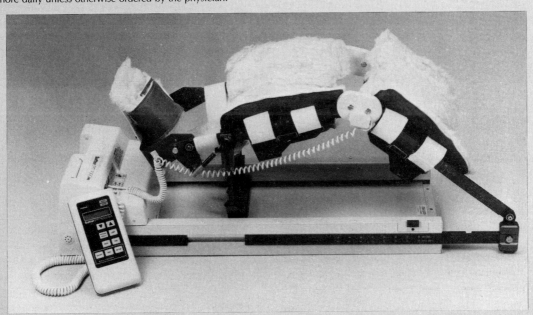

FIGURE 15-6 Continuous passive motion machine. (Courtesy Sutter Corporation.)

| **CRITICAL PATHWAY** | **Total Knee Replacement** |

DRG #: 209; expected LOS: 7

	Day of Surgery **Day of Admission** **Day 1**	**Day 2**	**Day 3**
Diagnostic Tests	Preoperative: CBC, UA, SMA/18,* PT/ PTT, chest x-ray, type and cross match, ECG, screen autologous blood, knee x-rays Postoperative: CBC	CBC, SMA/6,† PT/PTT q day until discharge, if coumadin prescribed	CBC SMA/6
Medications	Preoperative: IV antibiotic Postoperative: IVs; give autologous blood if necessary; IV antibiotic, IV analgesic	IV to saline lock; IV antibiotic; IV analgesic; stool softener; Rx for sleep; prophylactic anticoagulant	IV saline lock; IV antibiotic; PO analgesic; stool softener; Rx for sleep; anticoagulant
Treatments	Postoperative: vital signs; check dressing and neurocirculatory checks q hr × 4, then q 2 hr × 4, then q 4 hr; skin assessment and special care q 2 hr; empty and record drain output q 8 hr; I & O q 8 hr; elastic leg stocking (ELS) to unaffected leg; incentive spirometry q 2 hr; intermittent compression device (ICD) on both legs	Vital signs; check dressing and neurocirculatory checks q 4 hr; skin assessment and special care q 2 hr; I & O and drain output q 8 hr; ELS; incentive spirometry q 2 hr; ICD on both legs	Vital signs; discontinue drain; check dressing and neurocirculatory checks q 8 hr; I & O q 8 hr; change dressing; ELS both legs; ICD on both legs
Diet	NPO; clear liquids after nausea and/or if positive bowel sounds	Clear liquids; advance diet as tolerated	Regular diet
Activity	Bed rest at 40-degree flexion; trapeze; CPM‡ on affected leg at least 8 hr/day; ankle exercise q hr; T/Tilt-C-DB q 2 hr	Bed rest, CPM on affected leg; ankle exercise q 2 hr; T/Tilt-C-DB q 2 hr; advance CPM 5 degrees bid	Ambulate in room with help × 2; CPM on affected leg; ankle exercise q 2 hr; advance CPM by 5 degrees bid
Consultations		Physical therapy; up in chair as tolerated	Physical therapy, social service, rehab/ SNU/home health; up in chair as tolerated; encourage knee flexion

NOTE: Acknowledge that patients recover at varying rates; therefore specified daily actions should be based solely on patient need.
*Serum calcium, phosphorus, triglycerides, uric acid, creatinine, BUN, total bilirubin, alkaline phosphate, aspartate aminotransferase (AST; formerly serum glutamic oxaloacetic transaminase [SGOT]), alanine aminotransferase (ALT; formerly serum glutamic oxaloacetic transaminase [SGPT]), lactic dehydrogenase (LDH), total protein, albumin, sodium, potassium, chloride, total CO_2, glucose.
†Serum, sodium, potassium, chloride, total CO_2, glucose, BUN.
‡Continuous passive motion.

BACK DISORDERS
HERNIATED DISK/DEGENERATIVE DISEASE
Etiology/Epidemiology

Back pain is the second most common cause of physician visits and affects 8 to 10 adults during their life span. No definitive diagnosis can be found for up to 85% of these individuals. The pain may become chronic and unresponsive to usual therapies, including surgical intervention. Common causes of back pain include the following:

Muscle strains: overuse injuries to muscles from repetitive lifting, poor body mechanics and posture, and occupational hazards

Degenerative disk disease: replacement of the elastic and gelatinous disk with fibrocartilage, and narrowing of the disk space; occurs primarily in persons over 50 years.

Herniated nucleus pulposus: protrusion of the gelatinous disk through the surrounding cartilage, causing pressure on the spinal nerve roots; L4 to S1 vertebrae most vulnerable

Spinal stenosis: narrowing of the spinal canal or intervertebral foramina at any level; gradual development of symptoms

Rheumatoid/degenerative arthritis with osteophyte formation: inflammation or degeneration of the articular surfaces; osteophyte formation can result in vertebral fusion

Pathophysiology

Back pain may be produced by straightforward muscle strain or trauma or a more significant pathologic condition. Pain is the classic symptom and may be caused by nerve compression. It frequently follows the path of the sciatic nerve and radiates through the buttocks into the

| CRITICAL PATHWAY | | Total Knee Replacement—Cont'd | |

DRG #: 209; expected LOS: 7

Day 4	Day 5	Day 6	Day of Discharge Day 7
CBC SMA/7			
Discontinue saline lock and antibiotic; PO analgesic; stool softener; Rx for sleep; anticoagulant	PO analgesic; stool softener; Rx for sleep; anticoagulant	PO analgesic; stool softener; Rx for sleep; anticoagulant	PO analgesic; anticoagulant
Vital signs and neurocirculatory checks q 8 hr; I & O q 8 hr; ELS; dressing change PRN, ICD on both legs	Vital signs and neurocirculatory checks q 8 hr; disc; I & O; ELS; discontinue ICD	Vital signs q 8 hr; ELS	Vital signs q 8 hr; ELS
Regular diet	Regular diet	Regular diet	Regular diet
Ambulate in room with help × 4; CPM on affected leg; ankle exercise q 2 hr; advance CPM 5 degrees bid	Ambulate in hallway with help × 2; CPM on affected leg; ankle exercise q 2 hr; advance CPM 5 degrees bid	Ambulate in hallway with help × 4; advance CPM by 5 degrees bid	Ambulate in hallway with help × 4
Physical therapy; occupational therapy if self-care help needed	Physical therapy; occupational therapy if self-care help needed	Physical therapy; occupational therapy	Physical therapy; occupational therapy

posterior aspect of the thigh. Range of motion is impaired, and both motor and sensory involvement may be present along the affected nerve root. Paresthesias in the leg and foot, muscle weakness and spasm, and decreased reflexes may all be present. The pain is typically worsened with twisting movements, laughing, or coughing and is relieved by lying flat.

Medical Management

The diagnostic workup for back problems may include x-rays, myelography, and CT or MRI scanning. The initial treatment is usually conservative and includes bed rest with a firm mattress, muscles relaxants and analgesics, physical therapy for deep heat and massage, and pelvic traction to relieve spasms. A brace or corset may be prescribed to provide external support to the spine. If conservative management is successful the patient will then be instructed in a program of exercises to strengthen the back and abdominal muscles and increase flexibility.

Surgical management of back problems is frequently used but is controversial because of its relatively poor success rates in controlling pain. Surgery is indicated in situations where neurologic symptoms are progressive,

pain is intractable, or bony instability is present. Procedures include diskectomy, fusion, laminectomy, or limited procedures such as endoscopy or microdiscectomy. Chemonucleolysis is a procedure that involves injection of an enzyme to break down collagen fibers in the disk and relieve pressure. Its effectiveness is questioned. Bone grafts may be used in certain procedures, particularly fusions. They provide a scaffold for both mechanical support and the growth of osteogenic cells. Autografts produce the most consistent results and are usually harvested from the iliac crests and fibula.

NURSING MANAGEMENT

◆ ASSESSMENT
Subjective Data

    Pain pattern and extent, duration, and severity
    Presence of paresthesias or muscle weakness
    History of trauma or degenerative disease
    Actions that relieve or improve pain
    Patient's normal daily living, occupational, and leisure
        activities
    Patient's knowledge of surgery or therapy prescribed

CRITICAL PATHWAY	Laminectomy Without Complications or Fusion

DRG #: 214; expected LOS: 6

	Day of Surgery Day of Admission Day 1	Day 2	Day 3
Diagnostic Tests	Preoperative: chest x-ray film, CBC, UA, SMA/6,* PT/PTT, creatinine, MRI, myelogram, ECG, lumbar spinal x-ray films Postoperative: CBC, electrolytes		
Medications	Preoperative: IV antibiotic Postoperative: IVs, IV analgesic, stool softener	IV @ TKO, IV or IM analgesic, stool softener	IV to saline lock, PO analgesic, stool softener
Treatments	Preoperative: weight, VS Postoperative: I & O q 8 hr, VS q 4 hr, assess neurocirculatory systems to legs q 2 hr, T, C, & DB q 2 hr, incentive spirometry q 2 hr, elastic leg stockings (ELS)	I & O q 8 hr, VS q 6 hr, assess neuro-circulatory systems to legs q 4 hr, T, C, & DB q 2 hr, incentive spirometry q 2 hr, ELS	I & O q 8 hr, VS q 8 hr, T, C, & DB q 4 hr, incentive spirometry q 4 hr, ELS
Diet	NPO: advance to full liquids after nausea	Advance to regular diet	Regular diet
Activity	Bed rest, to bathroom with assistance; ambulate in room with assistance, no sitting	Ambulate in hallway with assistance, no sitting	Ambulate in hallway with assistance, no sitting
Consultations		Physical therapy	Physical therapy

NOTE: Acknowledge that patients recover at varying rates; therefore specified daily actions should be based solely on patient need.
*Serum sodium, potassium, chloride, total CO_2, glucose, BUN.

Objective Data

Gait or posture abnormalities

Pain or tenderness elicited by light palpation over lower back

Myelogram results showing disk protrusion or degenerative changes

◆ NURSING DIAGNOSES

Nursing diagnoses for the person with back problems being treated surgically may include, but are not limited to, the following:

Pain (related to surgical trauma, muscle spasm, and nerve irritation)

Injury, risk of (related to lack of knowledge of postoperative positioning restrictions and technique of log rolling)

Altered home maintenance management, risk of (related to insufficient knowledge of home care components)

◆ EXPECTED PATIENT OUTCOMES

Patient will experience steady reduction in the incidence and severity of back pain and spasm.

Patient will correctly discuss positioning restrictions and demonstrate the use of log rolling.

Patient will correctly describe wound care, activity precautions, and signs of complications to be reported.

◆ NURSING INTERVENTIONS
Promoting Comfort

Preoperative

Encourage patient to maintain bed rest with head of bed low and knees slightly flexed.

Establish and maintain pelvic traction if ordered.

Administer analgesics and muscle relaxants as ordered.

Use nursing measures to augment pain relief, such as diversion, application of heat, and back rubs.

Postoperative

Administer analgesics as ordered, and assess effectiveness.

Avoid all stress or strain on the operative incision.

Teach patient to use the arms and legs to transfer and support weight when getting in and out of bed.

Encourage an upright stance and good posture.

Preventing Injury

Teach patient about procedure and restrictions for postoperative positioning.

CRITICAL PATHWAY Laminectomy Without Complications or Fusion—Cont'd

DRG #: 214; expected LOS: 6

	Day 4	Day 5	Day of Discharge Day 6
CBC			
	IV saline lock, PO analgesic, stool softener	Discontinue saline lock, PO analgesic, stool softener	PO analgesic, stool softener
	I & O q 8 hr, VS q 8 hr, ELS	I & O, VS q 8 hr, ELS	VS q 8 hr, ELS
	Regular diet	Regular diet	Regular diet
	Ambulate in hallway with assistance, no sitting	Ambulate in hallway	Ambulate in hallway
	Physical therapy	Physical therapy	

Teach patient about log rolling, coughing, and deep breathing.

Obtain baseline preoperative neurologic assessment.

Check movement and sensation in lower extremities frequently in postoperative period.

Keep the head of the bed flat. Avoid use of prone position.

Encourage ambulation—patient should avoid sitting.

Administer stool softeners to prevent straining.

Monitor wound drains if present, and record output.

Inspect surgical area frequently for excess drainage or hematoma. Monitor donor sites if graft performed.

Teaching for Home Care

Teach patient principles of good body mechanics.

    Patient should do the following:

        Maintain broad base of support.

        Use large groups of muscles.

        Maintain good posture.

        Squat, not bend.

        Pull objects rather than pushing.

Teach patient back-strengthening exercises.

Continue to avoid prolonged sitting.

Avoid any twisting movements of the trunk.

Do not lift or carry weight in excess of 5 pounds.

Continue to monitor healing of incision(s) and any changes in mobility or sensation of the extremities.

Encourage weight loss if indicated.

Teach safe use of brace or corset if ordered—applied *before* the patient gets out of bed.

♦ EVALUATION

Successful achievement of expected outcomes for the patient with back problems being treated surgically is indicated by the following:

    Reports of decreased or absent back pain and spasm

    Demonstration of safe movement, presence of intact movement and sensation in the extremities, and a healing incision

    Correct description of activity restrictions to be observed after discharge and symptoms indicating the need for medical evaluation

NOTE: A "Critical Pathway" for the patient undergoing laminectomy without fusion is included.

RESTRICTIVE DISORDERS/SCOLIOSIS
Etiology/Epidemiology

Scoliosis, or spinal curvature, can be classified as structural or nonstructural. The nonstructural form is not progressive and rarely requires definitive intervention. The structural form involves a rotational deformity of the vertebrae and may be congenital, neuromuscular, or idiopathic in nature. Idiopathic forms account for 65% to 80% of all cases, and girls represent 90% of those affected.

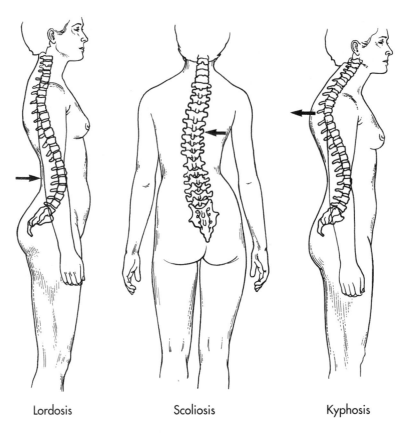

Lordosis   Scoliosis   Kyphosis

FIGURE 15-7 Curvatures of the spine.

Pathophysiology

Scoliosis may develop in a localized area or involve the entire spine. The curvature may be S or C shaped and is classified by magnitude, location, and direction (Figure 15-7). The deformity may range from slight to severe. The curve typically progresses rapidly during growth periods and then more slowly in the adult years as weight and mass continue their combined effects. Scoliosis may first be evident in uneven shoulder or hip height, scapular or rib prominence, and rib humps that are typically posterior and unilateral. In severe cases cardiopulmonary and digestive problems may develop from compression and displacement of vital organs. Pain is not usually a factor.

Medical Management

The diagnosis of scoliosis is established from the physical examination, x-rays, and calculations of the degree of curve and vertebral rotation. Specific treatment depends on the age and status of the patient and the degree of curvature. Flexible curves of less than 40 degrees may initially be treated with a combination of exercise and bracing, for example, a Milwaukee brace, Risser cast, or halofemoral traction. Nerves may be stimulated with electrical nerve stimulation (TENS) to induce flexion, strengthen the muscle, and help pull the spine into better alignment. Surgery is utilized when conservative management fails to halt the progression

when curves exceed 45 degrees. The surgical approach is usually posterior and frequently involves instrumentation with some type of rod (e.g., Harrington, Luque) that will fuse the spine to correct current curves and prevent future movement. The correction may need to be staged in severe cases.

NURSING MANAGEMENT

The nursing management is similar to the postoperative care described under back pain. The period of immobility is usually longer, and pain is more severe since larger areas of the spine are involved. Wound healing is critical, and the remobilization will occur on a more carefully phased basis. Many patients are fitted with braces postoperatively to secure the repair. Many of the patients undergoing scoliosis surgery will be adolescent or young adult women. Nursing attention must be focused on assisting the patient to deal with the challenges to body image and the effects of the surgery on creating social isolation from the peer group for prolonged recovery. The parents also frequently need significant support in dealing with the diagnosis and outcomes for their child. The ongoing regimen of bracing and exercise can create serious conflicts between parents and patients, and the family will need assistance to establish a satisfactory regimen that minimizes conflict between all parties.

INFECTIONS OF THE MUSCULOSKELETAL SYSTEM

OSTEOMYELITIS

Etiology/Epidemiology

Osteomyelitis is defined as infection of the bone. It is usually caused by bacteria but can result from invasion by viruses, fungi, and parasites as well. It typically occurs following trauma or surgery that creates an exogenous infection and can spread from the soft tissue to the bone. It can, however, also result from blood-borne pathogens that originate at another site in the body such as a genitourinary, respiratory, or sinus infection. This form begins in the bone and then spreads to the soft tissue, possibly eventually breaking the skin. This hematogenous form is more common in elderly persons.

Pathophysiology

Staphylococcus aureus is a common precipitating organism, but a wide variety of organisms may be responsible for the infection. Primary bone infection follows a pattern similar to infection in any other body tissue and is accompanied by edema, increased blood flow, and leukocyte activity. In exogenous forms the primary effects are initially in the soft tissue and muscle and may cause abscess formation. The symptoms vary with the organism and type of infection. Systemic symptoms may predominate with fever, malaise, anorexia, and fatigue. Local symptoms may be mild or severe.

Medical Management

The diagnosis is confirmed by the presence of an elevated WBC and ESR count, a positive bone scan, and cultures that grow the causative organism. Blood cultures are drawn to assess for septicemia. The treatment of osteomyelitis is difficult, protracted, and frequently complicated by recurrent infection and the development of zones of dead bone and scar tissue that can sequester organisms. IV antibiotic therapy for at least 6 weeks is a mainstay of treatment, followed by oral therapy for about 6 months. Irrigation and drainage may be employed to directly cleanse the infected area, and surgical debridement may be necessary if conservative measures fail. Bone grafting may be attempted if the amount of necrotic bone is extreme.

NURSING MANAGEMENT

The nursing role is largely collaborative and supportive. Long-term IV access will be needed, and comfort measures will be extremely important. Mobility is restricted during the treatment period, and interventions need to be planned to prevent associated complications. Home antibiotic therapy may need to be taught, as well as complex wound care regimens. The prognosis is uncertain with osteomyelitis, and it will be important for the nurse to provide encouragement and support for all of the patient's positive coping efforts.

TUMORS OF THE MUSCULOSKELETAL SYSTEM

OSTEOSARCOMA

Etiology/Epidemiology

Tumors may arise from any of the tissues of the musculoskeletal system, and they are classified according to their tissue of origin. They can be benign or malignant and occur in all age-groups although most develop in persons under 20 years or over 60 years. Osteosarcoma is the most common form of primary bone tumor, representing over 20% of the total. The bone is also a common site of metastasis for tumors originating elsewhere in the body, particularly in the prostate, breast, and lung.

Pathophysiology

Bone tumors create their principal destruction in the cortex of the bone through simple compression that weakens bone structure or through disruption of the blood supply and resorption. Malignant tumors are classified according to their growth patterns and sites of metastasis.

Osteosarcomas exhibit a moth-eaten pattern of destruction with poorly defined tumor margins. The erosion if unchecked eventually erodes the periosteum and soft tissue. Ninety percent develop in the metaphyses of the long bones. Dull, aching pain and swelling are among the most commonly reported early symptoms.

Medical Management

The diagnosis of osteosarcoma is established through x-rays, bone scan, CT or MRI, and bone biopsy. Because the growth rate is rapid, the prognosis is often poor. Treatment depends on the patient's general health and the size and location of the tumor. Surgery has been the mainstay of efforts to effect a cure. Amputation was the primary approach until recently, when limb salvage procedures coupled with aggressive adjuvant chemotherapy has been successfully developed. Survival rates for the two approaches are similar, but the technical difficulty of the surgery makes the incidence of complications much higher. Patient preference is a major consideration.

NURSING MANAGEMENT

The nursing care associated with treatment for osteosarcoma follows the guidelines established for chemotherapy (see Chapter 1) and the postoperative care outlined under amputation (see p. 376). Patients and families are attempting to cope with the diagnosis of a highly malignant form of cancer as well as the possibility of mutilating surgery and will need a great deal of teaching and support. The hospitalization may be protracted with limb salvage procedures, and it is important to ensure the patient's understanding of the risks, benefits, and potential complications involved. Patients should also have a very clear understanding of what their *functional* limb abilities will be like after surgery. No procedure preserves normal function. It is important to support self-care efforts and independence and yet encourage the patient to verbalize concerns and fears regarding the body image and functional changes resulting from the surgery.

AMPUTATION
ETIOLOGY/EPIDEMIOLOGY

Amputation involves surgical removal of a limb, usually as a result of trauma or disease. Ischemia of the limb is the most common predisposing factor, and it usually involves the lower extremity. The incidence of amputation has decreased over recent years, but the typical patient is still a late middle-aged or elderly diabetic man with a long history of smoking. The vast majority of nontraumatic amputations involve peripheral vascular disease, often as a result of diabetes that contributes to inadequate tissue perfusion.

PATHOPHYSIOLOGY

As circulation to the extremity gradually decreases the body attempts to compensate by laying down collateral vessels to maintain minimal perfusion. Intermittent claudication (cramping pain that occurs with exercise and is relieved by rest) develops when the collateral circulation fails to meet the perfusion needs. Ischemia can become so severe that the pain compromises the patient's mobility and is present even at rest. Tissue necrosis, ulceration, and gangrene are all possible complications of severe disease.

MEDICAL MANAGEMENT

The operative procedure and the level of the amputation are determined by the extent of damaged tissue and the adequacy of the arterial blood supply higher in the leg. It is a clinical judgment, although every effort is made to preserve knee joints if possible to allow for better prosthetic fit and a more normal walking gait. The level must ensure that adequate nutrition and blood supply are available for healing. The procedure can be performed by an open or a closed method and may be treated postoperatively with compression dressings or the immediate application of a cast with a temporary, prefitted prosthesis according to the patient's clinical status and the surgeon's preference.

NURSING MANAGEMENT

◆ ASSESSMENT
Subjective Data

History of disease and treatment
General health status
Medications in current use, adherence to regimen
Presence and severity of intermittent claudication
Smoking history, current usage
Knowledge of planned surgical procedure and outcomes
Psychologic response to need for surgery

Objective Data

Condition of affected limb
Presence of ulceration, skin breakdown, gangrene
Quality of peripheral pulses
Temperature, color, capillary refill, hair growth on affected extremity
Strength and mobility for crutch walking
Adherence to foot care regimen

◆ NURSING DIAGNOSES

Nursing diagnoses for the person undergoing amputation may include, but are not limited to, the following:
Pain (related to swelling, tissue injury, and phantom sensation)
Physical mobility, impaired (related to pain, decreased muscle strength, or decreased range of motion)
Body image disturbance (related to effects of limb loss)
Impaired home maintenance management, high risk for (related to insufficient knowledge of stump and prosthesis care)

◆ EXPECTED PATIENT OUTCOMES

Patient will experience a steadily decreasing level of pain and achieve relief with analgesic regimen.
Patient will maintain full range of motion in affected limb and utilize assistive devices as needed for ADL.
Patient will successfully incorporate amputation into a revised body image.
Patient will demonstrate appropriate care for stump and apply wrappings correctly.

◆ NURSING INTERVENTIONS
Promoting Comfort

Elevate stump for first 24 hours to reduce swelling.
Assess frequently for excessive bleeding.
Administer analgesics as needed.
Assess effectiveness of pain relief orders.

Explore use of PCA if approved.

Discuss concept of phantom limb sensation and reinforce that it is a normal occurrence.

Assess directly for incidence of phantom limb sensation and pain. Reassure patient that although phantom sensation is common, phantom pain is not.

Validate the reality of phantom pain if it occurs.

Supporting Range of Motion and Promoting Mobility

Begin active range of motion exercise, and encourage isometric exercise to gluteals, quadriceps, and triceps muscles for crutch walking.

Encourage patient to lie prone three or four times daily to prevent flexion contractures.

Reinforce crutch-walking regimen developed by physical therapy. Assist patient to compensate for altered balance and center of gravity.

Monitor stump carefully for signs of infection or irritation.

Change dressings as needed. Evaluate amount and nature of all drainage.

Rewrap the stump as needed using an upward spiral figure-8 type of wrap to help shape and shrink the stump.

Assess quality of all palpable peripheral pulses.

Promoting a Positive Body Image

Encourage patient to discuss concerns over losses. Reinforce importance of normal grieving for missing part.

Arrange for visit with rehabilitated amputee if patient approves.

Encourage patient to care for stump and view it during dressing change.

Encourage patient to explore changes in preferred life-style mandated by the amputation before discharge.

Encourage realistic goal setting based on general health and physical condition.

Involve physical therapy and prosthetics in all aspects of care planning.

Teaching for Home Care

Teach patient to provide skin care daily using a mild soap. Avoid use of creams or ointments that may excessively soften skin.

Instruct patient in proper technique for stump wrapping. Maintain appropriate wrapping at all times except for skin care.

Reinforce the importance of daily inspection of the stump for redness or irritation.

Teach patients to wash stump wrappings, and apply fresh ones daily.

Refer to prosthetist for fitting.

Encourage patient to utilize community support services.

◆ EVALUATION

Successful achievement of expected outcomes for the patient with an amputation is indicated by the following:

Reports of absent or managed pain

Full range of motion on operative extremity, independence in ADL with assistive devices

Verbalization of feelings concerning amputation and positive references to physical self

Correct description and demonstration of components of home care regimen

SELECTED REFERENCES

Barangan JD: Factors that influence recovery from hip fracture during hospitalization, *Orthop Nurs* 9(5):19-28, 1990.

Brosnan H: Nursing management of the adolescent with idiopathic scoliosis, *Nurs Clin North Am* 26(1):17-31, 1991.

Collo MCB et al: Evaluating arthritic complaints, *Nurse Pract* 16(2):9-20, 1991.

Dulin D: Facilitating early rehabilitation in limb-salvage patients, *Oncol Nurs Forum* 16(1):105, 1989.

Dunwoody CJ: Pelvic fracture care: reflections on the past, implications for the future, *Nurs Clin North Am* 26(1):65-72, 1991.

Feingold DJ et al: Complications of lumbar spine surgery, *Orthop Nurs* 19(4):39-57, 1991.

Gamron R: Taking the pressure out of compartment syndrome, *Am J Nurs* 88:1076-1080, 1988.

Hansell M: Fractures and the healing process, *Orthop Nurs* 7(1):43, 1988.

Herron DG, Nance J: Emergency department nursing management of patients with orthopedic fractures resulting from motor vehicle accidents, *Nurs Clin North Am* 25(1):71-83, 1990.

Hodge WA: Prevention of deep vein thrombosis after total knee arthroplasty: coumadin versus pneumatic calf compression, *Clin Orthop Re Res* 27(1):101-105, 1991.

Joseph N: Arthritis medications from A to Z, *Caring* 8(1):14-16, 1989.

Mims BC: Fat embolism syndrome: a variant of ARDS, *Orthop Nurs* 8(3):22-25, 1989.

Morris L: Nursing the patient in traction, *RN* 26, January 1988.

Piasecki PA: The nursing role in limb salvage surgery, *Nurs Clin North Am* 26(1):33-41, 1991.

Ross D: Acute compartment syndrome, *Orthop Nurs* 10(2):33-38, 1991.

Schoen D: Assessment for arthritis, *Orthop Nurs* 7(20):31, 1988.

Slye DA: Orthopedic complications: compartment syndrome, fat embolism syndrome, and venous thromboembolism, *Nurs Clin North Am* 26(1):113-132, 1991.

Sneed NV, VanBree KM: Treating ununited fractures with electricity: nursing implications, *J Gerontol Nurs* 16(8):26-31, 1990.

Valentine WA, Williams PA, Tafoya WL: Ilizarov external fixation, *AORN J* 51(6):1530-1545, 1990.

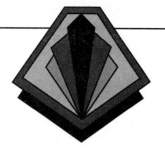

CHAPTER 16

Disorders of the Reproductive System

◆ ASSESSMENT

SUBJECTIVE DATA

Health history

Illness or surgery involving the reproductive organs, including sexually transmitted diseases (STDs)

Chronic diseases, such as HTN, diabetes, anemia

Use of diethylstilbestrol (DES) by mother during pregnancy

Understanding and practice of safe sex principles

Males

Immunization for mumps or history of the disease

Pain or swelling of testes or scrotum

Sores on or discharge from penis

Impotence, temporary or ongoing

Females

Immunization for rubella or history of the disease

Use of oral contraceptives or estrogen products

Gynecologic-obstetric history

Menstrual history

Age at menarche, interval and duration of periods, amount of flow

Problems with menstruation: dysmenorrhea, amenorrhea

Obstetric history

Pregnancies: dates, delivery type, complications

Abortions or miscarriages

Contraceptive history

Types used, duration, complications if any

Current complaint

Location, severity, duration, and self-treatment of all symptoms

Pain, bleeding, or discharge

Burning or itching of genitals

Sores on genitals

Swelling or masses

Urinary symptoms, such as urgency, frequency, dysuria, hematuria

Gastrointestinal (GI) symptoms, such as nausea, bloating, constipation

OBJECTIVE DATA

Physical Examination of the Female

Breast examination

Inspection for size, shape, color, contour, and symmetry

Palpation (using flat surface of three fingers)

Small concentric circles moving outward from nipple

Include tail of breast and axilla

Areola; gently squeeze nipple to check for discharge

Move nipples from side to side for mobility assessment

Abdominal examination

Inspection for symmetry, presence of masses; hair amount and distribution

GERONTOLOGIC PATIENT CONSIDERATIONS: PHYSIOLOGIC CHANGES IN THE REPRODUCTIVE TRACT

FEMALE

Mons pubis	Decreased fullness caused by redistribution of fat pad
Pubic hair	Becomes gray to white and thinner Curly hair becomes straightened
Labia majora/minora	Decrease in size Mucous membranes lining minora become dry and pale
Vagina	Decreased width and length; walls become drier and thinner Vaginal entrance (introitus) narrowed Vaginal secretions decrease and become more alkaline
Ovaries	Atrophy, with decreased size Nonpalpable 3-5 years after menopause
Uterus	Decreased size, lining thin

MALE

Pubic hair	Becomes gray to white and thinner Curly hair becomes straightened
Testes	Decreased size and firmness Change in position (lower)
Scrotum	More pendulous with fewer rugae
Seminal fluid	Decreased amount and viscosity
Prostate gland	Hypertrophy (enlargement)
Penis	Decreased size and sensation Easily retractable foreskin (if uncircumcised)
Ejaculation	Decreased force and volume
Bladder	Increase in bladder neck tone

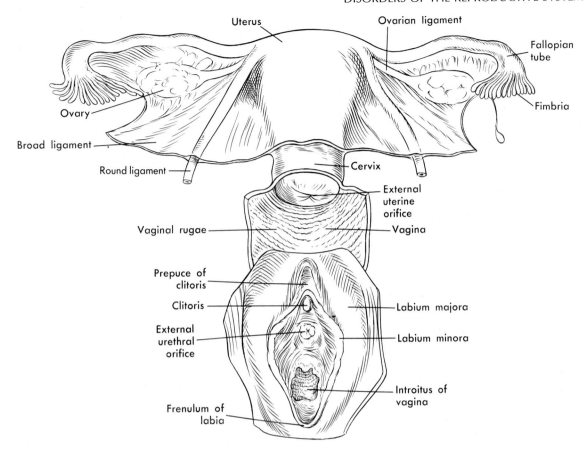

FIGURE 16-1 Female internal organs of reproduction. Major ligaments are shown.

Muscle tone, areas of weakness or herniation

Palpation for masses (NOTE: The reproductive organs are normally situated in the pelvis and are not palpable through the abdominal wall. Any mass is described by size, shape, tenderness, and relationship to pelvic or abdominal organs.)

Uterus: midline of lower abdomen

Fallopian tubes and ovaries: right and left lower quadrants

Pelvic examination

Lithotomy position with legs supported if possible

Inspection of external genitals for symmetry and presence of enlargement, lesions, exudates, scarring, or leukoplakia

Inspection of vagina and cervix following insertion of speculum

Cervix: color, contour, position, size, surface characteristics, patency of os, presence of discharge or erosion, polyps, scars

Vagina: color, consistency of mucosa and presence of ulcers, inflammation, rugae, odor, or discharge

Palpation of internal organs

Cervix: consistency and contour, free movement

Uterus: position; size, shape, and regularity of surface; free movement

Fallopian tubes and ovaries: fallopian tubes rarely palpable and ovaries may not be palpable, especially in obese women

Rectovaginal examination to confirm placement of the uterus and assess adnexal areas and rectal tone

Physical Examination of the Male

Inspection

Abdominal inspection as outlined above

Inguinal inspection for herniation

External genitals for structural abnormalities and visible evidence of discharge, infection, or masses

Palpation

Inguinal lymph nodes

Retractability of foreskin

Testes: size, shape, consistency, and presence of tenderness

Spermatic cords

Prostate gland (palpated rectally): size, shape, consistency, and presence of nodules

ASSESSMENT OF SEXUAL HEALTH

Human sexuality involves a complex interplay of biologic, psychologic, and sociocultural variables. It is now widely recognized that aging, illness, hospitalization, and surgery all can have a profound impact on an individual's sexual health. Pharmacologic effects, physiologic changes, structural changes, body image changes, and environmental factors can all affect sexual health, libido, and sexual functioning. It is generally accepted

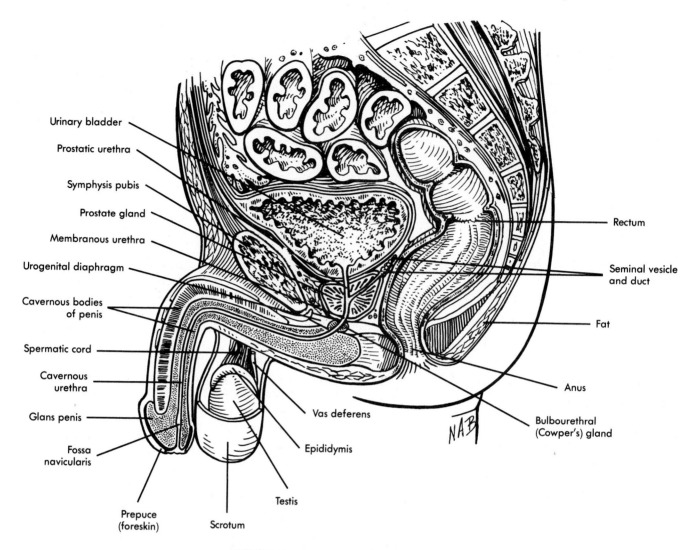

FIGURE 16-2 Male organs of reproduction.

that it is crucial for nurses to be sensitive and alert to the potential impact of illness and treatment on sexuality as assessment and care planning are conducted. However, many nurses remain unfamiliar with the techniques of sexual assessment and are uncomfortable about using them. The nurse should realize that no single approach to taking a sexual history is appropriate for every situation. General guidelines include the following:

Ensure privacy and establish an atmosphere of trust and confidentiality.

Begin sexual assessment with initial nursing assessment, use only language the patient understands, and clarify all terms.

Move from less sensitive to more sensitive areas.

Respect the patient's right to not participate in the process.

Encourage questions and comments.

Make questions all inclusive; for example, use "how" and "when" rather than "did you ever."

Indicate that practices are not unusual or shocking: for example, "many people experience. . . ."

A brief sexual assessment can be easily incorporated into the basic nursing assessment with the inclusion of three simple questions:

Has your (illness, hospitalization, etc.) affected your being a (wife, husband, mother, etc.)?

Has your (illness, surgery, etc.) affected the way you see yourself as a (man, woman)?

Has your (surgery, heart attack, etc.) affected your ability to function sexually (or your sex life)?

These questions are nonthreatening and place sexuality within its proper context of self-concept, self-esteem, and role performance. They invite patients to share their concerns. If concerns or problems are uncovered it is important to explore the following areas:

- Patient's understanding of the problem
- Onset, nature, duration, and severity
- Attempts at self-treatment explored
- Desires or expectations related to treatment

✍ DIAGNOSTIC TESTS

LABORATORY TESTS

Blood and Urine Tests

A variety of blood and urine tests (Table 16-1) may be used to evaluate problems of the reproductive system. They include tests of endocrine function, enzymes, and syphilis tests.

Cultures and Smears

Most infectious processes of the reproductive tract produce a purulent discharge. Secretions may be obtained for culture or smear from any orifice. The culture for *Neisseria gonorrhoeae* is one of the most important, since it is the only means of confirming a diagnosis of gonorrhea in asymptomatic women. The approach is also used for the evaluation of vaginitis, candidiasis, trichomoniasis, *Gardnerella,* and herpes simplex. Chlamydial infection is evaluated by analysis of cells obtained from the urethra or cervix rather than exudate. Various cultures, smears, and cytology examinations are summarized in Table 16-2.

RADIOLOGIC TESTS

Ultrasonography

Purpose—Ultrasonography is used primarily to detect foreign bodies and distinguish between cystic and solid masses; measure organ size; and evaluate fetal age, position, and viability. The transvaginal approach is being used increasingly to provide improved picture clarity, particularly of the structure of the ovary.

Procedure—The transducer is guided over the pelvic area, and the images are observed on an oscilloscope with the patient in a supine position. The transvaginal approach utilizes the lithotomy position, and the transducer is inserted a few centimeters into the vagina. A transrectal approach is used for prostate evaluation.

Patient preparation and aftercare—Patient education is the only real pretest requirement. The procedure is safe, noninvasive, and painless. A full bladder is needed to provide a landmark for defining pelvic organs, so the patient is instructed to increase her fluid intake before the test and not void. No aftercare is required.

Hysterosalpingography

Purpose—Hysterosalpingography involves visualization of the uterine cavity and fallopian tubes after injection of contrast material through the cervix. It is generally included in a fertility workup but also is useful in evaluating uterine and tubal tumors or other abnormalities.

Procedure—The patient is placed in the lithotomy position, and a plastic cannula is inserted into the cervix. Contrast medium is injected, and the uterus and fallopian tubes are viewed fluoroscopically. Serial x-rays are taken as the dye moves throughout the organs. The test takes about 15 minutes.

Patient preparation and aftercare—Patient education is the major pretest requirement. The procedure may trigger moderate cramping. The patient is also assessed for any known allergy to dyes, iodine, or shellfish. Mild analgesics may be used after the test if cramping persists. Some vaginal drainage of the dye is expected for 1 or 2 days. The patient is instructed to report the development of any signs of infection.

Computed Tomography

Purpose—Computed tomography (CT) scans are primarily used in gynecologic oncology to detect extension of pelvic cancer into the fat of the retroperitoneal space. CT is more useful in staging than in diagnosis, since surgical biopsy of all masses is still required.

Procedure—The patient is placed supine on the radiographic table, and serial x-rays are taken from a variety of perspectives, which are then computer regenerated into a detailed mapping of the organs. A contrast medium may be administered for improved visualization. A tampon may be inserted to help delineate the vaginal cavity in interpreting the films.

Patient preparation and aftercare—Patient education is provided before the test. Patients are carefully evaluated for allergy to iodine or shellfish. A mild premedication may be administered, particularly if the patient is claustrophobic. Patients who receive an oral contrast medium are kept NPO for 4 hours before the test. No aftercare is required.

Magnetic Resonance Imaging

Purpose—Magnetic resonance imaging (MRI) is used to achieve a better contrast between normal and pathologic tissue than can be obtained through CT scan. It is particularly effective in evaluating conditions associated with edema. It is used to monitor the spread of uterine and cervical malignancy.

Procedure—The patient is placed in a supine position on a narrow table, which slides into the desired position in the scanner. It generates a powerful magnetic field, and radiofrequency energy is directed at the pelvis. The images are shown on a monitor and transcribed on tape.

Patient preparation and aftercare—The test is painless and noninvasive, but careful teaching is required. The confined space can be frightening for any patient with claustrophobic tendencies, and loud noises are generated by the machinery that can be frightening. Earplugs may be provided. All metallic objects must be removed, and if the patient has a pacemaker, artificial valve, clip, or pin the test cannot be performed. No aftercare is required.

Mammography

Purpose—Mammography is a radiologic study of the soft tissue of the breast used to evaluate differences

TABLE 16-1   Blood and Urine Tests of the Reproductive System

TEST	DESCRIPTION	PRETEST AND POSTTEST CARE
BLOOD		
Endocrine Studies		
Prolactin assay	Detects pituitary dysfunction and causes of amenorrhea	Patient fasts before test
Serum androstenedione and testosterone levels	Ascertain whether elevated androgens are due to adrenal or ovarian dysfunction; serum testosterone also drawn to assess cause of amenorrhea	No special preparation needed
Serum progesterone radioimmuno-assay (RIA)	Used to detect functioning corpus luteum cyst; may also be used in determining adrenal pathologic conditions	Patient fasts before test; sample drawn around day 24 or 25 of menstrual cycle if possible
Serum estradiol RIA	Measures ovarian function; particularly useful in assessing estrogen-secreting tumors	Patient fasts before test
Enzyme Studies		
Acid phosphatase	Enzyme appears primarily in prostate gland and semen; high levels may indicate a prostate tumor with metastasis beyond prostatic capsule	No special preparation needed
Alkaline phosphatase	Enzyme reflects bone metabolism; high levels in known prostate cancer may indicate bony metastasis	Patient fasts before test
Prostate-specific antigen (PSA)	Enzyme appears in varying concentrations in normal and malignant prostatic tissue; used to monitor course of cancer and response to treatment; not useful for cancer screening at this time	No special preparation needed. Sample collected before digital prostate examination, which triggers enzyme release
Syphilis Studies		
General note: Check with the particular laboratory, regarding fasting requirements; some prefer patients to refrain from alcohol use for 24 hr before test		
Nontreponemal serologic tests Wassermann (complement fixation) Venereal Disease Research Laboratory (VDRL) (flocculation) Rapid plasma reagin (RPR) (agglutination)	Nonspecific antibody tests used to detect syphilis; positive readings can be made within 1-2 wk after appearance of primary lesion (chancre) or 4-15 wk after initial infection	No special preparation needed
Treponemal test Fluorescent treponemal antibody absorption (FTA-ABS)	Detects syphilis antibodies; also detects early syphilis with great accuracy; usually performed if results of nontreponemal testing are questionable	No special preparation needed
URINE		
Pregnancy testing (Pregnosticon Dri Dot [latex inhibition test], Gravindex, Pregnosticon Accuspheres [hemagglutination-inhibition])	HCG detected in urine to ascertain whether woman is pregnant; hydatidiform mole and chorioepithelioma (in men and women) may also be detected	Patient collects first morning urine specimen
Hormone testing Total estrogen levels	Urine estrogen levels used to detect ovarian pathologic conditions, hyperadrenalism, interstitial cell tumor of testes, liver disease, and ectopic pregnancy; 24-hr urine collection required; normal levels vary, depending on menstrual cycle	Urine collected and refrigerate for 24 hours
Pregnanediol levels	Progesterone levels assessed; most commonly used to detect corpus luteum cysts, and sometimes threatened abortions; may also be used to determine adrenocortical function and causes of amenorrhea; normal levels vary according to menstrual cycle or length of gestation	Urine collected and refrigerated for 24 hr
Testosterone levels	Tumors and developmental anomalies of testes can be detected	Urine collected and refrigerated for 24 hours

TABLE 16-2 Diagnostic Tests of the Reproductive System: Cultures and Smears

TEST	DESCRIPTION	PRETEST AND POSTTEST CARE
Dark-field microscopy	Direct examination of specimen obtained from potential syphilitic lesion (chancre) performed to detect *Treponema*	None
Wet mounts	Direct microscopic examination of specimen of vaginal discharge; determines presence or absence of *Trichomonas* organisms, bacteria, white and red blood cells (WBCs; RBCs)	Patient instructed not to douche before test
Cultures	Specimens of vaginal, urethral, or cervical discharge taken and used to assess presence of gonorrhea, chlamydia, or yeast	Patient instructed not to douche before test; urethral specimens obtained from male before voiding
Gram stain	Presumptive test used for rapid detection of gonorrhea	Same as cultures
Pap smear	Microscopic study of exfoliated cells via special staining and fixation technique detects malignancy; cells most commonly studied are those obtained directly from endocervix, cervix, vaginal pool, and endometrial lining of uterine cavity	Sample ideally taken at midpoint of menstrual cycle; patient instructed not to douche or tub bathe for 24 hours before examination; some physicians instruct patient to refrain from intercourse for 24 hours before test

in the density of the tissue and screen for malignancies that are too small to be palpated on physical examination.

Procedure—At least two radiographic views of each breast are taken while the breast is compressed between a platform and the x-ray cassette. The test is painless, but most women report some degree of discomfort from the chest compression. The test takes about 15 minutes.

Patient preparation and aftercare—Patient education is critical, especially if the test is being taken for the first time. The woman is advised that mammography has a high rate of false-positive results. The woman should avoid the use of deodorants, creams, or powders, which can mimic calcium clusters on x-ray. No aftercare is needed, although teaching may be provided concerning breast self-examination and the importance of regular screening after 50 years of age.

BIOPSIES
Cervical Biopsy

Purpose—A cervical biopsy is performed to obtain a tissue specimen for pathologic examination.

Procedure—A punch biopsy can be safely performed as an office procedure. Culdoscopic direction is standardly used. Conization involves the removal of a cone-shaped portion of the cervix and may be used therapeutically as well as diagnostically, and local anesthesia is used.

Patient preparation and aftercare—Patient teaching is the primary consideration. The woman is reassured that the cervix has few pain receptors, and discomfort with a punch biopsy is minimal. The woman is instructed to leave the tampon or packing in place for 8 to 24 hours and to report the incidence of excessive bleeding. Bleeding is more extensive after conization, and the woman is instructed to expect her menstrual flow to be increased for 2 to 3 months.

Endometrial Biopsy

Purpose—Endometrial biopsy is used primarily to diagnose cancer but can also evaluate bleeding or polyps and determine whether ovulation has occurred.

Procedure—A small curette is introduced into the uterus, and several strips of endometrial tissue are obtained for examination. It may be combined with a dilation and curettage (D&C) or other therapeutic procedure.

Patient preparation and aftercare—Patient teaching is the primary consideration. No special preparation is required. Some vaginal bleeding is expected after the procedure, but the woman is instructed to report excessive bleeding and any signs of infection. Douching and intercourse are restricted for 72 hours, and the woman should avoid any strenuous exercise or heavy lifting.

Breast Biopsy

Purpose—Breast biopsy is used to differentiate among fibrocystic lesions, fibroadenomas, and cancer.

Procedure—Fine needle aspiration, incisional, and excisional biopsy approaches may be used, and local anesthetic is usually sufficient.

Patient preparation and aftercare—Careful patient teaching is required, since this is usually an extremely stressful time for the patient. Aftercare involves monitoring the incision site for bleeding or infection. Numbness at the site may persist for months.

Prostate Needle Biopsy

Purpose—Needle biopsy of the prostate is performed to obtain cells for histologic study, usually to rule out cancer in the gland.

Procedure—The biopsy can be performed as an outpatient procedure with the patient under local anesthesia. Either a transrectal or transperineal approach is used. Ultrasound may be used to guide or evaluate the placement of the needle.

TABLE 16-3 Fertility Tests

TEST	DESCRIPTION	PRETEST AND POSTTEST CARE
Hormonal tests	See p. 382	
Semen analysis	Semen assessed for volume (2-5 ml), viscosity, sperm count (greater than 20 million/ml), sperm motility (60% motile), and percent of abnormal sperm (60% with normal structure)	Patient instructed to refrain from intercourse for 2-5 days and submit specimen within 2 hr of ejaculation
Basal body temperature	Indicates indirectly whether ovulation has occurred (Temperature rises at ovulation and remains elevated during secretory phase of normal menstrual cycle.)	Patient instructed to take and graph her temperature each morning before getting out of bed
Sims-Huhner test (postcoital cervical mucous test or cervical mucous sperm penetration test)	Mucus sample from cervix examined within 2-8 hr after intercourse, total number of sperm assessed in relation to number of live sperm; test performed to determine whether cervical mucus is "hostile" to passage of sperm from vagina into uterus	Couple instructed to refrain from intercourse for 3 days and then have intercourse at estimated time of ovulation; female instructed not to douche, bathe, or use supplemental vaginal lubrication and to remain in bed for at least 15 min after intercourse
Endometrial biopsy	See p. 383	
Laparoscopy	See below.	

Patient preparation and aftercare—Bowel cleansing may be ordered if a transrectal approach is used. The man is instructed to report the incidence of bleeding or any signs of infection, since sepsis is a potentially life-threatening complication. Prophylactic antibiotics are usually prescribed.

ENDOSCOPY

The pelvic organs and tissues can be visualized directly by endoscopy. Visualizations of the vagina and cervix (colposcopy), cul-de-sac of Douglas (culdoscopy), uterus (hysteroscopy), and fallopian tubes (fallopscopy) are variations often combined with other tests, but laparoscopy is the most sophisticated and extensively used test.

Laparoscopy

Purpose—Laparoscopy is used to inspect the outer surface of the pelvic organs as part of an evaluation of pelvic masses, endometriosis, or infertility, but it can also be combined with therapeutic interventions such as lysis of adhesions and tubal ligation.

Procedure—A needle is inserted through a small incision in the subumbilical area, and the peritoneal cavity is filled with 3 to 4 L of carbon dioxide to separate the abdominal wall from the viscera. The laparoscope is then inserted for inspection or treatment. The woman will receive a local or general anesthetic, and the test takes about 15 to 30 minutes.

Patient preparation and aftercare—The woman receives pretest teaching and is instructed to fast for 8 hours before the test. Referred pain to the shoulder is common from irritation of the gas, and the woman should be warned to expect its occurrence. Vital signs and urine output are monitored after the test, and the woman is encouraged to rest for about 24 hours before resuming her normal activities. She is instructed to report the presence of persistent abdominal pain, abnormal vaginal bleeding, and any signs of infections around the insertion sites.

INFERTILITY TESTS

The evaluation of infertility includes a battery of tests for the male and female partners. They are designed to establish a cause of infertility, determine a prognosis, and provide a basis for planning appropriate medical or surgical intervention, if any. Tests for the male focus on the number and viability of the sperm. Tests for the female determine the patency and functioning of the various organs and presence and regularity of ovulation and establish the adequacy of the hormonal balance to support pregnancy. The major tests are summarized in Table 16-3.

PROMOTING SEXUAL HEALTH

Annon (1974) presented a model for intervening with persons with potential concerns or problems related to sexuality that has been widely accepted in clinical practice. This PLISSIT model contains the levels of *p*ermission, *li*mited *i*nformation, *s*pecific *s*uggestions, and *i*ntensive *t*herapy. Nurses in general practice usually employ strategies from the first three levels.

Permission—The level of permission involves a wide variety of preventive and therapeutic interventions, including permission to (1) be concerned about sexual issues; (2) discuss alternative approaches to sexual pleasure when structural changes interfere with normal patterns; (3) grieve over losses, such as mastectomy; and (4) *not* engage in certain behaviors or activities. The process of assessment is often the most powerful form of permission. It validates sexuality as a legitimate topic of concern and indicates the nurse's willingness to serve as a resource.

Limited information—The limited information level provides the patient with information that is directly relevant to managing concerns about the particular situation. It again involves both preventive and therapeutic interventions. Examples include (1) basic education about sexuality and safe sex; (2) information about sexuality, pregnancy, aging, or menopause; and (3) information about sexuality adaptations following hysterectomy, myocardial infarction (MI), or ostomy.

Specific suggestions—The specific suggestions level directs interventions toward an actual or potential problem in sexuality and demands a specialty knowledge base from the nurse. Examples include suggestions for (1) positioning variations for intercourse for patients with arthritis, (2) incorporating sexual rehabilitation into cardiac rehabilitation, and (3) alternatives for sexual activity for spinal cord–injured patients. Open partner communication is often the most important suggestion that the nurse can offer.

Intensive therapy—The intensive therapy level is beyond the expertise of most nurses, but referral for management of sexual problems is as critical as referral for management of any other ongoing physical or psychologic problem.

DISORDERS OF THE FEMALE REPRODUCTIVE SYSTEM
DISORDERS OF MENSTRUATION

Almost all women experience problems with their menstrual cycle at some point in their reproductive years. Most problems are self-managed and rarely require medical intervention.

Dysmenorrhea

Dysmenorrhea, or menstrual cramps, affect about 75% of menstruating women to some degree and are the single most common cause of absenteeism among women in school and industry. Primary dysmenorrhea occurs in the absence of any demonstrable organic disease. Its severity typically decreases after pregnancy or 30 years of age. The pain results from a high concentration of prostaglandins, which stimulate uterine contractions, and is typically described as colicky, localized in the lower abdomen, and varying in severity from mild to incapacitating. Prostaglandin inhibitors such as aspirin and ibuprofen are the primary treatment. Local heat may also be helpful. Oral contraceptives may be prescribed in severe cases, although their mechanism of action is unknown.

Amenorrhea

Primary amenorrhea exists if the first menses has not occurred by 16 years of age. It is usually the result of a genetic or developmental defect. Secondary amenor-

rhea, when menstruation stops for more than 3 months, may result from stress, excessive exercise, or an acquired pathologic condition. It is relatively common among highly conditioned athletes. It is theorized to occur from hypothalamic/pituitary dysfunction related to excess dopamine levels coupled with failure to maintain the critical percentage of body fat needed to sustain menstruation. The primary adverse effects are infertility and excess bone resorption that may hasten osteoporosis. Counseling is the foundation of treatment, but hormonal therapy may be needed in certain situations.

Premenstrual Syndrome

Premenstrual syndrome (PMS) involves a cluster of physical and behavioral symptoms that occur in the second half of the menstrual cycle. About 40% of women are estimated to be affected to some degree. The etiology is unknown, but the symptoms are related to imbalances in various hormones such as estrogen, progesterone, and aldosterone. Classic symptoms include irritability and mood swings, water retention and bloating, headache, fatigue, and insomnia. Treatment may involve hormone therapy, diet modification, caffeine and sodium restriction, and life-style modification including regular aerobic exercise, rest, and stress management.

Dysfunctional Uterine Bleeding

Abnormal or irregular uterine bleeding can take many forms and be caused by a variety of factors, including systemic diseases and endocrine abnormalities. About 50% of all cases occur in perimenopausal women, in whom it is a significant warning sign of uterine cancer, which is diagnosed in 35% to 50% of cases. The diagnosis may involve endocrine studies or an endometrial biopsy. Treatment is guided by the cause and is usually conservative. Hormone therapy may be employed, and hysterectomy may be indicated if the bleeding cannot be controlled. Treatment for anemia may also be indicated.

Endometriosis

Endometriosis involves the seeding of endometrial cells, which normally line the uterus, throughout the pelvis. It affects women of childbearing age, and its etiology is unknown. It is a common cause of infertility. With each menstrual cycle the cells are stimulated by ovarian hormones and then bleed into the surrounding tissues, causing an inflammatory response. The classic symptom is dysmenorrhea that becomes progressively worse, and it is diagnosed through laparoscopy. Treatment is variable and may include hormonal therapy to suppress tissue growth and ovarian function. Pregnancy may be recommended if the woman desires children, since the fertility rate worsens over time. Hysterectomy may be required in severe cases. Menopause stops the progress of the disorder.

INFECTIOUS PROCESSES

Vaginitis

Etiology/epidemiology

Vaginitis is one of the most common gynecologic disorders. The cause is bacterial in most cases, and candidiasis and trichomoniasis account for about 40% of all cases. Viruses, parasites, and irritants are other potential causes. Risk factors include oral contraceptive use, low estrogen levels, poor hygiene, intercourse with infected partners, and treatment with broad-spectrum antibiotics.

Pathophysiology

The acid pH and normal flora of the vagina are effective barriers to infection. Any agent or event that alters the pH or lowers resistance can result in infection. Classic symptoms include tissue inflammation, discharge, and pruritus. Various forms of vaginitis and other infectious processes are summarized in Table 16-4.

Medical management

The diagnosis is usually established by culture of the discharge. Treatment is largely pharmacologic and administered orally, by ointment, by cream, or by vaginal suppository. Common treatments are also summarized in Table 16-4.

TABLE 16-4	Common Infections of the Female Reproductive System
CLINICAL MANIFESTATIONS	**MEDICAL MANAGEMENT**
NONSPECIFIC VAGINITIS	
Grayish white discharge Fishy or foul odor	Appropriate antibiotic applied locally or taken systemically, e.g., ampicillin or metronidazole (Flagyl)
CANDIDIASIS	
Vaginal itching and irritation Thick, white, cheesy discharge	Nystatin (Mycostatin) vaginal suppositories Miconazole (Monistat) vaginal cream
TRICHOMONIASIS	
Severe vulvar itching, burning, excoriation Yellowish to greenish discharge that is thick, foamy, and malodorous	Metronidazole (Flagyl) orally Symptomatic treatment
CERVICITIS	
Leukorrhea may be only external symptom Cervix edematous and erythematous	Appropriate antibiotic therapy after culture
BARTHOLINITIS	
Erythema around Bartholin's gland Severe swelling, edema, and pain Resolution of inflammation may produce a cyst	Appropriate antibiotics Surgical drainage or gland excision

NURSING MANAGEMENT

Women have self-managed mild infections for generations, and many folk or lay cures are in use. Nursing intervention focuses on teaching concerning proper perineal hygiene, appropriate use of pharmacologic agents, and the importance of refraining from intercourse until the infection is controlled. Male partners should be encouraged to use condoms to prevent reinfection, and referral for partner treatment may be important. Sitz baths and local heat may be comforting when symptoms are acute. Women are cautioned to avoid routine douching, which may alter the vaginal pH.

Pelvic Inflammatory Disease

Etiology/epidemiology

Pelvic inflammatory disease (PID) is a general term used to describe acute or chronic infection of the reproductive organs. About 1 million cases are diagnosed annually, primarily in young, sexually active women. The risk factors overlap those for STDs and include multiple sex partners and the use of intrauterine devices (IUDs).

Pathophysiology

Pathogenic organisms generally ascend from the cervical canal and invade the pelvis through the fallopian tubes. Gonococcus, chlamydia, and streptococcus are common pathogens. The inflammatory response causes purulent material to collect in the tubes, and both adhesions and strictures may form that can lead to sterility. Symptoms include abdominal pain and cramping, fever and chills, nausea and vomiting, and a foul-smelling vaginal discharge.

Medical Management

PID is diagnosed through blood studies, cultures of discharge, and possibly laparoscopy. Treatment involves broad-spectrum antibiotics and may necessitate surgery if abscesses are found or organs are compromised by the infection.

NURSING MANAGEMENT

The nursing role primarily involves support and comfort measures. Local heat may be comforting. Frequent perineal care may be needed if the drainage is copious. Fluids are encouraged, and both vital signs and intake and output are carefully monitored. Tub and sitz baths and the use of tampons are contraindicated until the infection is eradicated. The woman's sexual partner may also require treatment.

Toxic Shock Syndrome

Etiology/epidemiology

Toxic shock syndrome (TSS) is a severe disease triggered by certain strains of staphylococci that produce a unique toxin. It occurs in a variety of situations but is clearly associated with tampon use during menstruation. The overall incidence rate has dropped significantly since the link with tampon use was established.

Pathophysiology

The exact mechanism by which the organisms gain access to the circulatory system is unclear, and the role of tampons is only speculative. They are theorized to obstruct the vagina and cause a retrograde flow or increase the number of aerobic bacteria. Symptom onset is abrupt and includes high fever, vomiting, diarrhea, and general prostration. It can progress to hypotensive shock. A sunburnlike rash frequently develops over the face, extremities, and trunk.

Medical management

The diagnosis is confirmed by blood studies and cultures of the throat, urine, and vaginal secretions. Beta lactamase–resistant antibiotics are the cornerstone of care. Critically ill women may require shock management.

NURSING MANAGEMENT

The nursing role is largely supportive and involves careful monitoring of all physiologic parameters. Teaching for the general population includes the importance of scrupulous perineal hygiene, avoiding douching, limiting tampon use, particularly the superabsorbent varieties, and changing tampons every 2 to 3 hours when in use.

STRUCTURAL PROBLEMS: UTERINE DISPLACEMENT OR PROLAPSE

Etiology/epidemiology

The uterus may undergo minor displacement, which is of no real clinical significance, or it may be displaced in ways that involve other organs and create troublesome symptoms. Significant displacements include the following:

prolapse Uterus protrudes through the pelvic floor or vagina.
cystocele Bladder herniates into the vagina as the vaginal walls relax.
rectocele Rectal wall herniates into the vagina as the vaginal walls relax.

The conditions frequently occur in combination. Displacement occurs most frequently in multiparous women as a gradual response to childbirth injuries, relaxation of the muscles and ligaments with aging, and the prolonged effects of obesity and chronic constipation. Up to one half of all parous women develop some degree of structural relaxation, but only 10% become actively symptomatic.

Pathophysiology

Estrogen helps to maintain adequate blood flow and tone to the tissues, and menopause results in atrophic changes that render the tissues more susceptible to prolapse. The uterine prolapse may be contained within the vagina or prolapse entirely below the vaginal orifice. The woman may be asymptomatic or complain of backache that worsens with standing or walking. More severe prolapses create a distinct feeling of displaced mass. Leukorrhea, discharge, or bleeding may occur. Urinary stress incontinence typically accompanies cystocele, and chronic constipation may occur with rectocele.

Medical management

The diagnosis is readily established on physical examination. Asymptomatic problems are usually not treated, although estrogen therapy may be used for postmenopausal women. Conservative treatment may include the insertion of a pessary to support the uterus in a forward and balanced position by exerting pressure on the ligaments attached to the posterior wall of the cervix. Surgical intervention is usually planned when symptoms interfere with the woman's life-style. Hysterectomy is usually performed and may be supplemented by colporrhaphy, which tightens the vaginal wall, or a Marshall-Marchetti-Krantz type of urethrovesical suspension, which is used to correct stress incontinence.

NURSING MANAGEMENT

The Kegel perineal exercises are the mainstay of patient education. The exercises are repeated in sets of 10 at least 10 to 12 times per day. The nurse will also encourage and assist overweight women to lose weight and lessen intraabdominal pressure.

Women fitted with a pessary are taught how to insert or withdraw it if the device becomes displaced or uncomfortable. Pessaries need to be removed and cleaned every few weeks or months as established by the physician to prevent infection or fistula formation.

Surgical care is primarily related to the hysterectomy procedure (see p. 391). The nurse will assist the woman to perform perineal cleansing or douching as ordered. A Foley catheter is inserted after anterior colporrhaphy or bladder suspension and will be left in place for about 4 days. Stool softeners and laxatives are administered to prevent stress to the vaginal repair. Discharge instructions include avoiding heavy lifting, prolonged standing or walking, and sexual intercourse until healing is complete. A high-fiber diet and liberal amounts of fluids are encouraged to prevent infection. Vaginal sensation may be lost for several months after surgery, and the woman is reassured that this is a temporary problem.

BENIGN AND MALIGNANT NEOPLASMS
Cancer of the Cervix
Etiology/epidemiology

The incidence of invasive cervical cancer has declined steadily over the last 50 years at least partly in response to improved screening and early detection. Most lesions are now detected in their early precancerous stages

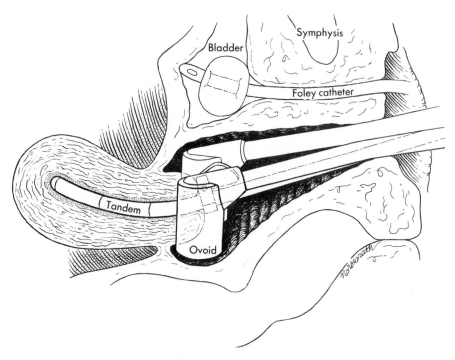

FIGURE 16-3   Placement of tandem and colpostats before vaginal packing.

when cure rates are 88% to 100%. Although the etiology remains unknown, clear association has been found with early and frequent sexual contact with multiple partners and viral cervical infection. Other risk factors include multiparity, low socioeconomic status, vitamin deficiencies, and possibly heavy smoking.

Pathophysiology

Ninety-five percent of all cervical cancers are squamous cell. Precursor lesions are classified by the degree of cell dysplasia from mild to severe, or carcinoma in situ. Dysplasia may regress but commonly progresses to carcinoma. The disease spreads by direct extension and blood and lymph invasion.

The disease is asymptomatic in its early stages. Progressive disease creates a watery discharge that may progress to bloody or foul smelling. Pain is a late sign as the growing tumor places pressure on the rectum, bladder, and lower back.

Medical management

The diagnosis of cervical cancer is confirmed by biopsy. The Pap smear is a screening tool but not a diagnostic test. Punch biopsy may be employed or conization, which combines treatment for early disease with preservation of reproductive capability. The disease is treated according to its stage, and treatment is typically aggressive to ensure a cure. Carcinoma in situ may be treated with conization, laser surgery, or cryosurgery to preserve fertility. More invasive disease is treated with simple hysterectomy with external or intracavitary implant radiotherapy (Figure 16-3), and extensive disease

is approached with radical hysterectomy or pelvic exenteration. Chemotherapy has traditionally not been very successful in disease management.

NURSING MANAGEMENT

◆ ASSESSMENT
Subjective Data

Pain: generalized abdominal discomfort; pelvic, back, or flank pain; pain with intercourse

Dysuria or constipation

Anorexia, fatigue, and weight loss

Objective Data

Vaginal discharge: thin and watery advancing to dark and foul smelling; spotting or intermittent metrorrhagia

Cervical erosion or enlargement, obvious lesion

Leg edema: late sign

◆ NURSING DIAGNOSES

Nursing diagnoses for the woman with cervical cancer being treated with intracavitary radiotherapy may include, but are not limited to, the following:

Anxiety (related to the fear of radiation, diagnosis of cancer, and the uncertainty of the outcome)

Self-care deficit: bathing, toileting (related to activity restrictions during treatment)

Social isolation (related to restrictions necessitated by the intracavitary implant)

Altered health maintenance, risk of (related to insufficient knowledge about home care management)

◆ EXPECTED PATIENT OUTCOMES

Patient will express less anxiety about treatment restrictions and communicate feelings about diagnosis and treatment.

Patient will adapt self-care activities to needed restrictions and accept help as needed.

Patient will utilize diversional activities within the established safety guidelines.

Patient will demonstrate competency in home care skills and correctly identify signs of complications.

◆ NURSING INTERVENTIONS

Reducing Anxiety

Encourage expression of feelings and concerns.

Provide privacy for expression of emotions.

Assess patient's understanding of the diagnosis and treatment options.

Provide careful teaching about intracavitary radiotherapy and its associated restrictions and safety precautions (see Guidelines box and Box 16-1).

Guidelines for Nursing Care of the Woman Undergoing Internal Radiotherapy

PREIMPLANTATION

Care before the insertion of the radioactive implant usually includes the following:

Cleansing enema to empty the bowel

Insertion of a Foley catheter to keep the bladder empty and small during treatment

Povidone-iodine (Betadine) douche and shaving of the pubic area if ordered

IMPLANTATION PERIOD

Care during the 24-72 hours of treatment includes the following:

Insertion of gauze packing into the vagina to separate the rectum and bladder from the irradiated area (One or two stitches may be taken in the labia to support the holder in position.)

Strict bed rest

Head of bed elevated no more than 20 degrees

Turning from side to side permitted

Low-residue diet and possibly antimotility agents to prevent bowel distension

Analgesics as needed for uterine cramping, which can be severe

Routine perineal cleansing if drainage is present; room deodorizer if discharge is foul smelling

A minimum fluid intake of 2500 ml daily

Emotional support, for example, visiting patient frequently from room doorway

Diversional activities appropriate to activity restrictions

Monitoring implant for proper placement

Long-handled forceps and a lead-lined container kept in the room in case of dislodgement

Monitoring for complications

Infection: increased vaginal redness or swelling; increasingly dark, foul-smelling drainage; cloudy urine; fever

Thrombophlebitis: painful leg swelling, positive Homans' sign

---

BOX 16-1	Radiation Precautions for Internal Radiotherapy

1. Time at the bedside is limited; each contact should last no more than 30 minutes.
2. Children and pregnant women/staff should not visit during treatment.
3. Staff members should wear a dosimeter during every patient contact to monitor radiation exposure.
4. Lead shield may be installed at the side and foot of the bed.
5. Staff should utilize the principles of distance, time, and shielding in all contacts with the patient.
6. Implant is always handled by means of long-handled forceps, never with the hands. A lead-lined container should be present in the room for use if the implant dislodges.
7. A sign that clearly identifies the radiation hazard is posted on the room door.
8. A contact number for the radiation safety officer of the institution should be posted on the warning sign.

Promoting Self-Care

Reinforce teaching concerning all activity restrictions.

Ensure that all self-care articles are within easy reach.

Provide assistance as necessary to support flat bed rest.

Encourage frequent turning and position changes.

Provide back care and massage.

Assist with needed perineal hygiene and pad changes; provide room deodorizer if foul smelling.

Administer analgesics for cramping as needed, and assess for effectiveness.

Encourage a liberal fluid intake, at least 2500 to 3000 ml daily.

Teach range of motion and leg exercises to prevent phlebothrombosis.

Preventing Isolation

Visit with patient frequently, maintaining prescribed distances for radiation safety.

Encourage family and friends to visit.

Explain rationale for all time and distance restrictions, and assist with monitoring.

Prevent visitation by children and pregnant women during the treatment period.

Provide a pleasant and odor-free environment.

Provide diversional activities that can be used during enforced bed rest.

Teaching for Home Management

Instruct patient about vaginal discharge:

Discharge may persist for weeks.

Frequent perineal hygiene is essential for odor control and prevention of infection.

Teach woman to douche as ordered, usually twice daily.

Mild vaginal bleeding is expected; excessive bleeding should be reported to the physician.

Instruct patient about vaginal narrowing and fibrosis resulting from the radiation:

  Regular gentle vaginal dilation is essential to prevent stenosis and needs to be continued for at least 1 year after treatment.

  Regular sexual intercourse (at least three times weekly) may be used for this purpose, or a manual obturator may be used.

    Obturator must be lubricated before use and washed thoroughly with soap and water after use.

  Sexual intercourse may be resumed about 3 weeks after treatment.

    A water-soluble lubricant will be needed for comfort.

    Include sexual partner in all teaching if possible and reassure him about the safety of sexual activity and absence of radiation hazard for himself from patient. The woman is *not* radioactive once the implant has been removed.

Instruct the patient about complications to monitor:

  Gradually increase activity, and monitor fatigue level.

  Maintain a liberal fluid intake.

  Adjust the diet to prevent constipation or diarrhea, which may occur in response to radiation.

  Report the incidence of heavy discharge, dysuria, fever, pain, or persistent bowel problems.

Provide the patient with written resource materials for home management.

Ensure that appointments are made for ongoing follow-up.

♦ EVALUATION

Successful achievement of expected outcomes for the patient with cervical cancer being treated by intracavitary radiotherapy is indicated by the following:

  Correct statements of rationale for all radiation and activity restrictions

  Verbalization of feelings and concerns

  Statements that anxiety is minimal or absent

  Performance of self-care with use of appropriate assistance

  Frequent interaction with family and friends

  Use of diversionary activities

  Correct description of home care regimen

  Demonstration of all skills needed for perineal care, douching, and use of obturator

  Correct identification of signs of complications

Uterine Leiomyomas (Fibroids)
Etiology/epidemiology

Uterine fibroid tumors, or myomas, are extremely common benign tumors of muscle cell origin. They typically occur in women in their 40s and can be found in one in four white females and one in two African-American

---

BOX 16-2	**Total Pelvic Exenteration**

Total pelvic exenteration is a radical surgical procedure that may be used in the attempt to control advanced cervical cancer or other malignancies that are still contained within the pelvis. The procedure involves removal of all of the pelvic viscera, including the bladder and urethra, rectosigmoid colon and anus, cervix and uterus, ovaries and tubes, and vagina.

A colostomy and ileal conduit will be constructed, and the woman may elect to undergo vaginal reconstruction. Omentum is used to keep the intestines out of the pelvis in the early postoperative period. Five-year survival rates range from 20% to 65%.

---

females. Their etiology is unknown, but the stimulus for growth appears to be estrogen, since they enlarge during pregnancy and with oral contraceptive use and often decrease in size after menopause. If untreated, the tumors can reach enormous size but rarely become malignant.

Pathophysiology

Myomas originate in the myometrium and are classified by anatomic location including submucous, intramural, and subserosal. Most are asymptomatic and may go undetected. Menorrhagia, usually in the form of premenstrual spotting or light bleeding following the menses, is the most reported symptom. Pain is rarely present, although large tumors may create circulatory congestion, backache, and constipation.

Medical management

The diagnosis of myoma is made on physical examination and confirmed by pelvic sonography or hysteroscopy. Small, asymptomatic tumors are simply monitored. Symptomatic tumors may be treated by hysteroscopic laser resection if they are submucous, drug therapy to reduce the levels of circulating estrogen and shrink the tumor, or hysterectomy. The decision for surgery is based on the degree of symptom severity, the woman's age, and her desire to preserve childbearing capability.

NURSING MANAGEMENT

♦ ASSESSMENT
Subjective Data

  History of condition

  Menstrual history

  Symptoms: presence and severity

    Menorrhagia

    Pain

    Constipation

  Knowledge of the planned procedure

  Feelings about hysterectomy

Guidelines for Preoperative Nursing Care for Hysterectomy

Provide simple explanation of effects of hysterectomy on sexual and reproductive functioning.

Teach patient concerning expected postoperative care, including early ambulation, diet restrictions, incisional care, use of TED stocking or pneumatic compression devices, and pain management.

Teach patient deep breathing exercises and use of incentive spirometer.

Teach patient leg and ankle exercises.

Provide preoperative care:
  Povidone-iodine (Betadine) douche
  Skin prep
  Bowel prep
  TED hose

Encourage patient to ask questions and express concerns about effects of hysterectomy.

BOX 16-3 Terms Related to Gynecologic Surgery

OOPHORECTOMY
Removal of an ovary

SALPINGECTOMY
Removal of a fallopian tube

BILATERAL SALPINGO-OOPHORECTOMY (BSO)
Removal of both ovaries and tubes

HYSTERECTOMY
Removal of entire uterus and cervix; may be performed vaginally or abdominally

TOTAL ABDOMINAL HYSTERECTOMY (TAH-BSO)
Removal of entire uterus and both ovaries and fallopian tubes

RADICAL HYSTERECTOMY
Total abdominal hysterectomy plus partial vaginectomy and dissection of the pelvic lymph nodes

---

Objective Data

Increased abdominal girth

Uterine displacement or palpable irregular nodules on uterine surface

Anemia: presence and severity

The nursing management of the patient undergoing hysterectomy for uterine leiomyomas is summarized in the "Nursing Care Plan." Preoperative care is summarized in the Guidelines box.

Cancer of the Endometrium

Cancer of the uterus primarily affects postmenopausal women between the ages of 50 and 65 years. Associated risk factors include obesity, nulliparity, late menopause (after 52 years of age), diabetes, and use of exogenous estrogens. The tumor is usually slow growing and responds well to treatment in early stages, but no reliable screening tool is available for early detection. There are few early symptoms, but dysfunctional uterine bleeding is the most significant. Any postmenopausal woman who develops dysfunctional bleeding should be carefully evaluated for uterine cancer.

Endometrial cancer is treated according to the stage of the disease, but treatment usually involves total abdominal hysterectomy with bilateral salpingo-oophorectomy. Radiation may be added as an adjunct, and hormonal therapy and chemotherapy are often used in advanced disease.

Ovarian Cysts and Tumors
Etiology/epidemiology

A variety of cysts, benign tumors, and malignant tumors may affect the ovary. Different types predominate at different points in the life cycle. Ovarian tumors and cancer may occur as early as infancy and childhood, but the risk increases after 40 years and peaks between 50 and 60 years. The vast majority are discovered during routine pelvic examination and are initially asymptomatic. Ovarian cancer accounts for only 4% of all cancers, but it is the most deadly form of reproductive cancer, with survival rates of only 19% to 39% if the disease is not diagnosed in its earliest localized stage. Various disparate risk factors have been identified but cannot yet be translated into workable suggestions for prevention.

Pathophysiology

Benign cysts and tumors may develop from a variety of physiologic imbalances, including hyperstimulation of the ovaries from gonadotropins. The size of the lesions can vary from a few millimeters to spectacular sizes that can fill the pelvis. Cancerous lesions also fall into a variety of categories depending on the cell type. Different histologic types seem to predominate at different ages.

Most benign tumors are asymptomatic for long periods or produce only nonspecific symptoms. When symptoms appear, they may include menstrual irregularities if hormonal imbalance is present, dull lower quadrant pain, fatigue, or a sense of heaviness in the pelvis. As malignant tumors increase in size they frequently cause pelvic, abdominal, and low back pain, anorexia and nausea, and weight loss.

Medical management

Palpation of the ovaries during pelvic examination can usually detect any mass or enlargement. Ultrasonography, CT scans, and laparoscopy may be used to refine or confirm the diagnosis and distinguish cysts and solid tumors.

Benign ovarian masses are managed conservatively if they are under 8 cm in size. They may resolve spontaneously, regress with oral contraceptive use, or require

NURSING CARE PLAN

WOMAN WITH LEIOMYOMA UNDERGOING ABDOMINAL HYSTERECTOMY

■ NURSING DIAGNOSIS

Pain (related to surgical incision and gaseous distention)

Expected Patient Outcomes	Nursing Interventions
Patient will experience steadily decreasing pain, resume normal activity, and state that she is successfully expelling flatus.	1. Provide adequate narcotic analgesic to control incisional pain. a. Encourage analgesic use before pain is severe and before ambulation or use of incentive spirometer. b. Monitor effectiveness of patient-controlled analgesia (PCA) use if ordered. 2. Encourage frequent position changes. 3. Encourage regular ambulation to support peristalsis.

■ NURSING DIAGNOSIS

Urinary retention, high risk for (related to loss of bladder tone, incisional discomfort, and pelvic congestion)

Expected Patient Outcomes	Nursing Interventions
Patient will void in sufficient quantities and resume a normal urinary elimination pattern.	1. Monitor intake and output for at least 48 hours; assess for urinary retention. Catheterize for residuals if ordered. 2. Use measures to facilitate voiding if urinary retention occurs. Monitor frequency and amount of voidings. 3. Encourage patient to void every 2 hours and to maintain a liberal fluid intake. 4. Provide catheter care if patient has an indwelling catheter. 5. Provide perineal hygiene after voiding and defecation. 6. Teach self-catheterization if ordered following radical hysterectomy, when bladder tone and sensation are compromised.

■ NURSING DIAGNOSIS

Altered tissue perfusion (peripheral), potential for (related to pelvic vessel congestion and venous stasis)

Expected Patient Outcome	Nursing Interventions
Patient will maintain adequate circulation without development of thrombosis.	1. Monitor patient for leg or chest pain or sudden dyspnea; assess for Homans' sign. 2. Apply thigh-high TED stockings or intermittent pneumatic compression devices. 3. Encourage leg exercises and frequent turning in bed during early postoperative period. Encourage ambulation. 4. Avoid elevating bottom of bed or placing pillows under knees; encourage patient to keep knees flat while in bed.

NURSING CARE PLAN—CONT'D

WOMAN WITH LEIOMYOMA UNDERGOING ABDOMINAL HYSTERECTOMY

■ NURSING DIAGNOSIS

Constipation, high risk for (related to surgical manipulation of the bowel and congestion)

Expected Patient Outcome	Nursing Interventions
Patient will successfully eliminate flatus and pass soft, formed stool.	1. Auscultate abdomen for return of active peristalsis. 2. Restrict food and fluid until patient passes flatus. 3. Encourage ambulation to stimulate peristalsis. 4. Offer rectal tube for excess flatus if ordered. 5. Administer stool softeners or other agents as ordered. 6. Monitor potassium level, because hypokalemia can contribute to ileus.

■ NURSING DIAGNOSIS

Self-esteem disturbance, risk for (related to loss of childbearing ability)

Expected Patient Outcome	Nursing Interventions
Patient will verbalize concerns related to loss of childbearing ability and maintain a positive view of self.	1. Give patient opportunities to express feelings and concerns about loss of uterus. 2. Be empathetic of patient's feelings that may include grief, guilt, shame, or remorse. 3. Offer support if depression occurs. 4. Help patient identify personal strengths. 5. Help partner understand rationale for behaviors expressed by patient and encourage him to demonstrate continued affection. 6. Correct any misconceptions about effect of surgery on sexual intercourse (normal relationships may be resumed after 4-6 weeks).

■ NURSING DIAGNOSIS

Knowledge deficit: home care restrictions and monitoring for complications

Expected Patient Outcome	Nursing Interventions
Patient will correctly describe home activity restrictions and symptoms indicating complications.	1. Teach the patient: a. To avoid driving a car for 2-4 weeks (especially with standard shift drive) b. To avoid heavy activities and active sports for 4-6 weeks c. To report to physician excessive or persistent vaginal drainage d. Physiologic effects of the hysterectomy e. That psychologic reactions may continue for a few weeks f. Possibility of slight vaginal discharge for 1-2 weeks g. That sexual intercourse may be resumed after 4-6 weeks; vaginal sensation may be decreased initially h. Importance of follow-up care

surgical removal. Surgery is also the primary treatment approach to ovarian cancer and is used to stage the disease as well. Total abdominal hysterectomy with bilateral salpingectomy and oophorectomy is usually performed. Adjuvant treatment includes both chemotherapy and radiotherapy.

NURSING MANAGEMENT

Nursing management with benign neoplasms includes reinforcing the importance of careful follow-up, providing routine surgical care, and reassuring the patient about her continued potential for normal childbearing as long as the second ovary is healthy. Removal of both ovaries does induce surgical menopause. Nursing care for ovarian cancer also includes routine surgical care plus support and teaching about the diagnosis, prognosis, and planned care.

Fibrocystic Disease of the Breast

The term *fibrocystic disease* has been used as an umbrella category for most benign breast disorders. Fibroadenomas are by far the most common example. Approximately 10% to 25% of women experience one or more of these tumors. They occur most often in young women under 25 years of age and may appear in the young teenage years. Breast cysts are most common in women between 40 and 50 years but can also occur at any age. The etiology of both types is unknown, but they are felt to be caused by hormonal imbalance in the cycle of changes that affect the breast.

Cystic lesions are soft, well demarcated, and freely movable. The process is usually bilateral, and the cysts may contain fluid. Breast tenderness is common, especially during or before menstruation. Fibroadenomas are firm, rubbery, and freely moveable and range in size from 1 to 3 cm. The primary clinical decision is the need for aspiration or biopsy. Cystic lesions are usually aspirated, and their fluid sent for cytology. Their presence makes the diagnosis of malignant lesions more complex, and periodic mammography may be ordered for monitoring changes. There is no evidence to suggest that cystic disease predisposes to the development of malignancy. Surgical removal with pathologic analysis is standard for fibroadenomas. Diet modification has been studied in cystic disease with no clear-cut positive results. Studies on the use of tamoxifen to reduce estrogen stimulation are ongoing with some early positive results in cyst regression and relief of discomfort.

Cancer of the Breast
Etiology/epidemiology

Despite significant research efforts in treatment and early detection, breast cancer remains the most common cancer in women, and the incidence has risen steadily since 1973. Breast cancer accounts for about one third of all cancers detected in women and 18% of

---

> **BOX 16-4** **Risk Factors for Breast Cancer**
>
> **Age:** over 50 years
> **Genetic factors:** cancer in first-degree relative (mother, daughter, sister)
> **Menstrual history:** early menarche or late menopause (over 55 years)
> **Reproductive history:** nulliparity or birth of first child after 30 years
> **Hormones and oral contraceptives:** link with oral contraceptive use is unclear, but they may cause increased risk in nulliparous women; link with postmenopausal estrogen use is clear
> **Diet and body weight:** a theorized link between high-fat intake and obesity has been proposed for years, but research to date does not support the link with either factor
> **Benign breast disease:** no link with fibrocystic disease has been found except when hyperplasia is present; the disease does make early detection more difficult
> **Radiation:** exposure during childhood and young adulthood does increase the risk
> **Race:** white although the rates for African-Americans are increasing, and they exhibit poorer survival rates

---

all cancer-related deaths, and women have a one in nine chance of developing the disease. The etiology remains substantially unknown, but research continues to uncover related elements. The incidence is increased with age, and women over 50 years are diagnosed most often. A hereditary link is clear, particularly with first-degree relatives who developed the disease premenopausally. Major risk factors are summarized in Box 16-4. The prognosis is related to the degree of axillary node involvement, size of the tumor, and the presence of a positive hormone receptor status.

Pathophysiology

Tumors of the breast arise in the epithelial cells of either the ductal or lobular tissue. If the tumor is confined to the duct or lobule, it is considered in situ. Infiltrative tumors have spread directly into surrounding tissue and may have metastasized. The majority of tumors are located in the upper outer quadrant.

The presence of estrogen or progesterone receptors indicates that the hormones are able to bind to the cell and affect cellular activity in some manner. Their presence is associated with an improved prognosis.

Breast tumors may present with a wide variety of signs and symptoms. Benign tumors generally have well-defined edges, are encapsulated, and are freely movable, whereas malignant tumors are harder to define and less mobile. As the tumor invades surrounding tissue it may cause retraction of the overlying skin, producing external dimpling. Nipple retraction or deviation may also occur. These symptoms are all related to advancing disease and will not be present in tumors diagnosed by mammography.

TABLE 16-5	American Cancer Society Guidelines for Breast Cancer Screening: Asymptomatic Patients	
TEST OR EXAMINATION	**AGE (yr)**	**RECOMMENDATION**
Breast self-examination	Over 20	Monthly
Breast physical examination	20-40	Every 3 yr
	Over 40	Yearly
Mammogram	35-40	One baseline mammogram
	40-49	Every 1-2 yr
	Over 50	Yearly

From Dodd DG: *CA* 42(3):177-180, 1992.

Medical management

The emphasis in breast cancer management lies in early detection, and the cornerstones of early detection are mammography and physical examination. Mammography screening guidelines are under constant revision, but the current recommendations are summarized in Table 16-5. A mammogram is able to detect breast lesions of less than 1 cm in size, the point at which tumors usually become palpable (Figure 16-4). Mammograms' value in early detection has been clearly demonstrated. Although breast self-examination is recommended by the American Cancer Society and 90% of all breast lesions are first detected by the woman herself, its true value in detecting *early*-stage breast cancer has not been determined. Guidelines for performing breast self-examination are outlined in the Guidelines box. Although the majority of breast lesions are not malignant, the diagnosis cannot be accurately made until the tissue is examined for histologic cell type. Therefore, when a mass is discovered, either a needle aspiration or biopsy will be performed.

A variety of treatment options exists for breast cancer, and the options have been strongly debated in the literature. Influencing factors include the stage of the disease at diagnosis, preference of the physician, and feelings of the woman concerning surgery versus other approaches. Early-stage breast cancer is usually treated surgically either with breast preservation procedures, such as lumpectomy, wedge resection, or partial mastectomy, or with modified radical mastectomy. Follow-up external or interstitial radiotherapy is often employed with tumors ranging from 1 to 4 cm in size. The risk of local recurrence is minimized with this approach. All procedures include lymph node dissection, but the number of nodes involved is determined by whether or not disease is identified in the axillary complex. Factors that influence the decision about which type of surgery to employ are summarized in Table 16-6.

Treatment for advanced or recurrent disease generally involves mastectomy (if not performed previously) and systemic chemotherapy or hormonal therapy. Most local recurrence occurs within 2 to 8 years, with 80% within

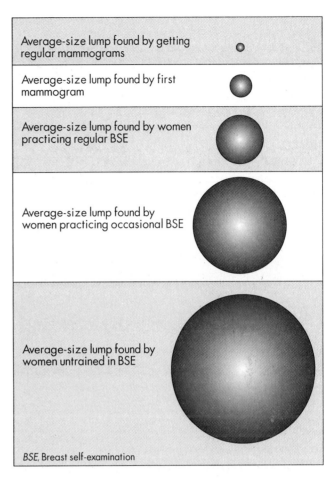

Average-size lump found by getting regular mammograms	
Average-size lump found by first mammogram	
Average-size lump found by women practicing regular BSE	
Average-size lump found by women practicing occasional BSE	
Average-size lump found by women untrained in BSE	

BSE, Breast self-examination

FIGURE 16-4 The importance of regular mammography screening in early detection of breast cancer.

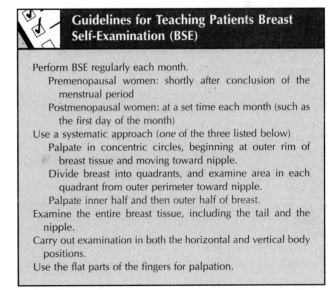

Guidelines for Teaching Patients Breast Self-Examination (BSE)

Perform BSE regularly each month.
    Premenopausal women: shortly after conclusion of the menstrual period
    Postmenopausal women: at a set time each month (such as the first day of the month)
Use a systematic approach (*one* of the three listed below)
    Palpate in concentric circles, beginning at outer rim of breast tissue and moving toward nipple.
    Divide breast into quadrants, and examine area in each quadrant from outer perimeter toward nipple.
    Palpate inner half and then outer half of breast.
Examine the entire breast tissue, including the tail and the nipple.
Carry out examination in both the horizontal and vertical body positions.
Use the flat parts of the fingers for palpation.

3 years. Systemic therapy has been shown to achieve long-term disease-free periods for women of all ages, but there is no accepted treatment protocol. The National Cancer Institute encourages physicians to consider adjuvant treatment for patients with early breast cancer,

TABLE 16-6 Factors Influencing Type of Surgery for Primary Breast Cancer

FACTOR	LUMPECTOMY	MASTECTOMY
Tumor size	Small	Large
Breast size	Average	Very small or very large
Tumor location	Upper outer quadrant	Near nipple
Type of cancer	Less aggressive	More aggressive or extensive intraductal
Number of tumors	One tumor present	More than one tumor present

From Ellerhorst-Ryan JM: *Innovations Oncol Nurs* 5(1):5, 1988.

BOX 16-5 Breast Reconstruction

IMPLANTS

Soft sacs filled with silicone gel are placed in a pocket beneath the pectoralis major muscle. The size is designed to match the remaining breast. An alternative type of implant is the tissue expander prosthesis. The expander sac is filled with 100-200 ml of sterile saline, and 30-100 ml is added weekly until the desired size is reached. The gradual expansion allows for stretching of the tissue and improved breast shaping. Complications include fibrous contraction around the implant, infection, and negative effects from the silicone.

AUTOGENOUS TISSUE FLAPS

Tissue flaps eliminate the need for implants unless inadequate tissue is available to achieve the desired size. Flaps may be taken from the latissimus dorsi or rectus abdominis myocutaneous tissue (TRAM). TRAM flaps are generally preferred, because the abdominal tissue is similar to that of the breast and usually available in sufficient quantity, and the surgical scar is easily hidden. Nipple reconstruction may use tissue from the opposite breast, tissue from the upper inner thigh, or a dermal tattoo.

but at present there is no sure way to identify which patients will benefit and for which it is completely unnecessary. Hormonal therapy is a useful adjunct in many situations in which the tumor cells are estrogen dependent. Tamoxifen, a nonsteroidal antiestrogen drug that has demonstrated antitumor effects, has shown excellent early promise and is now being researched for its potential role in prevention as well as treatment.

Reconstruction is an option offered to most women undergoing mastectomy surgery. The decision is a very personal one, because the female breast has meaning in U.S. society far beyond its lactation function. The reconstruction can be performed at the time of the initial surgery or at some future point. A delay of 3 to 6 months for initial healing and completion of therapy is often recommended. Options for reconstruction are summarized in Box 16-5.

NURSING MANAGEMENT

♦ ASSESSMENT
Subjective Data

Presence of risk factors, family history of breast cancer

Report of discovery of lump, time frame since discovery

Screening routines in use: BSE, mammography, physical examination

Knowledge of breast cancer and treatment options: surgery, radiation, chemotherapy, reconstruction

Feelings about surgery and diagnosis

Usual coping patterns

Response of spouse and other support systems

Objective Data

Breast physical examination
  Inspection: size, symmetry, skin signs, retraction
  Palpation: size and location of lesion, presence of palpable lymph nodes

The nursing management of the patient undergoing mastectomy is presented in the "Nursing Care Plan." A "Critical Pathway" for a patient undergoing lumpectomy is also included.

STERILIZATION
Etiology/epidemiology

Voluntary sterilization has become increasingly accepted as a method of preventing pregnancy and is now the most commonly used contraceptive method for married couples over 30 years of age. It is estimated that between 500,000 and 1 million men and 100,000 women elect surgical sterilization. The laws governing sterilization vary from state to state, but generally the surgery can be performed by a physician if written informed consent is obtained.

Pathophysiology

Tubal sterilization terminates a woman's ability to conceive but does not alter ovarian hormone or menstrual functioning. Artifical menopause is not induced, and sexual pleasure is not compromised. Bilateral vasectomy interrupts the continuity of the vas deferens and prevents sperm from being ejaculated, although sperm are still produced and the volume of ejaculate is not significantly altered. Sperm antibodies develop in about 50% to 60% of men. Again, there is no physiologic effect on either libido or erectile function.

Medical management

The procedure of tubal ligation has evolved over the last 70 years. The procedure may be performed by laparoscopy with electrocoagulation of a segment of the fallopian tube through a small abdominal incision or by open

NURSING CARE PLAN

THE PERSON WITH BREAST CANCER UNDERGOING MASTECTOMY

■ NURSING DIAGNOSIS

Fear (related to breast cancer treatment, unknown surgical outcome, and uncertain prognosis)

Expected Patient Outcome	Nursing Interventions
Patient will discuss fears about diagnosis, planned treatment, and the future.	1. Assist patient to verbalize feelings about meaning of impending surgery. Include husband and family as appropriate. 2. Encourage family to express fears and love to patient. 3. Support patient in whatever decisions she makes about treatment protocol. Repeat all teaching as needed. 4. Provide simple explanations of impending surgery and expected postoperative care. Describe size and appearance of postoperative dressing. Explain use of Hemovac if planned. 5. Insure that options for reconstruction have been presented.

■ NURSING DIAGNOSIS

Body image disturbance, high risk for (related to loss of breast)

Expected Patient Outcome	Nursing Interventions
Patient will gradually integrate loss into an altered but positive body image.	1. Continue to assist patient to explore and verbalize her feelings and grief. Prepare for easy fatigability. 2. Prepare patient for size and appearance of the incision. Provide support when incision is viewed for first time. 3. Help family show patient appropriate love and support. 4. Arrange visit by Reach to Recovery volunteer with patient's approval.

■ NURSING DIAGNOSIS

Impaired physical mobility, risk for (arm and shoulder) (related to pain, bulky dressings, and presence of drainage apparatus)

Expected Patient Outcome	Nursing Interventions
Patient will report minimal discomfort and begin to use her affected side for self-care activities.	1. Provide adequate analgesia to promote ambulation and exercise. Pain may be referred to arm and shoulder. 2. Encourage regular coughing and deep breathing exercises. 3. Place patient in semi-Fowler's position, with arm elevated on pillows. 4. Monitor Hemovac output. 5. Check dressing frequently for bleeding or excess serous drainage. 6. Check behind patient for bleeding. 7. Post signs warning against taking blood pressure, starting intravenous (IV) lines, or drawing blood on affected side.

Continued.

NURSING CARE PLAN—CONT'D

THE PERSON WITH BREAST CANCER UNDERGOING MASTECTOMY

Expected Patient Outcome	Nursing Interventions

	8. Initiate exercises to prevent stiffness and contracture of shoulder girdle.
	  a. Immediate:
	    (1) Flex and extend fingers.
	    (2) Pronate and supinate forearm.
	  b. Day 1 after operation:
	    (1) Squeeze rubber ball as tolerated.
	    (2) Brush teeth and hair.
	9. Teach special mastectomy exercises as prescribed. Exercise bilaterally, using both arms.

■ NURSING DIAGNOSIS

Impaired home maintenance management, risk for (related to inadequate knowledge concerning exercises, prosthesis, management of lymphedema, and prevention of complications)

Expected Patient Outcome	Nursing Interventions

Patient will correctly describe measures to control lymphedema, exercises to regain full range of motion, symptoms requiring medical follow-up, and use of breast prosthesis.	1. Provide patient with detailed information concerning breast prosthesis.
	  a. Fitting is not possible for 4-6 weeks.
	  b. A temporary prosthesis or lightly padded bra is worn until healing is complete.
	2. Teach patient to avoid constrictive clothing and report persistent edema, redness, or infection of incision.
	3. Tech patient to protect arm from minor injury, particularly if lymphedema is present.
	  a. Avoid leaving the arm in a dependent position for extended periods.
	  b. Contact physician if arm swelling persists for compression bandaging.
	  c. Limit sodium content of the diet.
	  d. Cleanse all cuts and scratches immediately and apply protective coverings.
	4. Inform patient that numbness and tingling and even phantom breast sensations are common but should resolve within a few months.
	5. Teach patient importance of continuing monthly breast examination on remaining breast and following recommendations for mammography.

CRITICAL PATHWAY   **Lumpectomy With Radium Implants for Breast Cancer**

DRG #: 258; expected LOS: 4

	Day of Surgery Day of Admission Day 1	Day 2	Day 3	Day of Discharge Day 4
Diagnostic Tests	*Preoperative:* CBC, UA, SMA/18*; radiologic needle localization			
Medications	IVs, IV/IM analgesic, Rx for rest/sleep	IV to saline lock, PO analgesic, Rx for rest/sleep	IV saline lock, PO analgesic, RX for rest/sleep	Discontinue saline lock, PO analgesic
Treatments	I & O q 8 hr including incisional Hemovac; VS q 4 hr; neurocirculatory assessment of affected side q 2 hr; elevate affected arm on pillow; T, C, & DB q 2 hr; incentive spirometry q 2 hr; check dressing	I & O q 8 hr; VS q 6 hr; neurocirculatory assessment of affected side q 4 hr; elevate affected arm on pillow; T, C & DB q 2 hr; incentive spirometry q 2 hr	Discontinue I & O; VS q 6 hr; neurocirculatory assessment of affected side q 8 hr; elevate affected arm on pillow; T, C & DB q 2 hr; incentive spirometry q 4 hr	VS q 8 hr; neurocirculatory assessment of affected side q 8 hr; elevate affected arm on pillow
Diet	NPO; clear liquids when nausea stops	Advance diet as tolerated; regular diet	Regular diet	Regular diet
Activity	Up in room with help; *no BP, IVs, injections, etc. in affected arm*	Up in room only with help; *no BP, IVs, injections, etc., in affected arm; establish and maintain radiation safety measures for patient, staff, visitors*	Up ad lib in room only; *no BP, IVs, injections, etc., in affected arm; maintain radiation safety measures for patient, staff, visitors*	Up ad lib in room only until radiation removed; *no BP, IVs, injections, etc., in affected arm; maintain radiation safety measures until radiation discontinued*
Consultations		Radiation and/or medical oncologist, physical therapist		

NOTE: Acknowledge that patients recover at varying rates; therefore specified daily actions should be based solely on patient needs.
CBC, Complete blood cell count; *SMA,* sequential multiple analysis; *T, C & DB,* turn, cough, and deep breath; *UA,* urinalysis; *VS,* vital signs.
*Serum calcium, phosphorus, triglycerides, uric acid, creatinine, BUN, total bilirubin, alkaline phosphate, aspartate aminotransferase (AST) (formerly serum glutamic-oxaloacetic transaminase [SGOT]), alanine aminotransferase (ALT) (formerly serum glutamate pyruvate transaminase [SGPT]), lactic dehydrogenase (LDH), total protein, albumin, sodium, potassium, chloride, total CO_2 glucose.

laparotomy, which allows for direct visual ligation of the tubes. Either local or general anesthesia may be used. A variety of procedures has also been developed for vasectomy, largely in response to the tendency of the vas deferens to rejoin spontaneously. The most common procedure involves making a small incision in the scrotum to expose the vas sheath and then removing a segment of 0.6 to 1.2 cm in length. The severed ends are then ligated. The procedure can be performed in an office setting with the patient under local anesthesia.

NURSING MANAGEMENT

The foundation of nursing care involves patient teaching for true informed consent. Federal guidelines are utilized (Box 16-6). Most men and women are very satisfied with the surgery, but occasional patients experience emotional difficulties and it is crucial to attempt to identify uncertain or ambivalent patients before the procedure is attempted. Questions are posed about the patient's motives and decision making, including cur-

rent methods of contraception and problems encountered and thoughts about the choice in the event of the loss of a child or spouse or remarriage.

It is important to emphasize that sterilization does not alter sexual performance or pleasure. It is frequently equated with a castration, and even men and women who clearly know the difference may appreciate the reassurance. Facts are also presented about the current status of reversibility for the procedures. Visual aids and models may be helpful.

Postoperative care for the female is straightforward. She is discharged when the effects of anesthesia have worn off and instructed to rest for about 24 hours and avoid all heavy lifting or strenuous exercise for about 1 week. Sexual activity may be resumed when the wound is healed. The woman is encouraged to report the development of any signs of infection or bleeding. Men are advised to expect slight swelling and minor discomfort. Ice and sitz baths usually are effective. The man must submit specimens for sperm counts 4 weeks after surgery, which are compared with a preoperative speci-

BOX 16-6	Informed Consent Guidelines (Federal) Relating to Sterilization

1. Choice is made by patient. No pressures are placed on choice (e.g., loss of welfare benefits, wrath of health care provider).
2. Benefits and risks of sterilization are described:
   a. Benefits: permanent, no further costs or decision making
   b. Risks: usual surgical risks, possibility of future pregnancy (i.e., not 100% effective)
3. Alternative contraceptive methods are described.
4. Patient is encouraged to ask questions.
5. Patient may withdraw from using the method without penalty.
6. Explanations are given about the entire sterilization procedure, costs, and possible side effects (effects of hormones, weight changes, menstrual changes, sexual response).
7. Written instructions and risk factors are given to patient.
8. A written consent to the procedure is signed by patient and witnessed.

men. Residual fertility persists because of existing sperm in the semen beyond the point of occlusion of the vas. Two sperm-free specimens are needed before the man is considered sterile.

DISORDERS OF THE MALE REPRODUCTIVE SYSTEM
INFECTIOUS AND INFLAMMATORY DISORDERS
Epididymitis
Etiology/epidemiology

Epididymitis is an acute inflammatory process that occurs most commonly in the young adult male, usually as a result of an ascending infection from the ejaculatory duct through the vas deferens into the epididymis. Sexual transmission is the most common means of infection, and the usual pathogens are *Chlamydia trachomatis* and *Neisseria gonorrhoeae*.

Pathophysiology

The acute inflammation of the epididymis and scrotal sac produces fluid accumulation in the scrotal sac, which can interfere with blood flow and damage nerves. The heat generated by the inflammatory process can negatively affect spermatogenesis. The classic symptoms include severe tenderness and pain in the scrotal area and noticeable swelling of one or both sides of the scrotum. The swelling and pain may be so acute that the man is unable to ambulate normally and waddles in a characteristic manner to protect the scrotum. A urethral discharge may also be present.

Medical management

Accurate prompt diagnosis is essential. It is critical to rule out the emergency condition of testicular torsion.

Urinalysis will usually show an increased WBC count and the presence of bacteria. Scrotal ultrasound may be used serially to monitor for any indication of reduced blood flow to the affected side. Radionuclide scanning may be performed if the diagnosis is unclear. Treatment involves oral antibiotics to eliminate infection and nonsteroidal antiinflammatory drugs (NSAIDs) to relieve swelling and pain. If the disease is sexually transmitted the man's partner should also receive diagnosis and treatment.

NURSING MANAGEMENT

The patient with epididymitis is generally treated as an outpatient. Nursing measures focus on instruction regarding comfort measures such as scrotal elevation and the application of ice. Bed rest is usually recommended until the patient is pain free. A scrotal support is recommended for about 6 weeks, and the man is encouraged to avoid any heavy lifting. Since STDs are the most common cause of epididymitis it is important for the man to receive instruction about prevention and the importance of early diagnosis. The importance of condoms is emphasized.

Orchitis

Orchitis involves inflammation of the testicle and may be caused by pyogenic bacteria or viruses. It occurs as a complication of mumps in 20% of cases that develop after puberty. The inflammatory fluid causes unilateral or bilateral swelling and may be severe enough to create a hydrocele. The symptoms are the same as those of epididymitis, but the infection is more systemic and causes fever, nausea, and vomiting in addition to the local pain. The inflammatory fibrosis may cause some degree of testicular atrophy but rarely leads to sterility unless both sides are seriously involved. Medical treatment involves ensuring that all males are vaccinated against mumps and aggressive treatment of bacterial infection with appropriate antibiotics. Nursing management again focuses on comfort measures and supportive care.

Prostatitis

The two major forms of prostatitis are bacterial and nonbacterial, and the disease may take an acute or a chronic course. It is one of the most common inflammations of the male reproductive tract and primarily affects young and middle-aged men. It is usually triggered by an ascending infection by an organism that causes a urinary tract infection. The gland becomes swollen and painful and may interfere with normal urination. Common symptoms include straining on urination, pain (particularly during or after ejaculation), and dysuria. Urine cultures are performed to isolate the causative organism, and treatment consists of appropriate antibiotic therapy. Inadequate treatment can result in chronic disease states. Nursing management focuses on comfort measures and teaching about antibiotic therapy, refraining from sexual activity until therapy is effective, and preventing constipation that can irritate the inflamed gland.

STRUCTURAL PROBLEMS

Testicular Torsion

Testicular torsion involves twisting of the spermatic cord, which acutely impairs the circulation of the testes. It can occur spontaneously or after activities that put a sudden strain on the cremasteric muscle. It is most common in the teenage years.

Torsion interrupts the blood supply, leading to ischemia and severe unrelieved pain that is aggravated by manual elevation of the scrotum. The scrotum is swollen and reddened and may be elevated from the shortening of the spermatic cord. Cessation of the pain can indicate infarction and necrosis. Testicular viability is directly related to the duration of the episode, with only a 20% salvage rate after 12 hours. Early diagnosis is critical.

Doppler studies and radionuclide scanning can measure the blood flow to the testis. Diminished or obstructed flow is the key feature. Manual detorsion may be attempted, but if detorsion is unsuccessful surgical intervention is planned immediately. Unless the testis is gangrenous it will be preserved and fixed to the scrotal wall to prevent recurrence. Postoperative care involves the application of ice and scrotal support. The man is instructed to avoid strenuous activity, heavy lifting, and sexual activity for about 6 weeks. Fertility may be affected by the torsion, but erectile function remains intact. The man should be reassured about any concerns over impotence.

Other structural problems involving the reproductive tract are summarized in Table 16-7.

Benign Prostatic Hypertrophy

Etiology/epidemiology

Benign prostatic hypertrophy (BPH) is a common problem that occurs in an estimated 75% of all men over 50 years of age and involves the enlargement of portions of the prostate gland, causing problems with urination. Benign hyperplasia is actually a more accurate term since only a portion of the gland enlarges while other portions may atrophy or become nodular. The changes in the gland are attributed to increased levels of androgens, particularly dihydrotestosterone. It is estimated that 10% of men who live to the age of 80 years will require some form of treatment to correct the symptoms of BPH.

Pathophysiology

The hormonal imbalance creates an adenomatous enlargement of the gland with an overgrowth of smooth muscle and connective tissue. The changes can create a variety of urinary problems. Compression on the urethra causes it to elongate, and urinary flow is obstructed. The bladder muscle thickens, and trabecula-

TABLE 16-7 Structural Disorders of the Penis, Testes, and Scrotum	
DESCRIPTION	**MEDICAL MANAGEMENT**
PHIMOSIS/PARAPHIMOSIS	
Phimosis: foreskin cannot be retracted behind glans. Paraphimosis: foreskin constricted behind glans and cannot be returned to its natural position	Attempts may be made to stretch foreskin to improve retractability, or circumcision may be performed; circumcision usually performed when paraphimosis is acute as well
HYDROCELE	
Benign, nontender collection of clear amber fluid within outer covering of testes; leads to scrotal swelling	Aspiration of fluid
SPERMATOCELE	
Benign, nontender cystic mass attached to epididymis; contains milky fluid and sperm	Usually no treatment needed—aspiration or excision may be done
VARICOCELE	
Dilation of spermatic vein, usually on left side	Ligation of vein

tion of the wall creates pockets for urinary retention. The bladder has less tone, and it is difficult for it to completely empty with urination. Stasis of the residual urine creates an alkaline medium that creates a fertile environment for bacterial growth. Symptoms include a decrease in the urinary stream, less force on urination, hesitancy, difficulty in starting the stream, straining, and urinary retention. Symptoms of irritation can include dysuria, nocturia, urgency, and hematuria.

Medical management

BPH is diagnosed from its classic symptoms and a rectal examination that reveals a smoothly enlarged prostate gland. Cystoscopy may be used to directly examine the lining of the bladder and rule out the presence of stricture, calculi, and malignancy, especially in the presence of hematuria.

The standard therapy involves surgery, but other alternatives are being researched. Drug treatment is being employed with finasteride (Proscar), a drug that inhibits the activity of 5-alpha reductase, thereby preventing the conversion of testosterone to dihydrotestosterone. The drug shrinks the prostate over a period of several months, but the long-term effectiveness is not fully known. Balloon dilation and laser resection are also under investigation.

Transurethral resection of the prostate (TURP) is employed most commonly, especially when the major glandular enlargement exists in the medial lobe that surrounds the urethra. A resectoscope with a cutting

TABLE 16-8 Comparison of Types of Prostate Surgery

REASON FOR SURGERY	LOCATION OF INCISION	DRAINAGE TUBES	BLADDER SPASMS	DRESSING	COMPLICATIONS
TRANSURETHRAL RESECTION					
Enlargement of medial lobe surrounding urethra	No incision; removal by way of urethra	Three-way Foley catheter with 30 ml bag in urethra; constant irrigation for 24 hr	Yes	None	Hemorrhage; water intoxication; incontinence
SUPRAPUBIC RESECTION					
Extremely large mass of obstructing tissue	Low midline abdominal incision through bladder to prostate gland	Cystotomy tube or drain through incision; Foley catheter with 30 ml bag in urethra	Yes	Abdominal dressing easily soaked with urinary drainage	Hemorrhage; wound infection
RETROPUBIC RESECTION					
Large mass located high in pelvic area	Low midline abdominal incision into prostate gland (bladder not incised)	Foley catheter with 30 ml bag in urethra, constant irrigation for 24 hr	Few	Abdominal dressing; no urinary drainage	Hemorrhage; wound infection
PERINEAL RESECTION					
Large mass located low in pelvic area	Incision between scrotum and rectum	Foley catheter with 30 ml bag in urethra	Few	Perineal dressing; no urinary drainage	Hemorrhage; wound infection
RADICAL PERINEAL RESECTION					
Cancer of prostate gland	Large perineal incision between scrotum and rectum	Foley catheter with 30 ml bag in urethra; drain in incision	Few	Perineal dressing; urinary drainage	Urinary incontinence; wound infection; impotence; sterility

and cauterization loop is inserted through the urethra. Tiny pieces of tissue are cut away, and the bleeding points are sealed by cauterization. The bladder and urethra are continuously irrigated during the procedure. TURP can be performed with the patient under general or spinal anesthesia. Most men remain symptom free for at least 8 to 10 years after the procedure, after which retreatment may become necessary. Other more invasive forms of prostatectomy are described in Table 16-8.

A three-way Foley catheter with continuous bladder irrigation is typically used after surgery. The large Foley facilitates clot removal and stabilizes the urethra. The 30 ml balloon is positioned in the neck of the bladder to exert pressure on the operative area and control bleeding. Traction may be applied by taping the catheter to the lower abdomen or thigh. Pressure on the internal bladder sphincter can create a significant urge to void or bladder spasm. These problems lessen in intensity over the first 24 hours. Irrigation is continued for about 24 hours, after which the catheter is removed and the man is discharged once spontaneous voiding is reestablished.

NURSING MANAGEMENT

◆ ASSESSMENT
Subjective Data

Patient's complaints of the following:
 Urinary frequency, urgency, nocturia

 Difficulty starting the stream, dribbling, weak stream
 Feeling of straining, incomplete bladder emptying
 Symptoms of dysuria
 Knowledge of purpose and function of the prostate gland, nature of the problem
 Knowledge of planned surgery, effect on sexual functioning and fertility

Objective Data

 Hematuria
 Urinalysis results showing infection
 Rectal examination showing enlarged prostate on palpation

The remainder of the nursing management is presented in the "Nursing Care Plan." A "Critical Pathway" for a TURP is also included.

CANCER OF THE MALE REPRODUCTIVE SYSTEM
Cancer of the Prostate
Etiology/epidemiology

The prostate gland is the most common site of cancer in American men, and it is the second leading cause of cancer death. The disease rarely occurs before 40 years of age, and the incidence increases with age. African-American men have the highest incidence rates in the world. Age is the most clearly identified risk factor along with the hormone changes associated with aging. Other

NURSING CARE PLAN

THE PATIENT WITH BPH UNDERGOING TURP

■ NURSING DIAGNOSIS

Urinary elimination, altered patterns of (related to obstruction of urine outflow or weakened muscles)

Expected Patient Outcome	Nursing Interventions

Patient will gradually return to a normal continent pattern of urinary elimination.	1. Maintain patency of continuous bladder irrigation if utilized (usually for first 24 hours).
	  a. Solution should run rapidly enough to maintain urinary drainage of light pink-red color.
	  b. Monitor carefully for clot information.
	  c. Maintain accurate intake and output records.
	  d. Maintain traction on catheter as prescribed.
	  e. Monitor vital signs frequently.
	2. Teach patient that 30 ml catheter balloon triggers constant urge to void and bladder spasms.
	3. Administer analgesics and antispasmodics as needed (belladonna and opium).
	4. Manually irrigate catheter if prescribed.
	5. Encourage liberal fluid intake by mouth unless contraindicated.
	6. Avoid use of rectal thermometer or tube and enemas.
	7. Provide or teach patient scrupulous catheter care. Monitor carefully for signs of infection.
	8. Assess for adequacy of voiding and bladder emptying when catheter is removed.
	9. Teach patient perineal exercises to aid in full return of urinary control. Dribbling is a common temporary problem.
	10. Assess patient for symptoms of hypertension, bradycardia, and confusion that could indicate water intoxication and hyponatremia from the irrigation.

■ NURSING DIAGNOSIS

Anxiety (related to poor understanding of prostate gland functioning and effects of surgery on sexuality)

Expected Patient Outcome	Nursing Interventions

Patient will verbalize concerns related to the outcomes of surgery and correctly state the alterations that occur in fertility from prostatectomy.	1. Encourage patient to express concerns about surgery and its impact on sexuality.
	2. Provide information as necessary:
	  a. TURP procedure does not affect sexual functioning but does cause sterility.
	  b. Retrograde ejaculation will occur, and urine may have a milky appearance.
	3. Avoid sexual intercourse for 4-6 weeks after surgery.

Continued.

NURSING CARE PLAN—CONT'D

THE PATIENT WITH BPH UNDERGOING TURP

■ NURSING DIAGNOSIS

Impaired home maintenance management, risk of (related to lack of knowledge concerning activity restrictions)

Expected Patient Outcome	Nursing Interventions

Patient will correctly state components of home care and symptoms to be reported to the physician.	1. Teach patient about postdischarge care.
	  a. Patient should refrain from lifting, vigorous exercise, driving, and sexual activity for 3-6 weeks.
	  b. Ambulation is encouraged.
	  c. Patient should use stool softener to avoid straining and avoid Valsalva's maneuver.
	  d. Patient should keep fluid intake high (at least 2500 ml).
	  e. Patient should contact physician if hematuria or signs of infection or cystitis occur. Rebleeding after 2 weeks is possible.
	  f. Instruct patient to avoid alcohol, which may cause burning during healing.
	  g. Encourage use of Kegel exercises to control dribbling.
	2. Fertility should be assessed once healing is complete to evaluate the ongoing need for contraception.

potential risks include viruses, a history of STDs and multiple sex partners, and exposure to varied industrial toxins.

Pathophysiology

Cancer of the prostate often begins in and occupies an area of senile atrophy in the gland. Most tumors are adenosarcomas and begin as discrete, localized, hard nodules in the peripheral or outer regions of the gland. Because the growth is generally on the outer portion of the gland, urinary symptoms are rarely present early in the disease. Sixty percent of men present with localized disease, but the tumor can metastasize through the blood and lymph to distant sites. Bony involvement is most common. The tumor may be extremely slow growing or very aggressive. There are few early symptoms. The man may complain of stiffness and back pain, urinary dysfunction or infection, and general malaise.

Medical management

Cancer of the prostate is frequently diagnosed as part of a general rectal screening examination. Tumors on the posterior portion of the gland can be palpated rather easily, but up to 40% of tumors develop on the anterior side of the prostate where they cannot be reached. The PSA (prostate-specific antigen) test measures the level of a glycoprotein secreted by the prostate that elevates with enlargement or inflammation. Acid phosphatase is secreted by epithelial cells in the prostatic ductal system, and a rise may also signal the presence of cancer. Transrectal ultrasound aids in the diagnosis of nonpalpable tumors. It may also be used to guide fine needle biopsy to obtain cells for examination (see p. 383).

A clinical staging system has been developed to guide treatment. The greatest treatment dilemma is determining how aggressively to treat early-stage prostate cancer in elderly men and even whether to treat it at all. Radical surgery and radiotherapy are the two primary treatment modalities. The radiation can be delivered by external beam or implant. Radiotherapy achieves results identical to radical surgery for at least the first 5 to 10 years, but the treatment is not curative and the outcomes drop off steadily after that time. Morbidity is significantly lower than for surgery, but radical surgery is generally curative in early-stage disease. The entire gland is removed, including the capsule and adjacent tissue. The urethra is anastomosed to the bladder neck. Perineal, retropubic, and suprapubic approaches may be utilized. Efforts are being directed at developing nerve-sparing techniques that preserve sexual potency when the need for wide-

	CRITICAL PATHWAY	TURP Without Complications		

DRG #: 336; expected LOS: 4 days

	Day of Admission Day of Surgery Day 1	Day 2	Day 3	Day of Discharge Day 4
Diagnostic Tests	Preoperative: chest x-ray film, CBC, UA, PT/PTT, ECG, SMA/18,* acid phosphatase Postoperative: CBC, electrolytes	CBC, electrolytes		
Medications	Preoperative: IV antibiotic Postoperative: IVs, IV antibiotic, IV or IM analgesic, B & O suppository PRN, stool softener	IV to saline lock, IV/PO antibiotic, PO analgesic, B & O suppository PRN, stool softener	Discontinue saline lock, PO analgesic, PO antibiotics, B & O suppository, stool softener	PO analgesic, PO antibiotics, stool softener
Treatments	I & O q 8 hr including Foley catheter and continuous GU irrigation; ? tension on Foley catheter; VS q 4 hr; assess neurocirculation to legs q 2 hr; elastic leg stockings (ELS)	I & O q 8 hr including Foley catheter; discontinue GU irrigation; Foley catheter to DD; VS q 6 hr; ELS	I & O q 8 hr; discontinue Foley catheter; VS q 8 hr; ELS; 7-bottle urine assessment	Discontinue I & O; VS q 8 hr; ELS; 7-bottle urine assessment
Diet	NPO, advance to regular diet as tolerated	Regular diet, force fluids	Regular diet, force fluids	Regular diet, force fluids
Activity	Flat for 6-8 hr after spinal anesthesia, then bed rest; assist with arising	Assist with arising	Assist with arising	Arise ad lib
Consultations		Social service, home health		

NOTE: Acknowledge that patients recover at varying rates; therefore specified daily actions should be based solely on patient need.
*Serum calcium, phosphorus, triglycerides, uric acid, creatinine, BUN, total bilirubin, alkaline phosphate, aspartate aminotransferase (ALT, formerly serum glutamic oxaloacetic transaminase [SGOT]), alanine aminotransferase (AST, formerly serum glutamic pyruvic transaminase [SGPT], lactic dehydrogenase (LDH), total protein, albumin, sodium, potassium, chloride, total CO_2, glucose.

spread lymph node removal or sampling is not great. Hormonal therapy may be utilized in widespread or recurrent disease.

NURSING MANAGEMENT

◆ ASSESSMENT
Subjective Data

Symptoms, if any: low back pain, urinary retention or dysuria, general malaise
Knowledge of disease and treatment options
Presence of risk factors, if any: viral infection, history of STDs, multiple sex partners
Understanding of effects of planned treatment on sexuality

Objective Data

Age over 40 years
Rectal examination showing hard, nodular areas in the prostate
Elevated PSA, acid or alkaline phosphatase
Positive biopsy specimen

◆ NURSING DIAGNOSES

Nursing diagnoses for the patient with prostate cancer being treated with radical perineal prostatectomy may include, but are not limited to, the following:

Knowledge deficit: planned surgery, postoperative care, effects on urinary continence and sexuality
Urinary or bowel incontinence, risk for (related to weakening of the sphincters and muscles necessary to control elimination)
Sexual dysfunction, risk for (related to surgically induced impotence)

◆ EXPECTED PATIENT OUTCOMES

Patient will correctly describe the planned surgery, expected postoperative care, and effects of surgery on elimination and sexuality.
Patient will reestablish adequate urinary and bowel control for continence.
Patient will verbalize concerns with sexual partner and explore alternative methods of sexual activity if impotent.

♦ NURSING INTERVENTIONS
Teaching About the Planned Surgery

Administer preoperative bowel prep: laxatives, enemas, and neomycin to cleanse the bowel.

Provide routine care for the perineal wound.

Monitor for urine leaks, hemorrhage, or signs of infection.

Avoid use of rectal thermometers, rectal tubes, and any hard suppositories that might injure the tissue.

Monitor the patency of all drains and evaluate the amount and character of drainage.

Position patient for comfort and utilize cushions when seated out of bed.

Provide a Fuller shield or jockey style of underwear to help hold the dressings in place.

Use sitz baths for cleansing once the drains are removed. NOTE: Wound is left open to drain and heal by secondary intention.

Promoting Continence

Maintain patency of Foley catheter. Monitor for bleeding. Frank bleeding is not expected.

Maintain irrigation if prescribed by physician.

Provide aseptic care to catheter as ordered. Catheter remains in place for 2 to 6 weeks to stabilize the urethra.

Monitor for signs of infection.

Teach patient how to apply and empty a leg bag for home use.

Monitor for bladder spasms, and administer antispasmodics if ordered.

Teach patient the following:

Dribbling and incontinence common after the removal of the catheter

Methods to ensure dryness and prevent embarrassing leaks

Pubococcygeal exercises to restore perineal tone

Options for controlling incontinence if conservative methods are unsuccessful

Reassurance that although residual stress incontinence may persist, normal daytime continence is an achievable goal for most otherwise healthy men over the period of a few months

Prevent constipation and straining with diet manipulation, a high fluid intake, and the use of stool softeners.

Relaxation of the perineal musculature may affect bowel sphincters, but the effects are usually temporary.

Promoting Sexual Function

Provide patient with accurate information about sexual functioning:

Ninety-five percent of patients who undergo nerve-sparing surgeries regain potency within 1 year.

Effects of radiotherapy are often permanent.

Genital innervation is initially disrupted, but the effects are not all permanent.

Encourage patient to explore nonintercourse sexual activity with sexual partner and verbalize feelings and concerns.

Clarify for patient that sterility is a permanent outcome of surgery.

Provide patient with information about reconstructive approaches for dealing with physiologic impotence.

Encourage patient to express grief over losses and concern for the future.

♦ EVALUATION

Successful achievement of expected outcomes for the patient with prostate cancer being treated with radical perineal prostatectomy is indicated by the following:

Patient correctly describes surgical procedure, postoperative care, and expected outcomes for continence and sexuality.

Patient regains urinary and bowel continence for normal activities.

Patient understands effects on sexuality and explores alternatives with sexual partner.

Testicular Cancer
Etiology/epidemiology

Testicular cancer is the leading cause of cancer death in men aged 15 to 35 years. It is 90% to 100% curable when detected and treated early, but it will result in death in 2 to 3 years if detected late. Its causes are unknown, but links have been found with cryptorchidism (undescended testicles), chemical carcinogens, and environmental influences. It occurs more commonly in the white population.

GERONTOLOGIC PATIENT CONSIDERATIONS FOR PROSTATE CANCER

Prostate cancer is primarily a disease of older men. Its usual slow-growing tendencies make treatment decisions difficult in elderly patients, especially if health is impaired. Radical prostatectomies do not necessarily prolong life in aged persons, and the complications occur more frequently and severely as recovery times are prolonged. Problems with wound healing and urinary continence may be severe and prolonged. Radiotherapy, which is accompanied by less morbidity, may be a more viable treatment alternative. Options and alternatives need to be carefully presented to the patient and family and their wishes concerning the aggressiveness of treatment respected. Research indicates that most elderly men with prostate cancer will die of something besides their disease.

Pathophysiology

Testicular cancers are divided into germinal (90% to 95%) and nongerminal classes. Treatment is based on cell type. The symptoms are usually vague and nonspecific until the man discovers a nontender lump or swelling in the testis or complains of a heaviness or dragging in the groin area. The tumor may grow in size very rapidly once established.

Medical management

Diagnosis of testicular cancer is established from the physical findings supplemented by CT scanning, blood tests, and lymphangiogram. Biopsy is contraindicated because of the risk of tumor seeding. Surgical removal of the testis is the prompt first step of treatment. Further treatment may consist of radiotherapy or chemotherapy depending on the stage of the disease, its cell type, and the presence and degree of any clinical marker of metastasis. Orchiopexy is recommended for all young children with undescended testes by age 1 to 2 years, because the condition increases the likelihood of testicular cancer by 40%.

NURSING MANAGEMENT

The nurse will provide the standard care associated with general surgery or radiation therapy. Although the normal testis is shielded during treatment, there will be some scatter damage, and it usually requires about 2 months to determine whether sperm production has been affected. Sperm banking may be performed before treatment. Orchiectomy has little effect on fertility or sexuality, because the remaining testis undergoes hyperplasia to compensate.

It is essential that teenaged and young adult men be instructed in the technique of testicular examination for routine screening for testicular cancer. This process is reviewed in Box 16-7.

Cancer of the Penis

Penile cancer accounts for about 1% of all male cancers and is more common in African-American and Asian men. It occurs most commonly in men over 50 years old but can occur in young men and even children. Its incidence is highly dependent on hygienic standards and practices and rarely occurs in circumcised males. The chronic irritation of the smegma produced under the foreskin is considered to be carcinogenic. The lesion typically begins on the prepuce and then may extend to include the entire glans or shaft.

Treatment is usually surgical. Circumcision may be sufficient in early cases, but partial penectomy or amputation may be necessary in advanced cases. Radiation therapy may be used as an adjunct, since fully one third of patients have metastases at the time of diagnosis. Chemotherapy is being used as an adjunct with some early success. Surgical outcomes are quite good, but the

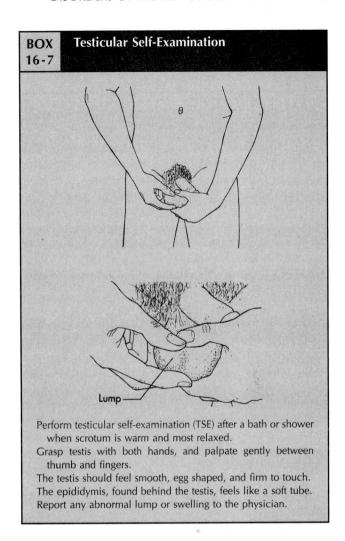

BOX 16-7 Testicular Self-Examination

Perform testicular self-examination (TSE) after a bath or shower when scrotum is warm and most relaxed.
Grasp testis with both hands, and palpate gently between thumb and fingers.
The testis should feel smooth, egg shaped, and firm to touch.
The epididymis, found behind the testis, feels like a soft tube.
Report any abnormal lump or swelling to the physician.

effects of surgery on sexuality, body image, self-concept, and urinary elimination can be profound. The man will need a great deal of support and encouragement to make a full recovery. Sexual counseling is recommended.

Male Breast Cancer

Less than 1% of the cases of breast cancer diagnosed each year occur in men. The incidence increases with age, with the average age at diagnosis being 60 to 66 years. A positive family history is an identified risk factor. Ductal infiltrating carcinoma is the most common form, and 80% of the tumors are estrogen receptor positive. Diagnostic measures are the same as those used with women, but advanced disease at the time of diagnosis is common because of long delays in seeking medical evaluation. The signs and symptoms are again similar to those in women. Modified radical mastectomy is the standard treatment, with radiotherapy, chemotherapy, or hormonal therapy with tamoxifen used to treat micrometastases or recurrent disease. The nursing care also reflects the general plan outlined on p. 397 with recognition of the unique psychosocial stressors of being afflicted with this highly publicized "female problem."

SEXUALLY TRANSMITTED DISEASES

Etiology/epidemiology

Sexually transmitted diseases (STDs) are disorders that are usually transmitted from one person to another during sexual contact with the genitals, mouth, or rectum. The category includes classic venereal diseases such as syphilis and gonorrhea as well as a wide variety of other diseases including genital herpes, nonspecific urethritis, scabies, and venereal warts. The addition of acquired immunodeficiency syndrome (AIDS) to the roster of STDs has refocused attention on these ancient health problems.

The true incidence of STDs is not known, because reporting requirements vary among the states and many clinicians who treat STDs do not report them. All states require that cases of syphilis and gonorrhea be reported to the state or local health office, but the other diseases are variously reported. Despite the requirements for reporting, it is still possible for adolescents to receive treatment for STDs without parental consent. It is estimated that almost 12 million cases of STDs occur yearly, with 46% of them in the 15 to 29-year-old age group. One out of every five persons has undergone treatment for an STD by 21 years of age. The medically underserved, poor, and racial and ethnic minorities are affected the most. The costs of STDs exceed $315 billion annually, and the problem is of such magnitude that it is well documented in the *Healthy People 2000* goals.

Much has been written about the rise in STDs over the last 50 years. Social permissiveness, particularly in regard to sexuality, is clearly considered to be the most significant variable. Studies do not confirm a pattern of promiscuous behavior among young people so much as they underscore a pattern of serial monogamous relationships, each of which lasts for a short period. Effective drug therapy is also theorized to have removed much of the fear and stigma traditionally associated with STDs. Decreased use of condoms in the 80s as IUDs and the "pill" dominated contraception is also discussed as a possible etiology.

Pathophysiology

The STDs are contagious diseases spread almost exclusively by the direct contact of mucus membranes during genital, oral, or anal sexual activity. Most organisms survive only briefly outside of a warm moist environment and cannot be transmitted by toilet seats, towels, or linens. A wide variety of disorders exists with a spectrum of etiologies and symptoms. The major disorders are summarized in Tables 16-9 and 16-10. Many diseases are asymptomatic during at least a portion of the cycle, particularly in women. This complicates the identification and treatment process, particularly when the toll on fertility, infant, and maternal morbidity is considered.

Medical management

The choice of treatment depends on the causative organism and is summarized in Tables 16-9 and 16-10. It is not unusual for individuals to be infected with more than one organism at the same time.

TABLE 16-9 Syphilis and Gonorrhea

INCUBATION PERIOD	SIGNS AND SYMPTOMS	MEDICAL MANAGEMENT
GONORRHEA		
Men: 3-30 days Women: 3 days to indefinite period	Men: purulent urethral discharge, dysuria, prostatitis, epididymitis; rectal and pharyngeal forms usually asymptomatic Women: asymptomatic in early stages; slight purulent discharge, aching or discomfort in pelvis or abdomen	Intramuscular penicillin G and probenicid by mouth or ampicillin and probenicid were traditional. More resistant organisms treated with ceftriaxone, cefixime, ciprofloxacin, or ofloxacin plus doxycycline for 7-10 days Salpingitis, PID, and sterility are potential complications in women
SYPHILIS		
3 weeks (9 days to 3 months)	Positive serologic tests Stage I: chancre (hard sore or pimple that breaks and forms painless, draining erosion on vulva, penis, mouth, or rectum) Stage II: fever, headache, malaise accompanied by sores or generalized body rash No signs during latent period Stage III: tumorlike masses, damage to heart valves and vessels, central nervous system (CNS) involvement with paresis, loss of judgment and memory	Penicillin G benzathine intramuscularly or tetracycline for 7 days Amoxicillin with probenicid as single-dose therapy

TABLE 16-10 Sexually Transmitted Diseases

CAUSES AND EFFECTS	TREATMENT
CHLAMYDIAL INFECTION Most prevalent STD in the United States; causes urethritis, epididymitis, cervicitis, PID, and lymphogranuloma venereum	Doxycycline for 7 days or a single doze of azithromycin
LYMPHOGRANULOMA VENEREUM Usually caused by chlamydia organism; affects lymph nodes, often in inguinal area, which may suppurate; often accompanied by urethritis symptoms	Tetracycline for 2 wk; erythromycin for 2-6 wk
CHANCROID Rare disease caused by gram-negative bacilli; produces lesions on genitals—ragged irregular ulcers that are highly infectious	Erythromycin for 10 days; local cleansing and comfort measures
CANDIDIASIS Monilial infection caused by a yeast form; produces thick white vaginal discharge	Fungicidal creams, ointments, and tablets—nystatin, miconazole; local measures to control itching
HUMAN PAPILLOMAVIRUS INFECTION Recently linked with development of cancer of cervix; characterized by single or multiple painless growths in genital area	Application of podophyllin in tincture of benzoin; several treatments may be necessary
HERPES GENITALIS Caused by infection with herpes virus type 2; 15-20% of Americans estimated to suffer from the disease; causes primary lesions that develop into clear fluid-filled vesicles that form ulcerations when they rupture; causes pain and local inflammation and may produce general symptoms of infection	Symptomatic treatment of lesions; acyclovir ointment to limit duration of initial attack (does not prevent recurrences)

NURSING MANAGEMENT

◆ ASSESSMENT
Subjective Data

History of sexual activity
    Number of partners
Homosexual or bisexual activity
Prior history of STD and treatment
Knowledge of disease—risks, mode of transmission
Complaints of the following:
    Vulvar or vaginal itching
    Dysuria and urgency
    Rectal symptoms
    Abdominal discomfort
    Sore throat

Objective Data

Vaginal or penile discharge
Genital lesions
Skin rashes
Rectal lesions or injury
Throat lesions or discharge
Postive cultures, smears, or blood tests

◆ NURSING DIAGNOSES

Nursing diagnoses for the person with an STD may include, but are not limited to, the following:

Knowledge deficit (related to transmission of STD and prevention)
Anxiety (related to consequences of STD on relationships and fertility)

◆ EXPECTED PATIENT OUTCOMES

Patient will accurately describe disease process, methods of transmission, and principles of "safer sex."
Patient will verbalize concerns related to the diagnosis and prognosis with staff and sexual partner.

◆ NURSING INTERVENTIONS
Increasing STD Knowledge Base

Teach patient about the etiology, transmission, and treatment of the STD.
Explain the nature and expected side effects of any drug therapy.
Encourage patient to complete full course of treatment.
Teach importance of refraining from sexual activity until treatment is complete.
Teach patient local care of skin lesions as appropriate:
    Frequent bathing
    Keeping lesions dry
    Use of cotton underwear to improve air circulation
    Local treatment as prescribed by physician
Reinforce importance of basic hygiene in prevention.
Encourage patient to inform sexual partners and help them seek appropriate treatment.

> **BOX 16-8**
>
> **Correct Use of Condoms to Prevent STD Transmission**
>
> Use latex condoms rather than natural membranes.
> Handle condom package carefully to prevent puncture.
> Store in cool, dry place away from direct sunlight.
> Apply condom *before* any genital contact.
> Leave space at the tip to collect semen.
> Use only water-soluble lubricants, not oil based.
> The use of vaginal spermicides in addition to condoms provides the best protection.
> Prevent slippage of the condom after ejaculation.
> Never reuse a condom.

Relieving Anxiety and Preventing Future Disease

Encourage patient to verbalize feelings about acquisition of the disease.

Teach patient principles of safer sex (Box 16-8).

Teach patient the correct use of condoms and their importance in preventing STD transmission (Box 16-8).

◆ EVALUATION

Successful achivement of expected outcomes for the patient with an STD is indicated by the following:

Correct description of disease process, planned treatment, and management of drug side effects

Verbalization of decreased disease-related anxiety and expressed commitment to prevention activities for the future.

SELECTED REFERENCES

Adamson GD: Surgical and medical treatment of endometriosis, *Contemp Obstet Gynecol* 36(7):48-63, 1991.

Andrist L: Taking a sexual history and educating clients about safe sex, *Nurs Clin North Am* 23:959-973, 1988.

Annon J: *The behavioral treatment of sexual problems,* Honolulu, 1974, Enabling Systems, Inc.

Berger PH, Saul HM: Radical hysterectomy: treatment for advanced cervical carcinoma, *AORN J* 52(6):1212-1222, 1990.

Bernhard LA: Consequences of hysterectomy in the lives of women, *Health Care Women Int* 13(3):281-291, 1992.

Blank B, Schneider R: Acute scrotal problems, *Patient Care* 24(11):152-155, 158, 1990.

Blesch KS, Prohaska TR: Cervical cancer screening in older women: issues and interventions, *Ca Nurs* 14(3):141-147, 1991.

Brucks JA: Ovarian cancer: the most lethal gynecologic malignancy, *Nurs Clin North Am* 27(4):835-845, 1992.

Chamorro T: Cancer of the vulva and vagina, *Semin Oncol Nurs* 6(3):198-205, 1990.

Corney R, Everett H, Howells A, Crowther M: The care of patients undergoing surgery for gynecological cancer: the need for information, emotional support and counselling, *J Adv Nurs* 17(6):667-671, 1992.

DeBow M: Safer sex. *Imprint* 35(1):33-34, 36, 1988.

Dulaney PE, Crawford VC, and Turner C: A comprehensive education and support program for women experiencing hysterectomies, *J Obstet Gynecol Neonatal Nurs* 19(4):319-325, 1989.

Eriksson JH, Walczak JR: Ovarian cancer, *Semin Oncol Nurs* 6(3):214-227, 1990.

Fishbein EG: Women at midlife: the transition to menopause, *Nurs Clin North Am* 27(4):951-957, 1992.

Fogel C, Lauver D: *Sexual health promotion,* Philadelphia, 1989, Saunders.

Fogel CI: Gonorrhea: not a new problem but a serious one, *Nurs Clin North Am* 23:885-897, 1988.

Gersham KA, Rolfs RT: Divergent gonorrhea and syphilis trends in the 1980s: are they real? *Am J Public Health* 81(10):1263-1267, 1991.

Hay EK: That old hip: the osteoporosis process, *Nurs Clin North Am* 26(1):43-51, 1991.

Heine P, McGregor JA: *Trichomonas vaginalis:* a reemerging pathogen, *Clin Obstet Gynecol* 36(1):137-144, 1993.

Hsia L, Long M: Premenstrual syndrome: current concepts in diagnosis and management, *J Nurse Midwifery* 35(6):351-357, 1990.

Hubbard JL, Holcombe JK: Cancer of the endometrium, *Semin Oncol Nurs* 6(3):206-213, 1990.

Jenkins B, Carbaugh C: Action stat: testicular torsion, *Nurs 89* 19(7):33, 1989.

Lamb M: Psychosexual issues: the woman with gynecologic cancer, *Semin Oncol Nurs* 6(3):237-243, 1990.

Liscum B: Osteoporosis: the silent disease, *Orthop Nurs* 11(4):21-25, 1992.

Lowdermilk D: Nursing care update: internal radiation therapy, *NAACOGS Clin Issues Perinat Womens Health Nurs* 1(4):532-541, 1990.

Maddox MA: Women at midlife: hormone replacement therapy, *Nurs Clin North Am* 27(4):959-969, 1992.

McCracken A: Sexual practice by elders: the forgotten aspect of functional health, *J Gerontol Nurs* 14(10):13-18, 1988.

McKenzie F: Sexuality after total pelvic exenteration, *Nurs Times* 84(20):26-28, 1988.

McMullin M: Holistic care of the patient with cervical cancer, *Nurs Clin North Am* 27(4):847-858, 1991.

Modica MM, Timor-Tritsch IE: Transvaginal sonography provides a sharper view into the pelvis, *J Obstet Gynecol Neonatal Nurs* 17(2):89-95, 1988.

Moore S et al: Nerve sparing prostatectomy, *Am J Nurs* 92(4) 59-64, 1992.

Nurata J: Abnormal genital bleeding and secondary amenorrhea: common gynecological problems, *J Obstet Gynecol Neonatal Nurs* 19(1):26-36, 1990.

Piver S et al: Epidemiology and etiology of ovarian cancer, *Semin Oncol* 18(3):177-185, 1991.

Rostad ME: The radical vulvectomy patient: preventing complications, *Dimensions Crit Care Nurs* 7(5):289-294, 1988.

Schumaker D: Preventing gynecologic cancer: every woman's guide, *Can Nurs* 87(9):23-24, 1991.

Secor RMC: Bacterial vaginosis: a comprehensive review, *Nurs Clin North Am* 23(4):865-875, 1988.

Smith D: Sexual rehabilitation of the cancer patient, *Ca Nurs* 12(1):10-15, 1989.

Sobel JD: Vaginitis in adult women, *Obstet Gynecol Clin North Am* 17(4):851-879, 1990.

Solomon M, De Jong W: Preventing AIDS and other STDs through condom promotion: a patient education intervention, *Am J Public Health* 79(4):453-458, 1989.

Thompson L: Cancer of the cervix, *Semin Oncol Nurs* 6(3):190-197, 1990.

Wickes S: Premenstrual syndrome, *Prim Care* 15(3):473-487, 1988.

Williams D, Riddle J: Understanding salpingitis: a pelvic inflammatory infection, *Prof Nurs* 6(4):217-220, 1991.

Williamson ML: Sexual adjustment after hysterectomy, *J Obstet Gynecol Neonatal Nurs* 21(1):42-47, 1992.

Wolenski M, Pelosi MA: Laparoscopic hysterectomy, *Today's OR Nurse* 13(11):23-29, 1991.

Wozniak-Petrofsky J: BPH: treating older men's most common problem. *RN* 7:32-37, 1991.

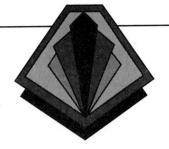

Disorders of the Immune System and Organ Transplantation

◆ ASSESSMENT

SUBJECTIVE DATA

Health history
  Infection history
    Recurrent infections
      Type, frequency, causes if known
    Skin rashes
      Location, type, severity, pruritus, factors that alleviate or exacerbate rash
    Pattern of fever or lymph node enlargement
      Location, number of nodes involved
      Severity, duration, time of day
      Presence of chills or night sweats
    Fatigue or weakness
      Effect on employment, social, and family life
  Allergy history
    Known allergies: food, medications, bites, environmental substances
    Type of physiologic response, severity
    Treatment used or attempted in the past
  History of autoimmune disorders
  Current or past medical problems and treatment
  Current medication use
    Prescription and over the counter (OTC)
Life-style factors
  Nutrition
    Diet pattern and nutrient adequacy
  Occupational exposure to chemicals, toxins
  Life stress: personal, occupational, financial
    Usual coping mechanisms, effectiveness
  Sexual relationships
    Risk factors for human immunodeficiency virus (HIV) exposure

OBJECTIVE DATA

General inspection
  Skin, hair, and nails
    Color and texture of skin
      Skin turgor
      Presence of rashes or lesions
    Hair texture, condition
    Presence of alopecia
    Nail color, configuration, brittleness
  Eyes, ears, nose, and throat
    Presence of tympanic membrane congestion
    Changes in conjunctivae
    Nasal obstruction, mouth breathing
    Presence of oral lesions
  Respiratory system
    Breath sounds
      Presence and quality
      Wheezing or dyspnea
    Work of breathing
      Use of accessory muscles
    Cough pattern
      Sputum volume and characteristics
  Palpation of lymph nodes
    Location, size
    Consistency, symmetry, and mobility
    Degree of discomfort if any

GERONTOLOGIC PATIENT CONSIDERATIONS: PHYSIOLOGIC CHANGES IN THE IMMUNE SYSTEM

NOTE: The extent of changes in the immune system varies significantly among elders. In general, however, the slow changes in organs and tissues result in a gradual imbalance of protective responses and leave the individual more susceptible to injury and infection. Specific immune system changes include the following:

Low rate of T lymphocyte proliferation in response to a stimulus

Decrease in number of cytotoxic (killer) T cells

Reduction in T cell response to certain viral antigens, allografts, and tumor cells

Reduced production of interleukin-2 by helper T cells; decreases stimulation of T lymphocytes and natural killer (NK) cells

Decreased relative proportion of CD4 (T4 or helper T cells) and CD8, affecting regulation of the immune system

Significant changes in thymus gland morphology

Some decrease in B cell responsiveness thought to be related to a decline in helper T cell functioning

Change in immunoglobulin balance with a marked increase in IgA and IgG antibodies

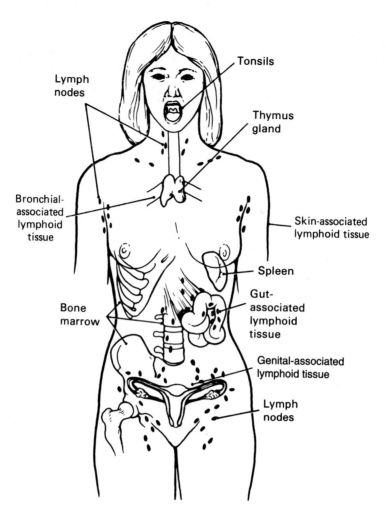

FIGURE 17-1 Organs and tissues of the immune system. (From Lewis SM, Collier IC: *Medical-surgical nursing,* ed 3, St Louis, 1992, Mosby.)

✍ LABORATORY TESTS
BLOOD TESTS

A variety of laboratory tests can measure aspects of nonspecific immunity as well as specific parts of the immune process. Nonspecific immunity is assessed through analysis of the inflammatory response and phagocytosis. Tests include white blood cells (WBCs) with differential, erythrocyte sedimentation rate (ESR), C-reactive protein, total complement activity test, and phagocytic cell function tests (Box 17-1).

Protein electrophoresis measures the relative concentrations of plasma proteins. The primary groups are albumin and globulin, which are further divided into alpha, beta, and gamma globulins. Chronic inflammatory diseases cause increases in alpha$_1$ and gamma globulins, whereas acute inflammation increases alpha$_2$ globulins. The gamma globulins can be further broken down by immunoelectrophoresis to show the relative quantities of each type. The clinical significance of each type is summarized in Table 17-1.

Antibody Screening Tests

Numerous tests exist for the detection of antibodies formed against specific bacteria, viruses, fungi, and parasites. Commonly used tests include the streptozyme, enzyme-linked immunosorbent assay (ELISA), and Western blot. Both the ELISA and Western blot are used in HIV antibody screening. The ELISA simply determines the presence of HIV antibodies and is vulnerable to false-positive results. The Western blot is more accurate and definitely confirms the presence of the virus.

Autoantibody and Antigen Tests

Tests are available to detect the presence of abnormal antibodies produced by the body against itself. Rheumatoid factor, anti-DNA antibodies, and antinuclear antibodies are common examples. Certain serum antigens can also be detected, including hepatitis B surface antigen. The most famous application is in ABO blood typing and direct and indirect Coombs' testing. ABO typing identifies types of naturally occurring antibodies

<table>
<tr><td colspan="2">**BOX 17-1** **Nonspecific Immune Function Tests**</td></tr>
</table>

WBCs

<50,000/cm³: leukopenia
>10,000/cm³: leukocytosis

DIFFERENTIAL (PERCENTAGE OF EACH CELL TYPE)

Neutrophils: Segs, Stabs, Bands

>70%: usually indicates bacterial infection
NOTE: reported on left side of most laboratory slips, so an increase in neutrophils is often referred to as a shift to the left

Lymphocytes

>40%: usually represents lymphocytosis, usually elevated, with viral infection
NOTE: reported on the right side of most laboratory slips, so an increase in lymphocytes is often referred to as a shift to the right

Eosinophils

Increase associated with allergic disorders

ESR

Increase seen when there are increased globulins or other substances causing blood to clump faster than usual; usually caused by infection, autoimmune disease, or malignancy

C-REACTIVE PROTEIN

Measures presence of an abnormal protein typically found after certain inflammatory processes

TOTAL COMPLEMENT ACTIVITY

Screening tool for complement cascade; high values indicate inflammation but do not determine source

TABLE 17-1 Classes of Immunoglobulins and Their Clinical Significance

CLASS OF IMMUNO-GLOBULIN	CLINICAL SIGNIFICANCE	
	INCREASED LEVEL	DECREASED LEVEL
IgG	IgG myeloma, bacterial infections, hepatitis A, glomerulonephritis, rheumatoid arthritis, systemic lupus erythematosus (SLE), acquired immune deficiency syndrome (AIDS)	Agammaglobulinemia, IgA myeloma, IgA deficiency, chronic lymphocytic leukemia, type I dysgammaglobulinemia, lymphoid aplasia, combined immunodeficiency, common variable immunodeficiency, X-linked hypogammaglobulinemia
IgM	Hepatitis A and B, Waldenström's macroglobulinemia, trypanosomiasis, chronic infections, type I dysgammaglobulinemia, hepatitis, SLE, rheumatoid arthritis, Sjögren's syndrome, AIDS	Lymphoid aplasia, hypogammaglobulinemia, chronic lymphocytic leukemia, IgG myeloma, IgA myeloma, agammaglobulinemia
IgA	SLE, rheumatoid arthritis, IgA myeloma, glomerulonephritis, chronic liver disease	Ataxia, telangiectasia, hypogammaglobulinemia, acute and chronic lymphocytic leukemia, IgA deficiency, combined immunodeficiency, common variable immunodeficiency, X-linked hypogammaglobulinemia, agammaglobulinemia, IgG myeloma, chronic infections (especially upper respiratory type)
IgE	Atopic disorders: allergic rhinitis, allergic asthma, atopic dermatitis, Wiskott-Aldrich syndrome with eczema, parasitic infestation, hyperimmunoglobulin E	Associated with IgA deficiency, intrinsic (nonallergic) asthma
IgD	Eczema, skin disorders	Unknown

toward red blood cells (RBCs). Indirect Coombs' testing is reported as the patient's Rh factor, and direct Coombs' testing detects antibodies coating the RBC not detected by other methods.

RADIOLOGIC TEST

Lymphangiogram

Purpose—A lymphangiogram involves evaluation of the lymphatic system after the injection of a contrast dye. It is used primarily to diagnose cancer or metastasis and to evaluate lymphedema.

Procedure—Contrast medium is injected intradermally into the webs between the toes where it infiltrates the lymphatic system. Within 15 to 30 minutes the lymphatic vessels are outlined on the dorsum of each foot. A transverse incision is made to expose a vessel in each foot, and the vessel is cannulated. An oil-based dye is injected by means of a pump over a period of about one-half hour. Fluoroscopy can be used to monitor the filling of the system. Films are taken at the completion of the injection and again in 24 hours when the lymph nodes are clearly outlined. The entire test takes about 3 hours.

Patient preparation and aftercare—No special preparation is required except careful education about this unusual test. The patient is instructed about the need for small incisions in the feet to inject the dye and is informed that the dye will discolor the urine and stool for about 48 hours and may give a bluish tint to the skin and vision during this time. Injection of the dye causes some discomfort, and it is important for the patient to lie completely still to avoid dislodging the small needles. The patient is carefully assessed for a history of allergy to iodine, shellfish, or any contrast medium.

The patient's vital signs are monitored every 4 hours after the test, and bed rest is maintained for 24 hours with the feet elevated. Ice packs are ordered to reduce swelling in the feet. Dressings are left in place for 2 days, and the sites are monitored carefully for any signs of infection.

SPECIAL TESTS
Skin Tests

Skin tests are a simple means to diagnose particular allergies or IgE-mediated reactions. The suspected allergen can be administered by intradermal injection or through a scratch, prick, or puncture of the skin. Intradermal injections are the most accurate, but they may cause a systemic reaction.

Skin testing can also be used to screen patients for T cell immunodeficiency. Specific antigens such as purified protein derivative (PPD), *Candida,* or mumps antigen are injected, and the response is read in 72 hours. Reactions indicate hypersensitivity and not disease. If an individual does not respond to any of the antigens, the individual is considered to be anergic. Anergy panels may be ordered when immunodeficiency is suspected.

LYMPH NODE BIOPSY

A lymph node biopsy may be taken to identify if inflammation or malignancy is present. The procedure is performed with the patient under local anesthesia. The site is covered with a sterile bandage and monitored for healing. The minor discomfort after biopsy can usually be effectively managed with mild analgesics.

DISORDERS OF THE IMMUNE SYSTEM
GAMMOPATHIES

The gammopathies represent elevated levels of serum gamma globulin. In the normal system an immunoglobulin is synthesized from the proliferation and differentiation of a single clone of B cells in response to a specific antigen. The gammopathies result when this single clone of B cells overproduces or when multiple clones overproduce any or all classes of immunoglobulins. The major triggers for polyclonal overproduction are the infectious diseases. Since the immunoglobulins are dysfunctional, the person is still extremely vulnerable to infection. The monoclonal gammopathies are also referred to as plasma cell dyscrasias, and the most common form is multiple myeloma.

Multiple Myeloma
Etiology/epidemiology

Multiple myeloma is diagnosed in approximately 4 of every 100,000 persons each year. It primarily affects elderly persons, and African-Americans are affected twice as often as whites. The etiology of the disorder remains unknown, but a higher incidence has been seen in farmers and individuals exposed to radiation or benzene.

Pathophysiology

The underlying pathologic condition involves the development of plasma cell tumors in the bone marrow that cause widespread destruction and gradually invade the hard bone tissue. Disorders of calcium and uric acid balance also occur. Greater than 95% of patients have monoclonal proteins in the serum and urine (Bence Jones protein).

The onset of symptoms is slow, and the disease is usually well established at the time of diagnosis. Compression fractures of the spine or pelvis are often the first noticeable occurrence. Compression can quickly lead to paraplegia or quadriplegia. The electrolyte imbalance of calcium can lead to renal failure, which may also be among the early symptoms. The overproduction of ineffective immunoglobulins results in frequent infections, particularly of the respiratory system, and bone marrow crowding leads to severe anemia and thrombocytopenia.

Medical management

Multiple myeloma is diagnosed from the results of x-rays and computed tomography (CT) scans that show "punched-out" lesions of the bone and generalized osteoporosis. These results are supplemented by laboratory studies showing increased serum calcium and uric acid; complete blood count (CBC) results confirming anemia, leukopenia, and thrombocytopenia; urine positive for Bence Jones protein; and elevated abnormal immunoglobulin and depressed normal immunoglobulin levels.

Treatment revolves around the administration of glucocorticoids and calcitonin to reduce bone destruction and reverse the hypercalcemia. The tumor burden is treated with chemotherapy administered orally or intravenously depending on response. Interferon may help to prolong remissions. Radiation may be used to shrink the bony tumors. Other interventions are aimed at correcting or compensating for the complications of the disease such as fracture and spinal cord compression. Dialysis may be necessary if the renal damage is advanced.

NURSING MANAGEMENT

Nursing intervention focuses on supporting independence in self-care while preventing further injury from fracture. Ambulation is important to prevent further bone breakdown and support osteoblastic activity, but safety is of primary consideration. Assistive devices to support balance and stability, and lightweight braces to support weakened parts will be implemented. The nurse assists the family to analyze the home situation and make modifications to improve the patient's safety. A fall can be disastrous.

Analgesics will be offered to control bone pain and support the patient's ability to ambulate. If the patient is on bed rest, extreme caution is used in assisting with turning and position changes. Lift sheets should be used, and there will need to be ample assistance to avoid any stress or trauma to the bones.

The nurse will encourage a liberal daily fluid intake of 3000 ml to assist with calcium elimination by the kidneys. The patient will be instructed in ways to reduce calcium intake in the daily diet. General measures are also implemented to balance activity and rest to avoid severe fatigue and to protect the patient from infection. Respiratory hygiene is emphasized.

HYPERSENSITIVITIES

The immune system functions to protect the body from foreign substances. At times, however, the response of the system is detrimental to overall body functioning. This response is typically a tissue-damaging overreaction to an antigen. Hypersensitivities then represent the normal responses of the immune system that take place in inappropriate sites, in excessive amounts, or involving unrelated tissues. Hypersensitivities can be broadly classified based on the involvement of either the humoral (B cell) or cellular (T cell) response systems. They are also typically further subdivided into types I to IV (Table 17-2).

Type I Hypersensitivities
Etiology/epidemiology

Type I reactions are characterized by an exaggerated response toward an external substance and range in severity from common allergic symptoms to life-threatening anaphylaxis. They include food allergies, hay fever, contact dermatitis, and venom hyperreactivity. Allergic responses are extremely common and occur in more than 15% of the population, but the occurrence of anaphylaxis is rare. The tendency to become hypersensitive is inherited, and allergic disease begins most commonly between the ages of 2 and 15 years. The underlying etiology involves a genetic predisposition to produce IgE antibodies in response to common antigens. Nonatopic responses are also mediated by the IgE antibodies but are not genetic in nature.

Pathophysiology

Type I hypersensitivity requires an initial contact with an allergen that serves to sensitize the B lymphocytes to produce specific IgE antibodies, which then attach themselves to the mast cells or basophils. Any subsequent exposure causes the allergen to be bound to the mast cell, which releases its internal agents, such as histamine, kinins, and prostaglandins. These mediators cause vasodilation, smooth muscle contraction, increased vascular permeability, and increased mucous gland activity, which combine to create the following classic symptoms:

- Respiratory: rhinorrhea, watery itchy eyes, sneezing, sinusitis; and in severe responses bronchospasm, dyspnea, wheezing
- Skin: hives, rash, angioedema
- Gastrointestinal: nausea, vomiting, diarrhea
- Other: fever, malaise, joint pain, anaphylaxis

The sequence of responses is outlined in Figure 17-2.

Medical management

Diagnosis of type I hypersensitivities is based primarily on the patient's health history supplemented by skin tests or radioallergosorbent test (RAST) tests as needed

TABLE 17-2	Hypersensitivity Reactions					
TYPE	ANTIGEN	ANTIBODY	COMPLEMENT INVOLVED	MEDIATORS OF INJURY	EXAMPLES	SKIN TEST
I. Anaphylactic	Exogenous pollen, food, drugs, dust	IgE	No	Histamine, SRS-A*	Allergic rhinitis, asthma	Wheal and flare
II. Cytotoxic	Cell surface of RBC, basement membrane	IgG, IgM, or IgA	Yes	Complement lysis, neutrophils	Transfusion reaction, Goodpasture's syndrome	None
III. Immune complex–mediated	Extracellular: fungal, viral, bacterial	IgG, IgM, or IgA	Yes	Neutrophils, complement lysis	Serum sickness, systemic lupus erythematosus, rheumatoid arthritis	Erythema and edema in 3-8 hr
IV. Delayed hypersensitivity (cell mediated)	Intracellular or extracellular	None	No	Lymphokines, T-cytotoxic cells, monocytes/ macrophages, lysosomal enzymes	Contact dermatitis, allograft or tumor rejection	Erythema and edema in 24-48 hr (e.g., TB test)

From Lewis SM, Collier IC: *Medical surgical nursing*, ed 3, St Louis, 1992, Mosby.
*Slow-reacting substance of anaphylaxis.

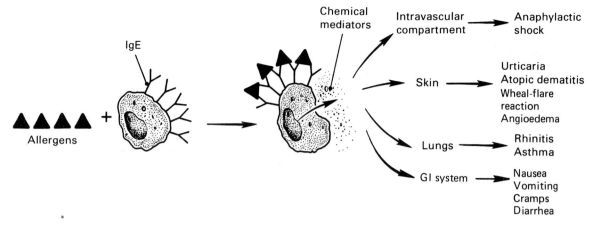

FIGURE 17-2 Steps in a type I hypersensitivity reaction. (From Lewis SM, Collier IC: *Medical-surgical nursing,* ed 3, St Louis, 1992, Mosby.)

to identify specific allergens and guide therapy. Drug therapy is primarily used for relief of specific symptoms and usually includes antihistamines and decongestants. Skin reactions are usually self-limiting and may not require specific treatment. The occurrence of anaphylaxis is managed with the administration of epinephrine to block the action of histamine and inhibit mast cell mediator release. Treatment may also include the use of antihistamines, hydrocortisone, and a bronchodilator such as aminophylline. Vasopressors may be needed if the patient goes into shock.

Immunotherapy may be used to achieve progressive hyposensitization of the immune system to the allergen. Treatment is individualized and involves injection of increasing amounts of allergen at weekly intervals, slowly diminishing symptomatic responses.

NURSING MANAGEMENT

Nursing management of type I hypersensitivity primarily involves helping the patient modify his or her life-style to reduce contact with the allergens in daily living. This may involve environmental changes in the home, reducing contact with animal dander and dust, limiting outdoor activities during seasons of high pollen counts, and modifying the diet to avoid contact with triggering foods. Some specific suggestions are summarized in Table 17-3.

Allergy assessment is critical in dealing with the hospitalized patient, and all patient records should be clearly marked to indicate sensitivities. Patients need to be monitored closely when starting on any new medications, particularly antibiotics, and with special attention to those drugs known to have high anaphylactic potential, such as penicillin, amphotericin, and streptokinase. Contrast media that are used in many diagnostic tests also have a high degree of allergic potential, and their administration needs to be closely monitored. Nursing responsibilities in the event of anaphylaxis include ensuring a patent airway, continuous monitoring, and the administration of any ordered medications.

TABLE 17-3   Methods of Decreasing Environmental Inhalant Antigens

AREA	METHOD
Floors	Do not use wool carpets or felt rug pads; washable throw rugs over wood or tile floors may be used.
Furniture	Do not use kapok stuffing; a minimum number of foam-stuffed furniture covered with leather or plastic is preferable.
Clothing	Do not wear wool; place closet garments in plastic bags.
	Use synthetic materials.
	Do not hang wash outside to dry.
Bedding	
Pillows	Do not use feathers or kapok; use polyester fiberfill.
Mattress	Use foam mattress over a covered box spring; use allergy-free covers.
Blankets	Use washable cotton.
Pets	Do not keep fur-bearing pets.
Cleaning	Do daily damp dusting with no shaking of articles.
Air	Use air conditioning, if possible; if not, try electrostatic filters.
	Run air conditioning in car for 10-15 min with windows open before driving.
	Keep windows closed during travel.
	Avoid being outdoors between sunset and sunrise, especially if windy.
Plants	Avoid dried plants.
	Limit house plants.
	Avoid gardening, raking leaves, and fresh-cut grass.
Furnace	Change filters monthly.

Type II Hypersensitivities

Type II hypersensitivities are cytotoxic and involve the direct binding of IgG or IgM to an antigen on the surface of the cell. This triggers a phagocytic attack that destroys the cells. Hemolytic reactions to a mismatched blood transfusion are a classic example of the reaction.

There are many antigens on the surface of the RBCs, but the ABO and Rh systems are the most significant.

Erythrocyte antigens are inherited, and an individual has formed antibodies to other blood types within 3 months of birth. The Rh system is more complex and involves over 27 different antigens. The D antigen is the most significant, and its presence is indicated by the term *Rh positive*. Multiple other antigens exist, but they tend to cause problems only for patients who undergo repeated transfusions.

Numerous types of transfusion reactions can occur, but adverse reactions occur in only 2% to 5% of all transfusions. Immunologic reactions are described in Table 17-4. The acute hemolytic reaction is by far the most serious, but it occurs in less than 0.5% to 1% of all transfusions. Nonimmunologic reactions to blood trans-

fusions can also occur. These include circulatory overload, sepsis, and the risk of disease transmission. Safe use and monitoring of blood component transfusions are presented in Chapter 7. The more often a patient has been transfused the greater the likelihood of some form of reaction occurring, regardless of the care taken in matching and screening. Routine, planned needs for transfusions, as before elective surgery, are increasingly being met by autologous blood transfusions.

Type III Hypersensitivities

The third type of hypersensitivity involves immune complexes. Soluble antigens and immunoglobulins of the IgM and IgG classes unite and form complexes that

TABLE 17-4   Immunologic Reactions to Blood Transfusion*

CAUSE	CLINICAL MANIFESTATIONS	MANAGEMENT
*ACUTE HEMOLYTIC		
Infusion of ABO-incompatible whole blood, RBCs, or components containing 10 ml or more of RBCs. Antibodies in recipient's plasma attach to antigens on transfused RBCs causing RBC destruction.	Chills, fever, low back pain, flushing, tachycardia, tachypnea, hypotension, vascular collapse, hemoglobinuria, hemoglobinemia, bleeding, acute renal failure, shock, cardiac arrest, death	Treat shock. Draw blood samples for serologic testing. To avoid hemolysis from procedure, use a new venipuncture (not an existing central line) and avoid small-gauge needles. Send urine specimen to laboratory. Maintain blood pressure with intravenous (IV) colloid solutions. Give diuretics as prescribed to maintain urine flow. Insert indwelling catheter, or measure voided amounts to monitor hourly urine output. Dialysis may be required if renal failure occurs. Do not transfuse additional RBC-containing components until transfusion service has provided newly crossmatched units.
*FEBRILE, NONHEMOLYTIC (MOST COMMON)		
Sensitization to donor's WBCs, platelets, or plasma proteins.	Sudden chills and fever (rise in temperature of greater than 1° C [2° F]), headache, flushing, anxiety, muscle pain	Give antipyretics as prescribed. Do not give aspirin to thrombocytopenic patients. *Do not restart transfusion.*
*MILD ALLERGIC		
Sensitivity to foreign plasma proteins.	Flushing, itching, urticaria (hives)	Give antihistamines as directed. If symptoms are mild and transient, restart transfusion slowly. Do not restart transfusion if fever or pulmonary symptoms develop.
*ANAPHYLACTIC		
Infusion of IgA proteins to IgA-deficient recipient who has developed IgA antibody.	Anxiety, urticaria, wheezing, tightness and pain in chest, difficulty swallowing, progressing to cyanosis, shock, and possible cardiac arrest	Initiate cardiopulmonary resuscitation (CPR) if indicated. Have epinephrine ready for injection (0.4 ml of a 1:1000 solution subcutaneously or 0.1 ml of 1:1000 solution diluted to 10 ml with saline for IV use). *Do not restart transfusion.*
DELAYED HEMOLYTIC		
Anamnestic immune response that occurs 7-14 days after transfusion. Sensitization to RBC antigen, not ABO system.	Fever, chills, back pain, jaundice, anemia, hemoglobinuria	Monitor adequacy of urinary output and degree of anemia. Treat fever with acetaminophen (Tylenol). May need further blood transfusion.

*Modified from the *National blood resource education program's transfusion therapy guidelines for nurses,* 1990, NIH Publication No. 90-2668.

BOX 17-2	Screening for Blood Donors

GENERAL REQUIREMENTS FOR BLOOD DONATION

Vital signs within normal range
Hemoglobin level
    Men: >13.5 g/dl
    Women: >12.5 g/dl

CONTRAINDICATIONS FOR BLOOD DONATION

Presence or history of infectious disease or malignancy, e.g., hepatitis, HIV, malaria, tuberculosis (TB), syphilis
Allergies or asthma
Current anemia or polycythemia vera, bleeding disorders
Current pregnancy or major surgery
Men with homosexual or bisexual contact since 1975
Blood transfusion during prior 6 months
Diseases of the heart, lungs, liver; history of jaundice
International travel to regions with high risk of malaria or AIDS
Immunization with attenuated viral vaccine for rubella or rabies

BOX 17-3	Examples of Autoimmune Disorders

TARGET ORGAN SPECIFIC

Hematologic	Hemolytic anemia
	Idiopathic thrombocytopenic purpura
Cardiac	Rheumatic fever
Nervous system	Multiple sclerosis
	Guillain-Barré syndrome
	Myasthenia gravis
Endocrine	Addison's disease
	Graves' disease
	Hashimoto's thyroiditis
Urologic	Glomerulonephritis
	Goodpasture's syndrome
Gastrointestinal	Ulcerative colitis
	Pernicious anemia

NONSPECIFIC

Systemic lupus erythematosus
Rheumatoid arthritis
Progressive systemic sclerosis

are incompletely cleared by the reticuloendothelial system because of their small size. The complexes bind complement and initiate the complement cascade with chemotaxis, vasodilation, and cell lysis. The release of chemotactic factors attracts phagocytes and worsens the inflammatory response. Immune complexes have been found in disparate autoimmune diseases such as multiple sclerosis, lupus, glomerulonephritis, and rheumatoid arthritis. The symptoms seen are the result of the quantity of antigens and antibodies present and the distribution of the complexes in the body. Serum sickness is another example of type III hypersensitivity that is important in the management of transplant.

Type IV Hypersensitivities

The type IV reactions are cell mediated and involve the T cells. Macrophages "pick up" antigens that they perceive as foreign and use them to sensitize the T lymphocytes. The next time the antigen is encountered the T cell can form cytotoxic cells to destroy it. In the normal individual this response is primarily responsible for organizing host defenses to chronic bacterial and fungal infection and in cancer cell surveillance. However, the mechanism is also theorized to underlie the process of contact dermatitis and allograft rejection.

Autoimmune diseases represent the most significant example of impaired type IV response. The formation of antibodies against self tissues is normal and necessary for the removal of dead cells and tissue debris. Autoimmune disease is present when these normal processes cause injury to normal host cells. The actual etiologic agent usually lies outside the immune system, but the immune response serves as the pathologic mechanism.

Autoimmunity is influenced by genetic, hormonal, viral, and environmental factors, and the diseases are often found to run in families. These diseases are also far more common in females for no known reason. The disorders are grouped according to their effects and may involve specific organs and structures or act nonspecifically throughout the body. Examples of autoimmune disorders are presented in Box 17-3.

IMMUNODEFICIENCIES
Primary Deficiencies

Primary immune deficiencies are congenital in nature. They are rare disorders seen mostly in infants and young children, and their underlying biologic errors in immune functioning are either poorly understood or unknown. A wide variety of disorders are possible, including antibody deficiencies, thymic hypoplasia, granulomatous disease, complement deficiencies, and severe combined immunodeficiency disease. The blockage in immune cell development is typically recognized by a pattern of chronic infections or treatment failure with common infections. The symptoms depend on the site of the infection and the specific organism. Without treatment most patients will die very early in their lives. The treatment depends on the specific nature of the deficiency but may include the administration of immune serum globulin or bone marrow transplant.

Secondary Deficiencies

Any factor that can interfere with the normal growth or function of the immune system can result in a secondary deficiency. Although the HIV retrovirus is by far the most important and recognized example, deficiency can also be the result of severe malnutrition, advanced liver disease, uremia, cancer, and the effects of chemical exposure, for example, asbestos, dioxin, heavy metals, and insecticides. Advancing age slowly impairs immune system function and places elders at particular risk for secondary problems. Immunosuppression may also be a planned goal in the treatment of autoimmune disorders and to suppress the rejection of transplanted organs. Drugs include glucocorticoids, cyclosporine, cytotoxic agents, and monoclonal anti–T cell antibodies (OKT-3). Treatment of secondary deficiencies focuses primarily on the underlying condition creating the deficiency and the management of concurrent infections. Adequate protein intake is ensured, and the importance of scrupulous personal hygiene is reinforced.

Human Immunodeficiency Virus (HIV) and AIDS
Etiology/epidemiology

The first cases of the illness that would later be termed *acquired immune deficiency syndrome (AIDS)* were identified in 1981. The retrovirus responsible for the underlying immune deficiency was not identified until 1985. Currently the disease has been responsible for over 1.5 million deaths worldwide and remains an incurable illness that is spreading steadily.

Five human retroviruses have been identified to date. HIV-1 and HIV-2 both cause depletion of T4 helper cells, resulting in a loss of cellular immunity. HIV-1 is the primary cause of AIDS in the United States and Europe, whereas HIV-2 is most prevalent in West Africa. It is estimated that over 18 million people are infected with

HIV throughout the world (1.5 million in the United States), a number that could increase to 40 million or more by the year 2000.

The infection was first identified in the homosexual population in the United States, but currently less than 50% of infections are found in this population. Those at greatest risk now include heterosexual women and their children and IV drug users. African- and Hispanic-Americans are at greatest risk. Worldwide the disease is primarily found in heterosexual men and women and their children. Mortality for AIDS reaches 80% within 3 years of diagnosis in the United States. It is suspected to be much higher in undeveloped countries, where treatment is nonexistent.

Pathophysiology

The HIV virus interacts with specific host receptors and then uses the host cell for replication of the virus. HIV interacts with the CD4 glycoprotein found primarily on the T4 helper lymphocytes (Figure 17-3). The core of the virus is injected into the cell's cytoplasm where the viral RNA is translated into DNA. Subsequent viral replication eventually depletes the host's T4 cells, causing a dramatic loss of the protective immune response.

HIV infection is associated with an extremely unpredictable disease course. Many persons experience a prolonged period of 10 or more years in which they are virtually asymptomatic. The virus is consistently detectable, however, and these persons are able to transmit the virus to others. Cofactors that influence disease

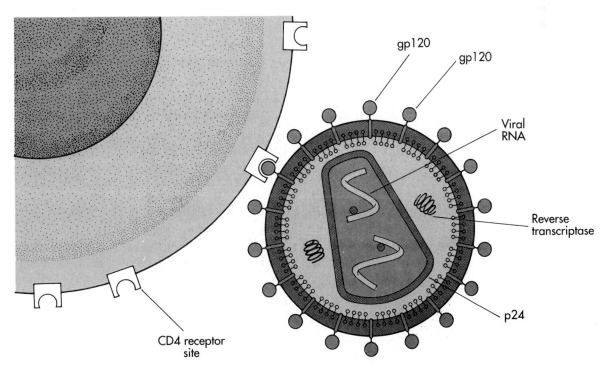

FIGURE 17-3 HIV virus attaching to CD4 receptors on surface of helper T cells. (From Lewis SM, Collier IC: *Medical-surgical nursing*, ed 3, St Louis, 1992, Mosby.)

BOX 17-4	Preventing the Spread of HIV

SAFE SEX COUNSELING

Vaginal, anal, and oral sex are all high-risk practices.

Use of latex condoms during sexual activity significantly reduces the risk of exposure to the virus.

Mutual masturbation, massage, and other activities that do not involve the exchange of body fluids reduce the exposure risk.

Exposure to multiple sexual partners increases the risk of infection.

Mutually monogamous sexual relationships minimize the risk of exposure.

REDUCING THE RISK OF INTRAVENOUS EXPOSURE

The use of contaminated needles poses a serious risk of exposure.

Use of bleach solutions to clean syringes and other paraphernalia is essential in reducing risk.

Substance abuse counseling is a critical long-term risk reduction strategy.

PROTECTION FOR HEALTH CARE WORKERS

Hand washing remains the most important principle of infection control.

Follow universal precautions:

Use gloves whenever direct care may involve hand contact with body fluids, such as drawing blood, starting lines, or doing finger sticks or dressing changes.

Use full protective garb (gowns, masks, goggles) appropriately when direct contact with blood or body fluid is expected or the risk of splashing is high.

Minimize needle stick injury by never recapping needles and using conveniently placed, puncture-proof disposal containers.

BOX 17-5	Laboratory Testing for HIV

ELISA TEST

The enzyme-linked immunosorbent assay test uses spectrophotometry to detect serum antibody reactions to HIV proteins. The test is highly specific and has a sensitivity of 93% to 99%, but it can detect only antibodies to HIV and not the viral antigen. Therefore it cannot detect infection in its earliest stages before the formation of antibodies. False-positive results are also common, and all positive tests are confirmed by Western blot.

WESTERN BLOT TECHNIQUE

Western blot is a second antibody detection test used to increase the reliability of a positive ELISA. It provides increased validity using the same blood sample, without the need to perform serial ELISA determinations over time.

• • •

NOTE: It is estimated that 90% of persons will form antibodies to HIV within 6 weeks to 3 months of exposure to the virus. A negative antibody test may occur during this initial period. In some individuals the time lapse may be as great as 6 months.

Newborn infants retain maternal antibodies for about 18 months after birth, and antibody testing during this time is unreliable.

TABLE 17-5 Antiretroviral Drug Therapy	
GENERIC AND TRADE NAMES	**SIDE EFFECTS**
AZT	
Zidovudine, ZDV, Retrovir, azidothymidine	Nausea, GI discomfort, malaise, fatigue, headache, red cell anemia, granulocytopenia
ddI	
Didanosine, Videx	Pancreatitis, peripheral neuropathy, liver failure, headache, diarrhea, asthenia, insomnia, nausea/vomiting, abdominal pain
ddC	
Dideoxycytidine, Hivid	Peripheral neuropathy, pancreatitis, esophageal ulcers, nausea, oral ulcers, abdominal pain, diarrhea, vomiting

progression are being explored, with viral, host, and environmental factors playing roles. Once viral replication increases, the number of T4 cells becomes depleted and the person is vulnerable to infections that were once easily controlled or eliminated by the immune system. Opportunistic infections include the following:

Viruses: herpes simplex, Epstein-Barr, cytomegalovirus (CMV)

Protozoans: *Pneumocystis carinii, Toxoplasma*

Fungi: *Histoplasma, Cryptococcus*

Mycobacteria: *Mycobacterium tuberculosis* and *avium*

Immune dysfunction also allows the development of various neoplasms, particularly Kaposi's sarcoma, non-Hodgkin's lymphoma, and cervical cancer. As the immunodeficiency progresses, any organ system of the body may be affected, and the signs and symptoms can vary substantially. Chronic fatigue, episodic diarrhea, and weight loss are common general early findings.

The methods of disease transmission are well identified. The virus has been identified in a variety of body fluids, but blood, semen, and vaginal secretions have been shown to be consistently infectious. The virus is transmitted by intimate sexual contact; by exposure to contaminated blood, blood products, and body fluids; and from mother to child in the prenatal period. It cannot be transmitted through casual contact such as sneezing or coughing, shaking hands, or contact with potential secretions on toilet seats, in bathtubs, or in swimming pools. Sexual transmission is estimated to represent over 95% of all exposures.

<table>
<tr><td>

BOX 17-6 **CDC Classification for HIV Infection**

STAGE I: ACUTE INFECTION

Occurs at the time of infection and lasts from days to weeks; characterized by flulike symptoms

STAGE II: ASYMPTOMATIC INFECTION

May last for years

STAGE III: PERSISTENT GENERALIZED LYMPHADENOPATHY

Characterized by palpable lymph node enlargement of 1 cm or greater at two or more sites that persists for more than 3 months

STAGE IV: OTHER DISEASES (STAGE III NOT A PREREQUISITE)

Group A: persistent fever and involuntary weight loss of >10% body weight, persistent diarrhea
Group B: neurologic disease, including AIDS dementia
Group C: secondary infectious diseases, e.g., *Pneumocystis carinii* pneumonia, herpes simplex, *Mycobacterium avium*, yeast
Group D: secondary cancer, e.g., Kaposi's sarcoma, non-Hodgkin's lymphoma
Group E: other conditions

</td></tr>
</table>

<table>
<tr><td>

BOX 17-7 **AIDS Complications: Mycobacterium Avium**

Mycobacterium avium is an atypical mycobacterium that is widespread in the environment, with high concentrations in the water and soil. It has a low pathogenicity in the normal host but is the most common bacterial infection in persons with AIDS. It presents with a tuberculosis-like process and often disseminates to multiple organs. Person-to-person transmission is not a source of infection, and airborne precautions are not necessary.

Diagnosis

The disease can usually be diagnosed by blood culture. Most patients also exhibit severe anemia.

Symptoms

Many patients are asymptomatic or experience general symptoms related to other infections and complications. Fever is common and may be persistent. Weight loss and diarrhea are also common.

Treatment

Combination drug therapy is most successful. Prophylactic drug therapy may be used in individuals with low CD4 cell counts. Commonly used agents include the following:

Clarithromycin	Rifampin
Azithromycin	Rifabutin (used for prophylaxis)
Clofazimine	Streptomycin
Amikacin	Ethambutol
Ciprofloxacin	

</td></tr>
</table>

Medical management

The presence of HIV is usually determined through antibody screening as outlined in Box 17-5. Once the presence of HIV is confirmed, the T4 helper lymphocyte count is monitored, usually every 6 months, to assess disease progression. T4 cells are also called CD4 cells, referring to the specific protein that binds the virus. A normal CD4 count is about 1000 cells/μl, although significant variations do occur. Most persons remain asymptomatic as long as their CD4 count remains above 500. Antiretroviral therapy is recommended for asymptomatic persons whose counts fall below 500 cells/μl. Research is ongoing as to the effectiveness of various drugs, some of which are summarized in Table 17-5. Antiretroviral therapy is believed to be effective in delaying the onset of opportunistic infections and prolonging survival, although study results are frequently inconsistent and contradictory to date.

The progression of HIV to AIDS has been described in a variety of ways as experience with the various manifestations of the disease has increased. The current U.S. Centers for Disease Control (CDC) classification system is presented in Box 17-6. The remainder of the medical management is driven by the presentation of the individual patient and involves management of opportunistic infections and complications and general supportive care. An overview of the most commonly encountered opportunistic infections and complications associated with AIDS is presented in Boxes 17-7 to 17-12.

NURSING MANAGEMENT

♦ ASSESSMENT
Subjective Data

Knowledge of the disease, transmission, diagnosis, treatment
Sexual history, knowledge and use of safe sex practices
History of recreational drug use, needle exposure
Exposure to blood products, equipment
Recent health and nutritional status
Complaints of the following:
  Persistent fatigue and lethargy
  Anorexia
  Headache
  Chills and night sweats

Objective Data

Abdominal discomfort and persistent diarrhea
Weight loss (usual weight)
Fever
Cough (dry or productive)
Lymphadenopathy
Skin rashes or lesions
Positive ELISA or Western blot antibody test
Decreased CD4 cell count

BOX 17-8	AIDS Complications: Fungal Infections

Fungal infections are a common problem among AIDS patients. Candidiasis, cryptococcosis, and histoplasmosis are the most common types.

CANDIDIASIS

Candida albicans is a normal organism of the mouth, GI tract, vagina, and skin. It produces infection only when the immune system is suppressed and is often an indication that significant immune decline is occurring. It typically presents as a mucocutaneous infection. The symptoms are troublesome but rarely create serious or disseminated disease.

Diagnosis

The infection is diagnosed from the classic white patches on the tongue or mouth, or creamy vaginal discharge.

Symptoms

The classic symptoms are creamy patches surrounded by an erythematous base that can be wiped off, leaving a reddened or bleeding surface. It can create anorexia or dysphagia.

Treatment

Drug treatment involves nystatin (swish and swallow), clotrimazole (lozenges), or fluconazole (tablets).

CRYPTOCOCCOSIS

Cryptococcus neoformans is found worldwide in pigeon droppings and is naturally acquired from the environment. It is not spread directly from animal or person. In severe HIV immunodeficiency the infection can present as meningitis.

Diagnosis

The organism can be identified in the cerebrospinal fluid and can be detected by antigen testing.

Symptoms

The disease is often insidious and nonspecific. Symptoms such as fever, chills, fatigue, and night sweats are common. Some patients experience stiff neck, nausea and vomiting, and altered mentation.

Treatment

The primary drug therapy is with amphotericin B administered either intravenously or intrathecally if no response is seen. Flucytosine and fluconazole may also be given in combination with amphotericin.

HISTOPLASMOSIS

Histoplasma capsulatum is present in the soil where bird or bat excrement collects, primarily in the mid central and south central states. It causes a common pulmonary infection that is usually benign in healthy persons. Acute, life-threatening pulmonary infection and disseminated disease can occur, however, in immunocompromised persons.

Diagnosis

Chest x-rays are often unreliable in the presence of disseminated disease, which can best be diagnosed through bone marrow biopsy and culture of blood, pulmonary secretions, and lung tissue.

Symptoms

Patients usually present with general symptoms of fever, weight loss, and fatigue. Enlargement of the liver and spleen is common, and the disease can progress to respiratory failure and disseminated intravascular coagulation (DIC).

Treatment

Disseminated disease is fatal without aggressive treatment, usually with amphotericin B. Fluconazole and flucytosine are also used as adjuncts. Long-term therapy is required, because current treatment does not cure the disease.

◆ NURSING DIAGNOSES

Nursing diagnoses for the person with HIV/AIDS may include, but are not limited to, the following:

Infection, high risk for (related to decreased immune response and frequent hospitalization)

Nutrition, altered: less than body requirements (related to anorexia, nausea, and chronic diarrhea)

Ineffective individual or family coping, high risk for (related to persistent stress of the diagnosis and prognosis)

Social isolation, high risk for (related to the stigma of the disease)

Impaired home maintenance management, high risk for (related to insufficient resources, lack of support, lack of knowledge)

◆ EXPECTED PATIENT OUTCOMES

Patient will not develop preventable secondary infections.

Patient will consume a balanced nutrient oral diet and maintain a stable body weight.

Patient and partner (family) will engage in open communication, strengthen usual coping patterns, and engage in constructive problem solving.

Patient will maintain social involvement with family and friends and seek out community support services.

Patient will seek out adequate resources to maintain home regimen effectively.

◆ NURSING INTERVENTIONS

Preventing Infection

Encourage patient to follow scrupulous personal hygiene. Emphasize the importance of good skin care and oral hygiene.

Teach patient to avoid contact with persons with infections and to avoid activities that can result in skin trauma.

Monitor patient for signs of new infection. Take routine vital signs. Monitor for fever.

Maintain scrupulous hand-washing regimen. Utilize protective isolation if indicated.

BOX 17-9 · AIDS Complications: Protozoal Infections

Protozoan infections can be caused by a wide variety of organisms. *Pneumocystis carinii* pneumonia and toxoplasmosis are among the most common protozoal infections affecting patients with AIDS.

PNEUMOCYSTIS CARINII PNEUMONIA (PCP)

Pneumocystis carinii, which has been classified as both a protozoan and a fungus, is found worldwide. It exists in the lungs and can be found in the air, on food, and in water, and it usually has infected an individual asymptomatically by 4 years of age. It causes aggressive disease in the immunosuppressed individual, however, and is typically regarded as the most common life-threatening infection associated with AIDS.

Diagnosis

Biopsies of lung tissue are usually performed to identify the organism in patients presenting with acute pneumonia. Chest x-rays will usually show a pattern of pneumonia, but some patients' x-rays appear normal. Pulmonary function tests reveal decreased vital capacity, and blood gases show hypoxemia and hypocarbia. A presumptive diagnosis is established based on the symptoms, chest x-ray, and blood gases.

Symptoms

Fever, fatigue, and weight loss may be present for weeks before definite respiratory symptoms develop. Dyspnea is fairly severe, particularly on exertion, and a cough (usually nonproductive) is also common.

Treatment

Drug therapy has been standardized to include either pentamidine isethionate or trimethoprim-sulfamethoxazole (TMP-SMX). TMP-SMX is better tolerated in most patients who are not sensitive to sulfa drugs. Aerosolized medication may be administered. Mechanical ventilation may also be necessary for patients who experience respiratory failure. Prophylactic treatment is now being recommended for patients whose CD4 counts fall below 200 and for all patients after a first bout with PCP. It consists of oral TMP-SMX or inhaled pentamidine administered monthly.

TOXOPLASMOSIS

Toxoplasma gondii occurs worldwide and affects both humans and animals. Cats have been identified as definitive hosts. Infection does not generally cause illness in healthy persons, but the organism is a major cause of encephalitis in patients with AIDS. Most people are unaware of a primary infection, but prevention of toxoplasmosis involves washing all fruits and vegetables carefully and wearing gloves for gardening and disposing of cat litter.

Diagnosis

A definitive diagnosis generally requires brain biopsy. Presumptive diagnosis is made from the symptom pattern, the presence of serum antibodies to toxoplasmosis, and CT or magnetic resonance imaging (MRI) scanning showing a lesion with mass effect.

Symptoms

Symptoms may be vague and nonspecific, but headache and altered mental status are common. Confusion, lethargy, delusion, frank psychosis, and coma are all possible. Focal neurologic signs are also possible and frequently include seizures or problems such as hemiparesis, aphasia, ataxia, cranial nerve palsies, or visual field losses.

Treatment

Drug therapy is the primary treatment and utilizes a combination of sulfadiazine and pyrimethamine. Symptom management may require phenytoin (Dilantin) or dexamethasone (Decadron). Pyrimethamine is also being used for prophylaxis in patients with extremely low CD4 levels and for maintenance after an initial episode of the infection.

CRYPTOSPORIDIOSIS

The cryptosporidium is a parasite known to be present in a wide variety of animals and is an acknowledged pathogen in both immunosuppressed and healthy persons. Person-to-person transmission and water-borne transmission are possible. The organism affects primarily the small intestine and produces profuse diarrhea.

Diagnosis

The oocytes of the parasite can be identified in fresh stool specimens.

Symptoms

Patients present with massive diarrhea accompanied by nausea and fatigue. The diarrhea volume may exceed 4 L daily and can easily lead to dehydration and electrolyte imbalance. Malnutrition and skin breakdown are extremely common and may be severe.

Treatment

No effective drug therapy exists for the infection. It is usually self-limiting in healthy persons but can be life threatening in persons with AIDS. Several drugs are currently in clinical trials, but none have proven clinical effectiveness. IV fluid management is essential, and total parenteral nutrition or other nutritional supplementation will probably be necessary. Skin care will become increasingly important if the diarrhea persists.

Institute a low microbial diet if neutrophil count falls below 500/cm³.

Encourage patient to wash all fresh fruits and vegetables carefully, and cook all meats thoroughly.

Encourage patient to keep home environment clean and damp mop daily to reduce dust.

Limit or eliminate fresh plants and flowers.

Use special precautions when caring for pet wastes.

Teach patient to seek immediate medical care in the event of signs of infection.

Promoting Nutrition

Monitor weight daily and maintain calorie counts if intake is poor.

Provide a high-calorie, enriched protein diet.

Offer six small meals per day.

Use supplements and protein powders if anorexia is severe.

Supplement potassium if chronic problems with diarrhea exist.

BOX 17-10	AIDS Complications: Viral Infections

Most viral infections in AIDS patients involve reactivation of various herpes viruses. Herpes zoster frequently erupts early in the course of HIV infection but typically responds well to acyclovir therapy. Herpes simplex eruptions occur with varying frequency and severity and again tend to respond well to acyclovir.

CYTOMEGALOVIRUS (CMV)

Infection with CMV is the most significant opportunistic infection of the herpes virus family. The organism is found worldwide and is usually asymptomatic in immunocompetent persons. Like other herpes viruses it can remain dormant for long periods after an initial infection and then be reactivated. CMV is one of the two known causes of mononucleosis. It can be acquired during the perinatal period, in the preschool years, or during the sexually active years.

Diagnosis

CMV infection is present in the majority of American adults. The diagnosis of CMV disease is based on identification of CMV inclusion bodies or through positive cultures from specific organs. Presumptive criteria may also be used.

Symptoms

Immunocompetent adults present with fever and fatigue, classic symptoms of mononucleosis. Patients with HIV are often asymptomatic but may develop clinical complaints indicating involvement of specific organs such as retinitis with progressive visual changes, adrenalitis with symptoms of adrenal insufficiency, or symptoms indicating pulmonary or GI involvement.

Treatment

Ganciclovir is the current drug of choice for treating the retinitis that can result in irreversible blindness. Foscarnet has also been approved for treatment, and a variety of other drugs are in current clinical trials. The combination of AZT and Ganciclovir significantly suppresses the bone marrow and requires the administration of colony-stimulating factors to compensate for the suppression.

BOX 17-11	AIDS Complications: HIV Encephalopathy

Invasion of the central nervous system (CNS) by the HIV virus can result in HIV encephalopathy or dementia. It is believed to be present to some degree in about 60% of patients.

Diagnosis

The diagnosis is primarily established from the pattern and progression of the patient's symptoms.

Symptoms

The organism can produce a progressive loss or decline in cognitive, motor, and behavioral functioning. The changes may be very subtle at first and mistaken for depression or grieving. Reduced concentration, slowed speech, and impaired memory are common. Advancing dementia can impair self-care abilities and progress to coma. Patients may be acutely aware of their losses and deficits or exhibit little insight into the changes. Aware persons are at high risk for suicide.

Treatment

Treatment is primarily palliative and supportive. AZT may effect some neurologic improvement in the early stages of the disease.

Provide oral hygiene before meals.

Use viscous lidocaine (Xylocaine) if mouth lesions are present.

Manipulate the environment to make it conducive to eating, for example, out of bed for meals, control of odors, involvement of family or friends at mealtimes, and obtaining favorite foods from home.

Explore home situation for obtaining and preparing food. Refer to community resources as needed.

Supporting Effective Coping

Establish a therapeutic relationship, and encourage the patient to express feelings.

Identify current coping mechanisms, and evaluate effectiveness with patient.

Reinforce all positive coping behaviors.

Provide opportunities for family and friends to express their concerns related to the diagnosis and prognosis.

Identify resources available to patient and family in the community, and facilitate involvement.

Explore new coping strategies.

Introduce relaxation and stress reduction techniques.

Preventing Social Isolation

Assist patient to deal with responses of family and friends to diagnosis.

Assist patient to identify current and potential sources of support.

Encourage involvement in community support group services.

Explore concerns of family and friends over their own risk of exposure to the disease.

Provide factual information about transmission.

Refer to social services and counseling as indicated.

Encourage patient to maintain realistic hope and share concern over the future.

Promoting Effective Home Maintenance

Encourage patient to be as active and independent as possible.

Teach energy conservation techniques and the importance of balancing activity and rest.

Explore the use of assistive devices as needed.

Modify the home to improve safety as needed.

Explore anticipated care needs and identify resources in the community for meeting them.

Initiate all needed referrals.

Encourage meticulous skin care.

Teach patient to use sitz baths and moisture barriers if diarrhea is present.

Reinforce principles to prevent disease transmission.

BOX 17-12 **AIDS Complications: HIV-Related Cancers**

The immunosuppression of AIDS leaves the patient with an increased vulnerability to malignancy.

KAPOSI'S SARCOMA

Kaposi's sarcoma is by far the most common neoplasm affecting persons with HIV. It affects the vascular epithelium and causes red-purple lesions on the trunk, head, neck, and extremities. The lesions can block the lymph flow and create severe edema.

Diagnosis

The diagnosis is established by tissue biopsy of the lesions.

Symptoms

The specific symptoms depend on the involved body systems. The cutaneous lesions are fairly classic and may produce no other symptoms, or the person may experience dyspnea and cough from pulmonary lesions or nausea and diarrhea from GI involvement.

Treatment

Radiation therapy may be used as a palliative measure, although the side effects of treatment may make this an unacceptable alternative. Supportive care is provided to the skin lesions and to prevent the tissue complications of severe edema. The patient needs assistance in dealing with the body image changes produced by the visible lesions.

LYMPHOMAS

Lymphomas are also common cancers in patients with HIV infection and are often associated with a poor prognosis. Non-Hodgkin's lymphomas are most common, but Burkitt's-like lymphomas also occur. When the tumors affect the CNS the symptoms of neurologic dysfunction may be severe. General symptoms include malaise, myalgias, and lymphadenopathies. Treatment is basically symptomatic and supportive. Radiotherapy may be used to shrink tumors that are affecting vital structures.

Teach patient to use household bleach to clean any articles or areas contaminated with blood or other body fluids.

Obtain disposable gloves for home care use.

Teach patient importance of telling all caretakers, such as dentists, about diagnosis.

Reinforce importance of informing all known sex partners about seropositivity or diagnosis.

♦ EVALUATION

Successful achievement of expected outcomes for the patient with HIV/AIDS is indicated by the following:

Absence of secondary infection: normal temperature, intact skin, lungs clear to auscultation

Maintenance of a stable body weight

Utilization of effective coping strategies; positive interaction with family and friends (partner)

Involvement with social, family, and support group activities

Maintenance of a safe and effective home environment

ORGAN TRANSPLANTATION

Organ and tissue transplantation has evolved in just a few years from an experimental procedure to a major therapeutic intervention for persons with end-stage organ failure who do not respond to conventional therapy. Since the demand for organs still far exceeds their availability, significant efforts are made to appropriately screen both potential donors and recipients to increase the likelihood of success for the transplant. Although standards vary from center to center it is generally agreed that recipients should be free of irreversible infection, malignancies, or high-risk concurrent illnesses. Ability to pay is another consideration, since insurance coverage for transplant procedures is inconsistent among major payers. A variety of legislation has been passed in the attempt to increase the supply of organs and ensure that available organs are fairly allocated. The general criteria of blood type, size, medical urgency, geographic location, and waiting time are used for most organs. A more definitive point system has been developed to guide the allocation of kidneys. Organ procurement organizations exist throughout the United States to provide 24-hour assistance and communication to the national transplant network.

Most transplants are allografts involving organs or tissue from another human being, usually a cadaver. The typical organ donor experiences brain death. Ideally this individual is free of disease in the affected organ, sepsis, transmittable disease, and malignancy. Successful allograft transplantation requires manipulation of the recipient's immune system. Although great progress has been made in both understanding and managing the process of organ rejection in the body, rejection remains the major ongoing threat to transplant success.

IMMUNOLOGY OF TRANSPLANT

All body cells and tissues have markers (antigens) on the surface of the cell membrane that are unique to that individual and allow the body to recognize components as either self or nonself. Since foreign substances have different markers they can be recognized as nonself by the B and T lymphocytes that act as surveillance cells for the immune system. Foreign cells activate the B and T cells, causing them to differentiate, proliferate, and attack the foreign substance. The ability of immune cells to recognize nonself is carried on chromosome 6. Each of the person's two number 6 chromosomes encodes seven specific human leukocyte antigens (HLA), one set from each parent. The ABO blood typing system is the other major antigen system that is crucial for transplant. The Rh system does not appear to influence survival or rejection of tissue.

A variety of histocompatibility tests can be performed on both the donor and recipient tissue depending on the time frame available and the tissue being transplanted (Box 17-13). Maximum testing is performed when a living donor is planned. Maximum compatibility

BOX 17-13 Tests Used for Tissue Typing and Matching

ABO COMPATIBILITY

Tests surface antigens on RBCs and other tissues; compatibility is same as for blood transfusions; recipient would have antibodies to any ABO antigens present on donor cells and not on recipient cells.

MINOR RBC ANTIGEN TESTING

Tests surface antigens on RBCs; transplant recipients who have had multiple transfusions may have antibodies to known minor RBC antigens.

MICROLYMPHOCYTOTOXICITY TESTING

Detects class I HLA antigens (A, B, C) and matches these antigens between recipient and donor.

MIXED LEUKOCYTE CULTURE OR MIXED LYMPHOCYTE CULTURE (MLC)

Detects class II HLA antigens (D, DR, DQ, DP); takes 4 to 5 days to complete test so performed only with living, related donors; there is a 24-hour HLA-DR typing test that may be used for cadaver kidneys.

WHITE CELL CROSS MATCH

Detects presence of preformed circulating cytotoxic antibodies in recipient to antigens on lymphocytes of donor; positive cross match is predictor of rejection.

MIXED LYMPHOCYTE CROSS MATCH

Also detects presence of preformed cytotoxic antibodies in recipient to antigens on lymphocytes of donor; used to test potential recipients against selected panel of donor lymphocytes; tells probability of finding cross match negative donor; response changes over time so potential renal transplant candidates are screened monthly.

is required for successful bone marrow transplant. Liver transplant allows the most flexibility in the match. The heart, lung, liver, and pancreas also have very short preservation times (3 to 5 hours for a heart), which makes extensive testing impractical. The minimum testing involves ABO compatibility and a mixed lymphocyte cross-match.

Tissue Rejection

The phenomenon of tissue rejection can be classified as hyperacute, acute, or chronic. *Hyperacute rejection* involves preformed cytotoxic antibodies, usually to incompatible ABO group antigens. It is controlled by the humoral immune system and occurs within 48 hours of transplant. The antigen-antibody reaction activates complement and clotting factors and causes massive intravascular coagulation and necrosis of the organ. Hyperacute rejection occurs exclusively in kidney transplants.

Acute rejection involves the trapping of foreign antigens by macrophages. The interaction stimulates T cell differentiation in the cellular immune system followed by direct or indirect destruction of the transplanted tissue. Acute rejection occurs from 1 week to 3 months after transplant and can recur after an initial episode. Acute rejection can be treated pharmacologically.

Chronic rejection occurs from 3 months to longer after transplant and involves both arms of the immune system. It causes slow but progressive destruction of organ function and does not respond to currently available drug treatment.

The survival of all types of organ transplants depends on the administration of immunosuppressive agents. Maintenance therapy at present combines the use of cyclosporine, azathioprine, and corticosteroids. Lymphocytic immune globulin and OKT-3 are added to treat episodes of acute rejection. The drugs must be taken for life and leave the person extremely vulnerable to infection. Good hand washing, aseptic technique for all procedures, and scrupulous personal hygiene are the best strategies for dealing with this long-term risk. Pulmonary hygiene, adequate fluids, and balanced nutrition are also long-term management goals.

TABLE 17-6 Drug Therapy to Prevent Organ Rejection

ACTION	SIDE OR TOXIC EFFECTS
CYCLOSPORINE	
Acts selectively on specific receptor sites of T lymphocytes; also suppresses macrophage activation	Multiple adverse effects, particularly nephrotoxicity; electrolyte imbalance, infection, and muscle weakness and tremor
AZATHIOPRINE	
Inhibits RNA and DNA synthesis and proliferation of immune cells	Bone marrow suppression: major toxic effect; GI distress also common
CORTICOSTEROIDS	
Decrease number of circulating lymphocytes and production of interleukin I and II	Multiple side effects, especially in high doses; e.g., sodium and fluid retention, osteoporosis, glucose intolerance, peptic ulceration, infection, and psychologic imbalance
LYMPHOCYTE IMMUNE GLOBULIN	
Animal products that contain antibodies to T lymphocytes	May trigger allergic response; administered with steroids, antipyretics, and antihistamines to reduce severity of reaction
OKT-3	
Monoclonal antibody to mature T lymphocytes	Can induce allergic response; headache and flulike symptoms common; careful monitoring during infusion is critical

NURSING MANAGEMENT OF THE TRANSPLANT PATIENT

Much of the care provided to patients undergoing transplant is similar to that provided to any patient undergoing complex surgery. *Infection* is one of the most common problems facing transplant patients. Nursing interventions include the following:

- Establishing an aseptic environment and protecting the patient from sources of nosocomial infection in the environment
- Monitoring the patient's vital signs frequently, particularly for the onset of fever
- Maintaining strict sterile technique for the management of all dressings, IV lines, and catheters
- Helping the patient maintain scrupulous personal hygiene including thorough mouth care several times daily

The nurse also institutes the immunosuppressive regimen and monitors the patient carefully for signs of organ rejection. Rejection is characterized by signs of organ failure and indications of increased immune system activity. Specific areas of concern for nursing care are outlined under the discussion of each transplant.

KIDNEY TRANSPLANT

Over 9000 kidney transplants are performed each year in the United States. Major advances have been made in surgical technique and tissue typing, but rejection continues to be a significant problem with cadaver transplants. Success rates after 1 year remain around 75%. Histocompatibility for both HLA and ABO antigens is essential.

The kidney is placed in the iliac fossa. Monitoring urine output and fluid and electrolyte balance is a critical aspect of postoperative care. Hemodynamic monitoring may be employed. The patient may have little or no urine output for hours or days following transplant, making fluid balance a critical concern. Possible surgical complications include anastomosis leakage, bleeding, occlusion of the renal artery or vein, and acute tubular necrosis. Monitoring for rejection is an ongoing concern (Box 17-14). General guidelines for care are summarized in the Guidelines box.

HEART TRANSPLANT

Heart transplant is used primarily for patients with end-stage ischemic heart disease or cardiomyopathy. The success rates exceed 80% after 1 year and 69% after 5 years. The donor and recipient need to be of comparable body weight and have ABO group compatibility. The donor heart, aorta, and pulmonary arteries are anastomosed. The postoperative care is similar to that required after other types of open heart surgery. Surgical complications may include leakage of the anastomoses, bleeding, hypovolemia, cardiac tamponade, hemodynamic instability, or decreased cardiac output. The nurse monitors all hemodynamic parameters and titrates

---

BOX 17-14	Signs and Symptoms of Acute Rejection in the Renal Transplant Patient

Decrease in urine output
Oliguria
Anuria
Fever greater than 37.7° C (100° F); may be masked by steroid therapy
Pain or tenderness over grafted kidney
Edema
Sudden weight gain: 2 to 3 pounds in a 24-hour period
Hypertension
General malaise
Increase in serum creatinine and blood urea nitrogen (BUN) values, proteinuria
Decrease in creatinine clearance
Evidence of rejection on renogram or other test

Guidelines for Nursing Care Following Kidney Transplant

FLUID AND ELECTROLYTE BALANCE

Maintain accurate intake and output.
Weigh patient daily.
Monitor for signs of fluid and electrolyte imbalance.
Regulate IV fluids per order (usually 1 ml of IV fluid for each milliliter of urine output, calculated hourly).

PREVENTING INFECTION

Take and record vital signs frequently; monitor and report fever.
Maintain good hand-washing practices.
Assess for signs of infection.
Maintain sterile technique for all wound care, IV care, and catheters.
Establish aseptic environment.
Restrict visitors and caretakers with colds or infections.
Encourage ambulation and pulmonary hygiene.

COMFORT MEASURES

Administer pain medications, and assess for effectiveness.
Encourage frequent undisturbed rest periods.
Assist with activities of daily living (ADL) as needed.

DISCHARGE TEACHING

Follow prescribed diet and any restrictions.
Follow prescribed medication regimen.
 Provide written data about immunosuppressives, side and toxic effects and their management, and signs to report.
Plans for ongoing follow-up and supervision.
Follow recommended preventive health care: dental; gynecologic; prevention of infection.

REJECTION

See Box 17-14.

---

fluid and medication administration per established protocol. Acute rejection and chronic rejection can occur and are usually confirmed by tissue biopsy (Box 17-15). Chronic rejection is insidious and characterized by development of atherosclerosis in the transplanted heart, which can result in ischemia, infarction, or failure.

BOX 17-15	Signs and Symptoms of Acute Rejection in the Heart Transplant Patient

SIGNS

Fluid retention, peripheral edema, crackles, jugular venous distention (JVD), S_3 gallop
Pericardial friction rub
Electrocardiogram (ECG) changes: arrhythmias and decreased voltage
Decreased cardiac output
Hypotension
Cardiac enlargement

SYMPTOMS

Fatigue, lethargy
Dyspnea
Decreased tolerance for exercise

BOX 17-16	Signs and Symptoms of Acute Rejection in the Liver Transplant Patient

Fever >38° C
Liver enlargement
Tenderness over transplant site
Fluid retention, hypertension
Tachycardia
Abnormal liver function tests (ALT, AST, bilirubin, albumin, clotting factors)
Abnormalities on scan or liver biopsy

BOX 17-17	Bone Marrow Harvest

PREPARATION

Thorough skin preparation through shower with antiseptic soap the evening before the harvest

PROCEDURE

Performed with the patient under general, spinal, or local anesthesia
 Posterior iliac crest is most commonly used site
 600-2500 ml of marrow collected
 Marrow transferred to a blood transfusion bag and administered immediately intravenously, although it can be stored frozen
 Pressure dressing applied to puncture sites

POSTPROCEDURE CARE

Pain controlled with analgesics
 Donor can be out of bed the night of the harvest
 Pressure dressing removed the day after the harvest
 Donor sites kept covered for 3 days, treated with povidone-iodine (betadine) ointment, and covered with an adhesive bandage

LIVER TRANSPLANT

Liver transplants are performed for a variety of conditions, including biliary atresia, chronic hepatitis, and end-stage cirrhosis. The procedure is technically difficult and requires the reconstruction of both the vascular and biliary drainage systems. ABO matching is preferred, but successful transplants have been performed with nonidentical blood groups. The complexity of liver function in metabolism can create a complex postoperative management challenge. Surgical complications include vascular thrombosis, biliary complications, coagulopathies, and pulmonary problems. Critical care management is standard for monitoring of all hemodynamic, fluid and electrolyte, neurologic, and pulmonary functions. The hospitalization is often prolonged and can produce multiple stressors for the family and support network. Immunosuppressive therapy is instituted before surgery and continued on a tight regimen. Signs of rejection are presented in Box 17-16.

BONE MARROW TRANSPLANT

Bone marrow transplant is being utilized as part of the treatment of patients with a variety of solid tumors and hematologic cancers. It is used as a "rescue" procedure that allows for the administration of doses of chemotherapy and radiation that would be incompatible with survival. Allogeneic transplants may be used, or the patient may serve as his or her own donor (autologous) if the marrow is disease free. A close HLA donor match is critical for all allogeneic transplants. Even so the body must be conditioned to accept the recipient tissue. This process usually involves irradiation and chemotherapy. Bone marrow harvest (from patient or donor) is performed to collect enough stem cells to reconstitute the hematopoietic system after transplant (Box 17-17). From 600 to 2500 ml of marrow is harvested from the posterior iliac crest with the patient under general or local anesthesia. After processing, the marrow is infused into the recipient intravenously. Marrow can be stored frozen for up to 3 years.

The complications of bone marrow transplant are frequently related to the high doses of chemotherapy with associated toxicity to the GI tract and other organs. The pancytopenia requires a sterile environment and reverse isolation as well as platelet transfusion if values fall to levels that might cause spontaneous bleeding.

Venoocclusive disease of the liver may occur from narrowing or obliteration of terminal hepatic veins from collagen deposits. The problem presents with liver insufficiency from 1 to 4 weeks after transplant.

Graft versus host disease is another acute complication of bone marrow transplant that may carry over and become a chronic problem. It may occur with allogeneic transplants where the immunocompetent cells of the recipient have been destroyed with irradiation. Once the donor cells engraft they can attack the recipient's tissues as nonself. The tissues most affected are the skin, liver, and GI tract. Chronic graft versus host disease may cause skin changes, hepatic dysfunction, structural changes in the esophagus and GI tract, and chronic inflammation of the vaginal mucosa. Patients are treated symptomatically as well as receiving immunosuppressive therapy that leaves them vulnerable to a variety of opportunistic infections.

Hospitalization for bone marrow transplant is long and stressful even when events move smoothly. The nurse plays a major role in ongoing patient assessment, administration of the complex regimen of drugs, and assisting both patient and family to cope with the rigors of the treatment and the uncertainty of the future. Recurrence of the initial malignancy is a constant threat. Patient teaching, particularly the prevention of infection during the protracted recovery period, is an essential component of the nursing role.

SELECTED REFERENCES

Agency for Health Care Policy and Research: *Evaluation and management of early HIV infection,* Rockville, MD, 1994, US Department of Health and Human Services.

Anastasi JK, Lee VS: HIV wasting: how to stop the cycle, *Am J Nurs* 94(6):18-25, 1994.

Anastasi JK, Rivera J: Understanding prophylactic therapy for HIV infections, *Am J Nurs* 94(2):36-41, 1994.

Brown ME: Clinical management of the organ donor, *Dimen Crit Care Nurs* 8(3):134-142, 1989.

Buckley RH: *Immunologic disorders,* St Louis, 1993, Mosby.

Centers for Disease Control: The HIV/AIDS epidemic: the first 10 years, *Morbid Mortal Weekly Rep* 40(22):357-375, 1991.

Chabelewski F, Norris MKG: The gift of life: talking to families about organ and tissue donation, *Am J Nurs* 94(6):28-33, 1994.

Clark JC, Webster JS: Bone marrow transplantation. In Smith SL: *Tissue and organ transplantation: implications for professional nursing practice,* St Louis, 1990, Mosby.

Cunningham NH, Boteler S, Windham S: Renal transplantation, *Crit Care Nurs Clin North Am* 4(1):79-88, 1992.

Davis FD: Organ procurement and transplantation, *Nurs Clin North Am* 24:823-836, 1989.

Flaskerud J, Ungvarski P: *HIV/AIDS: a guide to nursing care,* Philadelphia, 1992, Saunders.

Foccograndi JF, Clements KS: Managing AIDS related meningitis, *RN* 56(11):36-39, 1993.

Freedman SL: An overview of bone marrow transplantation, *Semin Oncol Nurs* 4(1):3-8, 1988.

Gibbs L: Assessment and management of the allergic patient, *ORL Head Neck Nurs* 10(3):10-16, 1992.

Hooks MA: Immunosuppressive agents used in transplantation. In Smith SL: *Tissue and organ transplantation: implications for professional nursing practice,* St Louis, 1990, Mosby.

Lancaster L: Immunogenetic basis of tissue and organ transplantation and rejection, *Crit Care Nurs Clin* 4(1):1-24, 1992.

Lange S: Psychosocial, legal, ethical, and cultural aspects of organ donation and transplantation, *Crit Care Nurs Clin North Am* 4(1):25-42, 1992.

Lavin J, Haidorfer C: Anergy testing: a vital weapon, *RN* 56(9):31-32, 1993.

Lockey RF: Future trends in allergy and immunology, *JAMA* 268(20):2991-2992, 1992.

Mann J: Global AIDS: further evolution of the pandemic and the response, *HIV Advisor* 7(3):3-8, 1993.

Mudge-Grout CL: *Immunologic disorders,* St Louis, 1993, Mosby.

O'Brien LM, Bartlett KA: TB plus HIV spells trouble, *Am J Nurs* 92(5):28-34, 1992.

Scherer P: How HIV attacks the peripheral nervous system, *Am J Nurs* 90(5):66-70, 1990.

Smith SL: Immunologic aspects of transplantation. In Smith SL: *Tissue and organ transplantation: implications for professional nursing practice,* St Louis, 1990, Mosby.

Smith SL: The cutting edge in organ transplantation, *Crit Care Nurs Suppl,* pp. 10-11, 26, June 1993.

Workman ML, Ellerhorst-Ryan J, Hargrave-Koertge V: *Nursing care of the immunocompromised patient,* Philadelphia, 1993, WB Saunders.

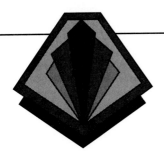

Index